Penetrating Trauma

George C. Velmahos • Elias Degiannis
Dietrich Doll
Editors

Penetrating Trauma

A Practical Guide on Operative Technique and Peri-Operative Management

Springer

Editors
Prof. George C. Velmahos
Harvard University Medical School
Massachusetts General Hospital
Division of Trauma, Emergency Surgery
and Surgical Critical Care
165 Cambridge Street, Suite 810
Boston, MA 02114, USA
gvelmahos@partners.org

Dr. Dietrich Doll
Department of Visceral
Vascular and Thoracic Surgery
Phillips-University of Marburg
Baldingerstraße
D-35043 Marburg
Germany
ddoll@gmx.de

Prof. Elias Degiannis
University of the Witwatersrand
Medical School
Chris Hani Baragwanath
Academic Hospital
Trauma Directorate
7 York Road, Parktown
2193 Johannesburg
South Africa (RSA)
degiannis@yebo.co.za

Illustrator
Peggy Firth
1816A Father Sky NE
Albuquerque, NM 87112
USA

ISBN 978-3-642-20452-4 e-ISBN 978-3-642-20453-1
DOI 10.1007/978-3-642-20453-1
Springer Heidelberg Dordrecht London New York

Library of Congress Control Number: 2011937718

Printed on acid-free paper

Springer is part of Springer Science+Business Media (www.springer.com)

To my parents, who lit my past, and to my wife and children, who light my present and future.

George C. Velmahos

To my patients, who taught me a lot, and to my teachers, who taught me everything.

Elias Degiannis

To my parents and family, my wife and my children, and to my teachers. Time is love.

Dietrich Doll

Foreword I

This ambitious textbook on "Penetrating Trauma: A practical Guide on Operative Technique and Peri-operative Management" is a significant addition to the body of published work on trauma. The editors are amongst the most experienced academic trauma surgeons in the world with unique experience in all types of penetrating injuries. This project represents many decades of collective experience in some of the busiest trauma centers in the world. The book is divided in 7 practical sections and 77 chapters, which cover all aspects of penetrating trauma, including prehospital care, penetrating injuries to the various body areas, specific organ injuries, orthopedic injuries, injuries to special group of patients, military injuries and many others.

The structure of the book makes it easy to read and provides clear and practical guidance on the evaluation, indications for operation, surgical techniques and perioperative problems. It is supported by numerous top quality photographs, illustrations and x-rays.

This book will be a great companion to residents and surgeons, in both civilian trauma centers and the military.

It will provide comfort and confidence to the surgeon who faces a catastrophic injury where a split second decision can make the difference between life and death, and good functional outcome and permanent disability.

Demetrios Demetriades, M.D., Ph.D., F.A.C.S.
Division of Trauma Surgery and Surgical Critical Care
Los Angeles County General Hospital
University of Southern California
Los Angeles, CA, USA

Foreword II

This book is directed toward the surgery and care of trauma, and is very timely. Over the past two decades, penetrating trauma wounds have decreased in most cities and experience in management of these injuries has declined as well. Thus, this book is a welcome addition to the trauma surgeon's library.

One of the major strengths of the book is how the authors articulate "how to do it." This makes it easy for the reader to find out what to do quickly. Despite this being an area of little Level I evidence, the authors offer reasonable approaches of how to manage difficult problems, based on personal experience and unequivocal expertise.

Another strength of the book is the geographical diversity of the authors representing many countries. This adds interest to the contents and challenges entrenched dogma. In the next edition I would welcome invited commentaries describing the multiple different alternatives.

Donald Dean Trunkey, M.D., F.A.C.S.
Professor Emeritus
Oregon Health & Science University
Oregon, USA

Preface

In the age of easy communication we are privileged to be bombarded by limitless bits of medical information. Textbooks, journals, tapes, and webpages rest at our fingertips. We can literally access everything and anything in our areas of interest. And exactly therein lurks the problem!

Penetrating trauma offers excitement, variety, and glory. It does not offer time. Decisions must be fast, solutions drastic. The patients bleed and ache and twist and turn and scream and do not cooperate. All happens when it is least expected – in the middle of the night, on a weekend, over a holiday. The surgeon is often alone with little help and even less resources. Questions need to be answered, actions to be taken. Not everybody is a trained trauma surgeon. How to repair a Grade IV duodenal injury? What is the best maneuver to stop the bleeding from the deep pelvis? How to control a bullet trajectory in the liver? Should this missile, lodged in the spine, be removed? Venous or synthetic graft for the arterial injury? Primary repair or a stoma after colectomy?

Suddenly, the endless sea of information becomes a liability. Confronted with an urgent scenario, the clinician does not have the time to study every possible alternative, to weigh in advantages and disadvantages of the available options. Punching on the keyboard the words "severe duodenal injury" produced 1,210,000 results. We argue that one does not have time to critically evaluate over a million of possibilities, when the duodenal hole is leaking. One needs to know a reasonable, safe, proven, and efficient way of managing the injury. This is what, we hope, this book offers. We assembled a group of experts who speak from personal experience. They describe how "I do this." Their approach is not the only one but is a good one! It paves a secure pathway to the end of the tunnel. It is an approach to remember, practice, and – with growing experience – even improve. It is a solid foundation on which one can comfortably rest and fearlessly build.

A picture is worth a thousand words! With multiple illustrations the steps of each operation are described in detail and with authority. We cannot appreciate enough the numerous authors who, yet again, responded to one more call for one more book chapter. They spent precious time to pass on their knowledge to the reader. We expect this book to be a useful first-aid manual for our colleagues who give the fight against the toll of penetrating trauma. Even if one life is saved because some surgeon, somewhere in the world scrolled through these pages and practiced a technique he read in this book, we have done our duty and fulfilled our promise of being responsible physicians and teachers.

Boston, MA, USA — George C. Velmahos
Johannesburg, South Africa — Elias Degiannis
Marburg, Germany — Dietrich Doll

Contents

Part I

Prehospital Care, Diagnostic Tools and Resuscitation Strategies

1 Prehospital Care in Penetrating Trauma

David Carlbom and Eileen M. Bulger

1.1 Planning a Systematic Approach

Prehospital care and movement of critically injured penetrating trauma patients are key components of an effective system of trauma care.

1.2 Scene Safety and Adequate Resources

The care of critically ill penetrating trauma patients begins before the time of injury. EMS leaders need to develop clear advance plans for the management of these challenging patients. Scene security and safety of EMS personnel is paramount, and you should give clear guidelines that should direct medical teams to stay out of dangerous situations until the scene is controlled by law enforcement. Even after law enforcement control is attained, providers should maintain situational awareness and strive for rapid departure from the location of the incident.

D. Carlbom
Emergency Services, Pulmonary Critical Care Harborview Medical Center,
325 9th Ave, Seattle, WA 98104, USA
e-mail: dcarlbom@u.washington.edu

E.M. Bulger (✉)
Department of Surgery, University of Washington,
Seattle, WA, USA

Emergency Surgical Services, Harborview Medical Center,
P.O. Box 359702, 325 Nineth Avenue,
Seattle, WA 98104, USA
e-mail: ebulger@u.washington.edu

There are no universally accepted guides or formulas regarding adequate staffing to care for a critically ill patient; one philosophy is to consider the time-critical nature of penetrating trauma to be akin to a building on fire. Severity of illness continues to grow and the time window for intervention continues to close with every minute. Thus, many medical providers are needed immediately, and it is better to assign more than the usual number of staff, with the option to reduce staff as able.

1.3 Dispatching Appropriate Resources

Emergency dispatchers face the challenge of deciding the most appropriate resources to send to the scene of a trauma based on telephone reports only. As time is the most critical factor in the prehospital management of trauma, dispatch centers should strive to expedite dispatching times and develop protocols that allow dispatchers to simultaneously send assistance while continuing to obtain information from callers. This "fast-dispatch" protocol should have a goal of achieving call answer to dispatch within 30 s.

While each trauma system should develop and constantly refine dispatch criteria to attain the best information on what resources to send to aid trauma patients, the new "Guidelines for Field Triage of Injured Patients" can provide some insight. These guidelines describe physiologic, anatomic, mechanism of injury, and special guides to triage trauma patients to high-level care.

Patients with absent respirations or pulse, those with tachypnea, and unconscious patients should be

G.C. Velmahos et al. (eds.), *Penetrating Trauma*,
DOI 10.1007/978-3-642-20453-1_1, © Springer-Verlag Berlin Heidelberg 2012

given highest priority and the most resources. Ringburg confirmed this in a systematic review of dispatch criteria. The criterion "loss of consciousness" had a sensitivity of 93–98% and a specificity of 85–96% in this review. The anatomic criteria of "penetrating injury to the torso, neck, head," should capture the highest risk victims of penetrating trauma. In a retrospective review of trauma deaths in the first hour, 31% of the penetrating trauma deaths were a result of gunshot wounds (GSWs) to the chest, and 21% from GSWs to the head.

The mechanism of injury may be more readily available to a witness, but the criteria described in the field triage document are primarily related to blunt trauma and are surrogates for significant energy exchange. As such, they are less useful for penetrating injuries. The same holds for the special considerations, which reflect age, anticoagulation use, burns, and "gut feeling."

1.4 ALS Versus BLS Care

Keep in mind that as with any subject area in medicine with little concrete evidence, prehospital care of injured patients is enveloped in controversy. It seems intuitive that only advanced prehospital care can benefit patients in extremis. However, due to a wide variation in prehospital systems, and the inability to randomize patients to advanced vs. basic life support model within any one system, there exist only limited data for the true benefit of ALS care, and some suggestion that any benefit may be negated by prolonged scene times.

When you are caring for critically ill trauma patients in the prehospital environment, time is the single most important factor. Historically, the first 60 min have been considered the window of time in which the patient must reach the trauma surgeon, but it may be even shorter. Thus, in all trauma patients, prehospital providers must balance the need for field-based interventions with prompt transport to definitive care, moving beyond the previously articulated binary systems of "rapid transport" vs. "stabilize on scene."

In a prospective study comparing ALS and BLS treatment of trauma patients cared for by the Scottish Ambulance Service and admitted to the hospital, Sukumaran and colleagues sought to describe the care provided and outcomes. Paramedics attended more severely injured patients and a higher proportion of patients with penetrating trauma, and had longer prehospital times. Patients managed by paramedics were more likely to be taken to the intensive care unit, operating theatre or mortuary, and had higher unadjusted mortality rates. No difference in mortality between the two groups was noted when corrected for age, Glasgow coma score and injury severity score.

An Israeli study of survival in severely injured trauma patients before and after the implementation of a prehospital trauma system demonstrated death rates decreased significantly from 21.6% to 14.7%.

Many authors have tried to find a relationship between survival and ALS care. Isenberg performed a review of articles that compared ALS to BLS care. Despite a wide variety of article types, there did not appear to be any benefit of ALS care in urban trauma patients. In a cross sectional investigation of the relationship of prehospital time to mortality, Baez and colleagues used logistic regression to demonstrate that longer prehospital time correlated significantly with hospital length of stay and complications, but not with mortality among young patients. In elderly trauma patients prehospital time had no significant predictive effect on length of stay, complications, or mortality.

Two before–after trials yield conflicting data on patient outcomes. One study examined preventable deaths during implementation of a prehospital trauma system. More patients were attended by Advanced Trauma Life Support paramedics and scene times increased after the implementation of the system. The combined preventable and potentially preventable death rates decreased from 36% to 28%. The Ontario Prehospital Advanced Life Support (OPALS) Major Trauma Study was a before-after study of the implementation of ALS care for trauma in Ontario; 400 paramedics (16 per 100,000 population) were trained and employed to care for all major trauma patients. Patients before the change received ALS care 2.5% of the time compared to 72.4% after. During the ALS phase, paramedics placed IVs in 63% of patients, but only gave an IV fluid bolus in 11.3%. They performed endotracheal intubation in only 6.8% of patients; one third via the nasal route. The number of attempts at intubation and success rates was not described. Scene times were longer in the ALS phase (16.8 vs. 15.0 min), as were transport times (7.2 vs. 6.1 min). Initial care upon hospital arrival was unchanged: 15% underwent intubation upon arrival in each group. Hospital length of stay was shorter in the ALS group by 5.7 days, and survival to hospital discharge was unchanged (81% in both groups). Thus, the authors concluded there was no evidence for better outcomes with ALS care. On subgroup analyses, they demonstrated that patients with a GCS < 9 had greater mortality in the ALS phase compared to the BLS phase. The authors speculate that intubation may be harmful, but do not provide enough data to further investigate any association for this possible relationship.

In the most exigently ill trauma patients requiring ED thoracotomy (EDT), one study reflects similar questions about ALS vs. BLS care. In a retrospective review of 180 consecutive penetrating trauma patients treated with EDT, survival differed by mode of arrival. Eight percent of patients arriving by EMS survived until hospital discharge compared to 17.4% of patients arriving by police or private vehicle. The authors were unable to calculate accurate prehospital times, but did identify prehospital procedures as an independent predictor of mortality.

Keep in mind that the experience of the paramedic is an unmeasured confounder in studies of ALS system. Bulger et al. showed a great deal of variability in prehospital procedures performed on critically ill trauma patients when examined in a large cohort across 15 metropolitan systems. The variation appeared in endotracheal intubation (5–48%), use of neuromuscular blocking agents or sedatives to facilitate intubation (0–100%), surgical airway access (0.1–3.5%), peripheral and central intravenous access (22–95%), and needle thoracostomy (0–5%). Some of this variation may reflect system design, such as the use of NMBA, but some may be a result of difference in experience. There is an inverse relationship between survival from ventricular fibrillation and number of paramedics per capita; cities in the US with the most medics per capita have the lowest survival. This is a reflection of the number of times per year each paramedic performs the procedure of resuscitation. A similar relationship may exist in trauma. Thus, systems need to be designed to ensure each paramedic can perform ALS skills with high accuracy and minimal time, and has ample exposure to critically ill trauma patients.

1.5 Selecting Appropriate Transport Destination

A recent comprehensive review of the 2006 American College of surgeons by a National Expert Panel on Field Triage provides a logical and evidence-based field triage schema. For trauma patients with penetrating injuries, the guideline is clear: "All penetrating injuries to head, neck, torso, and extremities proximal to elbow and knee," should be transported to highest level of trauma center available. In addition, physiologically unstable patients should also be transported to highest level of trauma care. Patients with penetrating abdominal injury (PAI) and shock benefit greatly from direct transport to a Level 1 trauma center. In a review of 478 patients with PAI and shock, investigators demonstrated that the relative odds of death was 0.02 (95% CI 0.002–0.25) at high-volume centers compared to low-volume centers. This is likely due to the severity of injury and the patients need for immediate operative intervention.

In the subset of patients who suffer cardiac arrest after penetrating trauma, the National Association of EMS Physicians and the American College of Surgeons recommend withholding resuscitation if there are no signs of life: pulse, respirations, pupillary reflexes, spontaneous movement, or organized ECG activity. They also cite a greater than 15 min transport time as an indication to withhold treatment. However, patients with penetrating injury do have better survival rates (8.8% survival) from ED thoracotomy than patients with blunt injury (1.4% survival), and better if injured by a stab wound (16.8% survival) compared to gunshot wound (GSW) (4.3% survival). Another study of 138 patients transported with traumatic arrest found a survival rate of 10.1%, despite 93% of the patients transported exceeding the recommended 15 min transport time. Further study is needed to refine these guidelines.

1.6 Treatment: Airway

1.6.1 Endotracheal Intubation

Airway management is one area of marked controversy in prehospital care. Failure to correctly control the patient's airway in trauma is a leading cause of preventable death. Early implementation of bag–valve–mask assisted ventilation with high-flow oxygen is a key step to initiating the resuscitation of the critically injured patient. This should be followed closely by the placement of a definitive airway with an endotracheal tube. However, prehospital intubation has been associated with impaired outcome in some studies.

The safest location for providers to perform endotracheal intubation remains unclear, as there is great variability in prehospital intubation success in trauma, ranging from 33% to 100%. Some authors argue that in systems with a high number of paramedics per capita and documented infrequent attempts at intubation, this procedure should be deferred until arrival in the emergency department. Lack of muscle relaxation remains one of the primary reasons for failed prehospital intubation. This factor can be eliminated by allowing paramedics to use neuromuscular blocking agents (NMBA) to facilitate intubation. The introduction of neuromuscular blockade to prehospital settings also is associated with higher rates of success at achieving endotracheal tube placement. When NMBA are utilized, there exists a small risk that the patient cannot be intubated easily with direct laryngoscopy. Paramedics must receive adequate training in rescue techniques, including the use of Combitube (Kendall-Sheridan Corporation, Argyle, New York), gum elastic bougie, or cricothyrotomy. Two recent studies have shown the need for this surgical technique in less than 1% of patients undergoing attempted endotracheal intubation, with a success rate of 90% in a system with organized continuing education in this technique.

1.7 Treatment: Breathing

1.7.1 Oxygenation

It is important to maximally saturate hemoglobin and ensure adequate oxygen content as oxygen delivery is impaired by shock or loss of hemoglobin with hemorrhage. There are no convincing data whether to use or not use oxygen, but a reasonable approach would be to use the highest concentration possible to maintain oxygen saturation (SpO_2) of >98% or to use maximal concentration (FiO_2) when SpO_2 is not measurable.

1.7.2 Ventilation

Prehospital providers should strive to maintain normocapnea during transport of intubated trauma patients; the assessment of arterial carbon dioxide tension ($PaCO_2$) is more challenging. A recent study demonstrated a $PaCO_2$ of 30–39 mmHg to be the ideal range for brain injured patients, but this is not possible without cumbersome laboratory equipment. Continuous waveform capnography has been identified as a method to confirm endotracheal tube placement; recent recommendations have suggested that end-tidal capnography ($EtCO_2$) may also be used to guide ventilation as a surrogate measure of $PaCO_2$. These recommendations are based on the observation of close $EtCO_2$ $PaCO_2$ correlation in healthy patients. It is commonly accepted that $PaCO_2$ measurements vary approximately 2–5 mmHg above $EtCO_2$ values.

Effective alveolar excretion of carbon dioxide is dependent on robust pulmonary circulation. Trauma patients with chest injury or hypoperfusion may not be able to effectively deliver CO_2 to the lungs or to excrete it appropriately. A recent study of the correlation of $EtCO_2$ and $PaCO_2$ in intubated trauma patients found poor correlation. Patients arriving at the trauma center with $EtCO_2$ in the recommended range of 35–40 mmHg were hypoventilated with $PaCO_2$ > 40 mmHg in 80% of the cases and severely under-ventilated ($PaCO_2$ > 50 mmHg) 30% of the time. This demonstrates that $EtCO_2$ should not be used to guide ventilation in intubated trauma patients, only to assure endotracheal tube placement, and that $EtCO_2$ tends to under-represent $PaCO_2$. Prehospital providers must use best judgment and ventilate at a reasonable physiologic rate (12–20), and avoid over-ventilation.

1.7.3 Pneumothorax Management

Paramedics need to have an effective means to treat tension pneumothorax in patients with penetrating trauma. Tube thoracostomy is clearly outside the scope of most prehospital providers, so needle thoracostomy should be taught and used for cases of tension pneumothorax with shock. A study of all trauma patients receiving CT imaging of the chest demonstrated a mean chest wall thickness at the second intercostal space of 3.5 cm, with one in five individuals having a chest wall thickness of >4.5 cm. A long, large-bore needle should be used, and placed in the second intercostal space in the mid-clavicular line. This procedure appears safe in one large review of paramedic-performed needle thoracostomies, and was associated with improved survival.

1.8 Treatment: Circulation

1.8.1 IV Volume Resuscitation

Intravenous fluid resuscitation is commonly used with the goal of restoring perfusion to critical end organs, thus ameliorating the injury caused by hypovolemic shock. There are many controversies revolving around this practice, and many questions remain regarding the use of IV fluids, what the resuscitation goal should be, and what route of IV access is most appropriate.

If the primary goal of prehospital trauma treatment is to minimize field time and expedite transportation to a trauma center, does the initiation of IV fluid therapy impede this goal? There exists great variation in the amount of time required to place an IV. Some authors report as little as 2–4 min and others much longer, 14–16 min. Paramedics need to place IVs during transport, and not delay transport for the initiation of IV fluid resuscitation. Due to brief transport times in the urban environment, the amount of fluid given prior to ED arrival is often quite small. In one review on this topic, the average amount of fluid given in 14 studies was 959 mL. Even though the amount of fluid may be inadequate, there is a non-statistically significant trend toward prehospital fluid being associated with 3.9-fold increase in survival. Fluid is the primary therapy that may account for improvement in blood pressure and heart rate in one comparison of prehospital and ED vital signs in trauma patients. In a series of 19,409 patients, Arbabi described 31% of patients having an increase in their systolic blood pressure in the ED compared to the field.

1.8.2 Hypotensive Resuscitation

Patients with uncontrolled hemorrhage represent a unique and special challenge when deciding how much IV fluid resuscitation to deliver. One working model is that the delivery of large volumes of non-oxygen carrying fluid cools the patient, impairs oxygen delivery, and dilutes clotting. There are also animal data that suggest partially controlled bleeding or temporarily clotted aortic injury in pigs re-bleed when the systolic blood pressure is raised above 94 mmHg. Cannon first described limiting IV fluid administration on the battlefields of WWI, "Injection of a fluid that will increase blood pressure has dangers in itself. Hemorrhage in a case of shock may not have occurred to a marked degree because blood pressure has been too low and the flow too scant to overcome the obstacle offered by the clot. If the pressure is raised before the surgeon is ready to check any bleeding that may take place, blood that is sorely needed may be lost." To prevent these deleterious effects, they established a goal systolic blood pressure of 70–80 mmHg.

There are many animal studies of hypotensive resuscitation with a myriad of endpoints, including inflammatory activation and even survival. In a systematic review of these trials, one author concluded, "hypotensive resuscitation reduced the risk of death in all of the trials investigating it."

Two randomized controlled trials of hypotensive resuscitation in penetrating trauma patients with uncontrolled hemorrhage have been performed. Bickell and group performed a prospective trial comparing immediate and delayed fluid resuscitation in 598 adults with penetrating torso injuries who presented with a prehospital systolic blood pressure of 90 mmHg. The immediate resuscitation group received an average of 870 mL of Lactated Ringer's solution compared to 92 mL in the delayed group. Twelve percent of the patients died before reaching the operative intervention, and the systolic blood pressure was improved on arrival to the operating room in both groups. Among the 289 patients who received delayed fluid resuscitation, 203 (70%) survived to hospital discharge, as compared with 193 of the 309 patients (62%) who received immediate fluid resuscitation ($P=0.04$). Intraoperative blood loss and complications were not different between the groups. There are several limitations to this study, most notably that it was unblinded, and that there may be survival bias: patients surviving (despite minimal fluids) to the OR were less sick than those surviving with fluid therapy to the OR. This study was also limited to an urban environment with short transport times to a Level 1 trauma facility. The effects of fluid restriction during longer transport times remain to be determined.

In a second study, patients presenting to a regional trauma center with shock in the prior hour were randomized to two different systolic blood pressure targets: >100 mmHg or 70 mmHg. One hundred and ten patients were enrolled over 20 months. Although there was a significant difference in observed SBP (114 mmHg vs. 100 mmHg, $p<0.001$), there was no difference in mortality and an improved survival versus the Bickell trial (overall survival 92.7%). This study included all patients, not just penetrating injuries of the thorax. Further randomized trials are underway, and we should have more information in the next decade.

Despite the lack of reproducible data, it makes sense to avoid over-resuscitating patients with uncontrolled hemorrhage, specifically penetrating trauma of the thorax. Prehospital providers should use physiologic measures of perfusion rather than a set SBP. The US and Israeli military have adopted this practice and administer IV fluids to patients with altered level of consciousness from shock and those who do not have a detectable radial pulse.

1.8.3 IV Access Options

When fluids need to be given rapidly, large-bore catheters should be used to facilitate flow rates. Since flow is related to the radius of the catheter raised to the fourth power, small increases in size (smaller Standard Wire Gauge numbers) dramatically increase flow. The flow rates quoted by manufactures often overestimate actual flow due to the standard testing procedure: flow into open container. McPherson recently described measured flow rates into a red rubber catheter vein simulation model with blood flowing through the simulated vein. The flow rates in the model were consistently less than those identified by the manufacture (Table 1.1).

Some EMS systems utilize central venous catheters when peripheral veins are not accessible. If they are of large bore and short, they will flow adequately, but should be reserved for times when peripheral IVs are not available, as they take longer to insert and have more associated complications.

Intraosseous infusion catheters are being employed as a safe and effective alternative to peripheral IV access. Little data exist regarding their flow; in one study the measured flow rate was between 70 and 85 mL/min, markedly less than the manufacture's claim.

Table 1.1 Comparison of flow rates

Size (SWG) 48 mm length	Standard flow (mL/min)	Model flow (mL/min)
20	59	49
18	103	92
16	224	184
14	290	209

Adapted from McPherson et al.

1.8.4 Alternative IV Solutions

Although there have been several promising preliminary trials of oxygen carrying solutions, no definitive and safe fluid has been found. Hypertonic saline has gained interest as a potentially beneficial fluid. It requires less volume, and many basic science studies have shown that it can modify the robust immune response stimulated by trauma that may be associated with significant morbidity. A recent large trial confirmed that treatment after trauma with hypertonic saline containing dextran reduced the levels of pro-inflammatory cytokines. A large multicenter prehospital randomized control trial has been terminated early after an interim analysis showed no difference in 28-day survival among treatment groups, and earlier, but not higher, mortality in the hypertonic saline group. Further exploratory subgroup analysis may guide researchers toward a specific group of patients that may benefit the most from hypertonic saline resuscitation.

1.9 Treatment: Hemorrhage Control

1.9.1 Hemostatic Agents

Several chemical hemostatic agents have been well tested in animals and are used in battlefield operations. These agents are of two primary classes: minerals and chitosan. Mineral formulations work by two primary methods; they absorb water rapidly, thus concentrating platelets and clotting factors and inducing rapid clotting. They also form a barrier over severed blood vessels that provides strength to in vivo clot. Minerals used include zeolite, magnesium, and potassium silicates. The major drawback of these compounds is the local heat generated which can raise wound temperature as high as 53.5°C. Chitosan formulations bind to RBCs due to their negative charge and activate the intrinsic pathway of clotting. They do not generate as much heat as some of the mineral formulations. Most of the hemostatic agents now come packaged in a dressing or porous bag, which helps contain the compound and facilitates operative repair by not contaminating the wound with powder.

Research groups have developed several animal models for investigation of effectiveness of these dressing materials. They range from low flow venous bleeding to large arterial high flow bleeding states. All hemostatic agents performed well, and in one study were associated with improved survival.

In case series of human use, primarily on the battlefield of Iraq, these dressings appear effective at hemorrhage control. In one series of 103 patients treated with hemostatic agents, bleeding was controlled in 92% of patients. In another review of 64 uses by the military, bleeding was controlled in 97% of cases.

Prehospital systems could consider these agents; however their use would likely be infrequent as the battlefield injuries caused by explosive devices and high-velocity missiles are markedly different than the typical injuries of the civilian world. Their use should be considered a low frequency event and receive special training or be limited to a select team of paramedics, such as a tactical medic group.

1.9.2 Tourniquets

Exsanguinating hemorrhage from injured extremities is a rare occurrence in civilian trauma, but still remains one of the leading causes of preventable death during wartime, typically as a result of explosions. There is ongoing debate regarding the role of emergency tourniquets in control of bleeding. As there is a paucity of human research in the use of tourniquets, most of the controversy regarding the capacity of tourniquets to save lives has been based on speculation.

The US Army Institute of Surgical Research recently published an observational study of trauma patients who had tourniquets applied and were cared for at the combat support hospital in Baghdad. They documented 232 patients who had 428 tourniquets applied to 308 injured limbs. The overall mortality was 13%, with a marked difference in mortality when the tourniquet was placed before the development of hemorrhagic shock. Patients in shock when the tourniquet was applied had a mortality of 90% compared to 10% for those patients not in shock. Prehospital use was also associated with better survival: 11% mortality in patients with tourniquet placed prehospital compared to 24% mortality when placed in the Emergency Department. The authors were able to identify a matched cohort of patients who meet criteria for tourniquet use but did not have one applied and compared to a group of similar injury pattern and severity who did receive a tourniquet for hemorrhage control. Mortality was 23% in the later group compared to 100% for those without a tourniquet applied. They also report only four transient nerve palsies for the entire cohort.

Based on these new data, tourniquets should be employed to control life-threatening exsanguination from severe extremity wounds as a result of explosions or high-velocity missiles. Further study is needed in the civilian trauma setting in other populations to confirm effectiveness and safety.

1.9.3 Conclusion

The prehospital care of the critically injured victim of penetrating trauma begins with systematic organization to place the proper staff, equipment, and other resources in position to aggressively treat these patients. Prehospital providers must fight the clock and be in a state of constant motion toward the definitive care offered by the trauma surgeon. The traditional treatment dichotomy of "stay and stabilize" vs. "scoop and go" should be modified to "treat during transport." Paramedics must be given adequate ongoing experience in caring for these exigently ill patients to facilitate rapid correction of deficiencies in the patient's airway, breathing, and circulation. New techniques, including tourniquets for life threatening extremity hemorrhage and hemostatic dressings, may play a role in the care of these patients. With rapid transport and simultaneous treatment, prehospital personnel can significantly change the outcome of their patients' disease, transitioning them from moribund to salvageable.

Important Points

1. Consider the critically ill patient akin to a burning house: interventions performed quickly and early have the greatest impact.
2. ALS interventions need to be performed without lengthening prehospital time.
3. Notification and transportation to highest level of care improves outcome.
4. Prehospital endotracheal intubation is feasible in a busy EMS system with focused continuing education and experience.
5. Providers should avoid over-resuscitation of penetrating trauma patients; a minimal perfusion blood pressure is adequate.
6. Hemostatic agents and tourniquets may serve a role in exsanguinating extremity trauma.

2 Airway Management in Penetrating Trauma

David A. Baker and Eileen M. Bulger

Airway management in patients with penetrating trauma can be one of the more challenging situations you will face. This is particularly true with penetrating neck and facial injuries, which have the potential to wreak havoc when you attempt to establish an airway: blood, edema, debris, and in rare cases, complete laryngotracheal transection. Airway management in such cases may involve direct laryngoscopy, fiberoptic intubation, the use of extraglottic devices, cricothyrotomy, tracheostomy, or direct intubation through a neck wound. Conversely, impressive neck lacerations may pose no immediate airway problem but distract you from life threatening injuries in the thorax or abdomen: one-third of patients with penetrating neck injuries have moderate to severe injuries elsewhere [1]. Facing a patient with penetrating injuries you must be skilled at evaluating the airway, be able to quickly determine the need for a definitive airway, and be familiar with the various techniques to do so. While some centers may have 24 h anesthesia support, there will be times when you are the most capable physician at establishing an airway, surgical or otherwise. Even when a skilled anesthesiologist is present, you, the surgeon, must decide what type of airway is most appropriate. Will oral intubation worsen a potential laryngotracheal injury? Will it be ineffective? Would fiberoptic intubation or a surgical airway make the most sense? In this chapter, we will review the pearls and pitfalls of airway management in penetrating trauma: who needs immediate intubation, how to do it, and what situations dictate a more creative means of establishing an airway.

2.1 Airway Assessment

Assessment of the patient with penetrating trauma begins with the airway, regardless of injury location. While this is a basic principle of Advanced Trauma Life Support (ATLS), it is remarkable how often we become distracted by an impressive injury distal to the chest and miss the fact that the patient has airway compromise. If the patient is not already intubated, begin your assessment by having the patient talk to you. The ability to speak conveys an intact airway; however, impaired quality of voice may predict subsequent compromise. A hoarse voice, especially in conjunction with other findings, portends impending airway obstruction. If they cannot speak, is it because they are obtunded (and hence unable to protect their airway)? Is there a mechanical cause (trismus from mandible fractures, laryngeal obstruction)? Or is it simply volitional (i.e., the patient does not want to talk due to pain)?

Visual inspection of the airway and neck should occur simultaneous with or soon after vocal assessment. Signs of respiratory distress, chest asymmetry, and agitation will usually be obvious. Take note of any entry or exit wounds, and look for expanding hematoma, air leaking through a neck laceration, and tracheal deviation. If tracheal cartilage is exposed, does it appear to be violated? Transected? If a cervical collar is present, do not delay in removing it to inspect the neck (with manual in-line stabilization, if appropriate): failure to do so

D.A. Baker (✉) • E.M. Bulger
Department of Emergency Services,
University of Washington/Harborview Medical Center,
Box 359702, 325 9th Ave, Seattle, WA 98104, USA
e-mail: davbaker@u.washington.edu;
ebulger@u.washington.edu

G.C. Velmahos et al. (eds.), *Penetrating Trauma*,
DOI 10.1007/978-3-642-20453-1_2, © Springer-Verlag Berlin Heidelberg 2012

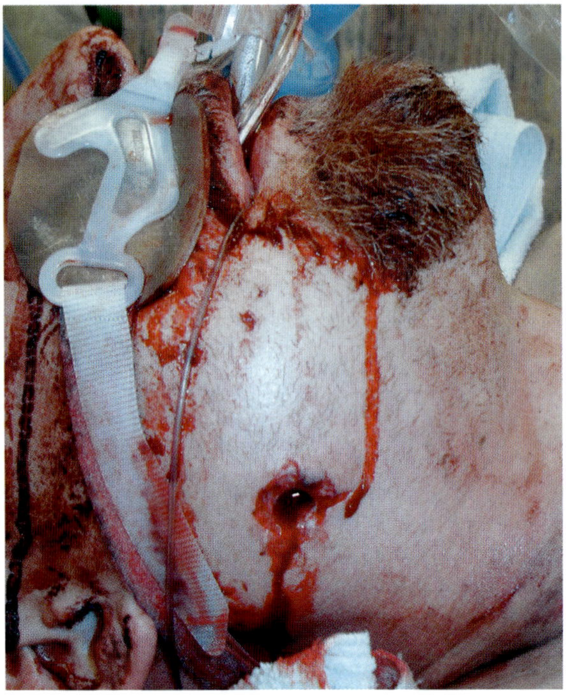

Fig. 2.1 The patient was shot with a high caliber rifle. The entry wound and exit wound demonstrate relatively little damage externally. When the patient was paralyzed, he proved very difficult to bag mask ventilate. CT scan revealed severe, comminuted mandibular fractures and soft tissue edema. This example reveals how, with penetrating facial and neck trauma, relatively benign appearing external wounds may mask significant airway damage

is a common cause of missed neck injuries. If facial injuries are present, you should pay special attention to ongoing bleeding which may lead to potential aspiration in the supine patient, especially massive epistaxis and oral lacerations. Always open the mouth and inspect: relatively benign appearing entry wounds in the neck, face, or head may cause significant injury to the oropharynx without obvious external damage (see Fig. 2.1). Mandible fractures, especially when bilateral, may cause trismus [2].

Auscultate both the chest and neck and focus on asymmetry and signs of airway edema. Stridor, a high-pitched, turbulent sound heard with respiration, indicates the development of airway compromise and impending obstruction [3]. Finally, palpation can offer insight into potential airway compromise. Palpate the face, neck, and chest closely for signs of subcutaneous emphysema, and closely feel along the cricoid and tracheal cartilages for signs of crepitus.

If the patient is already intubated, do not be lulled into complacency: confirm tube position with a CO_2 detector and auscultation of breath sounds. If these findings are equivocal, you should use a laryngoscope to confirm that the endotracheal tube (ETT) is going through the vocal cords. If it is not, replace the tube. If you are unsure and other clinical signs suggest an esophageal intubation (hypoxia, absent breath sounds, no change with the CO_2 detector), you should re-intubate. While many prehospital systems demonstrate remarkable success with intubation, there is obvious variability, and no ETT placed in the field should be considered secure until placement is confirmed [4].

2.2 Deciding Who Needs a Definitive Airway

A definitive airway is defined as a tube secured in the trachea with the cuff inflated. This can occur via three primary modes of tracheal intubation: nasal, oral, and surgical. The indications for intubation cannot be boiled down to a simple list of criteria, yet it is useful to consider a few broad categories. It should be stressed that determining who needs a definitive airway is a clinical decision and the use of objective criteria such as pulse oximetry, arterial blood gases (ABG), Glasgow Coma Scale (GCS), and vital signs, while useful, should not be relied upon alone. Patients with impending airway disasters may display no vital sign or laboratory abnormalities. Emergent intubation is common in patients with penetrating trauma and is influenced by the location and severity of injuries. Patients with penetrating neck injuries require emergency airway management in 46% of cases, and 60% require intubation at some point during their hospitalization [1, 2].

Indications for a definitive airway generally fall into one of the following broad categories:

1. *Obvious airway compromise or inability to protect the airway*: Airway obstruction can result from a variety of causes ranging from functional (i.e., in the obtunded patient) to mechanical (from edema, hematoma, or foreign body). Patients who are obtunded often lose the muscle tone of their posterior and oral pharynx, causing their tongue to drop back, leading to functional obstruction. While the obstruction may easily be relieved with simple maneuvers such as the jaw thrust, chin lift, or the placement of an oropharyngeal airway (OPA), the

patient remains at a high risk for aspiration. If a patient can tolerate an OPA, he cannot protect his airway and you should intubate him. If a patient displays signs of frank mechanical obstruction, simple basic life support (BLS) maneuvers are unlikely to help and therefore you should establish a definitive airway.

Even if the primary survey does not reveal obvious signs of airway obstruction, the patient may have lost their protective airway reflexes and be at risk for aspiration. This is particularly true in the patient with a depressed level of consciousness, which can result from a variety of causes: shock, intoxication, head injury, etc. The Advanced Trauma Life Support (ATLS) Program recommends that a patient with a GCS < 8 be intubated [5]. While a reasonable cutoff, this should not be a rigid one, and you should consider intubation if mental status appears to be declining rapidly even if the GCS is still above 8. The absence of the gag reflex is often cited as evidence of an inability to protect the airway, though there is scant literature to support this. Studies have noted the presence of the gag reflex across a broad spectrum of GCS scores, and the absence of a gag has been documented in individuals who are fully conscious [6, 7].

2. *Predicted airway compromise*: Patients with penetrating injuries, particularly of the neck, are at high risk for developing airway compromise, and an "intact" airway is not reassuring if early signs of obstruction are present. Early, mild signs of obstruction include subtle change in voice, cough, and mild neck hematoma [8]. These signs do not mandate immediate intubation but should be monitored closely. Stridor, expanding neck hematoma (especially in conjunction with other signs of obstruction), and obvious tracheal injury mandate early establishment of a definitive airway. The presence of stridor is a later stage of obstruction and indicates a 50% reduction in airway caliber [9]. Expanding neck hematomas, even when initially small, can lead to precipitous airway obstruction [10].
3. *Failed ventilation/oxygenation*: Consider the patient who cannot maintain adequate ventilation or oxygenation despite noninvasive measures such as supplemental oxygen as likely, but not necessarily, requiring intubation. The primary survey and adjuncts to the primary survey (respiratory rate, breath sounds, presence of cyanosis, pulse oximetry, arterial blood gases) will often make it clear whether or not a patient is in frank respiratory failure.
4. *Predicted clinical deterioration*: Even when a patient does not show hard signs of airway obstruction, inability to protect the airway, or respiratory failure, one should consider whether the likely clinical course will lead to one of these conditions. If this is the case, it is more prudent for you to intubate the patient early rather than waiting for clinical deterioration (which may occur in a less controlled environment such as the CT scanner). Is the patient extremely agitated, belligerent, and uncooperative? Will they be unlikely to tolerate diagnostic tests such as computed tomography (CT) without high doses of sedation? Is the patient in hemorrhagic shock and likely to require large volume fluid resuscitation?

2.3 Approaches to Establishing a Definitive Airway

There are numerous approaches to gaining a definitive airway, and the approach used will depend on the location of injuries, presence or suspicion of laryngotracheal injury, equipment available, and the experience of the clinician. In patients without obvious airway trauma, direct laryngoscopy generally is appropriate. In the past, it was common teaching that patients with penetrating neck injuries should proceed directly to a surgical airway. However, several retrospective studies suggest that direct laryngoscopy has a high success rate in such patients [1]. That said, if there are obvious injuries to the larynx or trachea, placement of an ETT through the cords might worsen a tracheal injury, or lead to intubation of a false passage. In patients with suspected tracheal injury, you should proceed to cricothyrotomy if the patient is unstable or, in the non-"crash" situation, go directly to the operating room (OR). In the OR, you can attempt fiberoptic intubation (when available), and be in a more controlled environment if a surgical airway is necessary. Fiberoptic intubation allows visualization of injuries below the vocal cords, and can help you to place the cuff of the ETT below the injury [11]. The different modes of obtaining a definitive airway are discussed briefly below.

Direct laryngoscopy: Appropriate initial approach for most emergent airways. Can be performed in patients with penetrating neck injuries but should be avoided if there are signs of laryngotracheal injury. May worsen injury below vocal cords or lead to intubation of false passage.

Fiberoptic intubation: If available and there is a clinician experienced in the technique, this is a good option when laryngotracheal injury is suspected but not obvious. It allows for identification of injuries below the cords, and placement of cuff distal to the injury site. Can be done awake in non-crash situation if the patient is cooperative.

Cricothyrotomy: Indicated in patients with obvious laryngotracheal injury above the cricothyroid membrane that demonstrate signs of significant airway compromise. Also an option when distortion of upper airway anatomy makes any form of laryngoscopy impossible or unlikely. This approach should be avoided if there is obvious tracheal injury below the cricothyroid membrane, or if underlying pathology (i.e., tumor or abscess) makes the approach impossible.

Direct intubation through neck wound: This should be considered in patients with obvious large defects of the trachea below the cricothyroid membrane, or in cases of complete tracheal transection.

Blind nasal intubation: There is no role for this technique if there is potential for injury anywhere in the airway. Blind passage may worsen underlying injuries and lead to complete obstruction.

Tracheotomy: This is generally avoided in the emergent setting as it is slower and carries a higher complication rate than cricothyrotomy. In cases where cricothyrotomy is impossible or there is obstruction or injury below the cricothyroid membrane it may be indicated.

2.4 Rapid Sequence Intubation

Once the decision has been made that a patient requires a definitive airway, and that direct laryngoscopy is appropriate, the next steps will depend on how emergent the situation is. A "crash" intubation essentially refers to the patient who is in frank cardiopulmonary arrest (or close to it) or in respiratory arrest [12]. In such cases, proceed to direct laryngoscopy, often without the need for induction agents or paralytics. If the patient needs a definitive airway emergently, but is not "crashing," take time to further assess the airway for potential difficulties, prepare equipment, optimize patient positioning, and formulate a backup plan in case the airway fails.

Rapid Sequence Intubation (RSI) is the near simultaneous administration of a sedative/hypnotic agent with a neuromuscular blocking agent to rapidly achieve unconsciousness and paralysis. Use this technique in emergent settings in which a patient has likely not been fasting and is at a higher risk of aspiration. If done with adequate pre-oxygenation it can often be performed without having to bag mask ventilate the patient at all, thus reducing gaseous distension of the stomach. While RSI generally improves intubation success, you should consider an alternate approach (such as awake fiberoptic intubation) in the spontaneously breathing patient who displays predictors of a difficult airway, especially if you predict they will be difficult to bag mask ventilate.

Predicting the difficult airway: Before you attempt intubation (in the non "crash" situation) you should ask these questions: Will the patient be difficult to bag mask ventilate (BMV)? Will the patient be difficult to intubate? Will it be difficult to perform a surgical airway? (Table 2.1).

2.4.1 Preparing for Intubation

Prior to intubation, it is important to make sure all equipment is laid out and working-laryngoscope with different sized blades, different sized ETT's with stylet, suction, end tidal CO_2 detector, airway adjuncts, alternative intubation device, and a rescue device (see below). While equipment is being gathered, the patient should be pre-oxygenated with 100% FiO_2 for at least 3 min. Keep in mind that 100% non-re-breather masks typically deliver only 65–70% FiO_2. It is preferable to pre-oxygenate with a well-sealed mask attached to an anesthesia bag or BMV system using 100% oxygen. During pre-oxygenation, you should attempt to place the patient in the most optimal position. Position the head of the patient as close to the end of the stretcher as possible, at a level high enough that you can get proper visualization without having to contort your body too much (usually around waist level). Pay attention to the alignment of the "airway axis": drawing an imaginary line the patient's external auditory canal should align with the sternal notch [13]. You can accomplish that with towels underneath the patient's head ("sniffing position") or by lifting the patient's

Table 2.1 Difficult airway predictors

Difficult BMV	Difficult laryngoscopy	Difficult surgical airway
• Beard	• Reduced mouth opening	• Obesity
• Elderly	• Receding chin	• Anterior neck hematoma
• Edentulous	• Obstruction (neck hematoma, stridor, tongue swelling)	• Surgical disruption (radical neck dissection, etc.)
• Perioral trauma that affects mask seal	• Large tongue	• Neck irradiation
• Mandible – fracture	• Obesity	• Overlying neck abscess
• Obesity	• Reduced neck mobility (C-collar, ankylosing spondylitis)	
• Significant tongue trauma/edema		
• Obstruction/debris/airway hemorrhage		

BMV bag mask ventilation

head with your right hand once they are paralyzed. Morbidly obese patients may need to be "ramped" up with blankets underneath their back and head in order to align the airway axis.

An important part of the intubation preparation process is choosing which RSI drugs you should give. A detailed discussion of induction agents and neuromuscular blocking agents is beyond the scope of this text, but one should have a broad understanding of the indications and contraindications of the agents available. There are several reasons for administering an induction agent: amnesia, sedation, and mitigation of the physiologic response to intubation (hypertension, tachycardia, increased intracranial pressure). Ideally, the induction agent chosen should have a rapid onset and a short half-life. In trauma, there is no one ideal agent, although etomidate is often used in patients with shock as it is hemodynamically stable and does not raise intracranial pressure (ICP). Unless there are contraindications, succinylcholine (SCh) is generally the preferred paralytic for RSI, as it has a rapid onset and is very short acting. If there are absolute contraindications for SCh, one of the non-depolarizing agents should be used. Rocuronium is perhaps the most attractive alternative as it has a rapid onset and is short acting. Furthermore, a reversal agent for rocuronium, sugammadex, has been approved for use in Europe and has been shown to recover muscle function quite quickly [8] (Tables 2.2 and 2.3).

Intubation adjuncts: At least one adjunct should be in place to help with intubation in case of poor airway visualization or inability to pass the ETT. Having several sizes of laryngoscope blades, both straight and curved, is the most basic necessary adjunct. The gum elastic bougie (Eschmann stylet) has also emerged as a simple and effective intubation adjunct (see below).

Alternative device: There are a plethora of alternative intubation devices on the market, all with different advantages and disadvantages. What you use as a backup will depend on institutional availability and your experience.

Rescue ventilation: In the case of intubation failure, especially if BMV is ineffective, you should have an extraglottic device (EGD) available. These devices rest above the vocal cords and may provide effective ventilation when BMV fails. The broadest clinical experience with EGDs has come from the laryngeal mask airway (LMA) and the esophageal tracheal combitube (ETC). EGDs do not provide a definitive airway but can be used in the rescue situation or as a bridge to cricothyrotomy (Fig. 2.2).

2.5 Orotracheal Intubation Technique

Bag mask ventilation: Anyone who performs endotracheal intubation needs to be proficient at BMV and be able to troubleshoot difficulties that arise when BMV is not effective. Effective use of the bag valve mask begins with a proper mask seal and airway opening maneuvers. The mask should be gently placed over the patient's face with the thumb and index fingers across the mask in a "C" shape, applying downward pressure. The remaining three fingers grasp the mandible, with the fifth finger hooking the mandible (see Fig. 2.3). These fingers should provide a jaw thrust and press the face toward the mask. Often, when clinicians have difficulty ventilating or encounter leakage around the mask, the tendency is to apply more pressure on the

Table 2.2 Commonly used induction agents for rapid sequence intubation

	Drug type	Clinical features	Precautions	Dosing
Etomidate	Imidazole derivative	Does not drop blood pressure appreciably	Causes transient adrenal suppression	0.3 mg/kg. Reduce dosing in hypotensive patients (mg/kg)
		Does not raise intracranial pressure	Recent concerns in sepsis and trauma (controversial)	Onset = 15–45 s
		Sedative, but no analgesic properties	May cause transient myoclonus (minimal clinical significance)	Duration = 3–12 min
		Should be followed up with sedative and/or narcotic once patient is intubated	Should not be used in repeated doses or as an infusion	
Propofol	Alkylphenol derivative	May have neuro-protective properties	Causes myocardial depression, peripheral vasodilation, and decrease in mean arterial pressure (MAP)	1.5–3 mg/kg
		Quick onset and short duration	Should be avoided in hypovolemic patients	Onset = 15–45 s
		Can be used as infusion		Duration = 5–10 min
Ketamine	Phencyclidine derivative	Provides both sedation and analgesia	May raise intracranial pressure ICP	1–2 mg/kg
		Preserves respiratory drive, raises MAP	Avoid or use with caution in head injured patients	Onset = 45–60 s
		Good choice if difficult intubation predicted in non-"crash" situation		Duration = 10–20 min
Midazolam	Benzodiazepine	One of best induction agents for providing amnesia (when dosed adequately)	In healthy patients induction dose drops MAP 10–25%	0.1–0.3 mg/kg
		Anticonvulsant properties	Caution in hypovolemic patients	Onset = 30–60 s
		Quickest onset of all benzodiazepines	Does not provide analgesia	Duration = 15–30 min

mask. Avoid this, as this may worsen airway obstruction. Instead, attempt to lift the mandible into the mask. In obtunded or chemically paralyzed patients, one can place an oropharyngeal airway to help relieve functional obstruction.

2.5.1 Intubation Technique

Various laryngoscopes are available for intubation, but the most commonly used are the curved blade (Macintosh) and straight blade (Miller). The curved blade laryngoscopes are advanced into the vallecula, engaging the hypoepiglottic ligament to indirectly lift the epiglottis and expose the laryngeal inlet. The straight blade is not inserted into the vallecula and instead is used to directly lift the epiglottis. There are advantages and disadvantages to both techniques, and ultimately the choice of technique will depend on your experience in performing the intubation (Fig. 2.4).

Always hold the laryngoscope in the left hand, regardless of whether you are left or right handed. With your elbow at a 90° angle, grip the laryngoscope handle near the base with your thumb pointed up slightly (see Fig. 2.5). You should maintain a relaxed posture, and your grip should be firm but not tense. Once the patient is completely relaxed, use the first and second fingers of your right hand to "scissor" open the incisors. Once open, insert the tip of the laryngoscope blade near the right corner of the patient's mouth and slowly advance the blade downward, attempting to sweep the tongue to the left. As you do this, gently move the blade so it is midline once the tongue moves out of the way (Fig. 2.6). As you advance, pay careful attention to identifying structures as you go, the most important of which is the epiglottis. If you insert "blindly" and go beyond the epiglottis, it can be extremely difficult to identify your location. Using a curved blade, the tip should be placed midline in the vallecula, which is the recess just anterior to the

Table 2.3 Neuromuscular blocking agents for rapid sequence intubation

	Drug type	Clinical features	Precautions	Dosing
Succinylcholine (SCh)	Depolarizing agent	Paralytic agent of choice when no contraindications exist	*Contraindications:* hyperkalemia, history of malignant hyperthermia, muscular dystrophy, rhabdomyolysis/crush injury, burns >72 h old	1.5–2.0 mg/kg
			Precautions: Raises intracranial pressure (unclear clinical significance)	Onset: 45–60 s
			Can cause bradycardia in pediatric patients (pre-dose with atropine)	Duration: 6–10 min
			Can cause bradycardia in adults, especially if given in repeated doses	
Rocuronium	Non-depolarizing agent	Primary alternative to SCh	Since it is long acting, it should be used with caution in patients with difficult airway features (though reversal agent may be available soon)	1.0 mg/kg
		Creates similar intubating conditions as SCh without the contraindications	Prolonged action will impair ability to monitor neurologic exam	Onset: 45–60 s
				Duration: 45–80 min
Vecuronium	Non-depolarizing agent	Primarily used in post-intubation management	Slow onset of action limits utility for intubation	0.1–0.3 mg/kg
			Prolonged action will impair ability to monitor neurologic exam	Onset = 1.5–3 min
				Duration: 45–90 min (higher dose = longer duration)
Pancuronium	Non-depolarizing agent	Primarily used in post-intubation management	Not a good agent for RSI	0.1 mg/kg
			Causes tachycardia and may cause arrhythmia	Onset = 3–5 min
				Duration = 60–90 min

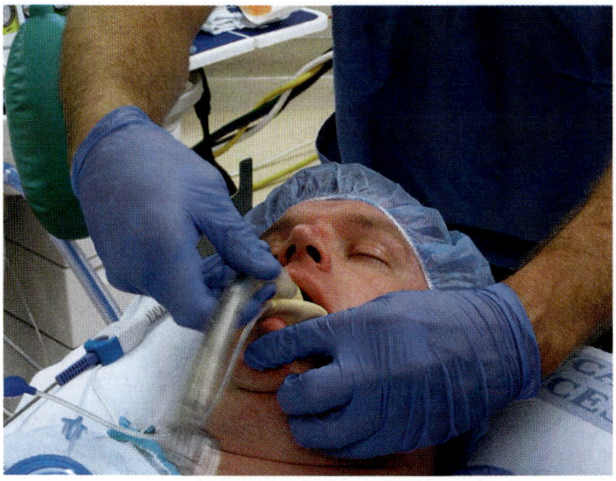

Fig. 2.2 The laryngeal mask airway (LMA): The LMA is one of several extraglottic devices (EGDs) that can be used for rescue ventilation when one cannot intubate a patient and cannot ventilate them with a bag valve mask. EGDs are not definitive airways

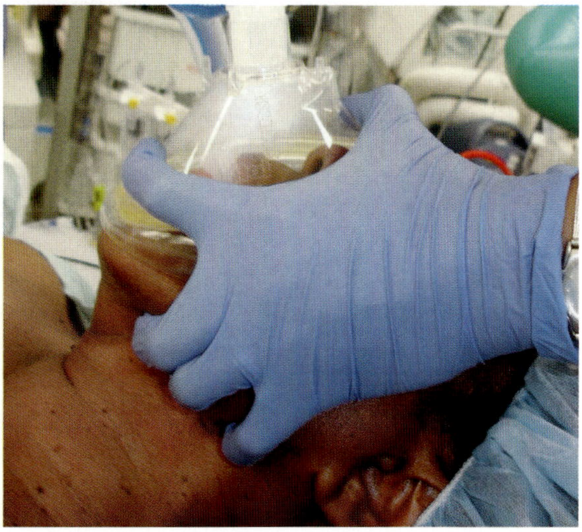

Fig. 2.3 Bag mask ventilation technique. Notice how the third, fourth, and fifth digits are used to lift the mandible into the face. Very little downward pressure is placed on the mask

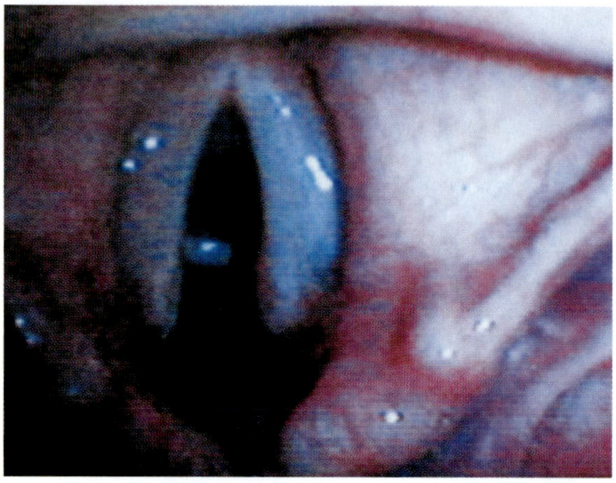

Fig. 2.4 Laryngeal anatomy: Ideal (grade 1) view of the laryngeal inlet. An important feature is the interarytenoid notch. If this can be visualized, one can be confident the endotracheal tube is directed correctly if it is above the notch. Below this, the ETT will enter the esophagus

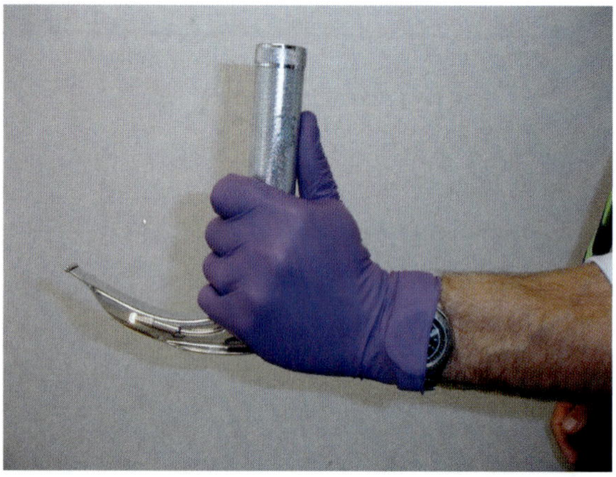

Fig. 2.5 Holding the laryngoscope: The laryngoscope should be held with the left hand close to the base of the handle. The elbow is held at a 90° angle to the intubator's torso

epiglottis. Once in place, lift the laryngoscope firmly away from the patient (carefully avoiding the tendency to lever back which can break teeth and supplies no mechanical advantage). This will lift the epiglottis and expose the vocal cords. Alternatively, advance the laryngoscope blade (if using a straight or a larger curved blade) directly lift the epiglottis.

Once the vocal cords are identified, keep your eyes on them! Have an assistant hand you an appropriate sized ETT, with a stylet in place. Having the ETT in the "straight to cuff" shape, with the tube bent at a 35° angle just distal to the cuff, has been shown to improve visualization of the vocal cords during ETT advancement [14]. Keep the ETT in a horizontal position, with the cuff deflated, and advance from the right corner of the mouth, making sure never to lose sight of the cords. When the ETT nears the cords, rotate counterclockwise about 45° and pass through. In cases where you cannot get full visualization of the cords, an endotracheal tube introducer (gum elastic bougie, or Eschmann stylet) can be introduced first, and the ETT passed over the stylet using the Seldinger technique (see Fig. 2.7). Once the tube has been advanced, inflate the cuff, attach a CO_2 detector, and ventilate. The best evidence that the ETT has been placed in the trachea is 100% confidence that it was seen passing through the cords. Other signs include color change with the CO_2 detector, misting of the tube, good breath sounds, and reinflation of an esophageal detector bulb device (Fig. 2.7).

2.6 Surgical Airways

There are several surgical approaches to obtaining emergency airways, including retrograde intubation, percutaneous transtracheal ventilation, cricothyrotome (using Seldinger technique), cricothyrotomy, and tracheostomy. Retrograde intubation, which involves insertion of a wire through the cricothyroid membrane, threading it into the oropharynx, then advancing an endotracheal tube over the wire, is a time consuming, multistep process that has had mixed results [15]. Percutaneous transtracheal ventilation does not provide a definitive airway, but may be the only airway option in children less than 12 years old in whom formal cricothyrotomy is extremely difficult due to small size of the membrane. Cricothyrotome incorporates the Seldinger technique in which a guide wire is thread through a locator needle and an airway catheter is then advanced through the cricothyroid membrane. Comparisons of cricothyrotome versus traditional cricothyrotomy have had mixed results, but a recent study using cadavers showed surgical cricothyrotomy to be superior to cricothyrotome in terms of success rate, time to ventilation, and complication rate [16].

There are several methods of performing a cricothyrotomy. Regardless of the technique used, it is important that you are familiar with one method, you

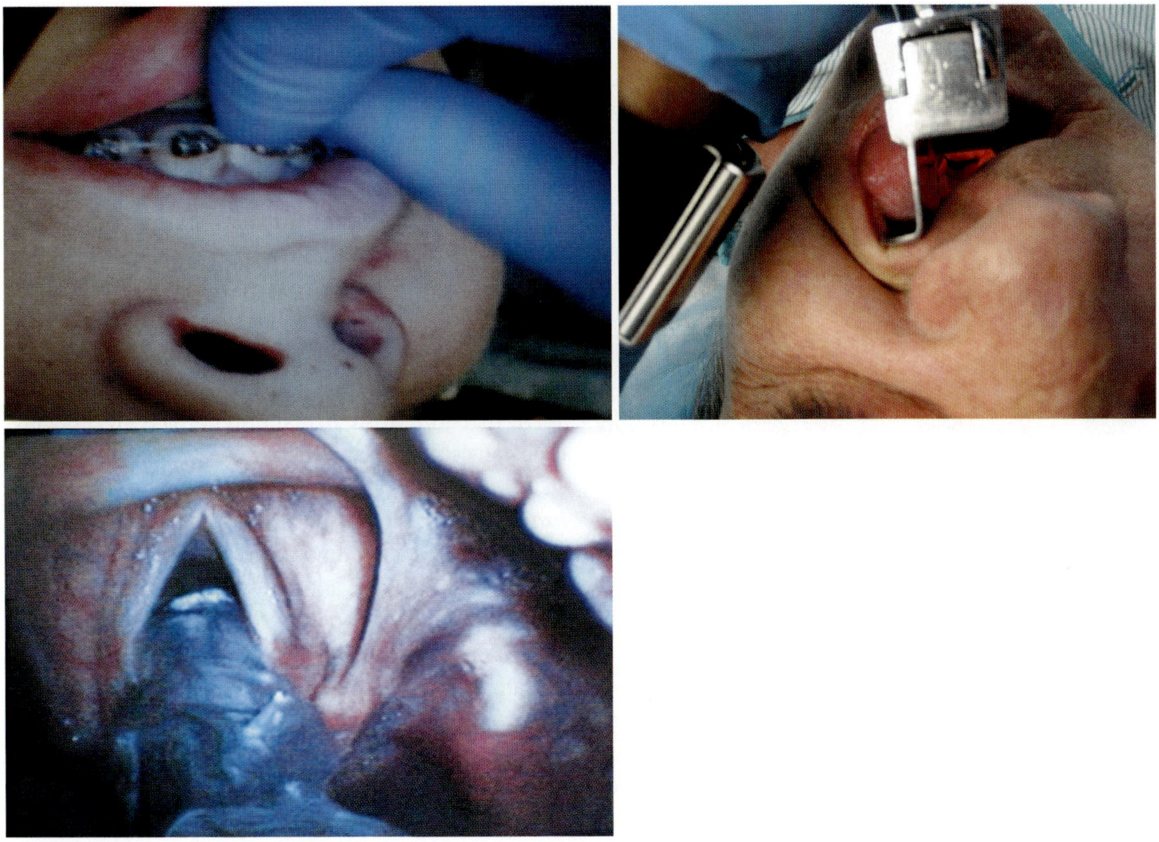

Fig. 2.6 *Upper left*: scissor technique for opening mouth. *Upper right*: laryngoscope inserted from right, sweeping tongue to left.

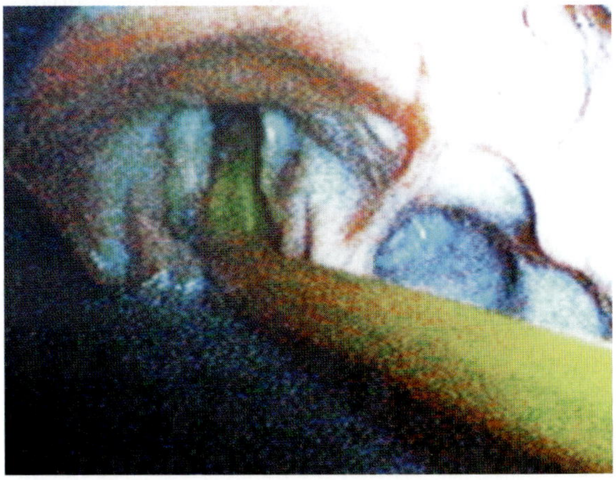

Fig. 2.7 The Eschmann stylet (gum elastic bougie): A useful intubation adjunct when unable to fully visualize the cords. The stylet is thread into the trachea and then the ETT is advanced over the Eschmann stylet using the Seldinger technique. Tracheal position of the stylet is suggested by a palpable "clicking" along the tracheal rings and inability to advance beyond about 20 cm as it enters the small airways. If it meets no resistance, it has likely entered the GI tract

are ready to use it, and you are able to make use of whatever equipment is immediately available. It must also be emphasized that in the crash situation one may not always be able to confidently identify all landmarks. This absolutely should not delay the quick establishment of an airway, even if this involves missing the cricothyroid membrane and opening the tracheal cartilage. While not ideal, the patient can later undergo formal tracheostomy under controlled circumstances but can ill afford additional minutes of hypoxia (Fig. 2.8).

Equipment: A traditional cricothyrotomy tray will contain the following: scalpel, Trousseau dilator, tracheal hook, skin retractors, hemostats, 4×4 gauze sponges, and either a #6 cuffed ETT or a #4 tracheostomy tube. What tools you actually use will depend on the patient, whether or not you have an assistant, and what is immediately available. In reality, most cricothyrotomies can be performed using a scalpel, hemostat, an endotracheal tube, and your fingers.

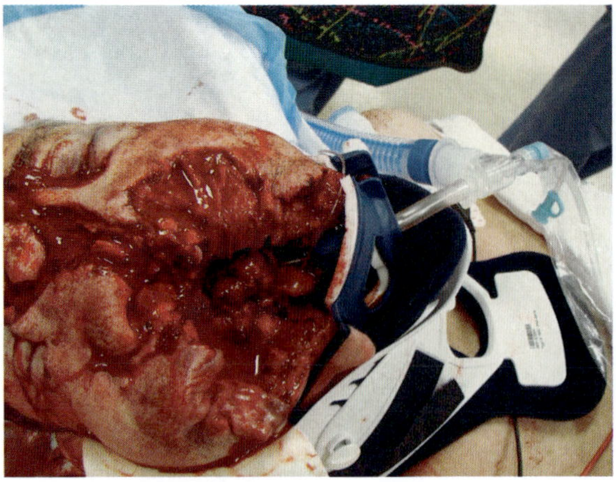

Fig. 2.8 Blast injury to the face: certain injuries may be so extensive that neither laryngoscopy nor traditional surgical airways are feasible. In this case, minor exploration revealed adequate visualization of the vocal cords leading to intubation

Landmarks: Once the decision is made to perform a cricothyrotomy, the first step is to identify landmarks. Feel for the notch of the thyroid cartilage and follow this inferiorly until you feel the soft depression, which is the cricothyroid membrane. Obviously, in cases of hematoma or obesity, these landmarks may be obscured. You can get a rough sense of the cricothyroid membrane's location by placing four fingers horizontally along the neck, with the fifth finger at the sternal notch. The cricothyroid membrane's approximate location will be under the index finger [12]. Also, if the thyroid cartilage is hard to appreciate, keep in mind that the cricoid cartilage is the first prominent cartilage palpated above the sternal notch. If it has been difficult to identify the cricothyroid membrane, consider using a surgical marker to indicate where you wish to incise. Once you have a reasonable feel for your landmarks, begin your preparations for the incision.

Preparation: If this is not a crash airway, take your time to position the patient. Extend the neck as much as possible (unless a cervical spine injury is expected) by placing a towel under the back of the neck. Infiltrate the skin overlying the cricothyroid membrane with 1% lidocaine with epinephrine, and anesthetize right through the membrane. This may briefly cause the patient to cough, but they will be better able to tolerate the ETT once placed. If the patient is awake, one should consider sedation. Clearly, this will not pertain to the crash situation, and caution should be used in the spontaneously ventilating patient still able to oxygenate. Ketamine is an attractive agent in this situation in that it preserves respiratory drive and blood pressure.

Incision: If you are right hand dominant, position yourself on the patient's right (opposite if you are left hand dominant). Before you incise, immobilize the larynx by grasping the posterior, superior aspect of the laryngeal cartilage with your non-dominant hand, using the middle finger and thumb. Now, you are in position to easily feel for the cricothyroid membrane with the index finger of your non-dominant hand. With the scalpel in your dominant hand, make a 2–3 cm, vertical incision. While some texts recommend using a transverse incision, this carries a higher risk of bleeding, especially if has been difficult to identify landmarks.

Identification and incision of the cricothyroid membrane: If the patient is obese, you may have to bluntly dissect through a fair amount of tissue before you reach the trachea. When available, have an assistant retract the skin laterally. Expect a fair amount of bleeding, even if you avoid major vessels, and rely on feel, not visualization, to identify the cricothyroid membrane. Do not concern yourself with hemostasis at this point: establish the airway first and then go back to control bleeding. While the middle finger and thumb continue to stabilize the larynx, use the index finger of the same (non-dominant) hand to palpate for the cricothyroid membrane. Once this is exposed and overlying tissue dissected, use your dominant hand to make a horizontal incision through the inferior aspect of the cricothyroid membrane. To avoid incising too superior (the cricothyroid artery and vein are more cephalad) you should keep your non-dominant index finger at the inferior border of the thyroid cartilage. Successful entry of the trachea will be obvious by the exiting of air, and often by reflexive coughing.

Preparing to place the endotracheal tube: Once the cricothyroid membrane is incised, it is important to stabilize the trachea. Overlying tissue can quickly obscure the incision site, and the trachea may drop down after incision, making successful airway cannulation difficult. Temporarily do this by placing the index finger of the non-dominant hand through the incision and grasp the inferior portion of the thyroid cartilage. If a tracheal hook is available, insert this into the incision, grasp the inferior border of the membrane, and pull the trachea caudally. Some authors recommend hooking the superior portion of the cricothyroid membrane, but we have found that securing the inferior border provides more secure traction when advancing the ETT. If a tracheal hook is not available, maintain the index finger of your non-dominant hand in the incision, securing the trachea. Alternatively, you can fashion a makeshift tracheal hook by bending an 18-gauge needle and clamping at the end of a hemostat.

Inserting the endotracheal tube: In most cases, one can proceed to inserting the endotracheal tube at this point, with no need for tracheal dilation. If the passage is too narrow to pass the endotracheal tube, try a smaller tube or use a Trousseau dilator. If you have incised directly through cartilage, it is usually necessary to use a dilator in order to pass the ETT. When using a Trousseau dilator, insert into the incision and dilate with the blades oriented vertically. Now, place the #6 cuffed ETT between the blades of the dilator and into the airway, rotate the dilator so the blades are oriented horizontally, and advance the ETT. While advancing the ETT, remove the dilator. Be sure not to advance the ETT too far so as to avoid right mainstem intubation. Inflate the cuff, check end tidal CO_2, and auscultate for breath sounds.

It must be emphasized once again that in the "crash" situation, when a patient is hypoxic and/or not ventilating, obtaining an airway quickly is essential. Do not become distracted by bleeding, or failure to quickly identify landmarks. If you do not find the cricothyroid membrane quickly, make your incision through the tracheal cartilage, dilate if necessary, and advance the tube. While not ideal, the timely establishment of an airway far outweighs the potential for a tracheal injury.

Important Points

1. Emergent intubation is often necessary in penetrating trauma, particularly when it involves the face and neck.
2. Orotracheal intubation of patients with penetrating trauma, even when involving the face or neck, has a very high success rate. It is rarely necessary to proceed directly to a surgical airway.
3. Be cautious about orotracheal intubation when there is suspected laryngotracheal trauma. The ETT may worsen a tracheal injury or intubate a false passage. When available, intubation should occur with a fiberoptic scope in the OR.
4. In cases involving slash wounds to the neck with large tracheal defects, one can intubate the trachea directly through the wound.
5. When performing cricothyrotomy, it may be difficult to identify landmarks clearly once the incision is made. One should rely as much on feel as visualization.
6. When performing cricothyrotomy, expect a lot of bleeding. Do not worry about hemostasis until the airway has been established.
7. If you have trouble identifying the cricothyroid membrane, it is okay to make your incision directly through the trachea. This can be repaired later.

References

1. Brywczynski JJ, Barrett TW, Lyon JA, Cotton BA (2008) Management of penetrating neck injury in the emergency department: a structured literature review. Emerg Med J 25:711–715
2. Pierre E, McNeer R, Shamir M (2007) Early management of the traumatized airway. Anesthesiol Clin 25:1–11
3. Lee C (2009) Reversal of profound neuromuscular block by sugammadex administered three minutes after rocuronium: a comparison with spontaneous recovery from succinylcholine. Anesthesiology 110:1020
4. Davis D, Fakhry S, Wang H, Bulger E, Domeier R, Trask A, Bochicchio G, Hauda W, Robinson L (2007) Paramedic rapid sequence intubation for severe traumatic brain injury: perspectives from an expert panel. Prehosp Emerg Care 11(1):1–8
5. American College of Surgeons Committee on Trauma (2008) Advanced trauma life support for doctors, 8th edn. American College of Surgeons, Chicago
6. Bleach N (1993) The gag reflex and aspiration: a retrospective analysis of 120 patients assessed by videofluoroscopy. Clin Otolaryngol 18:303–307
7. Moulton C, Pennybrook A, Makower A (1991) Relation between the Glasgow coma scale and the gag reflex. BMJ 303:1240–1241
8. Lee W, Eliashar R, Eliachar I (2006) Acute external laryngotracheal trauma: diagnosis and management. ENT Ear Nose Throat J 85(3):179–184
9. Mason RA, Fielder CP (1999) The obstructed airway in head and neck surgery. Anaesthesia 54:625–628
10. Keogh IJ, Rowley H, Russell J (2002) Critical airway compromise caused by neck hematoma. Clin Otolaryngol 27: 244–245
11. Desjardins G, Varon A (2001) Airway management for penetrating neck injuries: the Miami experience. Resuscitation 48:71–75
12. Walls R, Murphy M (2008) Manual of emergency airway management, 3rd edn. Lippincott Williams & Wilkins, Philadelphia

13. Kovacs G, Law J (2008) Airway management in emergencies, 1st edn. McGraw-Hill Companies, New York
14. Levitan R (2004) The airway Cam guide to intubation and practical emergency airway management. Airway Cam Technologies, Inc., Wayne
15. Warner K, Sharar S, Copass M, Bulger E (2009) Prehospital management of the difficult airway: a prospective cohort study. J Emerg Med 36(3):257–265
16. Schober P, Hegemann M, Schwarte L, Loer S, Noetges P (2009) Emergency cricothyrotomy – a comparative study of different techniques in human cadavers. Resuscitation 80:204–209
17. Tallon J, Ahmed J, Sealy B (2007) Airway management in penetrating neck trauma at a Canadian tertiary trauma centre. J Can Assoc Emerg Physicians 9(2):101–104

3 Hypotensive Resuscitation in Penetrating Trauma: Rules of the Game

Suresh Agarwal, Lejla Hadzikadic, and Peter Burke

Dr. William Halstead is attributed with the quotation, "The only weapon with which the unconscious patient can immediately retaliate upon the incompetent surgeon is hemorrhage." It is also a major weapon upon which patients involved in trauma present to the hospital. Thus, it is imperative for the competent surgeon to treat hemorrhage expeditiously in order to restore physiologic homeostasis and prevent the dire consequences of ongoing bleeding.

Unfortunately, for the surgeon taking care of the victim of a penetrating trauma, ongoing bleeding is often present prior to formal evaluation. The question of resuscitation, both type and extent, of these patients is a point of continuous debate and conjecture. Operative trauma surgery can be simplified into three basic steps: (1) stop the bleeding, (2) take out the bad, and (3) put the good back together. First and foremost, the cessation of bleeding takes precedent over all maneuvers once the abdomen has been opened. The question arises to what to do before the patient arrives in the operating room – aggressively resuscitate or permissively allow for hypotension and a degree of shock?

Historically, the field of trauma surgery has evolved with changing times and conflicts. Although the management of traumatic injury has been described in the Edwin Smith Papyrus found in Egypt and the Ayur Veda in ancient India, the term "shock" has been attributed to Samuel Gross who described it as a "rude unhinging of the machinery of life." Claude Bernard described the innate response to decreasing a disturbance of the "internal milieu" and Cannon expounded upon the "fight or flight" response that is seen with severe physiological disturbances. In 1919, Keith showed that hypovolemia was a mechanism for shock. Alfred Blalock's animal experiments demonstrated that blood loss was the primary cause of traumatic shock, and along with Wiggers, Cannon, and Scudder implicated that hypotension was its harbinger. Subsequently, Shires was able to beautifully demonstrate the response to resuscitation from hemorrhagic shock utilizing different fluid types: blood, blood and plasma, and blood and lactated Ringer's solution. His demonstration of an extracellular fluid deficit has been repetitively corroborated in human subjects. Accordingly, the Advanced Trauma Life Support Course from the American College of Surgeons Committee on Trauma developed a protocol of aggressive resuscitation for all trauma patients regardless of the mechanism of injury, with the end goal being the administration of crystalloid in a 3 to 1 ratio to the estimated amount of blood lost.

S. Agarwal (✉)
Surgical Critical Care, Boston Medical Center, Boston, MA 02118, USA

Department of Surgery, Boston University School of Medicine, 850 Harrison Avenue, Dowling 2 South, Boston, MA 02118, USA
e-mail: suresh.agarwal@bmc.org

L. Hadzikadic
Department of Surgery, Boston Medical Center, Boston, MA 02118, USA

P. Burke
Department of Surgery, Boston University School of Medicine, 850 Harrison Avenue, Dowling 2 South, Boston, MA 02118, USA

Trauma Services, Boston Medical Center, Boston, MA, USA

G.C. Velmahos et al. (eds.), *Penetrating Trauma*,
DOI 10.1007/978-3-642-20453-1_3, © Springer-Verlag Berlin Heidelberg 2012

Once this algorithm became accepted, the type of fluid administered has come under debate. Soon, it became clear that crystalloid resuscitation was not without its problems. Whereas the Korean Conflict introduced the world to the necessity of dialysis as a consequence of under-resuscitation and acute tubular necrosis, the Vietnam War ushered in the results of patients who had been over-resuscitated with the consequence being "DaNang Lung," which later became known as acute respiratory distress syndrome (ARDS), and increased incidences of abdominal compartment syndrome. Furthermore, as the costs of crystalloid administration upon the immune system and human genome have become better understood, adjuncts to traditional crystalloid solutions and techniques of genetic modification have become of increased interest [1].

3.1 Crystalloids and the Lethal Triad

In fact, it is now clear that aggressive crystalloid infusion may have the untoward effect of worsening the lethal triad of acidosis, coagulopathy, and hypothermia: all harbingers of poor outcome. The body has an outstanding capacity to compensate for physiologic instability following penetrating trauma. To the trauma surgeon, the lethal triad may portend the beginning of a whirlwind cascade of physiologic events that is very difficult, if not impossible, to overcome. Components of the triad have been targets of intense research aimed at looking for ways to prevent negative side effects of these compensatory mechanisms.

Coagulopathy has been thought to be mainly a dilution of clotting factors and platelets: a result of the aggressive crystalloid resuscitation of the trauma patient, due to endpoints aimed at restoring blood volume and central venous pressure. Growing evidence suggests that the trauma patient may arrive to the trauma bay with an existing coagulopathy which may be worsened by the rapid administration of lactated ringer's or normal saline.

Severe hypothermia, defined as a temperature less than 28°C, has been shown to correlate with 100% mortality. Moderate hypothermia, defined as a temperature between 28°C and 22°C, has been associated with mortality rates approaching 40%. It has also been shown to correlate directly to a reduction of coagulation factor activity by approximately 10% for each degree centigrade while affecting platelet function as well. With prolonged extrication times, heat loss, intoxication, and an open abdomen, trauma patients with hemorrhagic shock have an uncoupling of metabolic pathways resulting in loss of homeothermic ability.

Acidosis is the third leg of the lethal triad: a rising lactate indicates that the body's demands for tissue oxygenation are not being met, regardless of hemoglobin loss, poor oxygen diffusion, or poor pump capacity; a lactic acidosis indicates that anaerobic respiration exists. A pH less than 7.2 affects cell functions such as ATP generation, fatty acid biosynthesis, and enzymatic reactions, and correlates to a mortality approaching 80%. Oxygen delivery is vital to maintain proper tissue perfusion and organ function, and multi-system organ failure is difficult to reverse and often fatal. It is for this reason that acidosis has been linked with poorer outcomes in trauma patients and why lactate, base deficit, and mixed-venous saturation are followed as endpoints of resuscitation [2].

Correction of the lethal triad has guided our clinical judgment when it comes to the trauma patient. Unfortunately hypothermia, coagulopathy, and acidosis follow a cyclical pattern which is difficult to break. Both clinically and experimentally, attempts to block these three facets have been targets of intense interest. They include damage control surgery, warming of crystalloid fluids and blood products, the advent of Factor VII, and the emergence of hypotensive resuscitation as a treatment phenomenon.

3.2 Operative Control and Resuscitation

Bleeding cessation has been of considerable interest in the medical community and, particularly, with prehospital care. Mattox, et al. demonstrated that the utilization of medical anti-shock trousers (MAST), in order to increase venous return to the heart, improve systolic blood pressure, and improve cerebral perfusion, had no improvement upon survival and may increase mortality, particularly in penetrating injuries to the torso [3]. Nicholl, et al. in a meta-analysis showed that emergency medical technician attempts to increase systolic blood pressure in the bleeding trauma patient led to an increase in mortality [4].

With this in mind, Bickell et al. in 1994 published their results of a prospective trial examining resuscitation strategies in patients with penetrating torso trauma. They were able to demonstrate that patients who received immediate, preoperative resuscitation experienced a statistically significant increase in mortality and a strong trend toward increased morbidity and hospital length of stay, when compared with patients who received delayed, post-hemorrhage cessation resuscitation. Furthermore, Bickell was able to show that there was a significant increase in bleeding time, with respect to prothrombin and partial thromboplastin times, in the early resuscitation groups when compared to those patients who received fluid in a delayed manner [5].

Blair examined patients with gastrointestinal hemorrhage and was able to show a survival advantage in patients who received delayed resuscitation. Furthermore, he was similarly able to show a coagulopathy in those patients who were aggressively resuscitated prior to hemorrhage control. This study, however, lacked significant power with a total of 50 patients enrolled and a total mortality of 4% (all in the early resuscitation group) [6].

Despite this finding, the study, with respect to mortality, has not been able to be replicated in models of blunt mechanism or in patients who have not experienced a traumatic episode. Although Dutton, et al. were unable to confirm these findings in a patient group that included a preponderance of patients with blunt injuries, multiple animal studies have been able to clarify physiologic patterns regarding bleeding due to arterial injury [7].

Peitzman, et al. summarized multiple animal models of unresuscitated blood loss and showed that there are three phases to the bleeding patient: the first is a compensated phase in which the patient's intrinsic mechanisms maintain mean arterial pressure, the second a decompensated phase in which patients transition to a subacute lethal phase of shock, and, finally, an irreversible phase in which the patient becomes unresponsive to resuscitative efforts [8]. The period of time in which recovery is possible varies with respect to the innate response of individuals and the interactions of the systems involved, including: cardiovascular, neuroendocrine, and immunologic. As Kauver, et al. answered when asked about hypotensive resuscitation, "It is not a question of whether or not to do it (hypotensive resuscitation) the question is how low for how long [9]." Controlled intraoperative hypotension is a well established and widely used concept in anesthesia and can be achieved via delayed resuscitation and permissive hypotension. Mild to moderate hypotension allows for clot formation and slows bleeding from injured blood vessels until surgical hemostasis can be achieved.

Animal trials have concluded that the effect of fluid resuscitation on the risk of death in models of uncontrolled hemorrhage is related to the severity of hemorrhage. A combination of the patient's natural coagulation cascade, hypotension, and vessel spasm will temporarily arrest traumatic hemorrhage, thus conjuring up the theory of "popping the clot" with aggressive fluid resuscitation in uncontrolled hemorrhage [2, 10–12]. Keep in mind that injuries with faster rates of bleeding will achieve a faster intrinsic hemostatic plug at a lower MAP, therefore giving too much fluid to this group of patients delays innate hemostatic mechanisms. Injuries with slower rates of bleeding will achieve a slower innate hemostatic plug and therefore may appear as transient responders to a fluid bolus, as the patient will not become hypotensive within 15 or 30 min from injury [13, 14]. In operative management of penetrating trauma, as soon as you have a clamp on the bleeding vessel, you can use endpoints of resuscitation to give fluids. Once the bleeding has been controlled, the patient has a better ability to tolerate fluid administration.

It is the timing of fluid administration, with respect to intrinsic hemostasis, that shapes the hemorrhaging patient's hemodynamic response. Early boluses delay intrinsic hemostasis and, therefore, increase blood loss, while late boluses trigger re-bleeding. Therefore, fluid administration before and after intrinsic hemostasis may have entirely different hemodynamic consequences [13, 14].

Despite the advent and improvement of trauma systems, patients with injuries are still dying – however, now in the trauma bay instead of the field. Based on 40 years of data, trauma injury continues to have three peaks of mortality as initially described by Trunkey. Hemorrhage remains the leading cause of immediate death for patients who survive transport to the hospital [15].

3.3 Operative Control of Bleeding Has Been Established, Now What?

Now, you resuscitate.

Once you have controlled the bleeding vessel, either by clamp or suture, you should proceed with resuscitation. The focus of hypotensive resuscitation of the penetrating trauma patient is *after* definitive operative control. Patients with a full reservoir tank are better at tolerating fluid administration over hemorrhaging patients. This population needs damage control resuscitation, likened to the concept of damage control surgery, and fluid resuscitation should be aimed at preventing damage to the cardiorespiratory system leading to hypoperfusion and tissue hypoxia [2, 16]. You can accomplish that by low volume boluses of crystalloid or colloid (packed red blood cells, platelets, fresh frozen plasma) such as 250–500 mL given to maintain mean arterial pressure (MAP) to 65 mmHg. Fresh frozen plasma has the added benefit of restoring clotting factors as well as acting as a resuscitative fluid. It is important to keep in mind that colloids will stay intravascular for a longer period of time in a trauma patient likely to be experiencing edema from leaky capillaries after a highly inflammatory insult. Resuscitation continues until classic endpoints of lactate, base deficit, and mixed venous oxygen saturation have been met.

It would be negligence on our part to ignore modern day advances with fluid resuscitation. The military has contributed to many remarkable advances in low volume colloid materials aimed at assisting space-limited medics in the field and allowing them to temporize blood loss and shock until transfer to a definite care facility can be made.

Though not validated by prospective trials yet, several new fluid alternatives show promising advantages over conventional crystalloid fluids. HES (hydroxyethyl starch) and HDS (hypertonic saline dextran) have been shown to result in prompt recovery of tissue perfusion when compared to infusion with equal volumes of crystalloid [16, 17]. Hypotensive resuscitation with LR greatly reduced volume requirements when compared with normotensive resuscitation; however when HEX (hextend-6% hydroxyethyl starch in a balanced salt solution) was compared to both, it achieved an additional volume sparing benefit [18]. Aside from new fluid modalities, the military advocates use of fresh whole blood over the sum of its parts as the two are not equal; and though there is likely not to be much doubt that fresh whole blood is superior to component therapy, clearly a limiting factor for civilian use is availability and a supply/demand ratio [2].

Advances in low volume resuscitation therapy have been equaled only by advances in gene therapy. Though still in the experimental phase, studies show that conventional resuscitation fluids can actually worsen cellular injury caused by hemorrhagic shock and that hemorrhage and resuscitation affect the expression of approximately 7% of genes in a fluid specific fashion and alter down-stream cascades of acute phase proteins. One of the hot topics today lies in histone acetylation with hemorrhage being associated with histone hypoacetylation. An increase in histone acetylation is associated with enhanced transcription of acute phase reaction genes and adding a histone deacetylase inhibitor (HDACI) to resuscitation fluid increases histone acetylation and increases transcription of key regulatory genes [19]. Interestingly, an NIH sponsored study assessing the utilization of hypertonic saline in the resuscitation of trauma patients was terminated early due to an inability to show benefit when compared to traditional crystalloids.

Another hot topic lies in hemoglobin based oxygen carriers such as HBOC-201, where it has been found that hypotensive resuscitation with this oxygen carrier restored tissue oxygenation and reversed anaerobic metabolism at significantly lower volumes when compared with HTS, HSD, petastarch, or hetastarch solutions [20–22]. Other new areas of interest are focused on the endothelium and its role in reperfusion injury as well as mitochondria and cytopathic hypoxia and optimal delivery of oxygen compared to optimal utilization of this delivered oxygen [21].

Thus, as the idea of hypotensive resuscitation gets an overhaul, the age old debate of crystalloid vs. colloid becomes a less relevant discussion as new modalities of resuscitation are likely to make their way into the mainstream trauma bay.

3.4 Summary

Adaptation to a changing world and the need to revisit our philosophy of fluid resuscitation grew out of a practical necessity as studies have repetitively demonstrated that early and aggressive crystalloid resuscitation is not without consequence. Trauma surgeons were faced with the very real fact of the detrimental results of fluid overload, including ARDS; SIRS and MSOF have, for many, become the end product of over-resuscitation. An overwhelming amount of supportive studies have demonstrated that hypotensive resuscitation is likely beneficial in penetrating mechanisms of trauma. Thus, resuscitative efforts begin after surgical hemostasis, or temporizing methods, have been achieved. Once operative control of bleeding has been obtained, resuscitation to endpoints of adequate tissue perfusion should be achieved.

Important Points

- In penetrating torso trauma, hypotension is not a harbinger of death, but rather an opportunity to control bleeding prior to initiating resuscitative efforts.
- Aggressive crystalloid in penetrating trauma patients leads to a worsening of the lethal triad: coagulopathy, acidosis, hypothermia.
- Apply damage control resuscitation techniques to the hemorrhaging penetrating trauma patient until operative control can be established.
- Operate first, Resuscitate later.
- Once bleeding has been controlled, resuscitate to endpoints of adequate tissue perfusion: lactate, mixed venous saturation, base deficit.
- Immunomodulation and gene therapy are emerging as the future of patient resuscitation.

References

1. Alam HB, Shults C, Ahuja N, Ayuste EC, Chen H, Koustova E, Sailhamer EA, Li Y, Liu B, de Moya M, de Velmahos GC (2008) Impact of resuscitation strategies on the acetylation status of cardiac histones in a swine model of hemorrhage. Resuscitation 76:299–310
2. Beekley AC (2008) Damage control resuscitation: a sensible approach to the exsanguinating surgical patient. Crit Care Med 36(7 suppl):267–274
3. Mattox KL, Bickell WH, Pepe PE, Mangelsdorff AD (1986) Prospective randomized evaluation of antishock MAST in post-traumatic hypotension. J Trauma 26(9):779–786
4. Nicholl J, Hughes S, Dixon S, Turner J, Yates D (1998) The costs and benefits of paramedic skills in pre-hospital trauma care. Health Technol Assess 2(17):30
5. Bickell WH, Wall MJ, Pepe PE, Martin RR, Ginger VF, Allen MK, Mattox KL (1994) Immediate versus delayed fluid resuscitation for hypotensive patients with penetrating torso injuries. N Engl J Med 331(17):1105–1109
6. Blair SD, Janvrin SB, McCollum CN, Greenhalgh RM (1986) Effect of early blood transfusion on gastrointestinal hemorrhage. Br J Surg 73(10):783–785
7. Dutton RP, MacKenzie CF, Scalea TM (2002) Hypotensive resuscitation during active hemorrhage: impact on in-hospital mortality. J Trauma 52:1141–1146
8. Peitzman AB, Billiar TR, Harbrecht BG (1995) Hemoorrhagic shock. Curr Probl Surg 32:974
9. Kauvar DS, Lefering R, Wade CE (2006) Impact of hemorrhage on trauma outcome: an overview of epidemiology, clinical presentations, and therapeutic considerations. J Trauma 60(6):3–11
10. Capone AC, Safar P, Stezoski W, Tisherman S, Peitzman AB (1995) Improved outcome with fluid restriction in treatment of uncontrolled hemorrhagic shock. J Am Coll Surg 180(1):49–56
11. Krausz MM (2006) Initial resuscitation of hemorrhagic shock. World J Emerg Surg 1(14):1–5
12. Kreimeier U, Prueckner S, Peter K (2000) Permissive hypotension. J Suisse Med 130(42):1516–1524
13. Hirshberg A, Hoyt DB, Mattox KL (2006) Timing of fluid resuscitation shapes the hemodynamic response to uncontrolled hemorrhage: analysis using dynamic modeling. J Trauma 60:1221–1227
14. Hirshberg A, Hoyt DB, Mattox KL (2007) From 'leaky buckets' to vascular injuries: understanding models of uncontrolled hemorrhage. J Am Coll Surg 204(4):665–672
15. Hoyt DB (2003) Fluid resuscitation: the target from an analysis of trauma systems and patient survival. J Trauma 54(5):31–35
16. Ferreira ELA, Terzi RGG, Silva WA, Moraes AC (2005) Early colloid replacement therapy in a near-fatal model of hemorrhagic shock. Anesth Analg 101:1785–1791
17. Dubick MA, Atkins JL (2003) Small-volume fluid resuscitation for the far-forward combat environment: current concepts. J Trauma 54(5):43–45
18. Rafie AD, Rath PA, Michell MW, Kirschner RA, Deyo DJ, Prough DS, Grady JJ, Kramer GC (2004) Hypotensive resuscitation of multiple hemorrhages using crystalloid and colloids. Shock 22(3):262–269
19. Shultz C, Sailhamer EA, Li Y, Liu B, Tabbara M, Butt MU, Shuja F, de Moya M, Velmahos G, Alam HB (2008) Surviving blood loss without fluid resuscitation. J Trauma 64(3):629–640
20. McNeil JD, Smith DL, Jenkins DH, York GB, Josephs JD (2001) Hypotensive resuscitation using a polymerized bovine hemoglobin-based oxygen-carrying solution (HBOC-201) leads to reversal of anaerobic metabolism. J Trauma 50(6):1063–1075
21. Rushing GD, Britt LD (2008) Reperfusion injury after hemorrhage. Ann Surg 247(6):929–937
22. Sampson JB, Davis MR, Mueller DL, Kashyap VS, Jenkins DH, Kerby JD (2003) A comparison of the hemoglobin-based oxygen carrier HBOC-201 to other low-volume resuscitation fluids in a model of controlled hemorrhagic shock. J Trauma 55(4):747–754

4 BCLS Versus ACLS

Alasdair K.T. Conn

4.1 BCLS Versus ACLS

Prehospital providers can be divided into basic providers – in the United States, they are called emergency medical technicians or EMTs – and advanced prehospital providers – paramedics [1–3]. Although basic providers are restricted to splinting, bandaging, alignment of displaced limbs, and the administration of oxygen, many basic EMTs will have obtained an intermediate level (EMT-I) who can start intravenous fluids and in many states obtain a more definitive airway such as using a Combitube or even endotracheal intubation. Paramedics can initiate IVs, perform chest decompression for a pneumothorax, perform endotracheal intubation or a cricothyrotomy, and administer many medications [4]. These prehospital providers are licensed by the state usually for 2 years before relicensing is required (in a process similar to the licensing of nurses and physicians) and have defined codes of practice and standards of care. Many of these protocols are statewide; an example of such a protocol might be "Basic EMT protocol for the assessment and management of penetrating abdominal and thoracic injury."

A.K.T. Conn
Department of Emergency Services, Massachusetts General Hospital, 55 Fruit Street, Founders 114, Boston, MA 02114, USA

Department of Surgery, Harvard Medical School, Boston, MA, USA
e-mail: aconn@partners.org

4.2 The "EMS Paradox"

Paramedics are normally located in high volume (urban) environments when the transport times to hospitals are relatively short. In the urban setting, paramedics do not need to practice their more advanced skills if the transport time is only a few minutes. Indeed, if the patient has an airway that can be maintained by a bag mask valve, it may be more beneficial to transport the patient to a trauma center rather than to delay to initiate IV fluids or perform endotracheal intubation. Basic EMTs are more likely to be found in a rural environment where the transport times to definitive care might be an hour or more; the sparse population will only generate a small number of ambulance calls and response and transport times are much more likely to be prolonged. Skills maintenance is also an issue – although stimulation training might help – neither paid nor volunteer paramedics are likely to maintain skills that are only utilized once or twice a year. The paradox is that in a rural environment with a prolonged transport time, interventions such as needle decompression of the chest, endotracheal intubation, and intravenous resuscitation (all paramedic skills) might provide a better outcome for the patient with penetrating trauma than patients who have a BLS response.

4.3 Triage

It is to be assumed that the process of triage – which can be performed by both basic and advanced life support personnel – is already in place. The most recent

G.C. Velmahos et al. (eds.), *Penetrating Trauma*,
DOI 10.1007/978-3-642-20453-1_4, © Springer-Verlag Berlin Heidelberg 2012

revision of the triage guidelines [5] is now evidence based [6] and has the endorsement of the American College of Surgeons Committee on Trauma (ACS COT), the American College of Emergency Physicians (ACEP), and the national association of EMS physicians. (NAEMSP) Penetrating injury to the torso or abdomen – especially if the patient is hypotensive and tachycardic – should be triaged to a trauma center. It is also taken as given for the purpose of this chapter that the survival of severely injured patients is improved when managed at a trauma center [7, 8]. In most urban and suburban EMS systems, both BLS and ALS personnel can bypass non-trauma facilities to take appropriate patients to a designated trauma center.

4.4 The Process of Ambulance Response

Although the process of ambulance response may differ slightly from jurisdiction to jurisdiction, the following is a typical process [9]. A citizen dials the number to activate emergency response (in the USA, this is 911) and this is answered at a Public Service Answering Point (PSAP). Here the dispatcher will ask a series of protocol-driven questions to determine if fire, ambulance, or police dispatch – or a combination thereof – is required. If the EMS system has "enhanced 911," the dispatcher will have the exact location of the caller's telephone from a computerized directory. Many EMS system responses are tiered – the dispatcher will request the closest BLS ambulance to the scene to respond and simultaneously dispatch the closest ALS unit. Because there are more BLS responses required than ALS, a typical ratio for a Metropolitan area is to have four BLS ambulances to provide immediate response with a single ALS ambulance covering the same area. For example, a patient who has fallen but not lost consciousness and has a suspected ankle fracture will get a BLS ambulance only; a patient who has been hit by a car and is unconscious will get a BLS and an ALS response. A typical response would be 3–4 min for a BLS ambulance in an urban area with an ALS ambulance available in 4–8 min. Once on the scene, the patient will have to be evaluated, potentially placed on a backboard and have intravenous lines initiated, and then transported to the hospital. Occasionally, the ALS ambulance will rendezvous with the BLS ambulance during transport – the so-called ALS intercept – and provide additional care capability if needed. Recent data [10] suggest that the ALS intercept model provides little additional care to the patient; over 60% of intercepts provided no ALS treatment and in 11%, the only additional care was morphine administration. Transport times in urban areas are typically short, usually less than 10 min. In more sophisticated systems, the ambulances are equipped with GPS location equipment and the whole process is computerized – a computer-aided dispatch (CAD) system. In the United States, ambulance reporting is moving to a standardized format – the National Emergency Medical Services Information System (NEMSIS) – which will allow improved evaluation of the efficiency and effectiveness of prehospital care delivery [11]. Electronic reporting of NEMSIS compliant data is expected to become the norm over the next few years.

EMS personnel will not enter a scene that is potentially dangerous until it has been deemed safe – usually by the Police Department. This may mean that victims of penetrating trauma from gunshot wounds may not receive immediate treatment at the scene because this would place the EMS providers at risk.

For very severe injuries, a helicopter maybe dispatched to the scene; for distances less than 30 miles from the receiving hospital ground, ambulance transport is usually just as effective.

Chest decompression by needle thoracostomy might be considered a life-saving intervention that can only be performed by paramedic; however, the data suggest that this procedure may be overutilized [12]. It is also uncommon: In a retrospective review of the use of prehospital needle decompression of the chest by prehospital personnel [13] brought to a level 1 trauma center, of 20,330 ALS calls, only 39 patients (0.2%) had needle decompression for treatment of a tension pneumothorax, and of these, 22 patients (56%) were in circulatory arrest.

4.5 Three Options

For the injured patient, there are now three possible options. The first option is that the patient can be transported by private vehicle (or even taxi!) to the hospital; this allows a very rapid transfer response, but there is no prehospital notification to the emergency department, no interventions are performed (see Table 4.1 below), and there is the possibility of the patient being taken to a hospital that is not a trauma center. The second option is that the patient may be transported by BLS to the

Table 4.1 Interventions performed by Prehospital Personnel

Spinal immobilization	BLS, ALS	Takes a few minutes
Hemorrhage control	BLS, ALS	Extremity control only
Airway control (not intubation)	BLS, ALS	Not complete control, aspiration possible
Sucking chest wound	BLS, ALS	Occlusive dressing to chest wound
Oxygen administration	BLS, ALS	Usually high flow oxygen by protocol
Intravenous fluids	*BLS, ALS	Takes a few minutes
Airway control – Combitube, ET	*BLS, ALS	Complications documented in literature
Needle chest decompression	ALS	Not always successful, often performed when not indicated
Cricothyrotomy	ALS	Rarely utilized
Medication administration (including paralytics)	ALS	Paralytics improve intubation success rate.

Notes:
1. Prehospital intubation is controversial and probably related to the skills maintenance of providers; EMS prehospital esophageal intubations are probably under reported.
2. Prehospital intravenous fluid administration also controversial, often large volumes of fluids are administered. Recent animal data demonstrates a systolic pressure of about 93 mmHg will "pop off the clot" and promote further hemorrhage.

hospital; in this case, there is prehospital notification given to the emergency department, usually intravenous lines initiated, external hemorrhage may be controlled, airway control (but not intubation) performed, and the patient taken by protocol to the trauma center. The third option is an ALS response; endotracheal intubation, needle chest decompression, and medication administration are all possible, but this may entail a more delayed arrival for the patient at the trauma center. It is unlikely that any randomized trial utilizing these three options can be designed and implemented; we have to rely on retrospective data – with the reservations and caveats that this entails. There is another variable: As many EMS sages observe – if you train a prehospital provider to perform a skill, they are likely to use that skill (and delay the patient's hospital arrival) even under circumstances where rapid transfer to the hospital might be more important in the patient's best interest.

4.6 Discussion of the Data

In a study published in *Archives of Surgery* [14], a comparison of Emergency medical Services (EMS)-transported patients versus Non-EMS-transported patients was made; this was a prospective cohort-matched observation study. All non-EMS patients that arrived at a level 1 trauma center were matched with the next appropriate EMS trauma patient by an investigator who was unaware of the mode of transport and the outcomes of the patient; in addition, every tenth EMS patient with an injury severity score of more than 13 was also enrolled. An interview process with patients, witnesses, and friends was used to determine the time of injury and the study outcome designed to determine the time to hospital, mortality, morbidity, and length of hospital stay. A total of 103 patients were enrolled; deaths, complications, and length of hospital stay were similar in both groups purporting to suggest that prehospital EMS had little effect on patient outcome. An interesting analysis demonstrated that for the more severe trauma patients (defined as those with an injury severity score of equal to or greater than 13), the non-EMS-transported patients managed to arrive at the trauma center in less time than those transported by EMS (15 min vs 28 min; $P < 0.05$)

This study compared EMS versus Non-EMS – not BLS versus ALS; the study also included both penetrating and blunt injury patients; conceptually one would think that for penetrating trauma such as a gunshot wound or stab to the torso, there is little that the prehospital personnel can provide other than rapid transport to the appropriate trauma center. A notation within the article stated that in none of the patients with penetrating injury was spinal immobilization even theoretically warranted. It should be noted that this study was an analysis of patients taken directly to the level 1 center; there is no information on outcomes of those severely injured patients that might have been taken to non-trauma facilities by non-EMS transport.

Comparison of the BLS approach compared with the ALS approach has been extensively investigated by the Canadian group. In the *Journal of Trauma* [15], Lieberman and colleagues reported on a meta-analysis comparing BLS with ALS care in trauma patients; the author compiled statistics from 49 articles and found that the odds ratio of death was 2.59 times higher for the trauma patients receiving prehospital ALS compared with BLS. The ratio was adjusted for patient's severity. The same authors studied trauma care in urban areas served by level 1 trauma centers and published their results in 2003 [16] – patients who received ALS care had a mortality rate of 29% and those with BLS had a mortality of 18%.

There have been older studies examining the outcomes of ALS in more rural areas; it might be considered that in urban areas with a short transport time to a level 1 trauma center, the outcomes might be improved because of the immediate availability of operating rooms, surgeons, and the blood bank, and in many studies, the transport time was less than 15 min. There have also been concerns about the effectiveness of prehospital intubation and intravenous fluids – please see other chapters as to the current controversy – such that in an urban environment, these skills are not usually required and may be detrimental.

A comprehensive review of the question "does advanced life support benefit patients" has recently been published [17]. The article examines not only trauma patients but also medical conditions. The opinion of the authors is that there is poor evidence that ALS improves outcome for trauma patients in urban areas (indeed ALS may contribute to poorer outcomes), but it may be of benefit in rural areas with long transport times – hence the EMS paradox as noted above.

The most recent study was published in the *Canadian Medical Journal* [18] and would seemingly be now the definitive study on this topic. This was the Ontario prehospital ALS (OPALS) study – a before-and-after study involving 17 cities in Ontario, Canada; data on trauma patient outcome before and after ALS was collected. There were 2,867 trauma patients in the study, 1,373 had prehospital BLS and after initiation of ALS, a further 1,494 patients were enrolled. The primary outcome was survival to hospital discharge. Comparison of the two groups showed similar age, blunt and penetrating injury ratio, median injury severity score, and severe head injury as measured by Glasgow Coma Scale. After implementation of the ALS program, results showed that despite system wide implementation of ALS, there was no improvement in mortality or morbidity. Indeed in the patients with a Glasgow Coma Score of less than 9, survival was less with ALS (50.9% vs 60.0%; $P=0.02$) The authors conclude "Emergency medical services should carefully re-evaluate the indications for and the application of prehospital advanced life support measures for patients who have experienced severe trauma." This would seem to indicate that at least in the urban environment, BLS prehospital management of trauma – both blunt and penetrating – would have just as good outcomes as ALS and for severe head injuries better outcomes.

4.7 Conclusion

Based upon current literature, there is no evidence that ALS improves outcomes in trauma patients as compared with BLS; this is true in the urban environment but may need more study in the rural environment or in situations where transport times are prolonged (more than 30 min). In urban areas that are served by a level 1 or a level 2 trauma center, the goal should be to ensure that the airway is patent (and this does not always require endotracheal intubation) and then most rapidly transfer the patient to definitive care center for further evaluation and management. Prehospital interventions beyond the BLS level have not been shown to be effective and, in many cases, prove to be detrimental to patient outcome.

Important Points

- For trauma – particularly penetrating trauma – the main object of prehospital care is to get the patient to the trauma center in the shortest possible time, the number of meaningful interventions that can be made by prehospital providers is limited.
- Extremity hemorrhage control is one of the few prehospital interventions that will benefit the trauma patient.
- Prehospital fluid administration and endotracheal intubation are probably of value in only a limited number of patients and bring their own set of complications.
- Prehospital needle thoracostomy is rarely indicated and probably overutilized – about 0.2% of trauma patients will benefit from this procedure in the prehospital phase.
- Ambulance dispatch – although seemingly straightforward – has a complex administrative

structure and for a patient that is exsanguinating at the scene, it may take several minutes for an ambulance to be dispatched, arrive on the scene, and perform a patient evaluation. Further – they may attempt to "stabilize" the patient.

- If you teach a prehospital provider a skill such as intravenous fluid administration or endotracheal intubation, they are more likely to overuse the skill than underuse the skill. This may delay the arrival of an exsanguinating patient.
- All the published data so far indicates that advanced life support skills do not contribute significantly to an improved outcome of trauma patients. There may be subsets of patients that do benefit from specific prehospital interventions but these have yet to be identified.
- As computerized ambulance reports that are NEMSIS compliant become available, more data may be analyzed to specifically identify which prehospital interventions in which trauma patients can be proven to be of benefit.
- Direct feedback to prehospital providers is welcomed and should be performed on an ongoing basis.
- Trauma surgeons should be involved in the training of prehospital providers, establishment of prehospital trauma protocols, and have a working relationship with the medical directors of ambulance services to ensure that prehospital trauma patient care is optimal.

References

1. http://www.nhtsa.dot.gov/people/injury/ems/pub/emtbnsc.pdf accessed on April 15th 2011
2. http://www.nhtsa.dot.gov/people/injury/ems/EMT-I/disk1/Overview.htm accessed on April 15th 2011
3. http://www.nhtsa.dot.gov/people/injury/ems/EMT-P/disk_1%5B1%5D/Intro.pdf accessed on April 15th 2011
4. Pointer JE, McGuire TJ, National Association of EMS Physicians (2002) Levels of providers. In: Alexander E, Kuehl MD (eds) Prehospital systems and medical oversight, 3rd edn. Kendall/Hunt, Dubugue, pp 106–113, ISBN 0-7872-7071-7
5. American College of Surgeons (2006) Resources for the optimal care of the injured patient: 2006. American College of Surgeons, Chicago
6. Sasser SM, Hunt RC, Sullivent EE, et al., National Expert Panel on Field Triage, Centers for Disease Control and Prevention (CDC) (2009) Guidelines for field triage of injured patients recommendations of the national expert panel on field triage. MMWR Recomm Rep 58(RR01):1–35
7. MacKenzie EJ, Rivara FP, Jurkovich GJ et al (2006) A national evaluation of the effect of trauma center care on mortality. N Engl J Med 354:366–378
8. Cudnik M, Newgard C, Sayre M et al (2009) Level I versus level II trauma centers: an outcomes-based assessment. J Trauma 66(5):1231–1326
9. Clawson JJ, National Association of EMS Physicians (2002) Emergency medical dispatch. In: Alexander E, Kuehl MD (eds) Prehospital systems and medical oversight, 3rd edn. Kendall/Hunt, Dubugue, pp 106–113, ISBN 0-7872-7071-7
10. Myers L, Russi SC (2009) Characteristics of paramedic intercepts with basic life support services. Prehosp Emerg Care 13:145
11. http://www.nemsis.org/ accessed on April 15th 2011
12. Cullinane DC, Morris JA Jr, Bass JG et al (2001) Needle thoracostomy may not be indicated in the trauma patient. Injury 32:749–752
13. Warner KJ, Copass MK, Bulger EM (2008) Paramedic use of needle thoracostomy in the prehospital environment. Prehosp Emerg Care 12(2):162–168
14. Cornwell EE, Belzberg H, Hennigan K et al (2000) Emergency Medical Services (EMS) vs non-EMS transport of critically injured patients: a prospective evaluation. Arch Surg 135:315–319
15. Liberman M, Mulder D, Sampalis J (2000) Advanced or basic life support for trauma: meta-analysis and critical review of the literature. J Trauma 49(4):584–599
16. Liberman M, Mulder D, Lavoie A et al (2003) Multicenter Canadian study of prehospital trauma care. Ann Surg 237(2):153–160
17. Isenberg D (2005) Does advanced life support provide benefits to patients? A literature review. Prehosp Disaster Med 20(4):265–270
18. Stiell IG, Nesbitt LP, Pickett W et al (2008) The OPALS major trauma study: impact of advanced life-support on survival and morbidity. CMAJ 178(9):1141–1152

Prehospital Care and Transport

5

Michael A. Frakes, Heather A. Waden, and Suzanne K. Wedel

It is clear that trauma outcomes improve when patients are cared for in an organized trauma system. In a recent validation of trauma center benefit, Hess et al. demonstrated a specific advantage for patients with penetrating trauma taken to American College of Surgeons–verified trauma centers instead of to non-trauma hospitals, and suggested that the survival advantage may be greatest for younger and sicker patients [1]. The reasons for the outcomes differences are likely related, at least in part, to post-intervention care and systems. As the trauma care system does not end with resuscitation or injury repair, neither does it begin there: Trauma care begins with the emergency medical services (EMS) system and includes all out-of-hospital care components.

The out-of-hospital elements of the trauma system are important as drivers of notification and hospital selection, and they may be helpful in making resource utilization decisions. The system must also be designed to address access: Over one quarter of the American population can reach level I or II trauma care within an hour only with helicopter transport, and 15.9% of the population do not have 1-h trauma center access [2]. In addition to the systems providing initial care and transport, inclusive trauma systems must also integrate interfacility transport systems.

The prehospital emergency care system is largely operated by municipal agencies, with various public safety entities responding to about 95% of the initial requests for service and over two-thirds of patient transports from those requests in the 200 largest United States cities. Conversely, interfacility transport services, both ground and air, are primarily provided by commercial operators, including hospital-sponsored, for-profit, and not-for-profit organizations.

Transport providers are generally described as basic life support, advanced life support, and critical care clinicians. Basic providers, emergency medical technicians, represent about 70% of the over 200,000 working EMS providers in the United States. They offer stabilization and mostly noninvasive medical care. Paramedics are more advanced providers, with at least 1,200 h of training in the time-limited care of patients prior to their initial entry into the inpatient system. They provide protocol-driven care under the license of a physician, including invasive therapies such as medication administration and airway interventions.

Critical care transport teams are often part of air transport programs transporting patients to trauma centers from more remote injury sites or, more commonly, moving patients between facilities for higher levels of care. Increasingly, they also provide ground-based interfacility critical care transport. These teams are most commonly staffed by a nurse partnered with a paramedic to leverage the blend of EMS and in-hospital critical care expertise those providers offer, but some systems partner a nurse with an in-hospital provider such as a second nurse, a respiratory therapist, or a physician. The nurses, paramedics, and respiratory therapists on these teams typically have expanded training and a greater scope of practice than their non-critical care transport counterparts. There is no optimal out-of-hospital staffing pattern or system for either EMS or interfacility transport, due in large

M.A. Frakes • H.A. Waden • S.K. Wedel (✉)
Boston MedFlight, Robins Street, Hangar 1727,
Hanscom Air Force Base, Bedford, MA 01730, USA
e-mail: suzanne.wedel@bostonmedflight.org

G.C. Velmahos et al. (eds.), *Penetrating Trauma*,
DOI 10.1007/978-3-642-20453-1_5,

part to the diversity of environments in which medical transportation is provided. Systemic attention to provider quality and utilization is more important than provider or agency credentials.

The time to definitive care is likely an important factor in trauma outcomes. In the setting of urban trauma, there is increasing doubt about the benefit of on-scene advanced life support care, either by paramedics or physicians. In fact, transport of trauma patients in urban settings by non-medical providers is associated with equal, and perhaps better, outcomes than transport by EMS [3, 4]. The role of out-of-hospital care is less clear in non-urban areas or where patients are initially transported to non-trauma centers, but there is a suggestion that reduced times to definitive care are still beneficial.

When patients are taken to non-trauma centers or to non-tertiary centers, transfer to a higher level center improves outcomes. As patients increase in acuity and complexity, patient safety during movement requires providers with greater clinical and transport expertise. Even short in-hospital patient movements are associated with logistical and physiological complications [5–7]. The use of specialty critical care transport teams during interfacility transport is associated with reduced complication rates [8, 9]. Each trauma system must construct an appropriate model for both transport to the hospital and, as needed, transport between hospitals.

The EMS management of penetrating trauma outside the hospital is focused on accessing the patient safely, addressing immediately life-threatening injuries, and promptly transporting the patient to an appropriate destination. In parallel with well-established American College of Surgeons Advanced Trauma Life Support guidelines, care begins with assuring a patent airway. In the overwhelming majority of cases, this can be achieved with basic life support techniques such as positioning, suctioning, or the insertion of an oral airway. At the other end of the spectrum, emergent cricothyrotomy is rarely indicated: It is performed in 0.004% of all prehospital advanced life support (ALS) patients and 0.1% of helicopter EMS patients [10].

Patients with significant traumatic injury should receive high flow oxygen. There is essentially no downside to the short-term administration of high flow oxygen, especially when compared with the advantages of increased oxygen delivery. A patient on non-rebreathing facemask oxygen can be predicted to have near-complete oxygen saturation and an arterial pO_2 of over 400, optimizing blood oxygen-carrying capacity. This predictably high pO_2 makes identification of an abnormal PaO_2/FiO_2 ratio on the initial arterial blood gas easier than with a patient receiving an unpredictable amount of supplemental oxygen from some other device. High flow oxygen also facilitates a beneficial denitrogenation that prolongs the time to desaturation if airway management procedures are subsequently indicated.

Trauma guidelines emphasize the need empirically to restrict cervical spine motion until there is physician and, in patients with distracting injuries, radiologic evaluation. This may be overly dogmatic in some trauma populations. Cervical spine fracture or cervical spinal cord injury is rare with penetrating trauma, occurring in between 0.11% and 1.35% of patients, and is predictable by mechanism, presentation, and wound location. These injuries are over eight times more likely in patients with gunshot wounds than in those with stabbing injuries, and, in both situations, neurological deficit is almost always evident at the time of initial exam. The wounds associated with injury in gunshot wound patients are located between the ears and nipple, and stab wounds associated with cervical injury are those between the mandible and trapezius muscle [11]. Spinal motion restriction in penetrating trauma is associated with poorer outcomes (odds ratio of death 2.06, 95% confidence interval 1.35–3.13): The number needed to treat for potential benefit is 1,032, while the number needed to treat for potential harm is 66 [12]. There may be merit in trading time to definitive trauma care for *pro forma* attempts at spinal motion restriction in patients who do not have neurologic deficit or specific injury location.

The immediately life-threatening injuries associated with breathing addressed in the primary survey are tension pneumothorax and open pneumothorax. A tension pneumothorax can be managed easily in the out-of-hospital setting by needle decompression. The usual intravenous catheter is too short to reach the pleural space in up to a third of trauma patients, so providers should consider the use of a longer catheter that will optimize success rates [13]. An open pneumothorax can be covered with a three-sided dressing and the patient monitored carefully for the accumulation of air and subsequent development of a tension pneumothorax.

One significant controversy in out-of-hospital trauma care is the role of airway capture to assist breathing. It is clear that hypoventilating patients should have assisted ventilation, and mechanical ventilation in shock states beneficially redistributes the cardiac output consumed by work of breathing to increase mixed venous oxygen saturation independently of arterial oxygen content. The optimal timing and methods for achieving these goals, however, are less clear.

Endotracheal intubation is a core paramedic skill, but there is some suggestion that skill maintenance is difficult. Paramedics in large urban systems may have only a single intubation opportunity every year, and the overall success rate for paramedic prehospital intubation is about 74% for patients with vital signs who are intubated without the use of medications [14, 15]. While some systems perform intubation with great procedural success and few complications, there are reports of endotracheal tube misplacement rates up to 25% [16]. The addition of end-tidal carbon dioxide measurement devices for confirming endotracheal tube placement and for the ongoing monitoring of correct placement clearly improves out-of-hospital outcomes. It is a best practice that is becoming the standard of care [16, 17].

The question of ventilatory assistance becomes even more complicated when medications are used to facilitate airway capture. It is clear that specialty teams with high scrutiny, good quality improvement programs, and close supervision can be successful at the invasive airway capture [14, 16]. Procedure success rates by paramedics with sedation-assisted intubation are about 77%, rising to 96% with the use of neuromuscular-blocking agents [14].

Although procedural success can be achieved, there is little certainty of improved outcomes with routine and widespread paramedic out-of-hospital intubation. For example, the only subgroups of patients shown to have improved outcomes following out-of-hospital intubation for traumatic brain injury were those subsequently transported by a helicopter critical care transport team [18, 19]. There is no specific outcomes evaluation of out-of-hospital intubation in patients with penetrating trauma.

There is increasing focus on the risk of inducing secondary brain injury. The incidence of hypoxia during paramedic intubation may be as high as 56%, and there is some suggestion that true procedure success is not technical success, but rather the avoidance of that hypoxia [20]. Warner et al. showed increased mortality in more than two-thirds of intubated trauma patients, both with and without brain injury, delivered to a tertiary care center with an abnormal pCO_2 [16, 21]. It may be, ultimately, that the "benefit" of endotracheal intubation comes not from the procedure, but from the prevention of intraprocedure complications and careful post-procedure care [16].

There are a number of blind insertion airways, variations on an esophageal tube or a laryngeal mask, which can be used when patients are frankly hypoventilating. These devices, especially the esophageal tube airways, are designed to be used by providers trained to basic skill levels, to have high success rates, and to have few complications. An interesting paper showed that inexperienced providers using an intubating laryngeal mask airway could establish ventilation more quickly than with a traditional bag-valve-mask, and could intubate with greater success than with conventional laryngoscopy [22].

As the primary survey progresses to circulation, the life-saving intervention is to arrest hemorrhage. External hemorrhage is best controlled by direct pressure. Failing this, there is a role for the use of tourniquets to control limb bleeding when other means of hemostasis are inadequate. The military has deployed topical hemostatic agents and dressings on the battlefield, but they have not widely penetrated civilian EMS systems. The different nature of civilian wounds, in comparison with battlefield wounds, and the quasi-developmental nature of some agents are likely factors in this practice difference. It is conceivable that improved versions of these agents may become useful in civilian EMS for the control of otherwise unmanageable hemorrhage.

The question of prehospital fluid resuscitation for penetrating trauma appears to be well settled. For more than a decade, there has been a suggestion that survival and hospital discharge rates in hypotensive urban penetrating trauma patients improved when volume resuscitation was delayed until bleeding control was achieved. A recent National Trauma Data Bank review confirmed the absence of a benefit to prehospital volume resuscitation in trauma patients with bleeding, particularly noting increased mortality in the subgroups with penetrating trauma or hypotension [23].

Uncertainty about fluid resuscitation remains for patients who have associated brain injury or extended out-of-hospital times. For patients with brain injury, outcomes are clearly associated with the maintenance of cerebral perfusion pressure, with a goal of maintaining a mean arterial pressure of at least 80 mmHg [24]. Regarding patients with longer out-of-hospital times, there is a paucity of guidance about the point at which the deleterious effects of persistent shock from delayed resuscitation begin to outweigh the hemorrhagic and coagulopathic risks associated with volume repletion.

Once fluid resuscitation is initiated in a patient with penetrating trauma, the question becomes one of ideal fluid choice. Crystalloid fluid is the only option for most EMS providers. It appears that lactated Ringer's solution is less likely to produce coagulopathy and hyperchloremic acidosis than normal saline solution. Massive crystalloid resuscitation is clearly associated with coagulopathy, increased hemorrhage, and the development of the abdominal compartment syndrome. Investigation into the use of hypertonic saline solutions shows promise, but no clear outcome benefit has yet been demonstrated.

When available, blood products are optimal for patients with ongoing hemorrhage. Although not a completely settled question, it appears that early administration of platelets, fresh frozen plasma, and, perhaps, cryoprecipitate may be associated with improved outcomes when compared with traditional packed red blood cell and delayed component therapy. While this is not generally a prehospital option, it is a consideration for specialty care teams who respond to the site of injury with blood products and is also a consideration for those teams who transport trauma patients between hospitals. There has been little success to date in developing hemoglobin substitutes.

The other immediately life-threatening circulatory injury is pericardial tamponade. Classic management of pericardial tamponade is emergent pericardiocentesis. This skill is regularly taught to paramedics, but a recent consensus statement described the absence of evidence to support prehospital pericardiocentesis and the technical barriers to success [25]. Aggressive volume resuscitation in this setting may be a technique with greater likelihood for success outside of the hospital.

Although not a life-saving intervention, the provision of analgesia may be one of the most important out-of-hospital interventions [26]. Attention to analgesia has historically been poor in all aspects of the emergency system, from EMS care through trauma resuscitation. It is clear that out-of-hospital providers can safely administer short-acting opioid analgesics in systems with protocols and performance improvement systems, and this may be an area in which EMS systems should consider focused performance improvement efforts [26–28].

In addition to rapid, safe transport and the provision of life-saving interventions, the EMS role is to deliver patients to the best destination. The concept of direct point of entry into a trauma center hospital is well established in developed trauma systems. EMS may also have a beneficial role in determining resource utilization and in-hospital point of entry, as well. For patients with ST-elevation myocardial infarction, paramedic acquisition of electrocardiograms and the use of that information in activating the cardiac care system or catheterization suite is the standard of care [29]. For trauma patients, efforts at identifying helpful prehospital triage criteria are so far nonspecific and imperfect, but significant recent revisions to the recommended triage guidelines should improve both sensitivity and specificity [30]. The addition of technology and clinical expertise may offer improved results. For example, initial studies have shown that prehospital ultrasound is feasible during specialty care transport and can appropriately affect trauma patient management and in-hospital destination [31]. A 6-year case series similarly suggested that well-trained critical care transport teams can appropriately identify patients for direct operating room admission [32].

Verified trauma systems include comprehensive outcomes, performance improvement, and data collection components, but the out-of-hospital element of the system often lags in this area. Optimal system development, resource utilization, and patient care require that EMS and interfacility transport providers, in collaboration with hospital-based trauma systems, develop these elements [26].

The out-of-hospital elements of the trauma system offer opportunities not only to provide life-saving prehospital interventions, but also to optimize patient access, resource utilization, and safety. Mature trauma systems should integrate prehospital and interfacility transport components not only in clinical care, but also in research, outcomes, and quality management aspects of the system.

Important Points

- Time to definitive care is a key determinant of outcome for patients with penetrating traumatic injury.
- Integrated transport systems are essential in trauma care: Over one quarter of the American population can access a trauma center within 1 h only via helicopter transport, and interfacility transport to trauma centers also improves outcomes.
- The use of personnel with expertise in critical care and transport reduces complications during intra- and interfacility transport of critically ill patients.
- Cervical spinal cord injury is rare in patients with penetrating trauma and can be predicted by mechanism, wound location, and physical examination. There is increased mortality associated with the routine prehospital application of cervical spinal motion restriction devices in penetrating trauma patients.
- Prehospital endotracheal intubation for trauma patients is controversial and, if done, should be performed in systems with high procedure volume, attentive recurrent education and quality improvement processes, and that use continuous end-tidal carbon dioxide measurements and mechanical ventilation after intubation.
- There is minimal benefit to the prehospital volume resuscitation of trauma patients with penetrating trauma in most settings.
- There is no evidence supporting prehospital pericardiocentesis for cardiac tamponade.
- Transport systems have a proven role in determining destination choice and in-hospital resource activation. There may be opportunities to expand this role with trauma patients.

References

1. Hess B, Gregory J, Wang J, Rivara F, MacKenzie E, Nathens A (2008) Survival advantage in trauma centers: expeditious intervention or experience? J Am Coll Surg 208(1):28–36
2. Branas C, MacKenzie E, Williams J et al (2005) Access to trauma centers in the United States. JAMA 293(21): 2626–2633
3. Demetriades D, Chan L, Drornwell E et al (1996) Paramedic versus private transportation of trauma patients: effect on outcome. Arch Surg 131(2):133–138
4. Band R, Pryor J, Gaieski D, Dickinson E, Cummings D, Carr B (2011) Injury-adjusted mortality of patients transported by police following penetrating trauma. Acad Emerg Med 18(1):32–37
5. Gebermichael M (2000) Interhospital transport of the extremely ill patient. Crit Care Med 28(1):79–85
6. Indek M, Peterson S, Smith J, Brotman S (1988) Risk, cost, and benefit of transporting ICU patients for special studies. J Trauma 28:1020–1025
7. Becker A, Ipekoglu Z, Tureyen K (1998) Secondary insults during intrahospital transport of neurosurgical intensive care patients. Neurosurg Rev 21:98–101
8. Seymour C, Kahn J, Schwab C, Fuchs B (2008) Adverse events during rotary wing transport of mechanically ventilated patients. Crit Care 12(4):164
9. Orr R, Felmet K, Han Y et al (2009) Pediatric specialized transport teams are associated with improved outcomes. Pediatrics 124:40–48
10. McIntosh S, Swanson E, Barton E (2008) Cricothyrotomy in air medical transport. J Trauma 64(6):1543–1547
11. Rhee P, Kuncir E, Johnson L et al (2006) Cervical spine injury is highly dependent on the mechanism of injury following blunt and penetrating assault. J Trauma 61(5):1166–1170
12. Haut E, Kalish B, Efron D et al (2010) Spine immobilization in penetrating trauma: more harm than good? J Trauma 68(1):115–120
13. Zenegrink I, Brink P, Laupland K, Raber E, Zygun D, Kortbeek J (2008) Needle thoracostomy in the treatment of a tension pneumothorax in trauma patients: what size needle? J Trauma 64(1):111–114
14. Wang H, Yealy D (2006) How many attempts are required to accomplish out of hospital endotracheal intubation? Acad Emerg Med 13(4):372–377
15. Wang H, Kupas D, Hostler D, Cooney R, Yealy D, lave J (2005) Procedural experience with out of hospital endotracheal intubation. Crit Care Med 33(8):1718–1721
16. Wang H, Yealy D (2006) Out of hospital endotracheal intubation: where are we? Ann Emerg Med 47:532–541
17. Wang H, Davis D, O'Connor R (2006) Drug-assisted intubation in the prehospital setting. Prehosp Emerg Care 10(2): 261–271
18. Wang H, Peitzman A, Cassidy L, Adelson P, Yealy D (2004) Out of hospital endotracheal intubation: outcome after traumatic brain injury. Ann Emerg Med 44:439–450
19. Poste J, Davis D, Ochs M et al (2004) Air medical transport of severely head injured patients undergoing paramedic rapid sequence intubation. Air Med J 23(4):36–40
20. Dunford J, Davis D, Ochs M (2003) Incidence of transient hypoxia and pulse rate reactivity during paramedic rapid sequence intubation. Ann Emerg Med 42:721–726
21. Warner K, Cuschieri J, Copass M, Jurkovich G, Bulger E (2007) The impact of prehospital ventilation on outcome after severe traumatic brain injury. J Trauma 62(6): 1330–1338
22. Timmerman A, Russo S, Crozier T et al (2007) Novices ventilate and intubate quicker and safer via intubating laryngeal mask than by conventional bag mask ventilation and laryngoscopy. Anesthesiology 197:570–576

23. Haut E, Kalish B, Cotton B et al (2011) Prehospital intravenous fluid administration is associated with higher mortality in trauma patients: a National Trauma Data Bank analysis. Ann Surg 253(2):371–377
24. Foundation BT (2007) Guidelines for prehospital management of traumatic brain injury. Prehosp Emerg Care 12(Supp)):S1–S52
25. Lee C, Revelli M, Porter K, Steyrn R (2007) The prehospital management of chest injuries: a consensus statement by the faculty of prehospital care, Royal College of Surgeons of Edinburgh. Emerg Med J 24:220–224
26. Maio R, Garrison H, Spaite D et al (1999) Emergency medical services outcomes project: prioritizing conditions for outcomes research. Ann Emerg Med 33(4):423–432
27. Kanowitz A, Dunn T, Kanowitz E, Dunn W, VanBuskirk K (2006) Safety and effectiveness of fentanyl administration for prehospital pain management. Prehosp Emerg Care 10(1):1–7
28. Thomas S (2007) Fentanyl in the prehospital setting. Am J Emerg Med 25:842–843
29. O'Connor R, Brady W, Brooks S et al (2010) American Heart Association guidelines for cardiopulmonary resuscitation and emergency cardiovascular care. Part 10: acute coronary syndromes. Circulation 122:S787–S817
30. Sasser S, Hunt R, Sullivent E et al (2009) Guidelines for field triage of injured patients. Recommendations of the national expert panel on field triage. MMWR Recomm Rep 58(RR01):1–35
31. Walcher F, Welinlich M, Conrad G et al (2006) Prehospital ultrasound imaging improves management of abdominal trauma. Br J Surg 93(2):238–242
32. Shewakramani S, Thomas S, Harrison T, Gates J (2007) Air transport of patients with unstable aortic aneurysms directly into operating rooms. Prehosp Emerg Care 11(3): 337–342

6 Prehospital Monitoring During Transport

Heidi Frankel and Clinton J. Pace

The principal goal of EMS providers caring for penetrating injured patients in an urban environment is rapid transport to definitive care while delivering life-saving interventions. In most circumstances, this is accomplished by ground transport with Advanced Life Support techniques. Wound location and hemodynamic information should be communicated before arrival in a concise report to best prepare the trauma team to deliver rapid and appropriate definitive care. Depending on the trauma system, it may be beneficial to transport unstable patients to facilities with in-house trauma/general surgeons to address torso injuries and neurosurgeons to address brain injuries. Certainly, 24-h immediate access to the operating theater, transfusion services, interventional radiology, and CT scan (particularly for neurosurgical patients) are optimal in these patients. Hemodynamically unstable patients may benefit from resuscitative measures delivered while en route. These may include establishment and protection of the airway, decompressive needle thoracostomy, and judicious fluid administration and application of tourniquets for exsanguinating extremity wound. If definitive airway control is to be established for head-injured patients, tracheal intubation with care must be accomplished to protect against hypoventilation and elevations in intracranial pressure. Additional focus on resuscitative measures, including blood administration to maintain a perfusing pressure, may be required in penetrating injured patients in a rural environment or those with long transport times to the hospital. Air transportation may expedite delivery to definitive care.

H. Frankel (✉)
Division of Trauma,
Acute Care and Critical Care Surgery, Penn State Milton S. Hershey Medical Center, 500 University Drive, UPC I, Suite 3100, Hershey, PA 17033, USA
e-mail: hfrankel@hmc.psu.edu

C.J. Pace
Division of Burn, Trauma, Critical Care,
Department of Surgery, Nacogdoches Medical Center,
540 W. 5th Street, Suite 310, Odessa, TX 79761, USA
e-mail: clinton.pace@utsouthwestern.edu

6.1 Urban Environment

6.1.1 Goal of EMS Participation

The principal goal of EMS (emergency medical services) providers caring for penetrating injured patients in an urban environment is rapid transport to definitive care while administering life-saving interventions. The prehospital period involves expeditious evaluation of wounds and hemodynamics, stabilization and prevention of further injury, and rapid transportation of the patient to the closest appropriate facility where definitive care can be delivered. The care of the patient in the prehospital setting follows principles set out by the American College of Surgeons Committee on Trauma (ACS-COT) delineated in Advanced Trauma Life Support (ATLS) and the Prehospital Trauma Life Support (PHTLS), both of which are leading international programs of continuing education. The PHTLS course is taught to EMS providers in over 33 countries worldwide, and complements the physician ATLS course that is currently taught in 40 countries. Although useful for review, recent military experiences originate from an environment that differs from the civilian by the presence of a hostile setting, mass casualties, less

G.C. Velmahos et al. (eds.), *Penetrating Trauma*,
DOI 10.1007/978-3-642-20453-1_6, © Springer-Verlag Berlin Heidelberg 2012

available resources, and the foremost goal being completion of the current mission.

The benefits from extensive prehospital intervention for penetrating trauma, particularly in an urban environment, remain controversial. In critically injured patients, performance of other than life-saving interventions can delay arrival to a facility that will provide definitive care and can have a negative impact on survival. In general, the "scoop and run" paradigm should be the rule and not the exception for penetrating trauma. While stabilizing procedures should be undertaken before and during transport, any monitoring or intervention ("stay and play") that delays definitive treatment of penetrating injury – often an operation – is generally unhelpful.

6.1.2 Mode of Transportation

In most circumstances, the appropriate mode of transportation for penetrating injured patients in an urban environment is via ground ambulance. The benefit of Advanced Life Support (ALS) units may be questioned as noted above; however, most protocols call for this additional level of expertise "just in case." Use of whichever means gets the patient to the trauma center the soonest is optimal. Ambulance units should strive to keep the on-scene duration to 10 min or less to adhere to guidelines outlined by PHTLS. Depending on each particular region, the ground ambulance personnel who provide ALS may have similar interventional skills to that of the air transport crews, but knowledge and evaluation of local resources is necessary. Helicopter transport in urban settings is best utilized when the air transport time will be less than that of a ground ambulance. Within approximately 30 miles, ground transport is typically as fast as air when over favorable terrain in no traffic settings. Helicopter transport often flies in any inclement weather, including overcast skies with low ceilings.

6.1.3 Initial Assessment of the Patient by EMS

Wound location and hemodynamic information should be communicated in a concise report before arrival to best prepare the trauma team to deliver rapid and appropriate life-saving care. Initially, the injured patient should undergo assessment and management in an orderly, logical manner in a head-to-toe fashion. A patient with obvious penetrating trauma to the anterior torso can easily have a missed injury to the gluteal region if a careful inspection of all clothed areas is not performed. Such a missed injury can cause significant additional hemorrhage that may have been easily ameliorated by direct pressure. Few available devices offer diagnostic improvement over a thorough physical examination, including inspection, auscultation, percussion, and palpation by a well-trained medical provider. Additionally, data obtained from such additional devices must be verified as well, whether or not it is in a normal range.

6.1.4 Wound Assessment

There are three main pieces of information that data regarding the wounding should convey. First, the trauma team needs to know where the wound(s) is (are) to plan diagnostic and therapeutic maneuvers. Because the final destination of the missile or knifepoint may not be known from the external wound, it is key that EMS personnel not refer to wounds as affecting the "chest" or "abdomen" or "back." A wound at the sixth left intercostal space in the anterior axillary line may, in fact, involve abdominal structures and require a laparotomy for definitive treatment. Referring to it as a "chest" wound may set different expectations for the receiving trauma team. Similarly a "back" wound may involve chest or abdominal structures with different diagnostic and therapeutic maneuvers required. Although, the receiving team recognizes that rapid assessment on the spot may be flawed (particularly if the scene is not secured), it is most helpful to have identified all wounds prehospital and whether they appear to be tangential or superficial. Of course, it is safest to assume that no wound is an "exit" wound or infer trajectories without imaging or direct inspection that may not be possible in the field. Next, by conveying hemodynamic information as described below, prehospital providers can allow the trauma team to infer whether or not operative intervention might be warranted. This may result in alternate triage (i.e., some trauma centers might transport directly to the operating theater), activation of massive transfusion protocols, or release of other resources. Finally, by conveying information on wound location and hemodynamics in concert, the receiving trauma team may get a sense of what kind of operation (laparotomy versus thoracotomy) is warranted.

6.1.5 Hemodynamic Assessment

Prehospital hemodynamic assessment utilizes the rapid "ABC" approach of airway, breathing, and circulation adequacy determination. The airway should be examined while maintaining cervical spine protection and monitored for blockage with gurgling from vomitus, blood, or foreign body. Obtunded or nearly moribund patients may benefit from endotracheal tube placement en route as described below.

Breathing and ventilation are monitored by signs of full, symmetric chest wall movement, without crepitus or paradoxical motion. The patient should have a midline trachea with a normal respiratory rate and depth. A tension pneumothorax is a life-threatening condition that can be a cause of preventable death. Hyperresonance with percussion of the thoracic cavity and diminished breath sounds, especially in the face of a suspicious wound, are indications of a pneumothorax. Increased air pressure between lung parenchyma and parietal pleural in the thoracic cavity reduces venous return and causes tachypnea, dyspnea, air hunger, and eventual cardiovascular collapse. Tracheal deviation, hypotension, and distended neck veins are all late hallmarks. Diagnosis is often established by therapeutic decompression as described below.

Patients are also monitored for the status of their circulation with appropriate concomitant hemorrhage control. Signs of hemorrhagic shock include diaphoresis, cool clammy skin with peripheral vasoconstriction, and diminished peripheral pulses. Capillary refill may be normal or delayed. Systemic hypotension may be seen late or only with profound shock. Hemodynamic status can be evaluated by the presence and character of the radial pulse when other reliable means are not available. Manual assessment of a weak but present radial pulse correlates with a systemic blood pressure (SBP) of approximately 80 mmHg, but studies have shown that estimates of SBP tend to overestimate the actual pressure. Unfortunately, a change in the pulse, blood pressure, or mental status is a late sign of central hypovolemia and does not provide adequate warning of impending circulatory collapse. Both radial or arm pulses should be initially compared, as the occasional patient will have an asymmetric arm blood pressure in the pre-injured state from a subclavian artery stenosis, old injury, or atheroscleromatous plaque. The arm with the higher pressure should then be used for monitoring systemic blood pressure and circulation.

6.1.6 Monitoring and Resuscitation En Route

The ACS-COT, in conjunction with the American College of Emergency Physicians and the National Association of EMS Physicians, has published a pamphlet recommending certain equipment deemed essential on an ambulance unit. In general, the degree and level of monitoring should be individualized based on the availability of resources and training of individual municipalities. For example, if ALS is to be provided, then pulse oximetry, end-tidal CO2 (ETCO2) detection, along with electrocardiography, a defibrillator, and external cardiac pacemaking should be present and available. However, care must be taken not to delay transport beyond the benefit received by the intervention. It is up to the individual emergency medical director and local governing bodies to determine the practice guidelines to which the trauma system will adhere.

Patients with penetrating trauma should be transported to a trauma center on a standardized ambulance unit, optimally that provides ALS. Most units in urban and suburban areas provide ALS units that have the previously listed devices, as well as a thermometer and a sphygmomanometer. Other than standard vital signs and maintaining the ABCs of trauma care, there is a paucity of other useful prehospital monitoring currently utilized. Signs of internal hemorrhaging from a positive abdominal sonogram, for example, may alert one of a potential need to stop at a closer trauma center, but with penetrating trauma to the trunk, one assumes those injuries are present until proven otherwise.

Attention is given to addressing frequent causes of preventable penetrating trauma deaths, which are loss of airway control, tension pneumothorax, and exsanguination from extremity injuries. Monitoring principles should address these areas that are the foundations of ATLS and PHTLS, notably the ABCs airway, breathing, and circulation. Although electronics and mechanical devices aid in monitoring the status of the patient during transport, the time-honed skills of an experienced provider using inspection, auscultation, percussion, and palpation are invaluable. Specific monitoring can be organized by the familiar sequence of the ABCs of trauma care taught in many educational courses.

Initial assessment of the trauma patient requires the establishment of a functional airway as the paramount priority. Pulse oximetry and $ETCO_2$ detectors, either qualitative or quantitative, are recommended for ambulance units that provide ALS. Using infrared spectroscopy, quantitative detectors give an instantaneous numeric CO_2 value. In contrast, easily portable colorimetric devices change color in response to the presence of airway CO_2, but are unable to indicate hypo- or hypercarbia, and may falsely indicate loss of the airway by a low $ETCO_2$ in response to certain physiological conditions. While the quantitative $ETCO_2$ monitor can give feedback to prevent hypocapnia from vigorous ventilation in an intubated patient with a traumatic brain injury, the $ETCO_2$ detector is adequate for transportation of short duration and confirms tube presence in the airway. Constant surveillance is maintained, as even a secured airway may be lost. With endotracheal intubation, a mucus plug, blood, or dislodgment may necessitate reestablishing an airway that is believed to be secure. A high degree of suspicion is helpful to diagnose this potential change. An adverse change of the patient's condition en route necessitates reassessing from the beginning. If an endotracheal tube is inserted, condensation forming with each breath often confirms the correct placement across the larynx. With a difficult endotracheal intubation, two or three failed attempts should be the cause for reevaluation to see if other means can be used to secure the airway, such as bag valve mask, laryngeal mask airway, or a surgical airway. There exists much variability in the success rate of attempted prehospital intubation, ranging from approximately one-third to two-thirds. One of the primary reasons for a failed attempt at endotracheal intubation is because of trismus, or clenched jaw. While rapid sequence intubation (RSI) may increase the success rate in these particular patients, one only has to observe anesthesia providers in the operating room occasionally having difficulty under controlled, optimal circumstances to realize that an ambulance crew with only sporadic exposure to a patient who needs airway control may have serious hardships. When poor suctioning, mouth debris, facial trauma, and other complications are present, it is no wonder that securing an airway may be the most important responsibility and difficult-to-achieve goal of the ambulance providers.

If a tension pneumothorax is suspected, needle decompression with a long, large bore needle is performed by insertion in the second intercostal space at the midclavicular line. A rush of air upon entrance of the thoracic cavity confirms the diagnosis. ALS provides training to emergency medical technicians in proper placement of decompressive needle thoracostomy. Chest tube thoracostomy requires a higher level of training and skill and often is a cause of struggling in even junior level residents in a controlled emergency department setting.

Even subtle changes in standard vital signs may fail to predict mortality or the need for life-saving interventions prior to cardiovascular collapse, although an initial low pulse pressure may indicate central hypovolemia earlier than other changes in vital signs. Management of circulating blood volume relies on limiting the loss and restoration to maintain an adequate perfusion. Standard vital signs are often poor indicators of subtle changes or of early shock. Resuscitative hypotension is a strategy that aims to limit the amount of intravenous fluids in the prehospital arena by maintaining a mean arterial pressure of 60–65 mmHg. Most body organs can maintain viability with this level of perfusion, although patients with traumatic brain injury have a worse outcome using this approach.

6.1.7 Where to Transport Patients

As outlined by the triage decision scheme from the ACS-COT, all penetrating trauma should be taken to a trauma center with an activated trauma team, with the possible exception of penetrating extremity wounds distal to elbows or knees. Care should be taken to assess the presence of any special needs when determining which appropriate facility will receive the patient, such as the ability of the facility to provide neurosurgical, obstetrical, neonatal, or cardiovascular care.

Utilizing recent battlefield experience in Iraq and Afghanistan, Tactical Combat Casualty Care principles were developed to encourage life-saving damage control for penetrating trauma at a close facility before transporting to a facility with higher level of care that may be hours away. Although stabilizing the patient at a closer facility may be necessary, there is no point in diverting to a closer facility in the civilian arena that cannot provide the needed assets, such as a neurosurgeon in a patient with a neurosurgical emergency.

Triage requires evaluation of a patient to determine the appropriate facility to which the patient should be transferred. The ACS designates facilities from Level I to a Level IV trauma center. While Level I centers are usually affiliated with a university and provide the highest level of dedicated resources, a Level II trauma center is expected to provide initial definitive trauma care for injuries of all severities. The risk of death is 25% lower for a severely injured person if the patient receives care at a Level I trauma center. Part of this effect (not consistent in all studies) may be related to the presence of an in-house surgeon available in some Level I centers, although, once again, the benefit of in-house attendings is debated. Nonetheless, in a patient with exsanguinating torso injuries, seconds matter and having an experienced provider immediately available can only be expected to improve outcome. A Level III center provides resuscitation, emergency operations, and stabilization. A general surgeon is required to be available at Levels I, II, and III trauma centers. Specific patient needs should be anticipated when determining which receiving facility, such as injuries requiring neurosurgical, cardiovascular, neonatal, or pediatric intensive care.

6.2 Rural Environment

6.2.1 How and Where to Transport

For rural trauma care, a Level IV facility may be a clinic and not a hospital that provides advanced trauma life support without the presence of a physician. Air transportation may expedite delivery to definitive care. The Field Triage Decision Scheme was created by the ACS in 1986 and serves as a reference for developing triage protocols for EMS systems.

6.2.2 Additional Resuscitative Measures to Consider

Additional focus on resuscitative measures may be required in penetrating injured patients in a rural environment or those with long transport times to the hospital. Definitive control of the airway as well as blood administration to maintain a perfusing pressure are more likely to be needed in this setting.

Deterioration in the mental status as evidenced by a drop in the Glasgow Coma Scale, particularly in the motor or verbal component, has also been shown to correlate with central hypotension and impending demise. The eye component may be difficult to evaluate during transport because of poor lighting and motion during transport. In the intubated patient, the motor component alone is typically followed, since the verbal component score will stay at 1 T.

A pulse oximeter is included in the standard equipment on an ambulance providing ALS, and is used for continuous peripheral oxygen saturation monitoring in prehospital emergency medicine and transportation. The device measures hemoglobin saturation in a noninvasive fashion by passing a light between two surfaces of tissue. Forehead sensors may give more reliable readings, depending on the location of the injuries. Patient motion, hypothermia, and vasoconstriction can all interfere with accurate readings and cause aberrant results.

End-tidal CO_2 ($ETCO_2$) monitoring is a means of evaluating respiratory CO_2 levels during exhalation. It has become a standard component in an ambulance that provides ALS. Guidelines from the American Heart Association require exhaled CO_2 measurement following intubation for confirmation of accurate endotracheal (ET) tube placement. The qualitative measuring device fits between the Ambu bag and the ET tube and changes color in the presence of alveolar CO_2 when levels are near normal pulmonary artery CO_2 values. Inadvertent esophageal intubation reveals absent $ETCO_2$. Physiologic derangements such as shock, pulmonary embolism, and airway obstruction may produce a lower $ETCO_2$, while hypoventilation and exogenous bicarbonate administration may elevate the $ETCO_2$. Small reductions in $ETCO_2$ may give an early warning of cardiovascular collapse from hypovolemic hemorrhage, but small quantitative drops have not yet proved to be clinically useful in the prehospital setting.

In summary, monitoring during transport of penetrating trauma has been standardized with recommended devices found on ambulances that provide both Basic and Advance Life Support. A high degree of suspicion or even the expectation that the patient will decompensate en route will help limit adverse surprises. All penetrating trauma except that isolated to a distal extremity should be transported to a trauma center with an activated trauma team. On-scene delays should be avoided, including those from non-life-saving interventions, with ambulance durations of less than 10 min on-scene recommended. In general, physical examination of the patient using standard ABC sequence of trauma care should be followed. Preventable deaths en route are mainly from uncontrolled extremity hemorrhage, loss of the airway, and tension pneumothorax. Monitoring should closely evaluate for each of these causes. The emergency medical team should be capable of addressing each of these derangements, each of which can be rapidly lethal. Initial evaluation and survey is performed to determine the needs of the patient and which specific facility is most appropriate for treating the sustained injuries. Remaining cognizant of special needs of the patient, including the need for pediatric intensive care, availability of a neurosurgeon, or specialized critical care, helps determine the appropriate trauma facility. Logical, flowing patient evaluation sequences will help ensure that more occult injuries are not overlooked and optimal monitoring occurs during timely transport.

Important Points

- The principal goal of EMS providers caring for penetrating injured patients in an urban environment is rapid transport to definitive care – usually by ground without ongoing resuscitation.
- Wound location and hemodynamic information should be communicated in a concise prehospital report before arrival.
- It may be beneficial to transport unstable patients to facilities with in-house surgeons to address torso injuries and neurosurgeons to address brain injuries.
- Hemodynamically unstable penetrating injured patients in an urban environment may benefit from resuscitative measures delivered while en route (protection of the airway, minimal intravenous fluids, and tourniquets).
- If definitive airway control is to be established for head-injured patients, intubation must be accomplished while en route with care to protect against hypoventilation and elevations in intracranial pressure.
- Additional focus of resuscitative measures may be required in penetrating injured patients in a rural environment or those with long transport times to the hospital (e.g., air transport, securing of airway, administration of blood).

Suggested Literature

Bhende MS, LaCovey DC (2001) End-tidal carbon dioxide monitoring in the prehospital setting. Prehosp Emerg Care 5(2):208–213

Bulger EM, Maier RV (2007) Prehospital care of the injured: what's new. Surg Clin N Am 87:37–53

Carr ME Jr (2004) Monitoring of hemostasis in combat trauma patients. Mil Med 169(12 Suppl):11–15, 4

Convertino VA, Ryan KL, Rickards CA et al (2008) Physiological and medical monitoring for en route care of combat casualties. J Trauma 64(4 Suppl):S342–S353

Deakin CD, Low JL (2000) Accuracy of the advanced trauma life support guidelines for predicting systolic blood pressure using carotid, femoral, and radial pulses: observational study. BMJ 321(7262):673–674

Donald MJ, Paterson B (2006) End tidal carbon dioxide monitoring in prehospital and retrieval medicine: a review. Emerg Med J 23(9):728–730

Dretzke J, Sandercock J, Bayliss S et al (2004) Clinical effectiveness and cost-effectiveness of prehospital intravenous fluids in trauma patients. Health Technol Assess 8(23):iii, 1–iii, 103

Holcomb JB, Salinas J, McManus JM et al (2005a) Manual vital signs reliably predict need for life saving interventions in trauma patients. J Trauma 59(4):821–828

Holcomb JB, Niles SE, Miller CC et al (2005b) Prehospital physiologic data and lifesaving interventions in trauma patients. Mil Med 170(1):7–13

Mabry R, McManus JG (2008) Prehospital advances in the management of severe penetrating trauma. Crit Care Med 36 (7 Suppl):S258–S266

McManus JG, Ryan KL, Morton MJ et al (2008) Limitations of end-tidal CO_2 as an early indicator of central hypovolemia in humans. Prehosp Emerg Care 12(2):199–205

Nuhr M, Hoerauf K, Joldzo A et al (2004) Forehead SpO_2 monitoring compared to finger SpO_2 recording in emergency transport. Anaesthesia 59(4):390–393

Ryan KL, Batchinsky A, McManus JG et al (2008) Changes in pulse character and mental status are late responses to central hypovolemia. Prehosp Emerg Care 12(2):192–198

Sasser SM, Hunt RC, Sullivent EE et al (2009) Guidelines for field triage of injured patients. Recommendations of the National Expert Panel on Field Triage, Centers for Disease Control and Prevention (CDC). MMWR Recomm Rep 58(RR-1):1–35

Seamon MJ, Fisher CA, Gaughan J et al (2007) Prehospital procedures before emergency department thoracotomy: "scoop and run" saves lives. J Trauma 63(1):113–120

Shatney CH, Homan SJ, Sheck JP et al (2002) The utility of helicopter transport of trauma patients from the injury scene in an urban trauma system. J Trauma 53(5):817–822

Stockinger ZT, McSwain NE Jr (2004) Prehospital endotracheal intubation for trauma does not improve survival over bag-valve-mask ventilation. J Trauma 56(3):531–536

Sukumaran S, Henry JM, Beard D et al (2005) Prehospital trauma management: a national study of paramedic activities. Emerg Med J 22(1):60–63

Vajda P (2007) Prehospital care of the adult trauma patient. Bratisl Lek Listy 108(8):371–374

Trauma Resuscitation

7

Heena P. Santry and Marc de Moya

Hemorrhage, as both a disease of decreased perfusion and a disease of altered immunity, accounts for up to 40% of trauma-related deaths [1]. In both civilian and military settings, many of these deaths may be preventable [2, 3]. The majority of hemorrhage-related deaths occur in the first 6 h after injury. Hemorrhage leads to systemic hypotension, decreased end-organ perfusion, tissue hypoxia, and free-radical injury in the first few hours [4–7]. However, delayed deaths are due to hemorrhage-triggered secondary messenger modulation [8–10], gene expression [11, 12], and neutrophil activation [13] that make the host susceptible to the post-traumatic multiorgan failure and sepsis that account for the majority of late deaths after trauma [1, 2].

In the face of trauma, the means to improve survival is expeditious hemorrhage control and minimizing soft tissue secondary injury. Resuscitation is the key to minimize secondary soft tissue/organ injury but is not meant to be a surrogate for hemorrhage control. This chapter will focus on the resuscitation component of acute trauma care.

H.P. Santry (✉)
Trauma, Critical Care, University of Massachusetts Medical School, UMassMemorial Medical Center,
55 Lake Avenue North, Worcester, MA 01655, USA
e-mail: heena.santry@umassmemorial.org

M. de Moya
Division of Trauma, Emergency Surgery, and Surgical Critical Care, Massachusetts General Hospital, Harvard Medical School,
165 Cambridge Street, Suite 810, Boston, MA 02114, USA
e-mail: mdemoya@partners.org

7.1 Fluid Type

Historically, large volume crystalloid infusion was thought to improve survival through replacement of both intravascular losses and interstitial volume [14, 15]. However, newer research has identified the dangers of such an approach which has been shown macroscopically to cause edema of the gut, myocardium, and skeletal muscles, compartment syndrome, and acute respiratory distress syndrome and microscopically to cause derangements of cellular, metabolic, and immune functions that exacerbate the inflammatory cascade that ensues after hemorrhage [16]. Colloids (typically 5% albumin or 6% Hetastarch) were sought as an alternative to crystalloids for their higher oncotic pressure, but numerous studies failed to show any advantage of colloid over crystalloid in trauma patients [17]. More recently, hypertonic fluids (7.5% saline with 6% Dextran) were tested as low-volume alternatives to the traditional approach; and here, too, there was no mortality benefit with the new fluid in the prehospital setting [18].

Meanwhile, military experts, who arguably have the most experience resuscitating victims of penetrating trauma, have come together on several occasions to put forth consensus recommendations on optimal resuscitation strategies in combat environments. They have agreed that large volume resuscitation is deleterious and that aggressive fluid repletion should be avoided in the absence of hemorrhage control. Further, they have argued that hypotension is permissible as long as consciousness and a palpable radial pulse are maintained. When fluid is necessary due to altered consciousness or absent radial pulse (typically systolic blood pressure <80 mmHg), they recommend a low volume (250 mL)

G.C. Velmahos et al. (eds.), *Penetrating Trauma*,
DOI 10.1007/978-3-642-20453-1_7,

of hypertonic fluid (7.5% saline), hyperoncotic fluid (6% Dextran or 6% Hetastarch), or a combination (7.5% saline w/ 6% Dextran) [19–21]. These suggestions have not been rigorously supported by clinical data, and these solutions have not been proven to restore volume and microcirculation better than crystalloid.

7.2 Method of Fluid Administration

There is data that supports the safe use of small volumes of crystalloid such that the deleterious effects of volume overload are avoided while maintaining both macro- and microperfusion. However, if an injured patient has evidence of intact perfusion as measured by normal blood pressure or evidence of end-organ perfusion (intact mental status, palpable radial pulse), he/she does not need to be aggressively resuscitated. For these patients, hypotensive resuscitation, controlled resuscitation, and delayed resuscitation until the time of definitive hemorrhage control have been studied as means of low-volume crystalloid resuscitation. On the other hand, hypotensive patients, those with altered mental status, or those with a head injury (as hypotension at any point greatly worsens outcomes after head trauma), may benefit from additional resuscitation.

These strategies stem from an understanding that a return to normotension in the absence of hemorrhage control is dangerous [22–24]. Infusion rates are adjusted in hypotensive resuscitation to maintain a goal blood pressure (typically mean arterial pressure of 40–50 mmHg or systolic blood pressure of 80–90 mmHg). In the laboratory, this strategy has been shown to result in less acidemia, thrombocytopenia, and coagulopathy, decreased apoptotic cell death, and improved survival when compared to controls resuscitated to normotension [25, 26]. Controlled resuscitation is an alternative means of hypotensive resuscitation that is particularly useful in prehospital or austere environments where sphygmomanometry may not be available. In controlled resuscitation, the rate of fluid infusion is maintained at a predetermined rate selected a priori so that there is little chance of achieving normotension. Again compared to controls resuscitated to normotension, the data suggest that controlled resuscitation at a fixed rate of 60–80 mL/kg/h reduces organ injury, expedites recovery of cell-mediated immune function, and reduces mortality [27–29]. In delayed resuscitation, fluids are withheld until definitive hemorrhage control. This may be particularly useful in areas with short transport times and experimentally has resulted in reduction of blood loss and improved tissue oxygenation [24, 30]. A landmark prehospital study randomized hypotensive (systolic blood pressure <90 mmHg in the field) penetrating torso trauma patients in an urban US environment with short transport times to trauma centers to delayed ($N=289$) versus conventional resuscitation ($N=309$). The study showed that the delayed resuscitation group experienced higher survival than controls (70% vs. 62%, $p=0.04$) without any difference in complication rates [31]. This mounting data led to widespread clinical adoption of the so-called scoop and run approach toward prehospital care, wherein time to definitive care is not prolonged due to unnecessary attempts at intravenous access and fluid administration.

7.3 Blood Products

For patients in hemorrhagic shock who do not respond to these initial fluid resuscitation strategies or who have ongoing bleeding, blood component therapy can be life saving. However, the transfusion of blood products is not risk-free. Both human error and the presence of unmeasured antigens can lead to significant transfusion reactions ranging from mild fever to hemolysis and acute lung injury [32]. Despite modern testing for known blood-borne pathogens, the blood supply is not 100% free of infection risk [32] Furthermore, blood must be delivered in its individual components because, unlike fresh whole blood, components can be tested, processed, freeze-dried, irradiated, packaged, and stored. Unfortunately, in massive hemorrhage, the ratios of blood component delivery may lead to significant coagulopathy, electrolyte abnormalities, immunosuppression, and organ failure [32–36].

Historically, massive hemorrhage was treated with one unit of fresh frozen plasma (FFP) for every six units of packed red blood cells (pRBC) and one unit of platelets for every ten units of pRBCs. This strategy, however, often resulted in the so-called lethal triad for hemorrhagic shock-acidosis, hypothermia, and coagulopathy- wherein despite operative control at the site of injury, hemorrhage continues diffusely and often results in death [37]. Thus, more recently clinical studies in both the civilian and military literature have proposed optimum ratios for the transfusion of blood components in the face of hemorrhagic shock. These studies have focused on patients requiring massive transfusion (more than 10 units of pRBCs in the first 24 h) and have favored an FFP:pRBC ratio of 1:1 or 1:2 and a platelet:pRBC ratio of 1:2 or higher [38–41]. However, some have questioned the association between ratio of products and survival due to survivor bias. A recent study including time of blood component transfusion in the analysis found no survival benefit; the survival differences seen between patients receiving high and low ratios FFP:pRBC in the first 24 h were simply due to the fact that survivors lived long enough to receive additional components [42]. Despite some disagreement on optimal ratios of blood components, the research into these ratios has uniformly supported the implementation of Massive Transfusion Protocols (MTP) or Trauma Exsanguination Protocols (TEP) in order to optimize processes of care and possibly improve outcomes [38, 39, 43–45].

Given that blood component therapy suffers from lack of donors, storage issues, and risks of transfusion, much effort has been put into the design of blood substitutes that would provide the benefits of blood transfusion, in particular with regard to oxygen-carrying capacity, without the risks and with greater ease of use. Over the years, various hemoglobin solutions with long shelf-lives have been created and tested. Though more convenient and promising in the laboratory, none have shown the mortality benefit hoped for and some have caused significant adverse effects including higher mortality [46]. Although further research is ongoing, currently a safer alternative to blood component therapy does not exist for clinical use.

7.4 Technique for Resuscitation

Resuscitation is not a substitute for early hemorrhage control. From the moment of injury, all efforts to provide definitive control of hemorrhage as expeditiously as possible must be pursued. Due to the deleterious effects of large volume crystalloid on hemorrhage-induced inflammation and immune-modulation, lower volume resuscitation seems to be associated with a lower complication rate. When there is expected to be very minimal delay (on the order of minutes) in transfer to definitive care, resuscitation and time-consuming access procedures can be safely withheld for a patient with adequate cerebral perfusion (normal mental status in the absence of head injury) and a palpable radial pulse. For all other situations when the time to transfer to definitive care is longer than 10–15 min, goal-directed resuscitation with low-volume crystalloid should be implemented. Specifically, the goals should be either a SBP approximating 80–90 mmHg (MAP 40–60 mmHg) where sphygmomanometry is available, or the ability of the patient to mentate (in the absence of head injury) and the clinician to palpate a radial pulse when sphygmomanometry is not available. In the latter situation, an empiric rate of 60–80 mL/kg/h is typically appropriate. L-isomer lactated ringers solution is the most reasonable choice of crystalloid as it induces relatively less inflammation and immune dysfunction, causes fewer electrolyte abnormalities, is cost-effective, and is widely available for clinical use. If, after the infusion of 500 mL of crystalloid, hemorrhage control is not achieved, blood component therapy should be implemented under a well-defined system-wide protocol that streamlines component delivery. While the ideal ratio of blood components is also still under investigation, a 1:2 FFP:pRBC ratio and 1:5 platelet: pRBC ratio can be safely selected to minimize progression to the "lethal triad." Early and expeditious control of hemorrhage and modest, goal-directed resuscitation first with low-volume crystalloid, then with pre-selected blood component ratios is presently the optimal technique for trauma resuscitation.

Important Points

- Minimize time to definitive hemorrhage control.
- Candidates for resuscitation:
  - Hypotensive
    - SBP <90 mmHg
    - Absent radial pulse
  - Altered mental status
  - Head injury (even with intact mental status)
- Do not infuse large volume crystalloid
- Hypertonic and hyperoncotic fluids are not superior to crystalloid
- Anticipate transport time and choose a goal-directed resuscitation strategy
  - Short transport time (under 15 min)
    - Delay resuscitation until definitive hemorrhage control

  - Longer transport times with available monitors
    Titrate Ringer's lactate solution to MAP 40–50 mmHg (or SBP 80–90 mmHg)
  - Longer transport times without monitors
    Provide Ringer's lactate solution at 60–80 mL/kg/h
- Begin blood component therapy if 500 mL Ringer's Lactate does not show improvement or hemorrhage is ongoing.
- Blood components should be delivered in a protocolized fashion targeting the ratios of:
  - 1 unit of FFP to 2 units of pRBCs
  - 1 unit of Platelets to 5 units of pRBCs
- There are no blood substitutes at this time
- And again, STOP THE BLEEDING

References

1. Sauaia A, Moore FA, Moore EE et al (1995) Epidemiology of trauma deaths: a reassessment. J Trauma 38:185–193
2. Acosta JA, Yang JC, Winchell RJ et al (1998) Lethal injuries and time to death in a level I trauma center. J Am Coll Surg 186:528–533
3. Bellamy RF (1984) The causes of death in conventional land warfare: implications for combat casualty care research. Mil Med 149:55–62
4. Shackford SR, Mackersie RC, Holbrook TL et al (1993) The epidemiology of traumatic death. A population-based analysis. Arch Surg 128:571–575
5. Nunn JF, Freeman J (1964) Problems of oxygenation and oxygen transport during haemorrhage. Anaesthesia 19: 206–216
6. Abdelrahman M, Collin M, Thiemermann C (2004) The peroxisome proliferator-activated receptor-gamma ligand 15-deoxyDelta12,14 prostaglandin J2 reduces the organ injury in hemorrhagic shock. Shock 22:555–561
7. Abdelrahman M, Mazzon E, Bauer M et al (2005) Inhibitors of NADPH oxidase reduce the organ injury in hemorrhagic shock. Shock 23:107–114
8. McCloskey CA, Kameneva MV, Uryash A et al (2004) Tissue hypoxia activates JNK in the liver during hemorrhagic shock. Shock 22:380–386
9. Sato H, Tanaka T, Kasai K et al (2005) Role of p38 mitogen-activated protein kinase on renal dysfunction after hemorrhagic shock in rats. Shock 24:488–494
10. Sato H, Tanaka T, Kasai K et al (2007) Role of p38 mitogen-activated protein kinase on cardiac dysfunction after hemorrhagic shock in rats. Shock 28:291–299
11. Alam HB, Stegalkina S, Rhee P et al (2002) cDNA array analysis of gene expression following hemorrhagic shock and resuscitation in rats. Resuscitation 54:195–206
12. Chen H, Alam HB, Querol RI et al (2006) Identification of expression patterns associated with hemorrhage and resuscitation: integrated approach to data analysis. J Trauma 60:701–723
13. Xu DZ, Lu Q, Adams CA et al (2004) Trauma-hemorrhagic shock-induced up-regulation of endothelial cell adhesion molecules is blunted by mesenteric lymph duct ligation. Crit Care Med 32:760–765
14. Dillon J, Lynch LJ Jr, Myers R et al (1966) The treatment of hemorrhagic shock. Surg Gynecol Obstet 122:967–978
15. Shires GT, Canizaro PC (1973) Fluid resuscitation in the severely injured. Surg Clin North Am 53:1341–1366
16. Cotton BA, Guy JS, Morris JA Jr et al (2006) The cellular, metabolic, and systemic consequences of aggressive fluid resuscitation strategies. Shock 26:115–121
17. Rizoli SB (2003) Crystalloids and colloids in trauma resuscitation: a brief overview of the current debate. J Trauma 54:S82–S88
18. National Heart Lung and Blood Institute (2009) The NHLBI halts study of concentrated saline for patients with shock due to lack of survival benefit. In: NIH News. National Heart Lung and Blood Institute, Bethesda
19. Pope A, French G, Longnecker D (1999) Fluid resuscitation: state of the science for treating combat casualties and civilian injuries. Institute of Medicine, Washington, DC
20. Revell M, Porter K, Greaves I (2001) Fluid resuscitation in pre-hospital trauma care: a consensus view. J R Army Med Corps 147:147–152
21. (2001) Fluid resuscitation in combat. Defence and Civil Institute of Environmental Medicine, Toronto
22. Kowalenko T, Stern S, Dronen S et al (1992) Improved outcome with hypotensive resuscitation of uncontrolled hemorrhagic shock in a swine model. J Trauma 33:349–353
23. Stern SA, Dronen SC, Birrer P et al (1993) Effect of blood pressure on hemorrhage volume and survival in a near-fatal hemorrhage model incorporating a vascular injury. Ann Emerg Med 22:155–163
24. Holmes JF, Sakles JC, Lewis G et al (2002) Effects of delaying fluid resuscitation on an injury to the systemic arterial vasculature. Acad Emerg Med 9:267–274
25. Xiao N, Wang XC, Diao YF et al (2004) Effect of initial fluid resuscitation on subsequent treatment in uncontrolled hemorrhagic shock in rats. Shock 21:276–280
26. Lu YQ, Cai XJ, Gu LH et al (2007) Experimental study of controlled fluid resuscitation in the treatment of severe and uncontrolled hemorrhagic shock. J Trauma 63:798–804
27. Shah KJ, Chiu WC, Scalea TM et al (2002) Detrimental effects of rapid fluid resuscitation on hepatocellular function and survival after hemorrhagic shock. Shock 18: 242–247
28. Santibanez-Gallerani AS, Barber AE, Williams SJ et al (2001) Improved survival with early fluid resuscitation following hemorrhagic shock. World J Surg 25:592–597
29. Knoferl MW, Angele MK, Ayala A et al (1999) Do different rates of fluid resuscitation adversely or beneficially influence immune responses after trauma-hemorrhage? J Trauma 46:23–33
30. Sakles JC, Sena MJ, Knight DA et al (1997) Effect of immediate fluid resuscitation on the rate, volume, and duration of pulmonary vascular hemorrhage in a sheep model of penetrating thoracic trauma. Ann Emerg Med 29:392–399
31. Bickell WH, Wall MJ Jr, Pepe PE et al (1994) Immediate versus delayed fluid resuscitation for hypotensive patients

with penetrating torso injuries. N Engl J Med 331: 1105–1109

32. Alter HJ, Klein HG (2008) The hazards of blood transfusion in historical perspective. Blood 112:2617–2626
33. Spahn DR, Rossaint R (2005) Coagulopathy and blood component transfusion in trauma. Br J Anaesth 95:130–139
34. Aboudara MC, Hurst FP, Abbott KC et al (2008) Hyperkalemia after packed red blood cell transfusion in trauma patients. J Trauma 64:S86–S91; discussion S91
35. Hensler T, Heinemann B, Sauerland S et al (2003) Immunologic alterations associated with high blood transfusion volume after multiple injury: effects on plasmatic cytokine and cytokine receptor concentrations. Shock 20: 497–502
36. Silverboard H, Aisiku I, Martin GS et al (2005) The role of acute blood transfusion in the development of acute respiratory distress syndrome in patients with severe trauma. J Trauma 59:717–723
37. Kashuk JL, Moore EE, Millikan JS et al (1982) Major abdominal vascular trauma–a unified approach. J Trauma 22:672–679
38. Duchesne JC, Hunt JP, Wahl G et al (2008) Review of current blood transfusions strategies in a mature level I trauma center: were we wrong for the last 60 years? J Trauma 65:272–276
39. Holcomb JB, Wade CE, Michalek JE et al (2008) Increased plasma and platelet to red blood cell ratios improves outcome in 466 massively transfused civilian trauma patients. Ann Surg 248:447–458
40. Borgman MA, Spinella PC, Perkins JG et al (2007) The ratio of blood products transfused affects mortality in patients receiving massive transfusions at a combat support hospital. J Trauma 63:805–813
41. Gunter OL Jr, Au BK, Isbell JM et al (2008) Optimizing outcomes in damage control resuscitation: identifying blood product ratios associated with improved survival. J Trauma 65:527–534
42. Snyder CW, Weinberg JA, McGwin G Jr et al (2009) The relationship of blood product ratio to mortality: survival benefit or survival bias? J Trauma 66:358–362, discussion 362-354
43. Gonzalez EA, Moore FA, Holcomb JB et al (2007) Fresh frozen plasma should be given earlier to patients requiring massive transfusion. J Trauma 62:112–119
44. Malone DL, Hess JR, Fingerhut A (2006) Massive transfusion practices around the globe and a suggestion for a common massive transfusion protocol. J Trauma 60:S91–S96
45. Cotton BA, Gunter OL, Isbell J et al (2008) Damage control hematology: the impact of a trauma exsanguination protocol on survival and blood product utilization. J Trauma 64: 1177–1182
46. Natanson C, Kern SJ, Lurie P et al (2008) Cell-free hemoglobin-based blood substitutes and risk of myocardial infarction and death: a meta-analysis. JAMA 299:2304–2312

ABC Heuristics

8

Pantelis Vassiliu

Since the early years of evolution, oxygen released into the atmosphere permitted oxygen-dependent creatures to thrive. Humans are such creatures. A tube, an air pump, and a fluid pump, coded recently with the acronym ABC, extract oxygen from the environment and distribute it to the last cell, before any other functions occur. Disturb this fundamental process and human life, after a short period of vigorous compensation, expires. Thus, the management of A, B, and C injuries is considered crucial and this is preached worldwide. Most physicians (not only surgeons) have been taught and have practiced those techniques hands on. Less well known, owing to a lack of experience, is the sequence and time effectiveness with which these techniques need to be deployed in order to "buy time" for the patient, and to maximize the potential salvaging of life.

So "the name of the game is time." Brain oxygenation failure sends man on his ultimate 3-min trip (u3T), which ends in brain damage and "game over." This is the only path, whatever the underlying injury, to plunging a healthy individual headlong toward rapid death. It is fortunate that very few injuries lead to this death sprint; so, in this ultimate emergency, the focus is on identifying and treating, during primary ABC evaluation: Airway obstruction, Tension pneumothorax (tPTX), Cardiac tamponade, Massive hemorrhage. A couple more (i.e., cerebrocervical dissociation, neurogenic shock), although equally lethal, are irrelevant to penetrating injuries. The 3 min is an average estimation based on experience, and deviations from this limit do exist. The same applies for most of the occurrences mentioned in this chapter. The whole chapter runs fast-forward in order to emphasize the need to act time-effectively and to save every second possible. Real-life trauma is more gracious regarding time. However, to quote Sinatra: "If you can make it there [in less time] you'll make it anywhere."

P. Vassiliu
Department of Surgery, Attikon Hospital,
Kapodistrian University of Athens Medical School,
Athens, Greece
e-mail: pant_greek@hotmail.com

8.1 Airway

Let us first clarify the term. The airway starts from the mouth and nose orifices, and terminates at the end bronchiole before the alveolus. The airway is a tube that progressive diminishes in diameter. Complete obstruction equals a life-threatening situation. This happens at its narrowest location, the vocal cords, which are placed transversely, reducing drastically lumen's diameter. Objects small enough to pass through the vocal cords will obstruct minor bronchi, but are not life-threatening. The part of the airway sited at the neck is exposed to perforation, hematoma, edema, and also ends below the vocal cords. Distal from that, the trachea is protected deep within the mediastinum and although an injury may happen there, it can be managed surgically through B and C. So, the end of the airway, when we are dealing with the ABCs, is at the vocal cords. Obstruction, penetration, hematoma of A can be managed in an emergency within minutes, by bypassing the injury distal from the vocal cords, either with a tracheal tube or a surgical cricothyrotomy.

G.C. Velmahos et al. (eds.), *Penetrating Trauma*,
DOI 10.1007/978-3-642-20453-1_8, © Springer-Verlag Berlin Heidelberg 2012

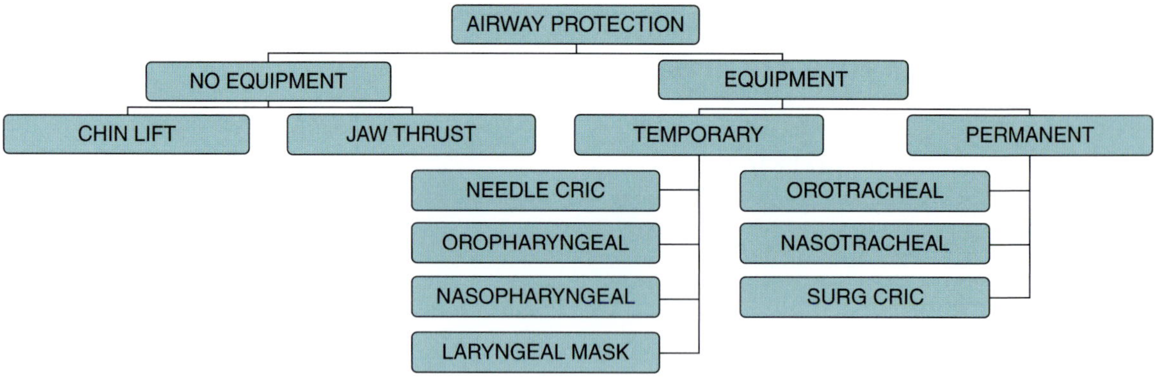

Fig. 8.1 Ways to re-establish patency or protect the airway [3]

8.1.1 Evaluation

The history (e.g., a penetrating neck injury) may alert you before you even see the patient and the clock starts to count down. The clinical examination, in a conscious patient (mumbling or hoarse vocals); physical signs in the unconscious (hearing, feeling, or seeing the air coming in and out of the mouth, observing the oral cavity for bleeding, emesis, and the neck for hematoma, a hole, bubbles, edema), and the combination of all these, answering definitively the three questions: *Patent*? *Threatened*? *Obstructed*? Mission should be accomplished within 10 s.

8.1.2 Treatment

A patent airway should indicate the green light to proceed to B. Easy and fast diagnosis … but would it remain patent in the near future? History/signs/clinical, if all negative, answer a definitive "yes" … and release the brake. Put on an oxygen facemask at 15 L/min and evaluate B.

You do identify a threat to A. This is the most time- and thought-intensive situation. You need permanent intubation, by an oro- or naso- or crico-tracheal tube with a balloon that fastens below the vocal cords. This action consumes a lot of time. In extremely experienced hands orotracheal intubation takes 2 min 30 s [1]. Offering this service in a hospital, where an anesthesiologist devotes his time to A, while you, although remaining alert to the need for surgical cricothyrotomy, take care of B and C, is okay. If you are dealing with this *alone* you need to think one more step ahead. What threat are you dealing with? An evolving threat (i.e., expanding hematoma) or a potential threat that may or may not ensue (i.e., GCS < 8 due to blood loss only, not head injury, risk of aspiration). In the first case do the intubation, immediately, whole-heartedly. In a potentially threatening situation, maybe it is better to conserve time. The >2 min 30 s needed for intubation will exhaust your patient's remaining lifetime if there is a coexisting problem from B or C. Instead, proceed to a rapid evaluation of B and C, and devote time to any real (not a potential) threat you may find there. After all it is better to have a living patient with aspiration pneumonia, than a dead one because of tamponade, with an intubated, safe airway [2].

An obstructed airway has an extremely dramatic clinical presentation in a conscious patient. Hand to throat, no vocal sounds, and extreme agony in the face are evident. Loss of consciousness, followed by loss of muscular tone may obstruct the airway because of the tongue dropping back, and can be treated easily within 10 s by a jaw thrust and chin lift. In all other cases of obstruction no contemplation, but time-consuming action is needed. Focus and devote the time required to re-establish patency and don't be concerned about B and C. Even if there are other injuries involved, you can offer nothing unless oxygen finds its way through A.

The ways to re-establish Airway patency are shown in Fig. 8.1.

Treatment of A with no equipment, chin lift and jaw thrust, can practiced "in the street," requires 10 s, works, and resolves almost all cases of airway obstruction due

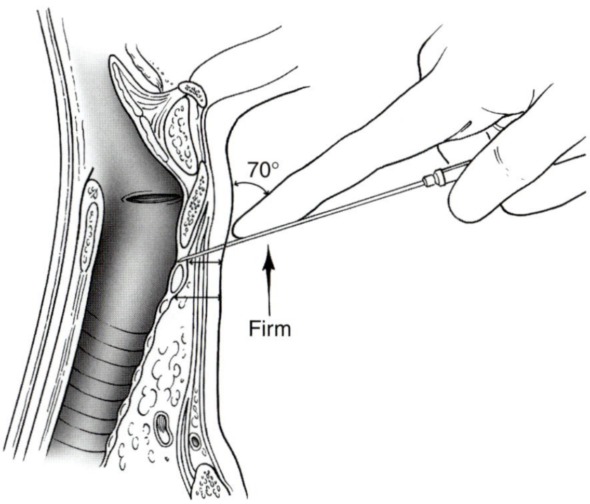

Fig. 8.2 Technique for needle cricotomy (lateral view)

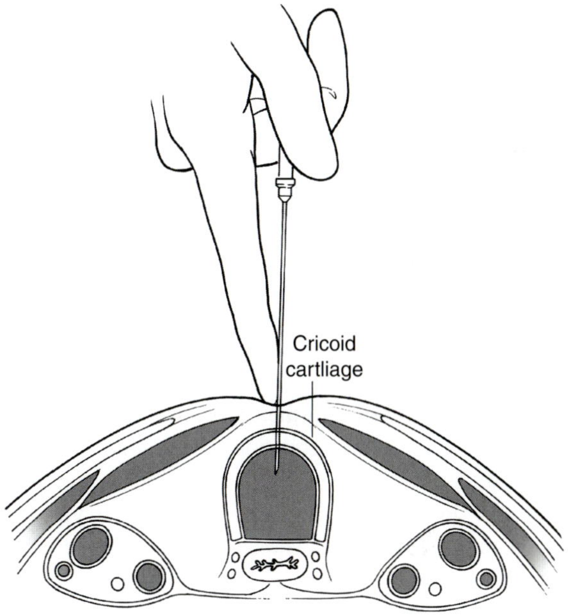

Fig. 8.3 Technique for needle cricotomy (craniocaudal view)

to the tongue simply dropping back. Remember to protect the spine.

Airway intubation with temporary measures is easier and faster than with permanent ones. It can be applied "in the street," but requires equipment. If you have to bypass an obstructed airway surgically with no means remember you can bail out with a needle cricothyrotomy (Figs. 8.2, 8.3). This takes 60 s and buys 30 min for your patient. If you are enthusiastic, confident, and courageous, and have common sense, have handy the pocket airway "Life-Stat"®: a metallic trocar with a large needle to penetrate the cricothyroid membrane, a connecting cannula, and a universal adapter matching the tubing diameter of any ventilator. The device is packed one tube within the other and you can carry it with your key holder. The only issue here is to convince airport authorities that you want this sharp instrument with you on board for a novel purpose.

Temporary airway tubing can become dislodged at any moment. Replacement with a permanent one is mandatory a.s.a.p. This requires an organized environment, equipment, more skill, and a lot of time [1]. A knife, a really helpful tracheal *hook*, a curved clamp, a tube, and your steady hand is all you need to perform an emergency cricothyrotomy (Fig. 8.4).

So, by now you have devoted something like 10 s, let's say, to evaluating your patient's airway and if it is *really* indicated, another 3 min (a lot of time) to securing it, and now you are ready to proceed to B.

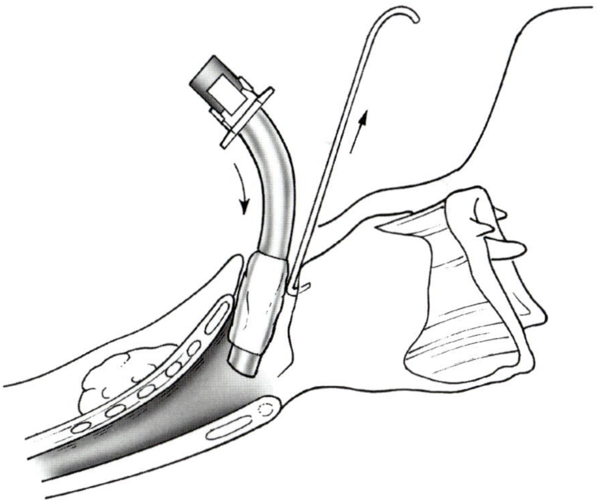

Fig. 8.4 Surgical cricotomy (notice the hook)

8.2 Breathing

8.2.1 Evaluation

Fifteen more seconds are needed to identify a life-threatening injury from B, and localize it R or L. Clinical presentation in a conscious patient is so impressive and typical that it strikes you from a distance. In extreme agony, combative, with swallowing, high-frequency breaths, speaking with sort, sharp phrases. "Doc, help I am dying." With every breath repeating exactly the same sentence, cutting the last word, because his breath volume is not enough to allow him to complete it. In such a "loud" case, are you allowed to bypass A and decompress the tPTX first? By all means. It's "ABC" vs common sense. A 15 s delay in A evaluation, to re-establish breathing and circulation, it's a bargain. If you are not "lucky" enough to see such a patient, a report of penetrating injury to the thoracic surface should alert you before you even see him. Observation of the respiratory movement of the two hemi-thoraxes, and bilateral auscultation at the 2nd intercostal, mid-clavicular, and 6th intercostal mid-axillary location, is diagnostic. At the initial evaluation a single breath or even less, one inspiration or expiration is enough to decide. If clear, proceed to C. If it sounds like there is a problem, do not waste a second, just treat. If you are inconclusive, given your clinician's common sense, it seems that your patient has enough respiratory reserve to undergo an on-table X-ray. Any second delay from radiology, should be invested in the next step, C.

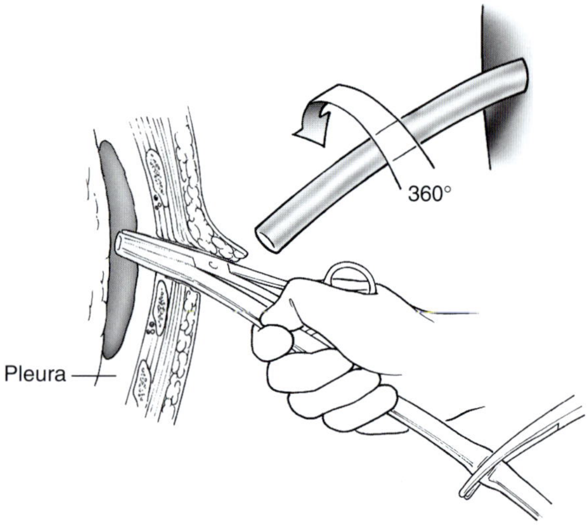

Fig. 8.5 Insert chest tube without its trocar on the upper boarder of lower rib. After insertion rotate tube by 360° at its longitudinal axis to avoid its entrapment in lung fissure

8.2.2 Treatment

Two life-threatening injuries in B need immediate action. In most cases, this action will solve the problem and only 15% [4] will need an operation.

- Tension PTX: Decompresses with a needle at 2nd intercostal space mid-clavicular line. Task should be completed within 15 s, … 14 of which are needed to find a large-caliber long venous catheter (a.k.a. needle) if you are not prepared. This will give time extension to a dying patient. During that time you now evaluate A. If this is already done you can put in a chest tube (Fig. 8.5), which takes a couple minutes if you are reasonably fast. If you anticipate needing more time for this task (skill confidence, where is the tube, collection system not ready) it is wise to complete a rapid evaluation of C (30 s and three answers away), to have an idea what waits you there and start preparing, and then come back and complete the job with B, adjusting your pace.
- Massive hemothorax (HTX): more than 1,500 cc drained as you put in a chest tube, or drain of 200 mL/h over 3–4 h [4]. Usually HTX is not massive, because vessels within the chest cavity are low-pressure/easily clotting and the issue is simply to drain the blood completely. The thoracic cavity/mediastinum contains high-pressure vessels, which, when bleeding, kill even before arrival at hospital. This could be one of the 15% of cases that will require immediate operative management, were you actually treat a problem from C located in a B area. While you transport the patient to the OR, evaluate C and prepare for additional surprises.

Two more injuries from B require immediate action although are less demanding regarding time.

- Flail chest: Infrequent in penetrating injury. Patient will have lung contusion that will become worst with aggressive fluid resuscitation, he will hypoventilate the injured area to diminish pain, and may have HTX or PTX. Manage them with oxygen, analgesia, and physiotherapy. If the FiO_2/PaO_2 ratio drops below 200, prolonged intubation is required until contusion resolves.
- Simple HTX or PTX: The issue here is to be sure that HTX is simple and not massive, and the easy way is an X-ray, most effective being a chest tube, both at least 2 min away. In simple open PTX a >3-cm defect at the wall affects respiration significantly and will press for immediate action (chest tube, dressing) [4]. In both cases, consider the vital signs, the time requirement for an X-ray/chest tube, and the stability of the patient, and you may choose to prioritize the chest tube over X-ray or even a rapid initial assessment to rule out lethal injuries from C.

The bare necessities you need for substantial management of B injuries: large caliber needle, chest tube, draining system with a Heimlich valve (sophisticated or simple), and the luxury of: X-ray, stethoscope. You will find them in every medical facility. In the extreme scenario where your services are needed in an isolated environment, develop them by being a bit innovative. A real example of chest tube placement during an airplane trip: whisky as antiseptic, a straightened wire from a dress hanger as a styleus and a straw as a chest tube.

8.3 Circulation

Common sense bypasses all principles/traditions. If you are facing the red-hot juice pouring out of the body, compress to stop it. Before B, before A. Devote 1 s and buy a *lot* of time. Applies to all compressible areas, from carotid to … digital artery. For uncompressible cavities (chest, abdomen) the patient needs an operation to contain the bleeding, so you follow time-effectively the ABC rules.

C is a little more complex than A and B. It has three components: the pump, the tubing, and the circulating fluid. This vignette raises more questions than need to be answered, but again rapidly fatal injuries are very rare.

Start vice versa, treating before evaluating. Two 18-gauge IV catheters give you access to the intravascular space, a bare necessity. Postponing this task narrows the chances of success because of volume depletion. You can accomplish this within 60 s, although much longer times have been reported [1]. Difficulties in venopuncture? Familiarize yourself with the intraosseous catheterization technique and its limitations and utilize power intraosseous "EZ-IO"®, which promises 30-s access to the intraosseous/intravascular space in adults, has been tested, and works [5–7].

8.3.1 Evaluation

Check first what kills most rapidly.

1. Pump

1a. Heart penetration: Suspect it if there is penetrating injury to the left chest. Blood pressure rapidly drops despite resuscitative efforts. An ideal indication for ER thoracotomy. Especially if the patient loses the pulse while retaining electrical heart function. You will need *only* six instruments, knowledge of the simple technique (see relevant chapter 11), boldness, and common sense. Within 4 min you have the descending aorta clamped, so you force the few circulating erythrocytes to perfuse the brain, repair the cardiac hole with traumatic and not elective techniques (see relevant chapter 11), and give IV blood at a rhythm of 1 L/min if you have a rapid infuser. This injury is unmanageable outside of a well-organized hospital.

1b. Tamponade: Clinical presentation looks a lot like tPTX. The differential comes from the story, penetrating injury to the left hemithorax, above the heart, instead of blunt chest trauma. Distended neck veins may be present or not if volume depletion develops, agony, blurry sounds heard. You are facing, as in cardiac penetration, this "crazy" type of shock that worsens with fluids! Occasionally diagnosis is difficult, but this is the less demanding case that gives more time. You should act immediately. The classical teaching of pericardiocentesis, although it applies for drainage of non-bloody pericardial effusion, is usually ineffective and potentially dangerous in trauma. It is your only option if you are not a surgeon. Preached and applied to assuage the doctor's conscience rather than to treat the problem itself. Remember that blood clots out of the vessels? Well, it applies here. And since clotting time is 6 min, it is logical to assume that this is the time you have to suspect, diagnose, target, and hit the pericardium with a needle to succeed. Narrow. The myth that pericardial blood does not clot is derived from elective cardiac surgery; where fully heparinized patients are treated with pericardiocentesis if they develop tamponade postoperatively. Five percent of trauma patients develop very early coagulopathy [8]. This group of patients may also contribute to the myth and may have a chance of effective tamponade evacuation with pericardiocentesis.

Practically the only chance of survival is operative drainage. This can be accomplished by a subxyphoid midline abdominal incision, through the diaphragm's abdominal surface (Fig. 8.6), or under the tip of the sternum after cutting its edge (Fig. 8.7; see relevant chapter 11). A left thoracotomy allows decompression and repair of the underlying heart injury so can also be applied. All techniques are easy, rapid (5 min), effective, and you can do them in the ER or OR, but not out of house.

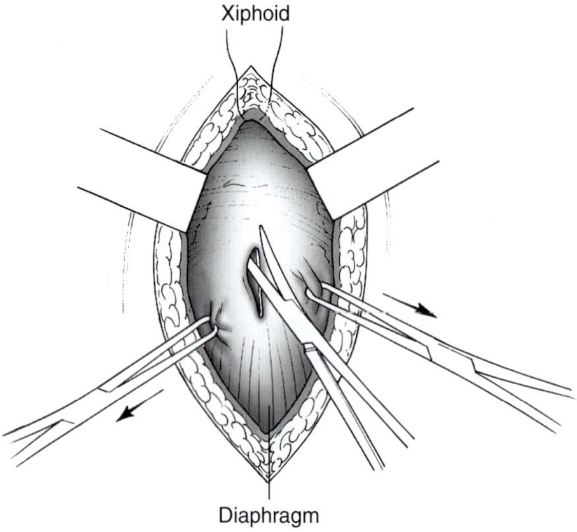

Fig. 8.6 Cut diaphragm between Allis clamps

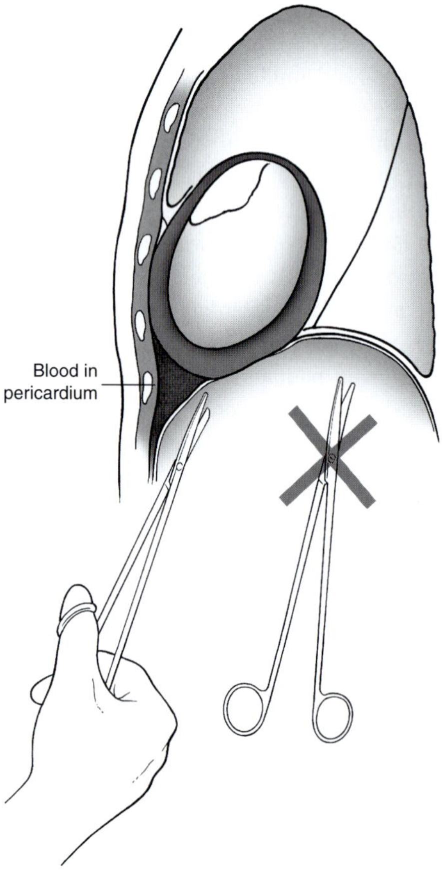

Fig. 8.7 Stay retrosternal to find your way to the pericardium

2. Fluid

The crux of the resuscitative effort is to preserve the minimal circulation necessary to keep the nervous tissue perfused until you control the bleeding. This is where hypotensive resuscitation comes on board. If you can retain an SBP of around 90 mmHg [9], you preserve brain perfusion, and avoid dislodging of the fresh clot that seals vessel injuries. Dislodging, rebreeding, and fatalities happen with elevation of SBP.

You estimate the percentage of missing blood through the vital signs. Vitals are examined in a specific order, prioritizing those that decline from normal first during hypovolemic shock development: pulse rate, mental function, breathing rate, pulse volume, skin color/temperature, urine volume, and blood pressure.

In the Iraq war, the US army effectively utilized just the first two clinical signs to resuscitate the injured soldier during transportation, with no equipment: the pulse rate, and mentation [7, 12]. Whenever the wounded lost either of the two (pulse, communication), they received an IV bolus or 100 cc of hypertonic saline 7.5% (HTS) combined with dextran 6% (HSD) [13]. This kept the patient alive during transportation to the closest surgical unit. HTS/HSD packs a lot of volume in a little box. 100 cc is infused, and another 300 cc is drawn into the vessels from the tissues because of the osmotic effect. Ideal for soldiers to carry into battle, where there are severe load limitations. The benefit of temporary expansion of intravascular volume is overpowered by time, and by the osmotic disturbance.

So which fluid is better? Normal/Saline is not exactly our electrolyte and osmolality composition so it's out. Dextrose 5% in water, gives sugar (which is not as essential as circulation at that time), and then metabolizes into electrolyte-free water, which dissolves electrolytes, adding this problem to all the others. Ringers Lactate is electrolyte- and osmolality-friendly, so this is what sells most. Colloids have been completely outmoded since the Iraqi war, where we realized that humans bleed whole blood and not "starch" [7, 8, 13]. In previous wars, we didn't have the technology to preserve blood so we broke it into components (red cells, platelets, plasma) or we tried to find substitute volume expanders, like colloids. In this last war, the survival rate rose dramatically with the utilization of whole blood, so now for the exsanguinating patient the issue is: either transfuse whole fresh blood, or for every unit of red blood cells give a unit plasma and a unit of platelets [14–18].

3. Tubing

You are facing a patient in hypovolemic shock due to a penetrating injury. Any compressible bleeding vessel should have been compressed on sight. But the patient's condition is deteriorating. Rule out tPTX, and cardiac tamponade/ penetration. What remains as a cause is vessel hole(s), either individual or within solid viscera.

As you are heading to the OR, you would like to know *one thing*: which cavity is bleeding. The "cavities" you target are few: chest (R or L), mediastinum, abdomen, retroperitoneum, the thigh and the environment.

Remember we are dealing with minimal time. Your time investment in B (clinical examination, chest tubes) would already have given a convincing answer for massive bleeding from the chest, so focus on the rest. The transmediastinal course of the injury and the injury located in the mid-thorax suggests mediastinal bleeding, although during evaluation of the heart you also shape an idea for the mediastinum. Before you decide to crack a sternum, remember that most preventable deaths from exsanguination come from the abdominal cavity, so devote your attention there first. Penetration of the abdominal wall and shock gives you a ticket for a xyphopubic incision, regardless of whether there is intra-abdominal or retroperitoneal bleeding. The only issue that you should think twice about is the fifth cavity. Exsanguination in the field that nobody informed you about (… "we found him in a lake of blood"), and a patient who remains in hypovolemic shock due to underescusitation. Think about it, ask the paramedics, before you hit empty from blood, one cavity after another. Don Trunkey, proud of his ability to save lives, suggests for such ultimate emergencies. "Two chest tubes within two minutes and then a xyphopubic incision, and you have all blood holding cavities handy for evaluation and treatment."

Vital signs (trend not just a measurement) will answer the other vital question: how much time you have? SBP of 80 mmHg, and after 2 min and 1–2 L of resuscitative effort, 70 mmHg, means red alert and the OR. If this is not the case you can deploy your close range diagnostic toys (FAST, X-ray) to locate the bleeding cavity, or if the patient is really stable you can use the long-range (p.e. CT) diagnostic equipment, and even think about non-operative management.

Literature exists on the rate of blood loss and the patient's remaining lifetime before expiration from penetrating injuries. Acute loss of >50% of blood volume equals death. Abdominal solid viscera (liver/spleen), bleeding at a rate of 25 cc/min, or 1,500 cc/h, hypotension occurring within an hour, and death in 2 h if untreated. Vascular injury, bleeding at a rate of 100 cc/min, hypotension occurring in 15 min, and death within 1 h [11, 19].

8.4 Cell Whisper

So you end up performing an emergency operation on a trauma patient. From the second you decide to embark on this trip, always remember another time restraint.

A specific range of temperature and pH allow biochemical reactions to proceed within our body. Prolonged hypoxia may not kill instantly, but makes cells function in an anaerobic way, creating metabolites (lactic acid, H^+, CO_2) that will drop outside of the normal range of the "milieu interieur." Loss of that warm red fluid will cause de facto hypothermia. The coagulation cascade, although all its factors are present, will not deploy because the biochemical reactions do not proceed in temperatures lower than 34°C and pH<7.2. YOU THE SURGEON, should at these initial steps confront the injured patient not as a broken doll that requires restoration of its anatomy, but as a severely disturbed internal *microscopic biochemical* environment. If you are not trained to hear the whisper of the gasping for oxygen cells, and prioritize the oxygen supply (control bleeding), and if you not actively re-warm (50°C water cavity lavage), the patient will soon (in a couple of hours) die, despite your novel effort to treat him with the classical principles of elective surgery, and for no obvious macroscopic reason.

Your anesthesiologist is there to translate the cell whisper into a language you understand. Just ask: pH, temperature, lactate. Ask every 5 min to readjust your speed [20]. Your goal in this OR is to stop bleeding and remove the septic factor. Anatomical restoration will follow after 48 h, when you have the luxury of a stable patient [8].

Important Points

1. Time is of the essence
2. Remember the injuries that put your patient on board for the ultimate 3 min trip, learn to suspect them, identify them, and treat them immediately, no matter where you are (trauma center or … airplane) otherwise the patient expires: airway obstruction, tPTX, tamponade, massive bleeding.
3. Common sense bypasses … tradition:
   (a) Tension PTX (B before A). Needle decompression.
   (b) Profound external bleeding (C before A and B). Compress.
   (c) Cardiac tamponade. To the OR. Intubate en route.
4. Hypovolemic shock that deteriorates with fluids: tPTX, tamponade, heart penetration, exsanguination in the field.
5. Before you reach the OR in an emergency (C will lead you there, to control hemorrhagic shock):
   (a) Be sure the causes in point 4 have been excluded as reasons for uncontrollable, but not surgically managed, hypovolemic shock.
   (b) Identify the cavity that is most probably bleeding.
   (c) If you really run out of time (and you do retain common sense) remember the bail-out rule of D. Trunkey: two chest tubes in and xyphopubic incision, within 5 min.
6. "If you encounter massive bleeding, remember this is *not your* blood." Raphael Adar, M.D., F.A.C.S [21].
7. Listen to the cell's whisper (pH, temperature, coagulopathy) during the damage control operation and complete your OR within 60–90 min. Your goal: control bleeding and sepsis. Re-warm (50°C in cavity lavage), close cavities rapidly (damage control technique), send to the ICU to normalize the milieu interieur. Come back after 12–48 h to restore the anatomy.

References

1. Carr BG, Brachet T, David G, Duseja R, Branas CC (2008) The time cost of prehospital intubation and intravenous access in trauma patients. Prehosp Emerg Care 12(3):327–332
2. Vassiliu P (2008) The name of the Game is …Time. In: ATLS annual meeting, ACS conference, San Francisco, 2008
3. Geranios A (2007) Airway management equipment. In: Athens
4. Cubasch H, Degiannis E (2004) The deadly dozen of chest trauma. CME Emerg Med 22(77):369–372
5. Davidoff J, Fowler R, Gordon D et al (2005) Clinical evaluation of a novel intraosseous device for adults: prospective, 250-patient, multi-center trial. JEMS 30(Suppl 10):20–23
6. Gillum L, Kovar J (2005) Powered intraosseous access in the prehospital setting: MCHD EMS puts the EZ-IO to the test. JEMS 30(Suppl 10):24–25
7. Holcomb JB (2003) Fluid resuscitation in modern combat casualty care: lessons learned from Somalia. J Trauma 54(5 Suppl):S46–S51
8. Holcomb JB (2007) Damage control resuscitation. J Trauma 62(6 Suppl):S36–S37
9. Sondeen JL, Coppes VG, Holcomb JB (2003) Blood pressure at which rebleeding occurs after resuscitation in swine with aortic injury. J Trauma 54(5 Suppl):S110–S117
10. Bickell WH, Wall MJ Jr, Pepe PE et al (1994) Immediate versus delayed fluid resuscitation for hypotensive patients with penetrating torso injuries. N Engl J Med 331(17):1105–1109
11. Demetriades D (2004) Hypotensive resuscitation in trauma patients. In: Hellenic Trauma Association conference, Athens, 2004
12. Holcomb JB, Salinas J, McManus JM, Miller CC, Cooke WH, Convertino VA (2005) Manual vital signs reliably predict need for life-saving interventions in trauma patients. J Trauma 59(4):821–828; discussion 8–9
13. Champion HR (2003) Combat fluid resuscitation: introduction and overview of conferences. J Trauma 54(5 Suppl):S7–S12
14. Borgman MA, Spinella PC, Perkins JG et al (2007) The ratio of blood products transfused affects mortality in patients receiving massive transfusions at a combat support hospital. J Trauma 63(4):805–813
15. Hess JR, Holcomb JB (2008) Transfusion practice in military trauma. Transfus Med 18(3):143–150
16. Spinella PC (2008) Warm fresh whole blood transfusion for severe hemorrhage: U.S. military and potential civilian applications. Crit Care Med 36(7 Suppl):S340–S345
17. Turner J, Nicholl J, Webber L, Cox H, Dixon S, Yates D (2000) A randomised controlled trial of prehospital intravenous fluid replacement therapy in serious trauma. Health Technol Assess 4(31):1–57
18. Malone DL, Hess JR, Fingerhut A (2006) Massive transfusion practices around the globe and a suggestion for a common massive transfusion protocol. J Trauma 60(6 Suppl):S91–S96
19. Demetriades D, Murray J, Charalambides K et al (2004) Trauma fatalities: time and location of hospital deaths. J Am Coll Surg 198(1):20–26
20. Moore EE, Thomas G (1996) Orr memorial lecture. Staged laparotomy for the hypothermia, acidosis, and coagulopathy syndrome. Am J Surg 172(5):405–410
21. Hirshberg A Mattox KL (2005) Top knife. The art & craft of trauma surgery. tfm Publishing Ltd, Harley, Nr Shrewsbury

Pediatric Trauma Resuscitation

9

Elizabeth S. Soukup and Peter T. Masiakos

The evaluation and treatment of traumatic injuries of infants and children requires specific knowledge of pediatric physiology and the physiological response to injury. Generally, the trauma resuscitation of children follows similar rules that have been described for adults by Advanced Trauma Life Support (ATLS) standards. However, there are several special considerations in the initial assessment and subsequent care for children and specific paradigms regarding ancillary studies that are different from those in adults. These special considerations will be discussed here.

9.1 Epidemiology

Pediatric Trauma significantly impacts the lives of children and families in the United States. In any given year, there are over 1.5 million injuries and close to 500,000 hospitalizations as a result of pediatric trauma [1]. Injury, both intentional and unintentional, accounts for over 50% of deaths in children younger than 18 years. Although there is a rise in the incidence of penetrating trauma, which now accounts for up to 10–20% of trauma activations, the vast majority of pediatric injuries result from blunt trauma with associated closed head injuries that require nonoperative management.

E.S. Soukup (✉) • P.T. Masiakos
Pediatric Surgical Services, Massachusetts General Hospital, 55 Fruit Street, Warren 11, Boston, MA 02114, USA
e-mail: esailhamer@partners.org; pmasiakos@partners.org

9.2 History

Blunt trauma is the most common mechanism after which children present for evaluation. However, the energy that is transmitted via blunt trauma through a thin and relatively amuscular abdominal wall may result in both solid organ injury and visceral perforation, often with only minimal signs of external injury. Therefore, a thorough history, mechanism of injury, and focused examination of the entire child are mandated so that signs of forceful impact can be elucidated. For example, a history of significant hemorrhage at the scene may instigate a more thorough investigation of the vessels in the proximity of injury in an otherwise hemodynamically stable patient who has no hard signs of vascular injury.

9.3 Initial Assessment, Resuscitation, and Stabilization

9.3.1 Primary Survey (A,B,C's)

As in adults, the primary survey should focus on the identification of acute life-threatening injuries. Attention to the airway, breathing, and circulation (A,B,C's) supersedes all other interventions in the initial resuscitation phase. All centers that care for children should have sequestered equipment designed for children, i.e., endotracheal tubes, laryngoscopes, catheters, and passive warming lamps. Room temperature should be kept warm to limit insensible heat losses in small children. The Broselow Pediatric Emergency Tape aides in estimating the weight of the child by measuring his/her length. A color-coded bar on the tape measures the

G.C. Velmahos et al. (eds.), *Penetrating Trauma*,
DOI 10.1007/978-3-642-20453-1_9,

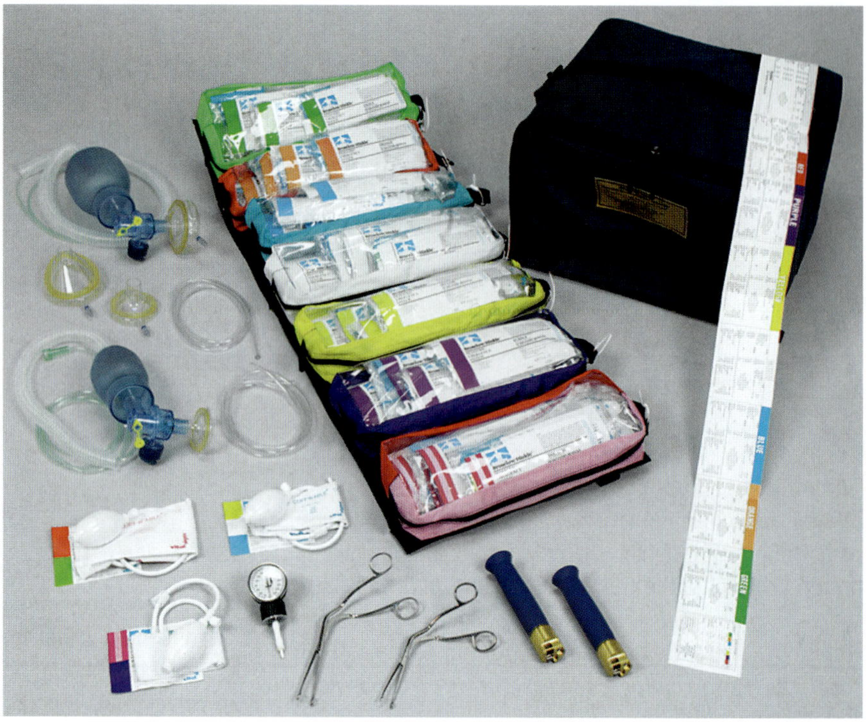

Fig. 9.1 Broselow Pediatric Emergency Resuscitation Tape

length of the child and indicates the appropriate equipment sizes and medication doses to perform emergency resuscitation on the child. Designated resuscitation equipment is contained in corresponding, color-coded equipment pouches or drawers (Fig. 9.1).

9.3.2 Normal Pediatric Vital Signs

Pediatric vital signs vary by age (Table 9.1). Children are able to maintain normal blood pressures until late hemorrhagic shock (>30% blood loss), and therefore subtle changes in heart rate and respiratory rate must be noted. As a general rule, the lower limit of acceptable systolic blood pressure (SBP) = (Age × 2) + 70 mmHg. For newborns, acceptable SBP is 60 mmHg or greater (Table 9.1).

9.3.3 A = Airway (C-Spine Immobilization)

Cardiac arrest in a child is most often of respiratory etiology. An injured child who is obtunded, unresponsive, or combative may need to be intubated. An uncooperative child who needs radiologic imaging may also need to be intubated. Intubation must be performed with the jaw thrust technique to maintain in-line cervical stabilization. Keep in mind these key anatomic differences for intubation in children: larger tongue, more anterior/superior glottis, shorter trachea. You may find that a straight Miller blade is easier than the curved because the epiglottis is floppy (less cartilaginous). The appropriate size of endotracheal tube (ETT) can be estimated by the size of pinkie finger (or the formula = [age + 16]/4). The Broselow Pediatric Emergency Resuscitation Tape is also a useful tool to estimate ETT (and other device) size and medication doses, given a child's height. Use an uncuffed ETT in a young child (<8 years old or approximately 60 lb), because the subglottic trachea is narrowed and provides a sufficient seal. However, cuffed ETT may be used (except in newborns), if appropriate cuff pressure are used. Rapid sequence intubation (RSI) is similar to adults, including preoxygenation with 100% FiO_2, medication administration (Table 9.2), cricoid pressure, cervical spine stabilization, laryngoscopy, and advancement of tube to 3 cm beyond the cords. Confirm exhaled CO_2 and secure the tube. In the rare event of acute airway obstruction, needle cricothyroidotomy with a 14 g catheter is preferential over open cricothyroidotomy because of the increased incidence of subglottic stenosis.

Table 9.1 Pediatric vital signs

	Pulse (beats/min)	Systolic blood pressure (mmHg)	Respiration (breaths/min)
Newborn (<1 month)	95–145	60–90	30–60
Infant (1 month–1 year)	125–170	75–100	30–60
Toddler (1–2 year)	100–160	80–110	24–40
Preschool (3–4 year)	70–110	80–110	22–34
School age (4–12 year)	70–110	85–120	18–30
Adolescent (>12 year)	55–100	95–120	12–16

Table 9.2 Common emergency medication doses in children

Medication	Dose
Adenosine	0.1 mg/kg IV first dose (max 6 mg) rapid push
	0.2 mg/kg IV second dose (max 12 mg)
Amiodarone (VF/VT arrest)	5 mg/kg IV (max 15 mg/kg/day)
Atropine sulfate	0.02 mg/kg IV (min 0.1 mg, max 0.5 mg)
	0.04 mg/kg IV for second dose
Calcium chloride (10%)	10–20 mg/kg IV
Calcium gluconate (10%)	15–60 mg/kg IV
Diazepam	0.5–1.0 mg/kg IV
Dobutamine	2–20 mcg/kg/min IV
Dopamine	2–5 mcg/kg/min IV (>15 mcg/kg/min for alpha effect)
Epinephrine (Asystole/PEA arrest)	0.01 mg/kg IV first dose (repeat Q3-5 min during CPR)
Epinephrine infusion	0.1 mcg/kg/min IV, then titrate (range: 0.1–1 mcg/kg/min)
Lidocaine	1 mg/kg IV push
	20–50 mcg/kg/min IV
Magnesium sulfate	25–50 mcg/kg IV over 10–20 min (max 2 g)
Morphine sulfate	0.1 mg/kg IV
Midazolam	0.1 mg/kg IV (max 5 mg)
Naloxone	0.1 mg/kg IV (if less than 5 year old or 20 kg)
	2 mg IV (if greater than 5 years or 20 kg)
Pancuronium	0.1–0.2 mg/kg IV
Sodium bicarbonate	1–4 mEq/kg IV
Succinylcholine	2.0 mg/kg (if < 10 kg)
	1.0–1.5 mg/kg (if > 10 kg)
Thiopental	4–6 mg/kg IV
Vecuronium	0.2 mg/kg IV

9.3.4 B = Breathing

Assess for potential life-threatening thoracic injuries: pneumothorax (open chest wound or tension pneumothorax), hemothorax, flail chest/pulmonary contusions, rib fractures with splinted breathing. The mediastinum of a child is very compliant and can lead to rapid decline from a tension pneumothorax Children are diaphragmatic breathers, and therefore, gastric distension can be an unrecognized contributor to respiratory distress, especially in the young child who is distended from swallowing air while crying. A nasogastric tube should be placed to decompress the stomach. (Use an orogastric tube in very young children who are obligate nose-breathers.)

9.3.5 C = Circulation (Hemorrhage Control)

Hemorrhage is the most common etiology of shock in trauma, but do not overlook obstructive etiologies (cardiac tamponade and tension pneumothorax), and distributive etiologies (neurogenic shock).

Assessment of volume status and shock is difficult in the child. Children have impressive physiologic reserve and can maintain SBP until late-stage hypovolemic shock (>30% blood loss). Tachycardia, tachypnea, altered level of consciousness, and poor peripheral perfusion (mottled cool extremities, weak thready pulses, narrowed pulse pressure, delayed capillary refill) are early but subtle signs of blood loss.

Establishing vascular access in an injured child is a priority and can be challenging. Peripheral IVs are ideal, but when they cannot be obtained, intraosseous

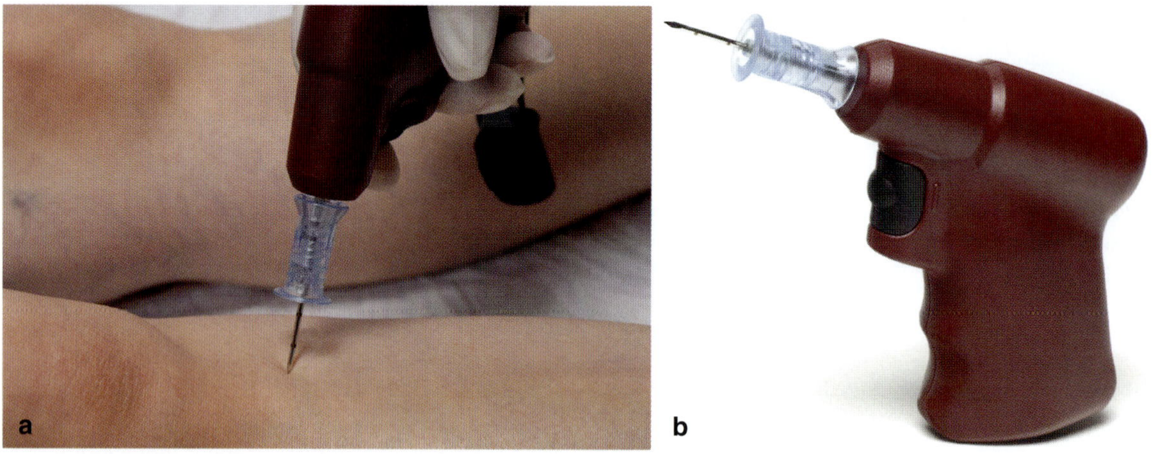

Fig. 9.2 (**a**) Intraosseus line placement. (**b**) EZ-IO drive

Table 9.3 Fluid management in children

Resuscitation fluids (NS or LR)	
If hypotension or signs of shock:	Bolus 20 mL/kg. Repeat if transient or no response, and then switch to blood transfusions (10 mL/kg).
Daily maintenance fluid requirements (D5 1/2NS or D10 1/2NS)	
Weight < 10 kg	100 mL/kg/day
Weight 11–20 kg	1,000 mL + 50 mL/kg/day (for every kg over 10)
Weight > 20 kg	1,500 mL + 20 mL/kg/day (for every kg over 20)

(IO) lines are quick, reliable, and allow high volume infusion of any fluid (crystalloid, blood products, and even medications, including pressors). An IO line is placed in the anteromedial tibia, 2–3 cm distal to the tibial tuberosity after a quick skin prep for sterility (Fig. 9.2). Avoid wounds, fractures, or infected areas. They should ideally be placed with a single attempt because multiple holes can lead to leakage of infusion fluids and resultant compartment syndrome. If contraindicated, definitive IV access can be obtained with a central line in the femoral vein, or a peripheral vein cutdown (i.e., saphenous vein).

Initial fluid resuscitation is indicated when there are signs of hypovolemic shock. Initial bolus consists of 20 mL/kg of warmed normal saline or lactated Ringer's solution. This may be repeated if there is no response or only a transient response. All subsequent volume resuscitation should be performed with blood products (10 mL/kg = "1 unit"). If there is no time for cross-matched, type-specific blood, "O-negative" blood is indicated. Once resuscitated, maintenance fluid requirements (Table 9.3) can be estimated using the "4-2-1" rule, and should be administered as D5 1/2NS (or D10 1/2NS for neonates). The "4-2-1" rule estimates hourly fluid requirements, and is calculated = 4 mL/kg/h (for the 1st 10 kg) + 2 mL/kg/h (2nd 10 kg) + 1 mL/kg/h (all subsequent kg).

As in adults, ongoing hemodynamic instability from blood loss in a child must be controlled expeditiously. Sources of bleeding include the chest, peritoneal cavity, retroperitoneum/pelvis, femur fracture/thigh compartment, and external injury (especially the scalp). In an infant, prior to suture closure of the skull, intracranial hemorrhage may produce hemodynamic instability.

9.3.6 D = Disability (Neurologic Assessment)

Head injury accounts for the highest degree of morbidity and mortality in children and is the principle determinant of outcome after trauma. However, children have the potential for more frequent and fuller recovery from even serious head injury, when compared to similar injuries in

Table 9.4 Modified Glasgow coma scale in children

	Infant	Child
Eye opening		
4	Spontaneous	Spontaneous
3	To verbal stimuli	To verbal stimuli
2	To pain only	To pain only
1	None	None
Verbal response		
5	Coos and babbles	Oriented, appropriate
4	Irritable cries	Confused
3	Cries to pain	Inappropriate words
2	Moans to pain	Incomprehensible sounds
1	None	None
Motor response[a]		
6	Moves spontaneously and purposefully	Obeys commands
5	Withdraws to touch	Localizes painful stimuli
4	Withdraws in response to pain	Withdraws in response to pain
3	Abnormal flexion posture to pain	Flexion in response to pain
2	Abnormal extension posture to pain	Extension in response the pain
1	None	None

[a]If patient is intubated, unconscious, or preverbal, the most important part of this scale is motor response and should be closely evaluated

adults [2]. Therefore, careful attention to preventing secondary injury and maximizing tissue perfusion to the brain can greatly improve outcome. The Glasgow coma scale is modified in young children who are preverbal to measure neurologic function and prognosis. The motor response scale tends to provide the most reliable assessment of function in a preverbal or intubated child (Table 9.4).

9.3.7 E = Exposure for Secondary Survey

In preparation for the secondary survey, the child must be exposed completely for a complete head-to-toe physical examination. Keep in mind they also have a larger body surface area ratio and therefore lose heat and water quickly and can become hypothermic. Use warm fluids, bare huggers, warming lights, and warm ambient room temperature to prevent heat loss in a child.

9.4 Secondary Survey

Children are more prone to multisystem trauma due to their small body size and more compliant body (less protective bones, muscle, and fat of the torso). They can sustain internal injuries without significant external signs of trauma. Careful attention to a bruise on the abdominal wall resulting from a bicycle handlebar should lead to a more thorough investigation of the abdomen. A lap belt mark across the abdomen may raise concerns of lumbar spine fracture (Chance fracture), with an associated risk of small bowel injury.

9.5 Diagnostic Modalities

Physical examination in a child can be technically challenging, and adjunct diagnostic modalities and imaging may be used to provide additional information in the evaluation of a pediatric trauma patient. Although diagnostic peritoneal aspiration (DPA) has been traditionally used to evaluate intra-abdominal injuries in the unstable patient, it has no role in the pediatric population where solid organ injuries are unlikely to require surgery. Focused assessment with sonography in trauma (FAST) exam has significant advantages over more invasive diagnostic maneuvers: The FAST examination can be performed quickly and exposes the patient to no potential harm from delay or ionizing radiation. However, children with intra-abdominal injuries are more frequently managed nonoperatively and, thus, the need for rapid decision-making regarding operative management is less common. Children also have a relatively higher incidence of solid organ injury without free fluid, and consequently a negative FAST exam may not obviate the need for an abdominal CT scan when there is a clinical suspicion of significant injury. Sensitivity of FAST is reported as 40–90% and specificity of 79–100% [3], and should not be relied on as a stand-alone screening tool in the pediatric population. Findings from CXR, AP Pelvis X-ray, and the FAST exam, along with the primary and secondary surveys, guide decisions regarding further radiographic examination, including CT scans or plain films.

9.6 Child Abuse (Non-accidental Trauma)

Non-accidental trauma is the leading cause of trauma in children and often goes unrecognized [2]. Suspect non-accidental trauma in certain specialized circumstances: Discrepancy between the reported history and physical exam findings; injuries are not consistent with an infant's developmental capability; injuries of different chronologic age (bruises or fractures at different stages of healing); delay in seeking medical care; sharply demarcated burns (scald); injuries related to bite marks, cigarette burns, rope marks, or involving perineal/genital region; multiple subdural, subarachnoid, or retinal hemorrhages without external signs of trauma (shaken baby syndrome); or multiple rib fractures (especially of different stages of healing).

Important Points

- ATLS is similar in adults and children, but there are some key physiologic and anatomic differences in children that are important to remember.
- Blunt trauma (i.e., handlebar) can produce injuries that resemble penetrating injuries (i.e., bowel perforation) in children with compliant abdominal walls.
- Broselow Pediatric Resuscitation Tape helps estimate a child's weight to determine device size and medication doses.
- Cardiac arrest is often of respiratory etiology in a child. Use a miller blade for intubation and an ETT the size of the child's pinky finger.
- Gastric distension can cause respiratory distress in children who swallow air while crying, because they are diaphragmatic breathers. Place nasogastric tube (orogastric in infants who are obligate nose-breathers) to decompress.
- Children have impressive physiologic reserve and maintain BP until severe blood loss (>30%). Lowest acceptable SBP = (Age × 2) + 70 mmHg.
- Intraosseous line may be placed for emergency vascular access if peripheral IVs are not possible.
- Crystalloid bolus = 20 mL/kg. Blood transfusion "unit" = 10 mL/kg.
- FAST exam has limited value in a pediatric trauma patient.
- Many solid organ injuries in children can safely be managed nonoperatively.
- Suspect non-accidental trauma when the story does not add up.

References

1. Tepas JJ III, Schinco MA (2004) Pediatric Trauma. In: Moore EE, Feliciano DV, Mattox KL (eds) Trauma, 5th edn. McGraw-Hill Companies, Inc, New York, pp 1021–1039, Chapter 45
2. Alterman DM, Daley BJ, Kennedy AP, Raju R, Lee S. Emedicine. Considerations in pediatric trauma. 8/18/08. URL: http://emedicine.medscape.com/article/435031-overview. Accessed 16 Dec 2009
3. Murphy R, Ghosh A (2001) Towards evidence based emergency medicine: best BETs from the Manchester Royal Infirmary. The accuracy of abdominal ultrasound in paediatric trauma. Emerg Med J 18(3):208–209

Fluids, Blood Substitutes, and New Tools

10

David C. Griffin and Raminder Nirula

Hemorrhage following trauma is one of the most common causes of trauma-related death, second only to head injury, making its management critical to patient survival. Control of hemorrhage is mandatory while resuscitation takes place. Appropriate fluid replacement in the penetrating trauma victim requires an understanding of the body's response to volume depletion as it relates to the depth of hemorrhagic shock and the body's capacity to shift fluid from different compartments.

10.1 Physiology

10.1.1 Fluid Compartments

The amount of total body water differs with age and gender. The "average" 70-kg male is approximately 60% or 42 L (since 1 kg = 1 L of water) of water. Two thirds of that water is intracellular and one third is extracellular. Of the 14 L of extracellular fluid, about one third of this volume, or 4.67 L, is intravascular volume [1].

It is this fluid that is referred to as the circulating blood volume. Most of the oxygen-carrying capacity is within erythrocytes rather than in the fluid itself, but without sufficient volume to distribute this red cell mass, effective delivery of oxygen ceases. As a result, adequate fluid resuscitation after hemorrhage is necessary to ensure adequate oxygen delivery (Fig. 10.1).

10.1.2 Response to Acute Hemorrhage

Each of these fluid volumes, the plasma, the interstitial and the intracellular, are in equilibrium; however, disturbances such as acute blood loss result in fluid shifts to maintain effective circulating volume [1]. Additionally, a complex neurohumoral response is generated to assist in the restoration of effective circulating volume [1]. Catecholamine release immediately stimulates increases in the peripheral vascular resistance and increases heart rate, thereby increasing blood pressure to the core circulation. Immediately, vasoconstriction of afferent arterioles results in decreased capillary hydrostatic forces driving less fluid from the intravascular space into the interstitium. Increases in plasma oncotic pressure secondary to reduced renal filtration increase the amount of water that diffuses from the interstitium into the intravascular space as well. Activation of the renin-angiotensin-aldosterone axis increases sodium retention which facilitates renal fluid retention. Angiotensin also increases systemic vascular tone which contributes to the reduced capillary hydrostatic forces. Decreased pressure in the atria and increased plasma oncotic pressure stimulate the release of antidiuretic hormone (ADH) from the posterior pituitary. ADH acts to increase renal distal tubule permeability to water through the production and placement of aquaporins in the luminal membrane and, as such, provides a delayed response to volume loss.

D.C. Griffin (✉)
Department of Surgery, University of Utah,
30 North 1900 East, Salt Lake City, UT 84132, USA
e-mail: david.c.griffin@hsc.utah.edu

R. Nirula
Section of Burns/Trauma/Critical Care, University of Utah,
50 North 1900 East, Salt Lake City, UT 84132, USA
e-mail: r.nirula@hsc.utah.edu

G.C. Velmahos et al. (eds.), *Penetrating Trauma*,
DOI 10.1007/978-3-642-20453-1_10, © Springer-Verlag Berlin Heidelberg 2012

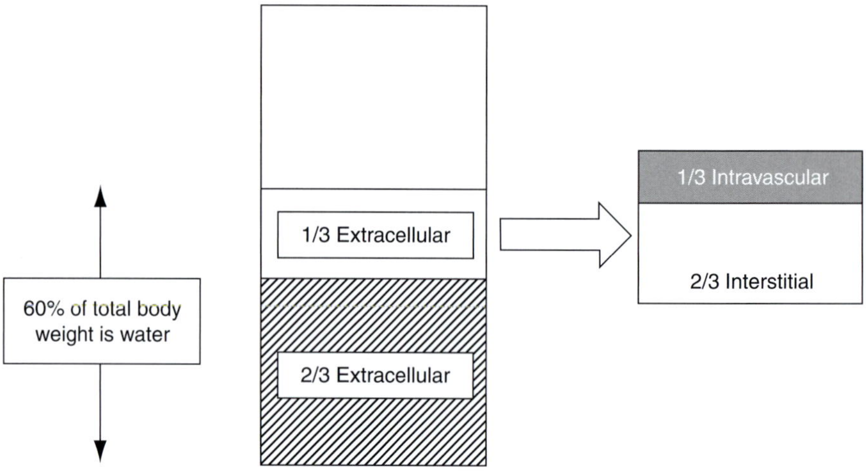

Fig. 10.1 Body fluid compartments. Distribution of total body water

Table 10.1 ATLS classification of hemorrhagic shock [2]

Parameter	Class I	Class II	Class III	Class IV
Volume of blood loss	≤750 mL	750–1,500 mL	1,500–2,000 mL	≥2,000 mL
% of total blood volume	≤15%	15–30%	30–40%	≥40%
Heart rate	>100	>100	>120	≥140
Systolic blood pressure	Normal	Normal	Decreased	Decreased
Pulse pressure	Normal or increased	Decreased	Decreased	Decreased
Capillary refill	Normal	Sluggish	Delayed	Delayed
Respirations per minute	14–20	20–30	30–40	>35
Urine output	≥30 mL/h	20– 0 mL/h	5–10 mL/h	Minimal
Mental status	Normal to slightly anxious	Mildly anxious	Anxious and confused	Confused and lethargic

10.2 Hemorrhagic Shock

Hemorrhagic shock is classified based on the volume of blood lost from the circulation and the resulting disturbances in hemodynamics observed [2]. It is important to remember that hemorrhage may be more than what is easily appreciated as blood lost into the environment. Blood loss into potential spaces such as the hemithorax, abdomen, and retroperitoneum can approach life-threatening levels without appreciable external loss (Table 10.1) [2].

10.3 Fluids

10.3.1 Crystalloids

Initial volume expansion with balanced electrolyte solutions such as normal saline or lactated ringers is the preferred therapy [2, 3]. Rapid infusion, either mechanically with a rapid infuser or through the use of a pressure bag, can quickly increase effective circulating volume. Fluids should be warmed to 39°C prior to infusion to reduce hypothermia and its effects [2]. Even isotonic crystalloid solutions rapidly leak out into the interstitium making their effect on circulating volume transient. Only about a quarter to one third of the volume will remain in the intravascular space, hence the 3:1 rule of crystalloids to volume of blood lost that is espoused in ATLS. Hyperchloremia is frequently observed with normal saline resuscitation and can lead to a hyperchloremic metabolic acidosis, which should not be mistaken for an acidosis secondary to decreased tissue perfusion [4].

Controversy exists regarding which fluid, lactated ringers versus normal saline, is the most effective for resuscitation. Animal models suggest that the same degree of resuscitation with normal saline will require more volume, cause more disturbances in coagulation and greater pulmonary edema than lactated ringers [5].

Lactated ringers can cause an insignificant increase in the lactate level.

Hypertonic saline has also been studied as a resuscitation fluid to restore effective circulating volume. Hypertonic saline, usually in small volumes, is often combined with a colloid product such as dextran to expand the intravascular volume. These hypertonic solutions required smaller volumes to expand the circulating volume as they draw interstitial and intracellular fluid into vascular space. Other effects of hypertonic solutions include small vessel vasodilation which can decrease afterload and increase preload resulting in improvements in cardiac output and tissue oxygenation.

Wade et al., examined hypertonic saline and dextran-based resuscitation in a prospective randomized sample of 230 victims of penetrating torso trauma. While no significant mortality difference was found in the overall sample, in the cohort that required surgical intervention for control of hemorrhage (about 2/3), they found a significant survival difference (84.5% compared with 67.1% in the control group ($p=0.01$)) There were no significant differences in coagulation or volume of resuscitation required between groups [6].

A recent multicenter randomized trial in the USA on "hypertonic saline versus isotonic solution use in traumatic shock" was stopped at a preplanned interim analysis for lack of overall survival benefit when compared to normal saline. They noted that more patients receiving hypertonic saline–based resuscitation died before or in the trauma bay than the saline patients, but overall mortality was the same at 28 days [7]. Therefore, at the present time, hypertonic saline cannot be advocated for initial resuscitation of uncontrolled hemorrhagic shock.

10.3.2 Colloids

Two large reviews of the use of colloids in hemorrhagic shock found the relative risk of mortality to be increased at least 30% compared to crystalloid infusion; however, these reviews were not limited exclusively to trauma patients [8]. There has been renewed interest in initial resuscitation of penetrating trauma victims with colloidal solutions following the war in Iraq. Difficulties related to the transport of large volumes of isotonic crystalloid solution into austere combat environments make small resuscitation with colloid solutions more attractive. Combat medics are now using colloids such as HEXTEND™ (6% Hetastarch solution) as first-line therapy for soldiers and other victims in shock with the rationale that it remains in the intravascular space longer, thus requiring less fluid use, particularly when long prehospital transport times are required. However, research into the use of colloidal solutions versus crystalloid solutions in civilian penetrating trauma is more controversial. A meta-analysis of colloid- versus crystalloid-based resuscitation trials in trauma patients demonstrated a trend toward improved survival in the patients receiving crystalloids [9].

10.3.2.1 Blood

Traditionally, blood products are added to the resuscitation after rapid expansion with crystalloids has been attempted. Ideally, like would be replaced with like, however, resuscitation with whole blood presents several challenges. Chiefly, whole blood does not preserve well. Separation into components improves the ability of blood banks to preserve and distribute this precious commodity. Current ATLS guidelines suggest replacement of lost blood volume in a 1:1:1 ratio of packed red cells to fresh frozen plasma (FFP) to crystalloid. This approximates the loss of whole blood in a wound (ASCOT 2004). FFP is often transfused both for volume expansion as well as for the clotting factors that have been consumed. There is some evidence that transfusion of FFP will improve coagulopathy but may not impact overall mortality [10]. Further study is warranted.

"Typed" or patient-matched blood products are available rapidly in most trauma centers but physicians are often faced with a symptomatic patient while the crossmatch is taking place. O negative "trauma" blood is usually available for immediate release and used in symptomatic patients with massive blood loss at the discretion of the physician.

Adverse events associated with any transfusion of blood products include transfusion reaction, transfusion-related acute lung acute injury, and immunosuppression that can contribute to multiple organ failure and infectious risks. While screening can reduce some of these risks, the risk is not zero. The most common infectious risks are with bacterial contamination of platelets, about 1 in 3,000. The risks of hepatitis C and HIV are approximately 1 in 2 million per unit transfused.

10.3.3 Massive Transfusion

Patients requiring massive transfusion are uncommon in civilian trauma centers, occurring in approximately 1–3% of admissions but are associated with significant morbidity and mortality.

The most feared complication of massive blood loss is the terrible triad of hypothermia, acidosis, and coagulopathy. Massive transfusion of component therapy can exacerbate this as stored products are refrigerated (except for platelets). In addition to the risk associated with blood therapy, massive transfusion requirements add the risk of hyperkalemia, hypocalcemia, and decreased effectiveness of oxygen delivery in tissues. Reduced effectiveness in the target tissues is related to depletion of 2,3-diphosphoglycerate in cells that reduces oxygen offloading and membrane defects that reduce the ability of the red cell to traverse smaller capillaries [11].

10.3.4 Iraq and Afghanistan Experience

Recently, military trauma surgeons have been renewing interest in transfusions of fresh whole blood for victims of trauma. Spinella found increased 48 h and 72 h survival in patients requiring massive transfusion treated with warm whole blood in comparison to those treated with component therapy. Others found that warm whole blood was a useful adjunct to component therapy in the most severely injured patients who were cold, acidotic, and coagulopathic [12]. These beneficial effects are likely related to the differences between stored blood and fresh whole blood. Retrospective research at a combat support hospital found minimal infectious risks, primarily Hepatitis C, with the use of fresh whole blood in combat casualties and postulated that these could be further reduced with the use of rapid screening modalities.

Others have found more liberal use of component therapy with a 1:1 ratio of packed RBC's to FFP and more liberal of platelets and cryoprecipitate before somewhat arbitrary thresholds have been reached to be associated with improved mortality.

10.3.5 Autotransfusion

Another potential source of blood products, usually packed red cells, is from the patient. Recovery of autologous blood lost either intraoperatively or through chest tubes can be processed and reinfused back to the patient without the use of donor blood. Several commercial devices are available and have been widely used in a variety of surgical procedures, including operative trauma for years. These devices process lost blood, remove excess cations, lipids, debris and other supernatant leaving washed autologous packed cells in a weak anticoagulant buffer solution. This is then transfused back to the patient as normally done. Generally, most physicians believe that the blood lost must be sterile, either in the operative field or within a closed system such as a chest tube; however, that is controversial. Hollow viscus injury has been listed as a potential contraindication to the use of red cell salvage methods; however, two small studies concluded that autotransfusion of contaminated blood in trauma did not result in significant change in the rate of infectious complications or death [13].

10.3.6 Effects on Coagulation

Too much crystalloid infusion, particularly saline, can exacerbate coagulation defects through hemodilution of coagulation factors and platelets [14]. It appears that hypertonic saline infusion may have even worse effects on coagulation when compared to isotonic fluids [14]. Furthermore, sodium citrate, one of the preservatives used in blood products, will bind calcium in circulation and lower levels of this cofactor for hemostasis. Colloids such as dextran and hydroxyethyl starch also impair normal coagulation, with hydroxyethyl starch impairing fibrin polymerization and dextran inhibiting platelet function [15].

10.4 Blood Substitutes

Given the problems associated with the use of allogeneic blood products, there has been extensive research into other methods of oxygen delivery. Most of the research has been focused on solubilized free hemoglobin or hemoglobin-based oxygen carriers (HBOC). In the United States, these products are only available on research protocols; however, Hemopure™ is available for use in South Africa. Recently, a meta-analysis of the available English language literature covering 16 separate trials, five different products, and a total population of approximately 3700 patients was published. Their analysis found an increased rate of adverse events, particularly acute myocardial infarctions with an increased odds ratio of 1.30 for mortality in patients treated with blood substitutes [16]. One of the main criticisms of this meta-analysis is that it considered several different types of HBOCs rather than each type as a separate entity. A recent US multicenter trial of Polyheme™ (Northfield Laboratories) of 714 mostly young males whose mechanism was approximately 52% penetrating found no statistically significant differences in 30-day mortality when compared to control groups but a slight increase in complications (93% versus 88% $p = 0.04$) including myocardial infarctions (3% versus 1%) [17]. The authors had an independent review of the patients with myocardial infarctions that did not find any appreciable difference between the groups. This study indicates that Polyheme™ was equally efficacious to the standard of care utilizing blood and that it had a reasonable safety profile. Therefore, in the absence of blood or during blood shortages, Polyheme™ may be a reasonable alternative for patients with an acute traumatic anemia.

10.5 Current ATLS Guidelines

10.5.1 Prehospital

Currently, emphasis is placed on early control of external hemorrhage and early transport to a trauma center (ASCOT 2004). Two attempts at IV cannulation can be made but should not slow down transport as mortality is increased when delay to definitive care occurs.

10.5.2 Trauma Bay

The ATLS algorithm mandates the ABCDE's of trauma evaluation. As part of Circulation, large bore intravenous (IV) access should be obtained immediately, if not accomplished in the field. Ideally, two peripheral IVs will be placed in either antecubital vein. Poisseuille's law regarding laminar flow shows that flow is inversely related to the length and the fourth power of the radius [1]. Thus, a large bore (18 gauge or larger), short IV catheter allows the rapid delivery of fluids and blood products if needed. If injuries or anatomy preclude IV placement, consider insertion of an interosseous (IO) line. IO catheters can be rapidly placed in one of several places with one of several commercially available devices and require minimal training and knowledge of anatomy. Any one of several commercially available products can be placed on the anterior surface of the tibia, the humeral head, and even the sternum with relative ease and minimal operator experience. Device studies have demonstrated rapid delivery of fluids to the central circulation. Should peripheral access be unable to be obtained or should the need for central access arise, a central venous line can be placed quickly with a low complication rate by experienced operators. We prefer placement of a percutaneous subclavian using Seldinger technique when we need central access as cervical collars are often present and blocking rapid access to the jugular veins. Preference should be given to the side where a chest tube is already present, if one is present. Femoral lines can also be placed as a third option, particularly when chest compressions are being performed, but we generally avoid placement in this area whenever possible to reduce the risk of infection and venous thrombosis.

Once access is obtained, infusion of 2 L of isotonic crystalloid is the usual starting point for a hypotensive patient. Determination of the severity of the blood loss, the ability of the individual patient to tolerate this insult, and the strategy for controlling ongoing hemorrhage guide further resuscitation and attempts to restore normal hemodynamic parameters as soon as possible. Control of the hemorrhage is the most important step as massive volume replacement is "not a substitute for manual or operative control of hemorrhage."(ASCOT 2004).

10.6 Permissive Hypotension

Some favor a more restrictive use of fluids for victims of penetrating trauma. This strategy is nothing new, it was espoused by surgeons treating soldiers wounded in World War One. The goal of this strategy is to maintain victims in a state of relative hypotension and minimally acceptable degrees of perfusion until definitive control of the site or sites of hemorrhage is obtained. Rationale for this strategy is rooted in the ATLS guidelines that hemorrhage control is the most important management strategy.

The concept of permissive hypotension is applied more extensively to trauma victims of all types in Europe but less so in the United States. Furthermore, there is a body of literature to support delaying definitive resuscitation until after source control of hemorrhage is obtained although most of it is animal models [18]. The best human studies concerning permissive hypotension are those involving permissive hypotension for patients with ruptured abdominal aortic aneurysms. Bicknell in 1994 prospectively examined almost 600 patients with penetrating torso trauma and found that patients who did not receive intravenous resuscitation until operative intervention had a statistically significant increase in survival and decrease in complication rates when compared to those that underwent standard resuscitation protocols [14]. This study has been criticized regarding selection bias as its randomization method of alternate days is suited to the difficult prehospital environment but is not really random. Several later studies have found no difference in mortality based on volume of prehospital resuscitation. A retrospective analysis from USC/LA County reexamined the question and found no difference in mortality based on volume of prehospital fluids administered [19]. Another series of mixed mechanism patients from Maryland Shock Trauma failed to find any difference in mortality between conventional resuscitation and a permissive hypotension group [20]. A cost-effectiveness meta-analysis from Britain found no benefit or savings to the use of prehospital fluids but only examined four clinical trials and found methodological flaws in most of them.

10.7 Conclusion

Fluid management in victims of penetrating trauma is one the most important and not surprisingly controversial topics in the field of traumatology. Mainstream guidelines favor stopping the hemorrhage as early as possible combined with early restoration of intravascular volume and the other fluid compartments as well as hemodynamics through the use of isotonic crystalloids initially and then colloid and blood products as necessary. Alternative resuscitation strategies exist and are currently being examined throughout the world. As with most things in medicine, individualization of treatment algorithms to particular situations such as long transport, and massive transfusion requirements will be needed. The use of blood substitutes may be warranted in austere environments and during blood shortages. Whole blood may return as a resuscitation strategy instead of component therapy for massive transfusion.

Important Points

- Initial resuscitation with isotonic crystalloids remains the cornerstone of fluid therapy.
- After 2 L of crystalloid infusion, hypotension should be treated with uncrossmatched blood if ongoing hemorrhage is suspected.
- Hypertonic solutions do not appear to be superior to isotonic solutions in terms of overall mortality.
- Blood substitutes provide similar outcomes to the current standard of care.
- Increasing the pRBC:FFP ratio to 1:1 may be associated with improved mortality.
- Whole blood may yield improved early survival in massive transfusion compared to component therapy.
- Autotransfusion devices are an important adjunct to massive transfusion to provide rapid restoration of red cell mass when blood supplies become exhausted.

References

1. Guyton AC, Hall JE (eds) (2000) Textbook of medical physiology, 10th edn. WB Saunders Co., Philadelphia
2. ATLS (2004) Advanced trauma life support for doctors, 7th edn. American College of Surgeons Committee on Trauma, Chicago
3. Carrico CJ, Canizaro PC, Shires GT (1976) Fluid resuscitation following injury: rationale for the use of balanced salt solutions. Crit Care Med 4(2):46–54
4. Scheingraber S et al (1999) Rapid saline infusion produces hyperchloremic acidosis in patients undergoing gynecologic surgery. Anesthesiology 90(5):1265–1270
5. Kiraly LN et al (2006) Resuscitation with normal saline (NS) vs. lactated ringers (LR) modulates hypercoagulability and leads to increased blood loss in an uncontrolled hemorrhagic shock swine model. J Trauma 61(1):57–64; discussion 64–65
6. Wade CE, Grady JJ, Kramer GC (2003) Efficacy of hypertonic saline dextran fluid resuscitation for patients with hypotension from penetrating trauma. J Trauma 54(5 Suppl): S144–S148
7. Communication (2009) NHLBI stops enrollment in study of concentrated saline for patients with shock for lack of survival benefit. NIH. http://public.nhlbi.nih.gov/newsroom/home/GetPressRelease.aspx?id=2632. Accessed on 7/11/2011
8. Alderson P et al (200) Colloids versus crystalloids for fluid resuscitation in critically ill patients. Cochrane Database Syst Rev (2):CD000567

9. Velanovich V (1989) Crystalloid versus colloid fluid resuscitation: a meta-analysis of mortality. Surgery 105(1):65–71
10. Kashuk JL et al (2008) Postinjury life threatening coagulopathy: is 1:1 fresh frozen plasma:packed red blood cells the answer? J Trauma 65(2):261–270; discussion 270–271
11. Perkins JG et al (2008) Massive transfusion and nonsurgical hemostatic agents. Crit Care Med 36(7 Suppl):S325–S339
12. Spinella PC (2008) Warm fresh whole blood transfusion for severe hemorrhage: U.S. military and potential civilian applications. Crit Care Med 36(7 Suppl):S340–S345
13. Ozmen V et al (1992) Autotransfusion of potentially culture-positive blood (CPB) in abdominal trauma: preliminary data from a prospective study. J Trauma 32(1):36–39
14. Bickell WH et al (1994) Immediate versus delayed fluid resuscitation for hypotensive patients with penetrating torso injuries. N Engl J Med 331(17):1105–1109
15. Innerhofer P et al (2002) The effects of perioperatively administered colloids and crystalloids on primary platelet-mediated hemostasis and clot formation. Anesth Analg 95(4):858–865; table of contents
16. Natanson C et al (2008) Cell-free hemoglobin-based blood substitutes and risk of myocardial infarction and death: a meta-analysis. JAMA 299(19):2304–2312
17. Moore EE et al (2009) Human polymerized hemoglobin for the treatment of hemorrhagic shock when blood is unavailable: the USA multicenter trial. J Am Coll Surg 208(1): 1–13
18. Holmes JF et al (2002) Effects of delaying fluid resuscitation on an injury to the systemic arterial vasculature. Acad Emerg Med 9(4):267–274
19. Yaghoubian A et al (2007) Reanalysis of prehospital intravenous fluid administration in patients with penetrating truncal injury and field hypotension. Am Surg 73(10):1027–1030
20. Dutton RP, Mackenzie CF, Scalea TM (2002) Hypotensive resuscitation during active hemorrhage: impact on in-hospital mortality. J Trauma 52(6):1141–1146

Emergency Department Thoracotomy

11

Carlos V.R. Brown and D.J. Green

Emergency Department Thoracotomy (EDT), also known a resuscitative thoracotomy, can be used as an adjunct during the resuscitation of penetrating trauma patients who have sustained a cardiac arrest. EDT should be performed liberally in penetrating trauma patients, particularly those with a suspected cardiac injury. Appropriate preparation of personnel and equipment is required to perform EDT in a safe and efficient manner. EDT provides the opportunity to release cardiac tamponade and repair cardiac injuries, cross-clamp the descending thoracic aorta to improve cerebral and coronary perfusion during resuscitation, control hemorrhage within the chest, and perform internal cardiac massage and defibrillation [6]. This chapter will focus on the indications, preparation, and technique for EDT in penetrating trauma patients.

11.1 Indications

Though there is some controversy surrounding the application of EDT [7, 8], there are clearly select patients who will benefit from liberal application of EDT. In 2001, the American College of Surgeons – Committee on Trauma developed practice management guidelines for EDT and published several evidence-based Level II recommendations [2]. The committee recommended that EDT should rarely be performed in blunt trauma patients due to low survival rate and poor neurologic outcomes. Furthermore, EDT should be reserved only for blunt trauma patients who sustain a witnessed cardiac arrest [4]. However, recommendations regarding EDT for cardiac arrest after penetrating trauma were much broader and stated that EDT is best applied to patients sustaining penetrating cardiac injuries, and should also be applied to patients with penetrating noncardiac thoracic injuries and patients with exsanguinating abdominal vascular injuries.

Though some surgeons would argue for restricted indications due to poor outcomes and risk of occupational exposures to the health care provider [11], there are several reasons to apply EDT liberally, particularly in the setting of penetrating trauma [10]. First, though overall survival is quite poor following EDT (usually 5–10%), mortality after EDT is largely dependent on mechanism and location of injury, as well as of evidence prehospital or hospital of signs of life [9, 12]. Though survival after EDT for blunt trauma is dismal and usually <1%, survival after penetrating trauma is about 10% and higher for stab wounds (~15%) than for gunshot wounds (~5%). Furthermore, while patients with injuries to multiple body regions have a survival close to zero, patients with abdominal, thoracic, and particularly cardiac injuries have reasonable survival rates of about 5%, 10%, and 20%, respectively, after EDT. The presence or absence of signs of life (palpable pulse, blood pressure, spontaneous respirations, pupillary reaction, extremity movement, or electrical

C.V.R. Brown (✉)
Department of Surgery, University of Texas Southwestern – Austin, Austin, TX, USA

Trauma and Surgical Critical Care, University Medical Center Brackenridge, 601 East 15th Street, Austin 78701, TX, USA
e-mail: cvrbrown@seton.org

D.J. Green
Trauma and Surgical Critical Care, Navy Trauma Training Center, University of Southern California, 1200 North State Street, Los Angeles, CA 90033, USA
e-mail: donaldgr@usc.edu

G.C. Velmahos et al. (eds.), *Penetrating Trauma*,
DOI 10.1007/978-3-642-20453-1_11, © Springer-Verlag Berlin Heidelberg 2012

cardiac activity) clearly has a major impact on survival for patients undergoing EDT, with patients exhibiting signs of life immediately prior to EDT having better outcomes than those with remote or absent signs of life. However, the hectic nature of prehospital transport and the trauma resuscitation room during the care of a patient in extremis can make determination of signs of life difficult and unreliable.

11.2 Preparation

EDT requires preparation of both personnel and equipment. EDT cannot be performed in a vacuum or in isolation, and requires a team approach in order to be carried out in an organized and efficient manner [1]. All health care providers (technicians, nurses, emergency medicine physicians, and surgeons) involved in the care of a patient requiring an EDT need to be familiar with the basic maneuvers required before and during the procedure. This preparation may come in the form of didactic education, patient simulations, or potentially with experience during previous EDT's. Furthermore, the individual performing the EDT must be prepared to identify and repair injuries within the chest as well as provide resuscitative maneuvers required during EDT. If personnel and resources are not available and/or there is no individual willing or able to perform maneuvers required during EDT, then this procedure should not be part of the resuscitative plan.

If the personnel are available and capable of performing an EDT, then the necessary equipment should be readily accessible in the trauma resuscitation room. Equipment for EDT should be stored within a single operative tray and all instruments should be loose within the tray for easy handling. Though a standard thoracotomy tray would suffice to perform EDT, a scaled-down version should be prepared to remove unnecessary instruments [13]. An EDT tray should be stocked with a #10 scalpel blade (already secured to a handle), a *pre-assembled* retractor (Finochietto or Balfour retractor), curved Mayo scissors (short and long), several forceps (short and long, toothed and smooth), needle drivers (short and long), a variety of large clamps (Satinsky clamps, Debakey aortic aneurysm clamps, Duval lung clamps), and an instrument to perform a transverse sternotomy (heavy shears, Lebsche knife, Gigli saw). Consideration should be given to having at least one additional EDT tray available should a right thoracotomy be required during resuscitation. Suture should be readily available for cardiac or vascular repair; the author prefers a 2-0 Prolene suture on a large tapered needle. Furthermore, the resuscitation room should be equipped with adequate lighting, laparotomy pads or towels, and wall suction, all to allow adequate visualization during the procedure.

11.3 Technique

Prior to patient arrival, the trauma team should be assembled and don universal precautions for personal protection. Once the decision to perform an EDT has been made, you should quickly evaluate the location of penetrating wounds, as right-sided thoracic wounds may prompt a simultaneous right thoracotomy during EDT (discussed later). As you perform the EDT, the remainder of the trauma team should concomitantly secure a definitive airway with endotracheal intubation, establish large bore intravenous access for fluid and blood resuscitation, and place a right tube thoracostomy to better evaluate for a potential source of hemorrhage in the right chest. Though most operative procedures require sterile technique, the life-saving and emergent nature of EDT does not allow time to perform a sterile procedure. Splashing iodine onto the chest prior to incision provides no anti-infective efficacy and merely makes the instruments wet and slippery, making the procedure more difficult. As time is crucial and patient cannot be prepared in the usual sterile fashion, EDT should be performed without preoperative antibiotics, complete surgical skin prep, or standard wound draping.

To begin the EDT, you should place the patient in the supine position with the left arm abducted, widening the rib spaces and allowing optimal access via a left anterolateral thoracotomy. You begin the procedure with a generous curvilinear skin incision over the left chest, extending from the left lateral edge of the sternum medially to the anterior edge of the latissimus dorsi laterally. In a female, you should retract the breast superiorly and the incision should follow the inframammary crease. In a male (Fig. 11.1a, b), the incision should be centered over the fourth or fifth intercostal space, which you can achieve by positioning the curvilinear incision just inferior to the left nipple–areolar complex. You make the initial incision through the skin, subcutaneous fat, much of the thoracic

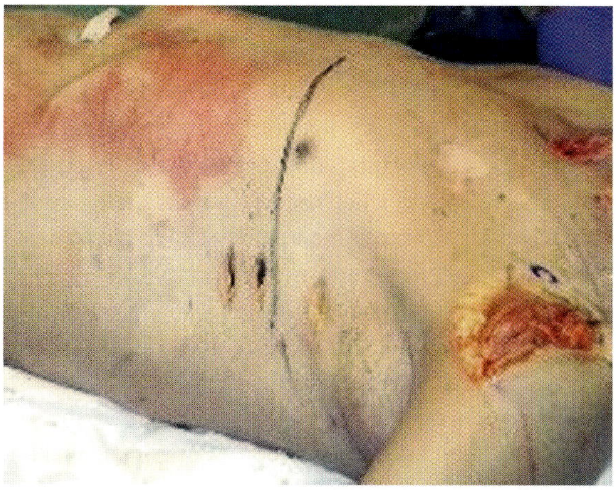

Fig. 11.1 Skin incision for emergency department thoracotomy in a male patient

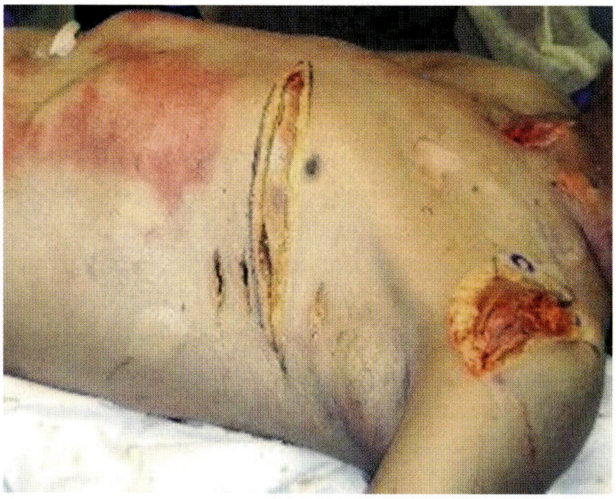

Fig. 11.2 Incision extended through skin, subcutaneous tissue, and most thoracic musculature

musculature (Fig. 11.2), and should be down to the intercostal space and ribs with the first (or at the most second) pass of the scalpel. Once you reach the intercostal space, use the curved Mayo scissors to puncture the intercostal muscles and parietal pleural, just superior to a rib as you would for a tube thoracostomy, then spread the scissors widely. Once you have created a large pleural opening, use the scissors to enlarge the incision medially and laterally, taking care to avoid the neurovascular bundle and allowing enough space to place a thoracic retractor. Place your thoracic retractor and open widely (Fig. 11.3). Keep in mind this is an emergent procedure done relatively quickly, so fracturing ribs while opening the retractor may be unavoidable. While fractured ribs should not alter

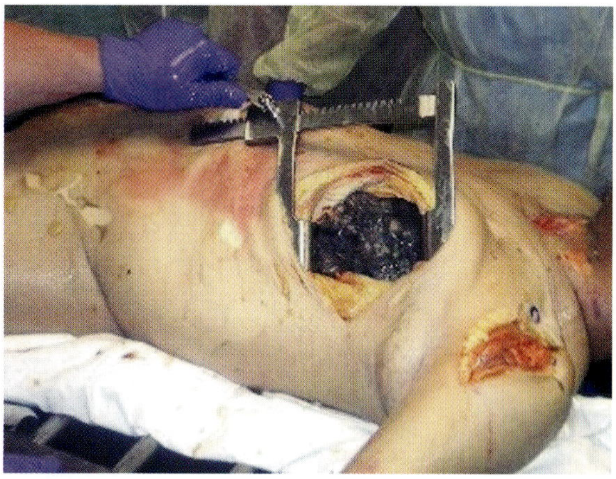

Fig. 11.3 Left anterolateral thoracotomy with retractor in place and opened widely

the course of your EDT, make sure to protect yourself and your assistant from sustaining injury from the sharp edges of the fractured ribs. Once you place and spread the retractor, you will likely be limited somewhat and will need to extend your incision with Mayo scissors through all muscular layers and parietal pleura medially and laterally, to include the full length of your skin incision. Now you should be able to fully open retractor and adequately visualize the left pleural cavity.

Once you have completed positioning your retractor and adequately lengthening the incision, you should first turn your attention to the pericardium [3]. Your assistant should retract the left lung posteriorly, allowing you to easily visualize the anterior mediastinum and pericardium. You should easily visualize the phrenic nerve following its cranio-caudal path along the lateral aspect of the pericardium (Fig. 11.4). While taking care not to injure the phrenic nerve, you use forceps to grasp the pericardium 1 cm anterior to the nerve and make an incision with scissors. The initial incision should allow you to confirm the presence of pericardial blood. Occasionally, a tense cardiac tamponade will be present, making it difficult to grasp the pericardium with forceps. In these cases, you may make the initial pericardiotomy with a small stab incision using a scalpel. Next, you should lengthen the pericardiotomy cranially and caudally with scissors, about 1 cm anterior and parallel to the path of the phrenic nerve (Fig. 11.5). By enlarging the pericardial incision, you can evacuate pericardial tamponade and deliver the heart into the wound. This will allow you to repair any cardiac injury that may be present.

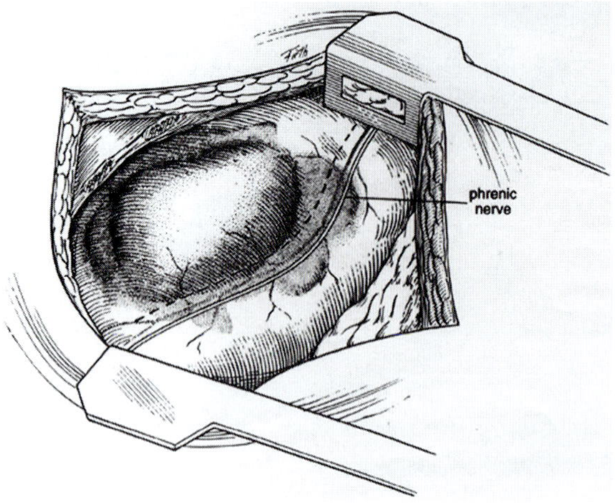

Fig. 11.4 The phrenic nerve following its cranio-caudal path along the lateral aspect of the pericardium

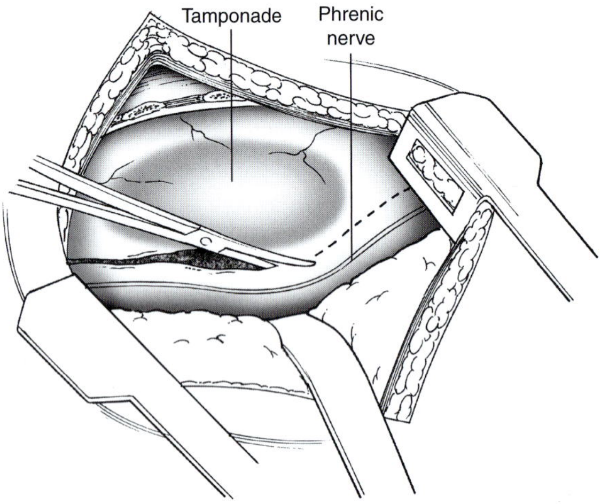

Fig. 11.5 Extension of pericardiotomy with scissors

If the heart is in asystole, then repair is obviously quite easy. However, if there is an organized cardiac rhythm, you will need to gently stabilize the heart in order to perform the repair. You should be able to fix most cardiac injuries with a simple interrupted suture repair; the author usually uses a 2-0 polypropelene suture on a tapered needle. You do not need to use pledgets during the initial repair, but if the tissue tears during repair, you may consider adding pledgets to reinforce the repair. You may also use a running stitch, figure-of-eight, or horizontal mattress. If the cardiac wound is approximate to a coronary artery, you may need to alter your approach. If the injury is near a distal coronary artery, then a repair that ligates the artery distally should be well tolerated by the myocardium. However, if the injury is near the proximal portion of a coronary artery (particularly the left anterior descending artery), the ligation will surely lead to a massive myocardial infarction and death. In these cases, you should perform a horizontal mattress suture around the laceration and the coronary artery, so as not to ligate the myocardial blood supply (Fig. 11.6).

If the repair proves difficult or you are not accustomed to performing cardiac repairs, a few optional approaches exit. You may temporize bleeding from a cardiac wound by placing a urinary catheter into the laceration and inflating the balloon (Fig. 11.7), making sure you clamp the proximal part of the catheter to prevent bleeding. Rather than placing sutures, you may able to repair the laceration with a skin stapler and perform the definitive suture repair in a delayed fashion in the operating room. You may also control the bleeding from a cardiac laceration using a Satinsky clamp, particularly for right atrial lacerations (Fig. 11.8). Finally, if the wound is on the posterior surface of the heart, you can elevate the heart by grasping the apex with a Duval lung clamp to allow visualization (Fig. 11.9). If the heart is beating while elevating the apex, venous return to the heart may be impeded and lead to cardiac arrest, so you should perform this maneuver gently and only elevate the enough to complete the repair. If no cardiac wound is identified or at the completion of cardiac repair, attention should be turned to the descending thoracic aorta.

The left lung should now be retracted anteriorly by your assistant. You should evacuate any significant hemothorax to allow you to visualize the descending thoracic aorta. The descending thoracic aorta lies quite posterior and medial in the left chest, running along the left, anterior thoracic spine. With the left lung retracted anteriorly and the left chest evacuated of blood, you should recognize the thick, white, muscular descending aorta (Fig. 11.10). Remember, the esophagus lies anterior and medial to the descending thoracic aorta and you should keep its position in mind when cross-clamping the thoracic aorta in order to avoid iatrogenic esophageal injury. You may consider placing a nasogastric tube to make it easier to identify the esophagus in the chest. Before you can reliably apply a cross-clamp, you must incise the parietal pleura that covers the descending thoracic aorta. You should grasp the parietal pleura with forceps and make the initial incision with scissors. You can perform the remainder of the exposure bluntly with finger dissection of the

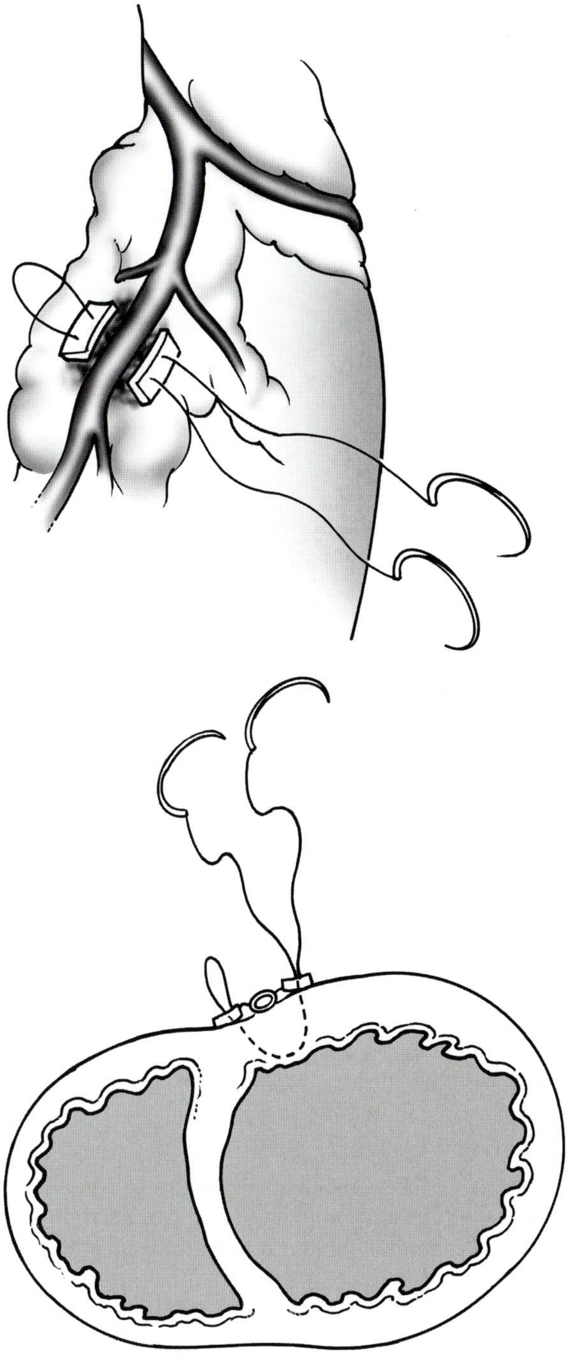

Fig. 11.6 Horizontal mattress repair of laceration adjacent to a coronary artery

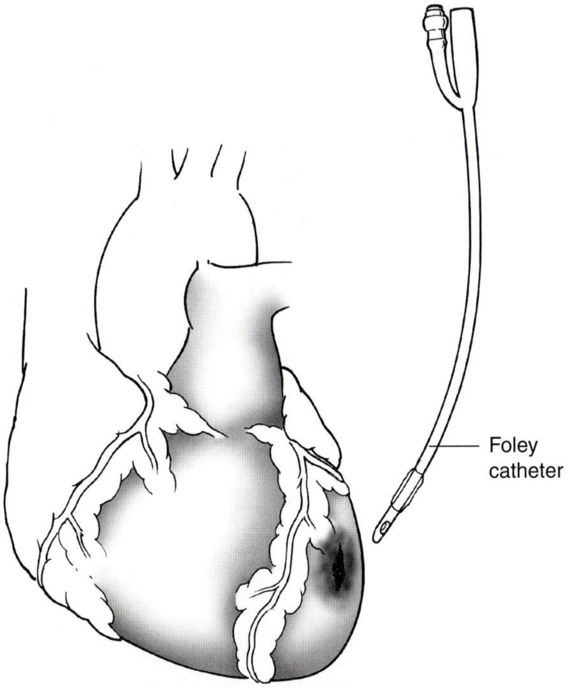

Fig. 11.7 Temporary control of cardiac laceration using a urinary catheter

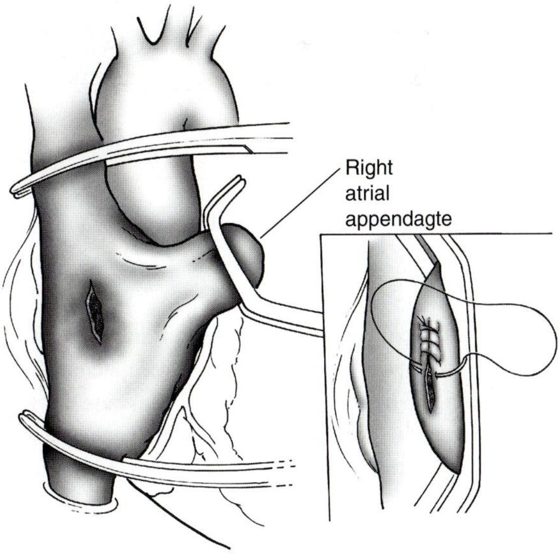

Fig. 11.8 Temporary control of right atrial laceration with a Satinsky clamp

parietal pleura off of the aorta, both in a cranial and caudal direction. Keep in mind you do not need to circumferentially mobilize the descending aorta, as this wastes precious time and may cause iatrogenic injury to intercostal branches. Once you have swept away the parietal pleura, you should cross-clamp the descending aorta with a Debakey aortic aneurysm clamp or Satinsky clamp (Fig. 11.10).

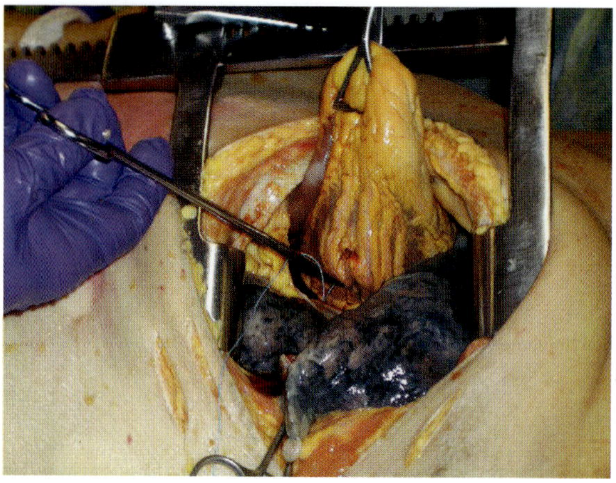

Fig. 11.9 Elevation of the tear with a Duval clamp grasping the apex in order to repair a posterior cardiac laceration

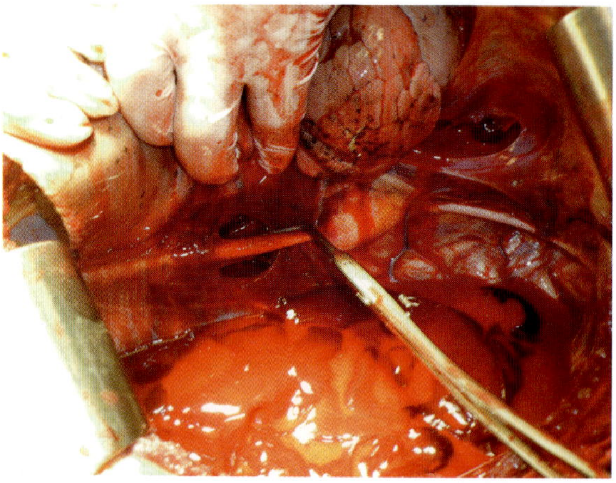

Fig. 11.10 Cross-clamp of the descending thoracic aorta with a Satinsky clamp

Cross-clamping the descending thoracic aorta during EDT improves resuscitation via three mechanisms. First, when you begin internal cardiac massage, having the thoracic aorta cross-clamped will improve cerebral blood flow and perfusion pressure during systole. Similarly, the coronary arteries, which fill during diastole, will receive better perfusion during internal cardiac massage. Finally, aortic cross-clamping will slow down intra-abdominal hemorrhage until a definitive abdominal operation can be performed. You should cross-clamp the thoracic aorta as distally as possible in order to maintain adequate perfusion to the spinal cord during the cross-clamp time. Furthermore, you should remove the aortic cross-clamp as soon as possible and preferably within 30 min. Once you have successfully applied the aortic cross-clamp, you can turn your attention to internal cardiac massage.

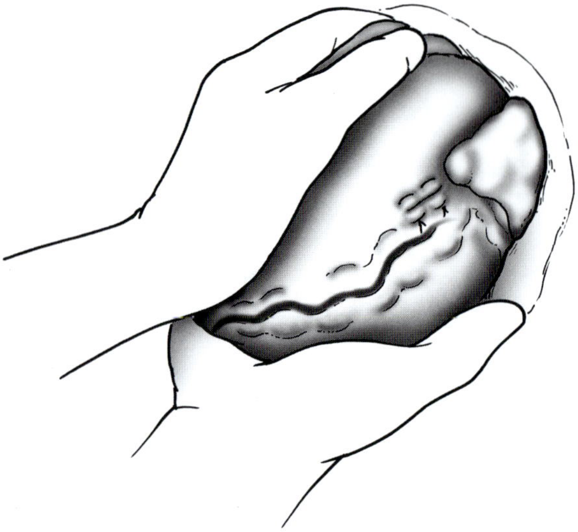

Fig. 11.11 Internal cardiac massage

With the pericardium already opened widely and the heart delivered into the wound (with or without a previous cardiac repair), you should be able to easily evaluate the heart's rhythm and contractility. Patients with an organized rhythm and adequate contractility do not need internal cardiac massage, but may require intravenous drugs such as atropine and epinephrine to support heart rate and blood pressure. Patients with asystole should receive internal cardiac massage. You can provide internal cardiac massage by cupping your hands and placing one anterior and one posterior to the heart (Fig. 11.11). Using the palm of each hand, you may begin internal cardiac compression at a rate of about 100 beats/min, compressing the heart from its apex to its base. You should take care to use only your palms, to avoid iatrogenic injury from point pressure on the heart from your fingers or thumbs. Simultaneously, the patient should receive intravenous ACLS drugs to assist with resuscitation. Drugs should be allowed to circulate for at least 1 min of internal cardiac massage. If the patient develops ventricular fibrillation, you may use internal paddles and defibrillate with an initial setting of 10–15 J. The internal paddles should be positioned with one paddle anterior and one paddle posterior to the apex of the heart (Fig. 11.12). You may continue with internal cardiac massage, defibrillation, and ACLS protocols until the patient has a return of spontaneous cardiac activity or you decide the care is futile.

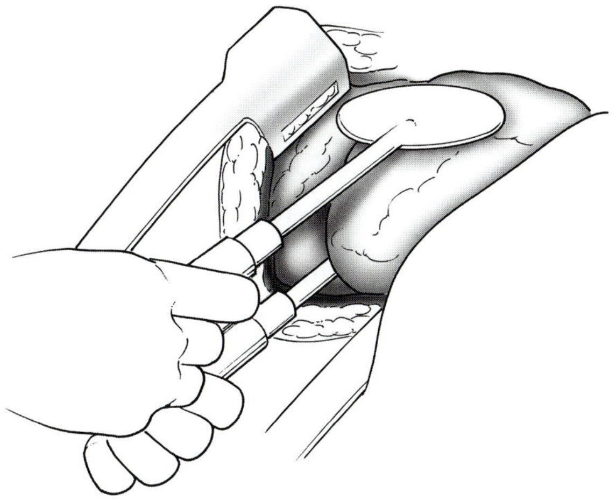

Fig. 11.12 Internal defibrillation paddles

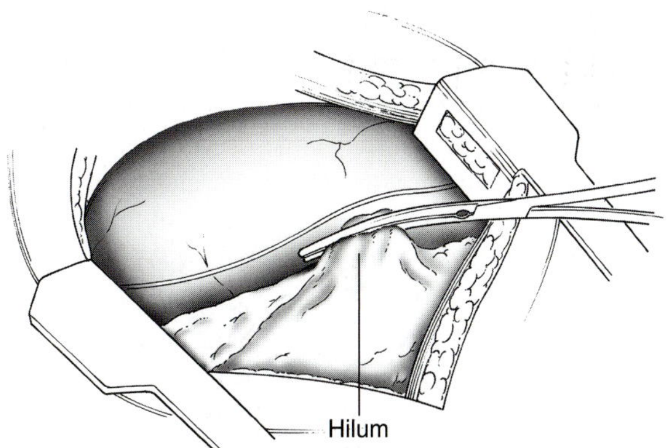

Fig. 11.13 Cross-clamp of the pulmonary hilum

At any point during the EDT, you may be required to control hemorrhage from a variety of sources including the chest wall, spine, heart, lungs, or pulmonary vasculature. Repair of cardiac injuries has been previously described in this chapter. You can usually control bleeding from the chest wall or its associated vessels (intercostal, internal mammary) like anywhere else in the body, with simple clamping and ligation with nonabsorbable sutures or vascular clips. Occasionally, you may encounter bleeding from the chest wall that is not amenable to usual techniques of hemostasis. Similarly, bleeding from the thoracic spine can be quite difficult to control and a bleeding vessel is not usually obvious. In both of these circumstances, you may consider packing the chest wall with laparotomy pads, the spine wound with bone wax, using any available topical hemostatic agents, inserting a urinary catheter to provide balloon tamponade, and return to the site of bleeding for definitive hemorrhage control later in the operation.

Bleeding from the lung parenchyma is not usually significant due to its low pressure and intrinsic ability to form clot from a high local concentration of tissue thromboplastin. You can usually leave lacerations from the pulmonary parenchyma alone until definitive operation, or you may apply a Duval lung clamp to temporize troublesome bleeding. While bleeding from the pulmonary parenchyma does not usually present a significant problem, bleeding from the pulmonary vasculature can be torrential and quickly result in exsanguination. Furthermore, significant disruption in the pulmonary venous system (with or without associated bronchial disruption) can lead to air embolism to the left-sided cardiac circulation [5]. You can control bleeding from pulmonary vasculature within the substance of the lung parenchyma using suture ligation. If the bleeding is too heavy to allow visualization or the bleeding is emanating from the pulmonary hilum, you may need to obtain control of the hilum either manually or with a vascular clamp. You may gain control of the pulmonary hilum by first temporarily halting ventilation to allow adequate visualization. Next, while retracting the lung posteriorly, you may bring your hand or a Satinsky clamp from above and grasp or clamp the entirety of the pulmonary hilum, including the pulmonary artery, pulmonary veins, and mainstem bronchus (Fig. 11.13). It is important that you approach the hilum from above, as an inferior approach will be impeded by the inferior pulmonary ligament and may not allow hilar control. Some authors have advocated dividing the pulmonary ligament to mobilize the lung, but in our opinion, this is an unnecessary maneuver for several reasons. Dividing the inferior pulmonary ligament takes valuable time, may lead to iatrogenic injury of the inferior pulmonary vein, may be quite difficult in the emergent setting with ongoing hemorrhage, and the pulmonary hilum can be easily controlled with a superior approach while leaving the inferior pulmonary ligament intact. Despite control of the pulmonary hilum, you may suspect an air embolism (or confirm the diagnosis by seeing air bubbles in the coronary arteries). In these cases, you may aspirate the left ventricle with a needle and syringe in an attempt to evacuate any intra-ventricular air.

Though you can perform most required maneuvers during an EDT through a left anterolateral thoracotomy, you may occasionally be required to convert the left thoracotomy into a bilateral or clamshell thoracotomy. You may perform the bilateral thoracotomy through two separate incisions, or you may extend your left thoracotomy onto the right chest via transverse sternotomy. You should consider adding a right thoracotomy to the left anterolateral EDT in a few situations. First, if the patient presents with primarily right-sided wounds, you may consider performing the usual EDT but have an associate start a right thoracotomy simultaneously. A left thoracotomy is still necessary, as access to the right chest will allow you to perform pericardiotomy, control intrathoracic hemorrhage, and perform internal cardiac massage, but does not allow you to cross-clamp the descending aorta. Another indication for right thoracotomy is based on the output of the right tube thoracostomy placed concomitant with EDT. If the initial right chest tube output is more than 500–1,000 cm^3, you may consider performing right thoracotomy in an attempt to control the source of hemorrhage in the right pleural cavity.

The most common reason for extending a left-sided EDT is to improve your visualization of the mediastinum in order to allow repair of the heart or great vessels. In this case, you will always need to perform a transverse sternotomy and will usually extend your left thoracotomy into a clamshell thoracotomy. You can perform the right thoracotomy portion of the bilateral or clamshell thoracotomy as a mirror image of the left thoracotomy already described. You can perform the transverse sternotomy with a variety of techniques. The skin incision is simply a transverse incision connecting the right and left thoracotomy (Fig. 11.14). You should carry this incision through the subcutaneous tissue and thoracic musculature until you reach the anterior portion of the sternum. You can then perform the transverse sternotomy with heavy shears, Lebsche knife, or a Gigli saw. Once you perform your transverse sternotomy, you may need to adjust your thoracic retractor or add a second retractor to optimize visualization. Next, you will need to extend your pericardiotomy across the anterior pericardium, taking care not to injure the right phrenic nerve. Keep in mind that during transverse sternotomy, you will divide both internal mammary arteries. This may not be readily apparent if the patient is pulseless, but you should ligate or clip both internal mammary arteries as they will bleed significantly during cardiac massage or if the patient regains a pulse.

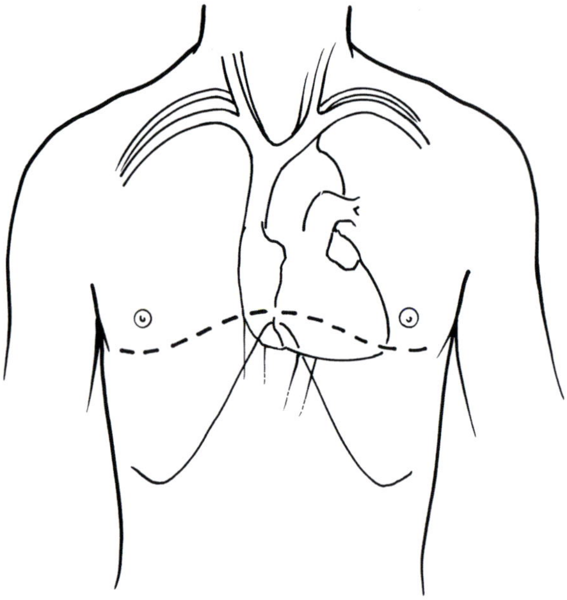

Fig. 11.14 Skin incision for clamshell thoracotomy

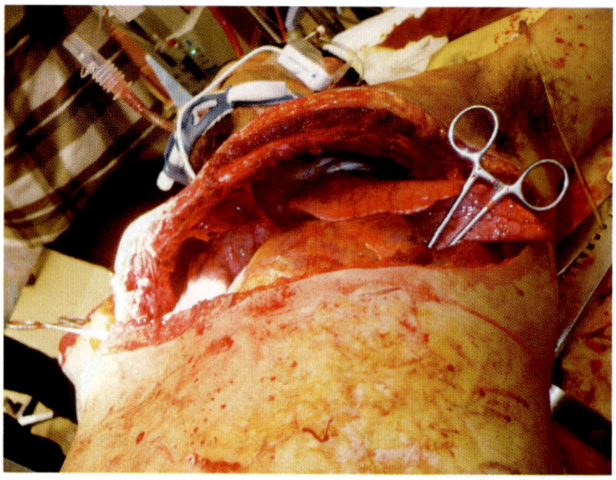

Fig. 11.15 Exposure obtained to both pleural cavities and mediastinum via a clamshell thoracotomy

The clamshell incision provides spectacular exposure to both pleural cavities and all mediastinal structures, which should allow you to perform any and all maneuvers required during emergency department thoracotomy (Fig. 11.15).

Before patient arrival and throughout performing EDT, you must consider what the plan will be if the patient has a return of organized cardiac activity or if cardiac arrest persists despite all resuscitative efforts. If at any time during EDT, the patient has return of a sustained pulse and blood pressure, they should be transported to the operating room for definitive operative procedures. Furthermore, you should try to remove the aortic cross-clamp as soon as possible if the patient's physiology will tolerate it. If cardiac arrest persists during EDT, then you must determine if ongoing resuscitative efforts should be continued or if the care is futile. Futility in the setting of EDT for penetrating trauma is dependent on several factors including patient age and comorbidities, location of injuries identified during EDT, and local resources including personnel and blood bank availability.

Important Points

- An emergent thoracotomy tray with all necessary instruments and retractors needs to be prepared and quickly available in the emergency department.
- As you perform the EDT, the remainder of the trauma team should concomitantly secure a definitive airway with endotracheal intubation, establish large bore intravenous access for fluid and blood resuscitation, and place a right tube thoracostomy to better evaluate for a potential source of hemorrhage in the right chest.
- In a female, you should retract the breast superiorly and the incision should follow the inframammary crease. In a male, the incision should be centered over the 4th or 5th intercostal space, which you can achieve by positioning the curvilinear incision just inferior to the left nipple–areolar complex.
- Occasionally, a tense cardiac tamponade will be present, making it difficult to grasp the pericardium with forceps. In these cases, you may make the initial pericardiotomy with a small stab incision using a scalpel.
- Before you can reliably apply a cross-clamp, you must incise the parietal pleura that covers the descending thoracic aorta.
- The descending aorta should *not* be circumferentially mobilized to apply a cross-clamp, as this unnecessary maneuver takes time and may lead to iatrogenic injury of intercostal vessels.
- Bleeding from the chest wall or spine may require packing, topical hemostatic agents, or balloon tamponade to temporarily control hemorrhage.
- Dividing the inferior pulmonary ligament during EDT is unnecessary as it wastes valuable time, may lead to iatrogenic injury of the inferior pulmonary vein, may be quite difficult in the emergent setting with ongoing hemorrhage, and the pulmonary hilum can be easily controlled with a superior approach while leaving the inferior pulmonary ligament intact.
- During transverse sternotomy, you will divide both internal mammary arteries. This may not be readily apparent if the patient is pulseless, but you should ligate or clip both internal mammary arteries as they will bleed significantly during cardiac massage or if the patient regains a pulse.

References

1. Aihara R, Millham FH, Blansfield J et al (2001) Emergency room thoracotomy for penetrating chest injury: effect of an institutional protocol. J Trauma 50:1027–1030
2. Asensio JA, Wall MJ, Minei J, Working Group, Ad Hoc Subcommittee on Outcomes, American College of Surgeons – Committee on Trauma et al (2001) Practice management guidelines for emergency department thoracotomy. J Am Coll Surg 193:303–309
3. Grove C, Lemmon G, Anderson G et al (2002) Emergency thoracotomy: appropriate use in the resuscitation of trauma patients. Am Surg 68:313–317
4. Hall BL, Buchman TG (2005) A visual, timeline-based display of evidence for emergency thoracotomy. J Trauma 59:773–777
5. Hunt PA, Greaves I, Owens WA (2006) Emergency thoracotomy in thoracic trauma: a review. Injury 37:1–19
6. Mejia JC, Stewart RM, Cohn SM (2008) Emergency department thoracotomy. Semin Thorac Cardiovasc Surg 20:13–18
7. Miglietta MA, Robb TV, Eachempati SR et al (2001) Current opinion regarding indications for emergency department thoracotomy. J Trauma 51:670–676
8. Powell DW, Moore EE, Cothren CC et al (2004) Is emergency department resuscitative thoracotomy futile care for the critically injured patient requiring prehospital cardiopulmonary resuscitation? J Am Coll Surg 199:211–215
9. Rhee PM, Acosta J, Bridgeman A et al (2000) Survival after emergency department thoracotomy: review of published data from the past 25 years. J Am Coll Surg 190:288–298

10. Seamon MJ, Fisher CA, Gaughan JP et al (2008) Emergency department thoracotomy: survival of the least expected. World J Surg 32:604–612
11. Sikka R, Millham FH, Feldman JA (2004) Analysis of occupational exposures associated with emergency department thoracotomy. J Trauma 56:867–872
12. Søreide K, Petrone P, Asensio JA (2007) Emergency thoracotomy in trauma: rationale, risks, and realities. Scand J Surg 96:4–10
13. Wise D, Davies G, Coats T et al (2005) Emergency thoracotomy: "how to do it". Emerg Med J 22:22–24

Intensive Care: Principles and Therapy

12

Terence O'Keeffe

As technology has advanced over the last 20 years, the field of critical care has expanded enormously to meet the challenges of the sick and injured patient, from changes in invasive and noninvasive monitoring to advanced modes of ventilation as well as the pharmacologic manipulation of sepsis, all of which now incorporate more of an evidence-based approach.

While the format of this book does not allow us to adequately cover even the smallest fraction of the breadth and scope of current surgical critical care, we will attempt to summarize some of the more important areas, focusing on basic principles and current therapies, with the emphasis being on penetrating trauma.

12.1 Metabolic Response to Trauma

The body's response whether due to a traumatic or surgical insult is the same, namely, an activation of the sympathetic nervous system and an increase in circulating catecholamines. Endocrine stress hormones are also released from the pituitary, as well as changes in the immune system including production of inflammatory cytokines in addition to a leucocytosis.

These neurohormonal changes cause tachycardia and fever, which taken together with tachypnea and leucocytosis form the Systemic Inflammatory Response Syndrome (SIRS) [1]. Metabolic changes lead to the retention of sodium and water, in addition to hyperglycemia that is compounded by insulin resistance, proteolysis of skeletal muscle, lipolysis of fat stores, and cytokine release all contributing to a catabolic state.

It is presumed that this proinflammatory response is of overall benefit to the body as it responds to the insult and aids in recovery. However, in some patients, the degree of trauma is so great that despite adequate resuscitation, it overwhelms the capacity for recovery and severe SIRS develops. A second "activating" event may also occur after the initial injury, which leads to a rapid downward spiral into multiorgan failure. The majority of modern critical care is designed to decrease the likelihood of this second event and/or to abrogate its effects on the patient.

12.2 ICU Monitoring

The last decade has seen the pendulum swing away from aggressive invasive cardiovascular monitoring, with more emphasis now being placed on increasingly sophisticated noninvasive devices.

Arterial catheterization is standard practice in most ICUs, not only to monitor arterial blood pressure, but also to facilitate blood gas monitoring in ventilated patients. Complication rates are low, but thrombosis, pseudoaneurysm formation, and infection may all occur. The radial or femoral routes are preferred for ease of placement and degree of complications. Some sophisticated monitors can now be attached to the arterial line, which can give real-time estimates of the cardiac output.

Although there is some data that pulmonary artery (PA) catheters may have benefit in younger patients and those with more severe injuries, there has been a

T. O'Keeffe
Division of Trauma/Critical Care and Emergency Surgery, University of Arizona, 1501 N Campbell Avenue, Rm 5411, P.O. Box 245063, Tucson, AZ 85724-5063, USA
e-mail: tokeeffe@surgery.arizona.edu

G.C. Velmahos et al. (eds.), *Penetrating Trauma*,
DOI 10.1007/978-3-642-20453-1_12, © Springer-Verlag Berlin Heidelberg 2012

significant decrease in the use of these devices in recent years [2]. No randomized controlled trial has to date shown benefit in their use, and at least, one study has shown that the fluid status of severely ill patients can be adequately managed using simple central venous catheters [3]. Therefore, the use of PA catheters should be reserved for those patients who are refractory to adequate volume resuscitation without obvious cause, or who have cardiac dysfunction, either acute or chronic, where monitoring of cardiac output is necessary to guide clinical care.

Echocardiographic and noninvasive monitoring of cardiac output in the ICU patient have been suggested as alternatives, but either require sophisticated equipment or a degree of technical skill that is not available in most ICUs. Other specialized monitors have been developed that can monitor hemoglobin levels in real-time, assess muscle bed oxygenation, and even continuously monitor glucose levels. It is likely that these devices will replace some of our more traditional methods in the near future.

12.3 Neurological System, Pain Control, and Traumatic Brain Injury

One of the biggest challenges in the ICU is appropriately managing pain and agitation in postoperative or critically ill patients. There are a number of considerations that you must take into account when choosing medications, not least of which are comorbidities that may affect the pharmacokinetics of the various agents. It is preferable to use short-acting intravenous narcotic analgesics as infusions for initial pain control, an example of which would be fentanyl. The choice of a benzodiazepine or other agent such as propofol as a sedative depends to a degree on the preference of the treating physician, as well as their hemodynamic stability. Both propofol and dexmetomedine infusions have deleterious effects on blood pressure and so you should not use them in patients who are actively being volume resuscitated. Conversely, benzodiazepine infusions have long half-lives, and you should avoid them as maintenance sedation over many days. Sedation should be individualized and tailored to a specific goal, which should involve a sedation scale using a specific target range for that patient.

An early transition of patients to oral analgesia (e.g., Oxycodone) via the enteral route is recommended, as soon as the GI tract is available for use. If your patient requires sedation in the longer term, intermittent bolus dosing of a medium-length half-life benzodiazepine such as Lorazepam (Ativan) works well. Whatever form of sedation you use, the patient should undergo daily "sedation vacations" to allow the medication to wear off, which will allow you to make an accurate assessment of the patient's level of consciousness.

Traumatic Brain injury is another major problem seen in the ICU. Unfortunately, the prognosis of most penetrating brain injuries is poor, especially if it is due to a missile that crosses the midline. The principles of management are similar to blunt trauma, but there may be a role for debridement of devitalized tissue in the initial phase of the illness. The subsequent care that is required will be dictated by the patient's neurological exam, CT scans, and/or intracranial pressure. The initial Glasgow Coma Scale remains the most important prognostic factor in these patients.

12.4 Respiratory Failure, Acute Lung Injury, and ARDS

Many trauma patients suffer respiratory failure following injury and need to be maintained on invasive ventilation. Daily sedation vacations and spontaneous breathing trials have both been shown to facilitate earlier extubation. Weaning protocols that directly involve the nursing staff or respiratory therapists in the process are highly effective. Computer-driven weaning protocols have also been developed and may be directly incorporated into ventilators in the future. The key is to extubate patients as soon as possible, as this minimizes the risk of ventilator-associated pneumonia, which is one of the more serious nosocomial infections that patients develop in the ICU. These infections are associated with significant mortality, morbidity, and cost. Noninvasive ventilation may also have a role either as a means to avoid intubation while still providing ventilatory support, or as a bridge following extubation to allow the patient time as their respiratory function improves.

Each clinician has his or her own strategy to deal with patients who have acute lung injury or are difficult to oxygenate. Airway Pressure Release Ventilation (APRV) in patients with acute lung injury appears to be effective in reversing atelectasis and improving oxygenation, without requiring the deep sedation or paralysis that is usually necessary in the other mandatory forms of ventilation [4].

As we have come to better understand the consequences of excessive crystalloid administration and the pendulum has swung away from supranormal resuscitation, there has been a noted decline in patients developing the acute respiratory distress syndrome [5]. The mainstay of treatment for this condition remains ventilation with low tidal volumes, but certain patients will continue to require prone positioning, high-frequency oscillatory ventilation, inhaled nitric oxide, or even extracorporeal membrane oxygenation, although none of these modalities have been conclusively proven to improve mortality.

12.5 Cardiac Failure

Cardiogenic shock is a relatively rare complication following penetrating trauma and is usually due to direct lacerations of the heart itself or secondary to underlying baseline cardiac disease.

In cases of direct trauma to the heart, take care to avoid damage to the coronary arteries and veins if at all possible during surgical repair, as this will lead to infarction of the cardiac muscle distal to the injury. Pay attention to the possibility of damage to the cardiac valves, papillary muscles, and septae following penetrating injury, which is best evaluated by echocardiography; either via the transesophageal route during the initial operation, or via the transthoracic method once the patient is in the ICU. It is good practice to routinely perform echocardiography postoperatively following cardiac stab wounds, and this should be done urgently if there are signs of cardiac dysfunction.

It is not unusual for the trauma surgeon to be dealing with elderly patients who have multiple cardiac comorbidities such as coronary artery disease, valvular problems, or arrhythmias. Patients frequently have stents in place and are on Plavix (Clopidogrel), Aspirin or are anticoagulated with Warfarin. The risk of thromboses in these patients needs to be carefully weighed against the risk of ongoing hemorrhage if the anticoagulation is maintained.

The choice of vasopressor to use in cardiogenic shock will depend on the exact cause of the shock, Dopamine being most beneficial in those cases where the patient needs inotropic support and when they are not tachycardic. Dobutamine is a better choice for the patient with a history of congestive cardiac failure. Rarely, agents such as epinephrine or milrinone for right heart failure may be required. In the most severe cases, an intra-aortic balloon pump may be required to maintain left ventricular function. Patients with cardiogenic shock are one of the few situations where one should strongly consider placing a pulmonary artery catheter.

12.6 Surgical Nutrition

While the exact indications for and benefits of specialized enteral formulas remain to be elucidated, it is clear that early enteral feeding carries significant benefits. Place the patient on enteral feeding as soon as is feasibly possible after admission to minimize the catabolic effects of their trauma and/or surgery. There is little data to support the time-honored practice of transitioning patients from sips to clears to soft to regular diet, and unless there are obvious contraindications, a regular diet should be established as soon as possible.

For those patients who are intubated or otherwise unable to take a PO diet, enteral feeding access should be obtained, preferably post-pyloric. Calculation of the metabolic requirements of the patient using the various nutrition formulas (e.g., Ireton-Jones energy expenditure) has been shown to be accurate, and a detailed metabolic cart assessment is not normally required. Tube feeds can be given either continuously or as bolus feeds, with the later approach being slightly more effective at delivering the daily nutritional goals. Unless the patient has specific indications (e.g., ARDS, sepsis, renal, or hepatic failure), use simple enteral formulas (e.g., Promote, Jevity). The immune-enhancing or specialty formulas should be reserved for those cases where there is likely to be maximal benefit. Intolerance to enteral feeds can usually be successfully managed with promotility agents, such as Erythromycin, which is somewhat more effective than Metoclopramide. Both agents can also be used together for a synergistic effect, but it should be remembered that tachyphylaxis often develops within a week, independent of the agent used.

Total parenteral nutrition (TPN) retains a place in surgical nutrition, particularly in those patients who cannot tolerate enteral feeds or who have enteral fistulas. Use of a PICC line for administration rather than a central line decreases some of the mechanical complications, but patients are still at risk for metabolic and infectious problems. Close monitoring of electrolyte and glucose levels is mandatory and the patient should be transitioned as soon as possible to enteral feeds. It is preferable to use it only in those cases where the patient will be unable to tolerate enteral feeds for at least 7 days.

12.7 Fluid, Electrolytes, and Renal Failure

Trauma patients often require the administration of significant amounts of intravenous fluids following injury due to blood loss, shifts of sodium and water from the interstitium, and/or fluid losses from wounds. Although there is no perfect measure for assessing adequacy of resuscitation, a mixture of base deficit, serum lactate, and urine output works well (although none of these measures are adequate taken in isolation). As mentioned before, in certain circumstances with persistent hypotension, further invasive monitoring may be required, which may help guide the endpoint of resuscitation.

The choice of intravenous fluid has been hotly debated since the 1960s and remains contentious. Both normal saline and lactated ringer's are usually used in the acute phase. The proinflammatory effects of excessive crystalloid use have been well documented, and in this new era of "hemostatic resuscitation," the goal is to minimize injudicious use. Care should be to taken to monitor for hyperchloremic acidosis if normal saline is used as the primary resuscitation fluid; lactated ringers may therefore be preferable to eliminate this potential complication.

Hypertonic saline has a number of advocates, and although to date there is no large randomized controlled trial in humans showing benefit in hypovolemic shock (one recent large community trial was halted due to lack of efficacy and possible harm), there is some data suggesting benefit in patients with traumatic brain injury. Its use should probably be reserved for these patients until and if clearer data emerge regarding its overall benefit in the trauma patient.

Many hospitals have protocols for electrolyte replacement on standard order sets, although in the asymptomatic patient who is tolerating a diet, most of these electrolyte abnormalities are of little consequence. In contrast, the intubated patient in the ICU with arrhythmias should have electrolyte levels closely monitored and aggressively corrected. Hypo- or hypernatremia may be a result of an underlying serious diseases such as the syndrome of inappropriate ADH secretion (SIADH) or diabetes insipidus, and needs to be appropriately investigated and treated. Hypophosphatemia and hypomagnesemia are two other conditions which are common in the ICU and should be looked for and treated aggressively as the consequences can be serious.

Renal failure is not uncommon in the trauma ICU for a number of reasons; it may be related to underlying disease, age, nephrotoxin exposure (i.e., IV contrast), or hypovolemic shock. Adequate and early resuscitation is the best method of prevention, as once established, there are few effective treatment options. The most likely type of renal failure in the trauma patient is prerenal, but renal and postrenal causes still need to be excluded. A fractional excretion of sodium (FENA) should be calculated, and the Foley catheter must be checked for obstruction. Central venous pressure monitoring is warranted to assess volume status. Although dopamine will increase urine output temporarily, it will not influence the need for dialysis or mortality and has therefore been abandoned due to deleterious side effects. Similarly, the administration of loop diuretics has not been shown to improve outcomes and should not be used. In those cases where renal failure becomes established, nephrology consultation for dialysis (either continuous renal replacement therapy or hemodialysis) may be necessary. There is some emerging data that patients who receive early, aggressive dialysis have improved outcomes, but this has yet to be universally adopted.

12.8 Endocrine: Glucose Control and Steroids

One of the most controversial topics in surgical critical care has been the purported benefit of so-called tight or intensive glucose control in the intensive care unit. The landmark study in 2001 by Van den Berghe on cardiac surgery patients, showed improved outcome with glucose levels kept at between 80 and 110 mg/dL, and led to the large-scale adoption of this therapy despite its single-center study design [6]. Subsequent studies by the same group failed to show similar benefits in broader surgical patients, and higher rates of morbidity particularly related to hypoglycemia led many to question the benefit of this approach. In a more recent, larger randomized controlled trial, the target range of 80–110 mg/dL was shown to increase mortality, whereas a target of less than 180 was shown to improve it [7]. Although glucose monitoring and control is indeed important in the intensive care unit, it is likely that a target of 150–180 is more reasonable and achievable without the morbidity associated with hypoglycemia.

Another area of controversy has been the use of steroids in sepsis. Since the publication of a trial which showed improved mortality using low-dose corticosteroids in patients with septic shock, there has been renewed interest in the use of steroids in the ICU [8]. This study used a rapid ACTH stimulation test to decide whether the patients needed steroids, using a cutoff of less than 9 mg/dL increase in serum cortisol following ACTH stimulation. A subsequent study failed to show such benefit although it did show more rapid resolution of symptoms of shock [9]. At this point, the recommendations of the surviving sepsis campaign (revised 2008) are to use hydrocortisone only in patients who are unresponsive to fluid resuscitation and vasopressors, and the ACTH stimulation test should not be used to identify patients for steroid therapy [10]. More study will be needed to help identify those patients, if any, who will truly benefit from this therapy.

12.9 Transfusions and Blood Products

Since the advent of solid organ transplantation, the transfusion of blood has been recognized as having an immune suppressive effect. Study after study has shown an increase in infectious complications in the critical care setting, but it was really the landmark TRICC trial in 1999 that set the stage for a reduction in unnecessary and ineffective blood transfusions. Patients were randomized into either a restrictive blood transfusion arm (Hemoglobin of 7–9 g/dL) or a liberal transfusion arm (10–12 g/dL). The investigators found clinical equipoise in the two transfusion strategies, which when given the side effects, time, cost, and infectious risks associated with blood transfusion obviously favors a restrictive transfusion strategy. Interestingly, in subgroup analysis, patients who were younger and more severely ill had improved survival in the restrictive transfusion arm, although there was no difference between groups in those patients suffering trauma. Therefore, in the intensive care unit, practice has changed to closely follow the hemoglobin in the asymptomatic patient and transfuse only if the levels fall close to or below 7 g/dL.

It should nevertheless be remembered that for entry into this trial, these patients were required to be euvolemic and not actively hemorrhaging. The treatment for a trauma patient with hemorrhagic shock is still aggressive blood product transfusion until the source of hemorrhage is controlled either surgically or by other means. In fact, the concept of "hemostatic resuscitation" has been developed to denote aggressive blood and blood product administration in the early hours after injury in a patient with massive blood loss [11]. This has also led many centers to develop transfusion protocols in those patients with massive blood loss, to address the coagulopathy that results from the aggressive resuscitation that is required.

Correction of coagulopathy in the ICU is another area of controversy. Many clinicians are unaware that fresh frozen plasma (FFP) is not as efficient as fresh, whole blood in improving coagulation. Indeed, the international normalized ratio (INR) of the average unit of FFP lies between 1.3 and 1.4, and will therefore be ineffective at correcting any coagulopathy to below this level. These patients may need an adjunctive agent if correction of the INR to 1.0 is required such as Factor VIIa, cryoprecipitate, or a prothrombin complex concentrate (PCC). As there is a paucity of data regarding the need to reduce the INR to an absolutely normal number, it is safe not to treat patients with an INR of 1.6 or less with transfusions of coagulation factors unless the patient is actively hemorrhaging and/or it is anticipated that this coagulopathy will worsen. Similarly, there is very little data to support the prophylactic administration of platelets or treatment of a platelet count unless it is below 50×10^6, or the patient is currently bleeding, although there are increasing number of patients being prescribed antiplatelet agents. It is to be hoped that we will soon have some studies that will provide some guidance on the effectiveness of platelet transfusion on outcomes in trauma patients who are receiving antiplatelet therapy.

12.10 Infectious Disease Inc. Nosocomial Infections

Sepsis in the ICU remains a significant problem with mortality rates ranging from 25% to 40% despite advances in antibiotics and critical care. The reader is referred to the 2008 campaign for surviving sepsis guidelines for a full breakdown of ICU measures designed to minimize mortality from sepsis and septic shock [10].

Source control remains an important part of the fight against infection in the surgical patient, which may require surgical drainage, aggressive debridement of soft tissue infections, and multiple operations to obtain final control of the infection. Although the tissue defects created may be large, an aggressive initial debridement will serve the patient much better than leaving a continued source of sepsis behind.

A guiding principle for antibiotic use in the ICU should be the early use of empiric antibiotics in suspected cases of infection. Numerous studies have shown that early use of appropriate antibiotic therapy is associated with a survival advantage [12, 13]. In those cases where infection is suspected and not proven, it appears that the use of 72 h of empiric antibiotics followed by cessation if the cultures are negative is not associated with increased resistance patterns [14].

Nosocomial infections remain the bane of ICU care, with ventilator-associated pneumonia (VAP) and catheter-related bloodstream infections (CRBSIs) being the most serious and difficult to treat. Nursing measures such as head of bed elevation and oral care as well as avoiding the use of proton-pump inhibitors for GI prophylaxis have all been shown to help reduce the rate of VAPs. Modifications to the endotracheal tube to allow for subglottic suctioning, and/or impregnation with silver ions, have also shown promise in reducing these serious infections [15, 16].

In a recent study on CRBSIs, five simple measures were found to drastically reduce the incidence of this nosocomial infection: hand-washing prior to line insertion, use of a chlorhexidine skin prep, full barrier precautions including full body sterile draping, avoidance of the femoral and internal jugular routes, and daily assessment for line removal. Using this approach, the investigators showed a 66% drop in CRBSI rates, which was maintained for at least 18 months following the intervention [17].

Prevention of urinary tract infections (UTI) also remains a problem area, with many patients requiring indwelling Foley catheters due to the severity of illness, the need to accurately monitor urinary output, or an inability to spontaneously void. UTI's are the second most common nosocomial infection, and can prolong length of stay as well as lead to unnecessary morbidity. As the risk for development of an UTI increases with length of time that a Foley is in place, patients should have their need for an indwelling catheter reviewed daily, and it should be removed as soon as possible to minimize the risk of infection. Early removal of catheters is the only proven intervention to reduce the risk of UTI.

12.11 Prophylaxis in the ICU: DVT, Ulcer Prophylaxis

Trauma patients should receive both mechanical and chemical thromboprophylaxis as soon as is feasible after injury, although this will have to be tempered by the patient's injuries, e.g., brain injury, liver laceration, etc. The weight of evidence suggest that low molecular weight heparin in the form of Lovenox at a dose of 30 mg every 12 h is a more effective agent than unfractionated heparin. Despite the aggressive routine use of inferior vena cava filters in trauma patients who cannot initially be anticoagulated, there is very little data to prove that they are effective and this cannot be recommended at this time as an effective strategy to reduce the incidence of serious or fatal pulmonary emboli. Use of IVC filters may need to be considered, however, in patients with pelvic fractures and moderate-to-severe traumatic brain injuries.

There remains confusion regarding the need for prophylaxis against stress ulceration in intensive care unit patients. Absolute indications for prophylaxis include: intubated patients, coagulopathy, active upper GI hemorrhage or known gastritis, and current steroid use. The following are relative indications: traumatic brain injury, major burn injury, poly-trauma or sepsis. H2-antagonists are typically used for stress ulcer prophylaxis, and proton-pump inhibitors (PPIs) are reserved for those patients who were being previously treated with these medications, those who develop thrombocytopenia after introduction of H2-antagonists or patients who have interactions with another medications. PPIs have been shown to increase ventilator-associated pneumonia in the ICU and so should be avoided as first-line therapy.

12.12 Multiple Organ Failure

This is a devastating consequence of our improved ICU technology and ability to keep patients alive, and has remained one of the hardest challenges for the intensivist, even as its incidence has decreased over the last decade [18]. This syndrome is characterized by sequential progressive organ dysfunction involving the lungs, kidneys, liver, gastrointestinal tract, and coagulation cascade. Mortality has been reported to be as high as 80%, but more recent studies have suggested mortality rates of 30–50% [19, 20]. Nevertheless, the challenge appears to be in abrogating the initial inflammatory response that led to the development of this syndrome. To date, there are no effective pharmacological agents for therapy and the focus remains on early and adequate resuscitation (with much recent research focusing on more aggressive use of blood and blood products in the early phases) as well as avoiding secondary insults.

12.13 Complications of ICU Care

The clinician needs to remain acutely aware of sudden complications, which can occur at any time in these critically ill patients. Two iatrogenic complications in particular, tube dislodgements and self-extubation, can result in serious consequences.

With the multitude of invasive devices, drains, and catheters, one must be continuously vigilant to prevent them from becoming dislodged. It is important to ensure that they are adequately secured after insertion with sutures, the liberal use of adhesive tape or securing devices. Simple measures such as a note at the head of the bed will communicate to all members of the team looking after the patient which tubes are vital and/or tenuous.

Self-extubation is usually a consequence of inadequate sedation. Reported rates range from 6.6% to 14% with few consistent predictive risk factors [21, 22]. Although the ICU length of stay is longer in these patients, this does not seem to come with a mortality disadvantage. Self-extubations often occur during nursing care and special attention should be paid at this time. Approximately 35–50% of these patients will require re-intubation within the ensuing 48 h and any patient self extubating should be watched carefully in the ICU for signs of respiratory distress.

12.14 Ethical and Family Issues

One of the hardest aspects of dealing with the critically ill patient is interfacing with the family. This interaction can vary from being conducted entirely long distance by telephone with relatives, to trying to control an excessive number of visitors to the patient's bedside, all of whom are emotional and some of whom may not be on good terms with the patient. One of the most important roles of the intensive care physician is to help the family negotiate this difficult time by providing timely information, support, and enough time to visit with their family member. This can sometimes require infinite patience, but can also be intensely rewarding.

Futility of care is often a source of conflict between the family and the clinician when there is a difference of opinion regarding the possibility of a successful outcome. Although this needs to be approached in a sensitive manner, it usually requires time on the part of a family to adjust to the reality of the situation. It is recommended that an ethics consult be obtained in these difficult situations, after all other approaches by the family have proven unsuccessful. Rarely, a legal approach may be necessary in the case of intransigent or belligerent families where consensus simply cannot be reached.

12.15 Conclusions

Intensive care has become increasingly complex and technology-driven, such that it has become a multidisciplinary specialty in its own right. While most surgeons enjoy the challenge of managing their own patients through the period of their critical illness, it is clear that a dedicated critical care service is necessary to provide the minute-to-minute care that these patients require. A thorough and up-to-date knowledge of the medical literature is also vital. These are the sickest patients in the hospital, and the most demanding of our attention, but the rewards are immense whether it is saving a life or helping a family come to terms with the death of their loved one. There is no better reward than to meet a patient who returns to the ICU many months after their illness, walking tall and fully recovered from their critical illness.

Important Points

- PA catheters can be safely omitted in most patients.
- Avoid benzodiazepines as drips.
- Low tidal volume ventilation for ARDS.
- Do daily spontaneous breathing trials to assess patients for extubation.

- Early enteral feeding should be started whenever possible.
- Dopamine and Lasix do not help renal failure.
- Aim for a target glucose of less than 180 mg/dL.
- Keep Hgb 7–9 mg/dL.
- The INR of FFP is 1.3–1.4 – you cannot correct lower than this using FFP.
- Get central lines out as quickly as possible.
- Not every patient needs an H2-blocker.
- Treating the family is an important part of ICU care.

References

1. American College of Chest Physicians/Society of Critical Care Medicine (1992) Consensus conference: definitions for sepsis and organ failure and guidelines for the use of innovative therapies in sepsis. Crit Care Med 20:864–874
2. Friese RS, Shafi S, Gentilello LM (2006) Pulmonary artery catheter use is associated with reduced mortality in severely injured patients: a National Trauma Data Bank analysis of 53,312 patients. Crit Care Med 34:1597–1601
3. Wheeler AP, Bernard GR, Thompson BT et al (2006) Pulmonary-artery versus central venous catheter to guide treatment of acute lung injury. N Engl J Med 354:2213–2224
4. Habashi NM (2005) Other approaches to open-lung ventilation: airway pressure release ventilation. Crit Care Med 33:S228–S240
5. Martin M, Salim A, Murray J, Demetriades D, Belzberg H, Rhee P (2005) The decreasing incidence and mortality of acute respiratory distress syndrome after injury: a 5-year observational study. J Trauma 59:1107–1113
6. van den Berghe G, Wouters P, Weekers F et al (2001) Intensive insulin therapy in the critically ill patients. N Engl J Med 345:1359–1367
7. Finfer S, Chittock DR, Su SY et al (2009) Intensive versus conventional glucose control in critically ill patients. N Engl J Med 360:1283–1297
8. Annane D, Sebille V, Charpentier C et al (2002) Effect of treatment with low doses of hydrocortisone and fludrocortisone on vmortality in patients with septic shock. JAMA 288:862–871
9. Sprung CL, Annane D, Keh D et al (2008) Hydrocortisone therapy for patients with septic shock. N Engl J Med 358:111–124
10. Dellinger RP, Levy MM, Carlet JM et al (2008) Surviving Sepsis Campaign: international guidelines for management of severe sepsis and septic shock: 2008. Crit Care Med 36: 296–327
11. Duchesne JC, Islam TM, Stuke L et al (2009) Hemostatic resuscitation during surgery improves survival in patients with traumatic-induced coagulopathy. J Trauma 67:33–37; discussion 7–9
12. Leone M, Bourgoin A, Cambon S, Dubuc M, Albanese J, Martin C (2003) Empirical antimicrobial therapy of septic shock patients: adequacy and impact on the outcome. Crit Care Med 31:462–467
13. Kumar A, Roberts D, Wood KE et al (2006) Duration of hypotension before initiation of effective antimicrobial therapy is the critical determinant of survival in human septic shock. Crit Care Med 34:1589–1596
14. Namias N, Harvill S, Ball S et al (1998) Empiric therapy of sepsis in the surgical intensive care unit with broad-spectrum antibiotics for 72 hours does not lead to the emergence of resistant bacteria. J Trauma 45:887–891
15. Dezfulian C, Shojania K, Collard HR, Kim HM, Matthay MA, Saint S (2005) Subglottic secretion drainage for preventing ventilator-associated pneumonia: a meta-analysis. Am J Med 118:11–18
16. Kollef MH, Afessa B, Anzueto A et al (2008) Silver-coated endotracheal tubes and incidence of ventilator-associated pneumonia: the NASCENT randomized trial. JAMA 300: 805–813
17. Pronovost P, Needham D, Berenholtz S et al (2006) An intervention to decrease catheter-related bloodstream infections in the ICU. N Engl J Med 355:2725–2732
18. Ciesla MFDJ, Moore EE (2008) Multiple organ failure. In: Feliciano M, Moore EE (eds) Trauma, 6th edn. McGraw Hill, New York, pp 1359–1380
19. Ciesla DJ, Moore EE, Johnson JL, Burch JM, Cothren CC, Sauaia A (2005) A 12-year prospective study of postinjury multiple organ failure: has anything changed? Arch Surg 140:432–438; discussion 8–40
20. Cohn SM, Nathens AB, Moore FA et al (2007) Tissue oxygen saturation predicts the development of organ dysfunction during traumatic shock resuscitation. J Trauma 62: 44–54; discussion 5
21. Chevron V, Menard JF, Richard JC, Girault C, Leroy J, Bonmarchand G (1998) Unplanned extubation: risk factors of development and predictive criteria for reintubation. Crit Care Med 26:1049–1053
22. Boulain T (1998) Unplanned extubations in the adult intensive care unit: a prospective multicenter study. Association des Reanimateurs du Centre-Ouest. Am J Respir Crit Care Med 157:1131–1137

Plain X-Rays for Penetrating Trauma

13

Marko Bukur and Donald J. Green

With the advent of new and sophisticated imaging technology, one may rightfully question whether there is still a role for conventional radiography in penetrating injuries. Though there is no question that advanced imaging provides superior resolution and diagnostic capability, there is still great utility in using plain x-rays for rapid assessment of penetrating injuries. Despite the limitations of x-rays, they can provide a wealth of rapid information to those experienced in their interpretation. We have presented several scenarios in which plain film imaging can be used for the initial evaluation in the patient sustaining penetrating trauma. In conjunction with physical examination, conventional radiography allows for more judicious use of adjunctive imaging studies, which in turn can reduce health care costs and resource utilization.

M. Bukur
Division of Trauma and Surgical Critical Care, Department of Surgery, Cedars-Sinai Medical Center, 8635 West Third Street, Suite 650, Los Angeles, CA 90048, USA

D.J. Green (✉)
Department of Surgery, University of Arizona, 1501 N Campbell Ave, Tucson, AZ 85724, USA
e-mail: azsurg@gmail.com

13.1 Plain X-Rays for Penetrating Trauma

With the advent of new and sophisticated imaging technology, one may rightfully question whether there is still a role for conventional radiography in penetrating injuries. Rapid, helical, multi-slice computed tomography is readily available and steps away from the resuscitation bay. Its "routine" use has been adopted as protocol in many centers, including our own [1]. Though there is no question that advanced imaging provides superior resolution and diagnostic capability, there is still great utility in using plain x-rays for rapid assessment of penetrating injuries.

13.2 Rationale for the "Plain Film"

You should become facile with interpretation of plain diagnostic x-rays for a multitude of reasons. Adjunctive imaging studies are readily available in most civilian centers, but may be unavailable in more austere environments, and subject to technical failures. Additionally, patients in critical condition after sustaining penetrating injury are not the ideal candidates to be transported away from the resuscitation bay. The infamous "death in CT Scan" is a topic that is typically "hotly" debated in the Morbidity and Mortality session and one that is best avoided. The "plain film" may be the only feasible study in a decompensating patient. Furthermore, screening of asymptomatic patients with diagnostic x-rays has been shown to decrease time spent in the Emergency Department [2], provide substantial cost savings to the patient and institution [3], and decrease the amount of

G.C. Velmahos et al. (eds.), *Penetrating Trauma*,
DOI 10.1007/978-3-642-20453-1_13, © Springer-Verlag Berlin Heidelberg 2012

radiation exposure to those that do not require further workup [3].

13.3 Limitations of "Plain Film" Imaging

With the aforementioned advantages in mind, you must also acknowledge some limitations with conventional x-rays. The portable chest x-ray is the most common image acquired in the trauma patient. The trauma patient is often in a supine or semi-recumbent position when films are acquired. This image is taken as a single anteroposterior (AP) view that can produce pseudo-cardiomegaly, mediastinal enlargement, and deceiving increases in pulmonary vascularity [4]. In abdominal images, the AP view cannot distinguish superimposed soft tissue/bony structures from underlying viscera. Additionally, since the x-ray beam is perpendicular in orientation to the bowel, air-fluid levels are not well demonstrated. Abdominal and upright x-rays are also highly variable in their accuracy to diagnose free intraperitoneal air [5, 6]. In addition, radiographs only provide imaging in one dimension. At least two (sometimes more!) views are needed to present anatomical information in two dimensions. Despite these limitations, when analyzed appropriately by an experienced clinician, plain films can be invaluable with respect to the information they readily provide.

13.4 Chest Radiography

Thoracic injuries account for a significant number of traumatic deaths [7]. Penetrating injuries to the thorax account for 4–15% of admissions to major civilian trauma centers [8]. A high percentage of these patients will have injuries involving the chest wall, pleura, or lung that are identifiable on chest x-ray. The portable chest radiograph is the screening test for the majority of patients with penetrating thoracic trauma. It allows for detection of major life-threatening thoracic injuries and can assist in triage of these patients. We will discuss the utility of thoracic plain films as well as imaging findings for specific injuries in the sections that follow.

13.4.1 Soft Tissues and Bony Thorax

Subcutaneous hematomas present as nonspecific radiodense opacities overlying the chest wall due to blood accumulation in the soft tissues. This can result from damage to muscular structures, underlying rib fractures or thoracic vessels themselves. Foreign bodies (either a missile or other sharp object) can also be present after becoming lodged in the soft tissue.

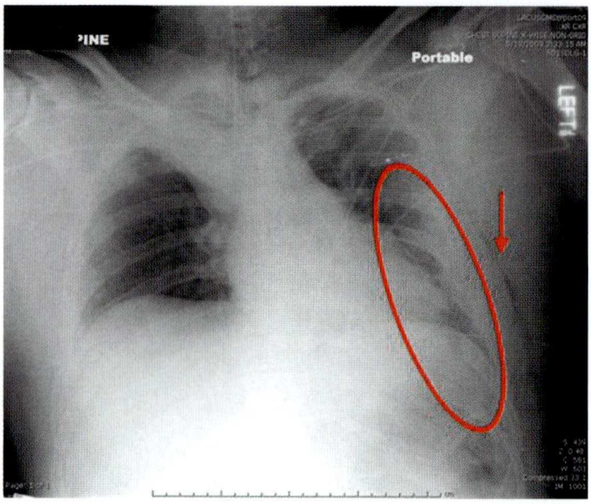

Fig. 13.1 Image of a left flail chest (*red ellipse*) with associated subcutaneous emphysema (*red arrow*)

Rib fractures are the most common injury identified on the x-ray (Fig. 13.1) and are important to identify clinically since they are markers for other pleural and parenchymal findings [9]. Once a rib fracture is found in the penetrating setting, you should also suspect and vigilantly look for a possible hemothorax, pneumothorax, or pulmonary contusion as the sharp edges may cause damage to the underlying intercostal vessels or lung parenchyma.

Soft tissue emphysema is another common abnormality that is often identified on radiographic imaging (Figs. 13.1 and 13.2). The presence of soft tissue gas should alert you to look for additional intrathoracic pathology. The most common scenario is subcutaneous air with ipsilateral rib fractures. This constellation of findings should be presumed to signify a pneumothorax, even if not readily identifiable on the radiograph.

13.4.2 Pleura and Lung Parenchyma

Pneumothoraces are common complications after penetrating thoracic injury and occur secondary to disruption of the alveoli and lung parenchyma leading to leakage of gas into the interstitial space. The most

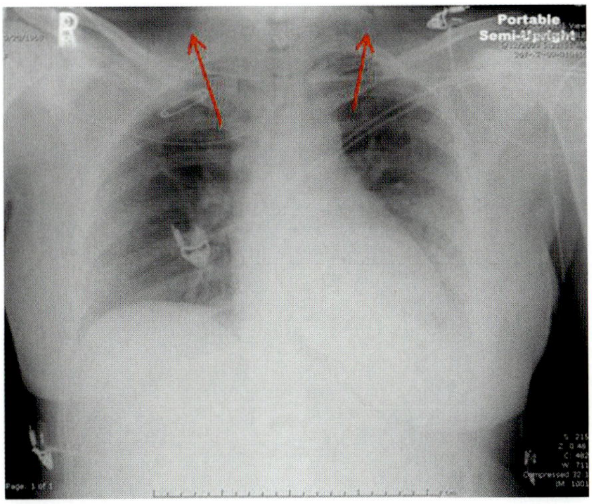

Fig. 13.2 Subcutaneous emphysema (*red arrows*) in a patient with no other radiographic findings

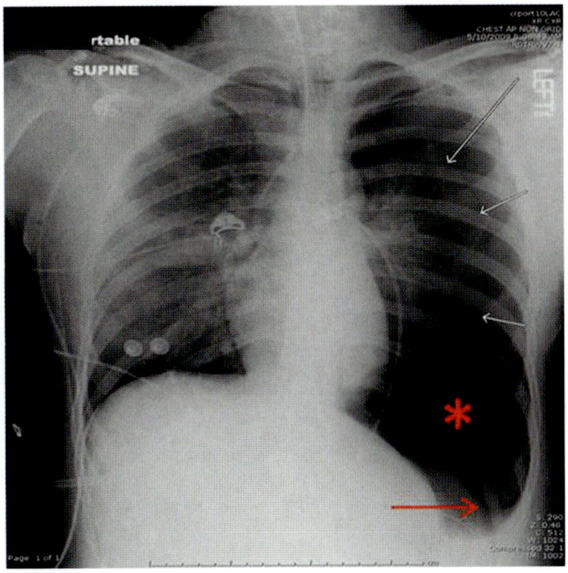

Fig. 13.3 Image of a large left pneumothorax after line placement. Visceral-pleural line clearly seen (*white arrows*), with a hyperlucent upper abdomen (*red asterisk*), and deep sulcus sign (*red arrow*)

frequent radiographic finding is the "visceral-pleural line" (Fig. 13.3) in the apical-lateral lung field representing separation of the normally apposed visceral and parietal pleura. Pneumomediastinum is also frequently encountered, and is most commonly due to pulmonary-alveolar rupture [9]. These radiographic signs can vary from subtle findings to gross abnormalities. Trauma patients are often in the supine or semi-recumbent position when the portable chest x-ray is acquired. In these positions, it has been reported that up to 30% of pneumothoraces are not visualized [10]. Patient positioning can be changed to increase radiographic sensitivity but is often not feasible in the trauma setting. Instead you should be aware of other places that the pneumothorax may be visualized, namely the antero-medial and subpulmonic recesses (Fig. 13.4). Other less common imaging findings present with a pneumothorax include: a hyperlucent upper abdomen, sharply demarcated diaphragm, demarcation of the inferior surface of the lung, and the "deep sulcus sign" [9] (Fig. 13.3).

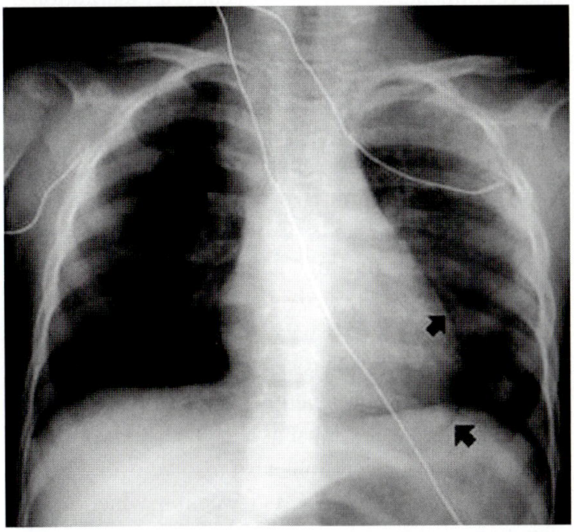

Fig. 13.4 Subtle anterior pneumothorax in antero-medial (*superior black arrowhead*) and subpulmonic (*inferior black arrowhead*) recesses

Hemothorax is another common pleural abnormality after penetrating trauma. The source of bleeding may be from the chest wall, intercostal arteries, internal mammary arteries, lung parenchyma, heart, or mediastinal vessels. Typically, a volume of 200–300 mL is necessary to be picked up on conventional chest x-ray. These radiographic findings are due to radiodense blood collecting in the pleural space. Presentation may vary from an opacified hemothorax (Fig. 13.5) to a subtle blunting of the involved costo-phrenic recess. Because blood serves as an excellent culture medium for bacteria, drainage is important for significant collections. Often after tube thoracostomy, "follow-up" chest x-rays are obtained daily to judge adequacy of drainage. We caution against this practice as they are often misleading in determining the amount of residual blood in the thoracic cavity. Computerized tomography is much more accurate in evaluating which patients

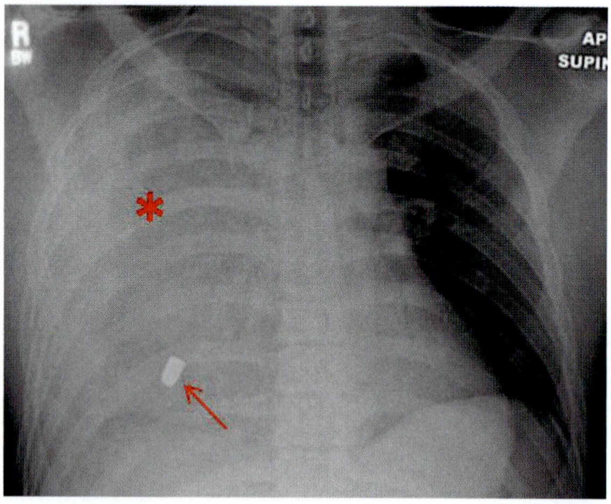

Fig. 13.5 Large right hemothorax (*red asterisk*) after penetrating trauma (*red arrow*)

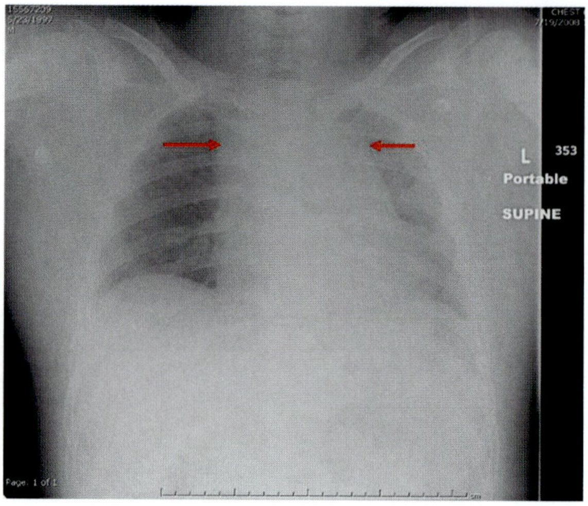

Fig. 13.6 Widened mediastinum (*red arrows*) after penetrating injury to thorax

will require further evacuation and has been proven in a prospective trial [11].

Parenchymal injuries to the lung itself are also regular findings on chest radiography after penetrating injury. Pulmonary contusions occur after disruption of the alveolar capillaries and interstitial blood vessels along the tract of injury. This leads to hemorrhage into the surrounding lung tissue and edema. Contusions appear as "ground glass" peripheral air space opacities, which may not be apparent on the initial radiograph [4]. These infiltrates typically develop within 6 h of injury and begin to resolve over the next several days [12]. Contusions may take up to 2 weeks to completely clear from the patients chest x-ray. Pulmonary lacerations often may have the same radiographic appearance as contusions. However, blood may fill a laceration cavity incompletely, resulting in a clot with a small air crescent known as the "air-meniscus" sign [12]. Pulmonary lacerations also resolve over a longer period of time (generally 3–5 weeks), which allows them to be distinguished from contusions radiographically [12].

13.4.3 Mediastinum

Cardiac injuries are difficult to diagnose on plain films, but can be associated with subtle imaging findings. Irregular convexities of the heart border or marked shift of the cardiac silhouette can signify underlying heart injury or cardiac herniation [4]. A globally enlarged heart ("water-bottle" sign) can signify a pericardial effusion in rare cases.

Great vessel injury is predominantly secondary to penetrating injury and often presents as a widened mediastinum (>8 cm) on chest x-ray (Fig. 13.6). Rather than pulling out a measuring tape, a quick method that we find useful is to hold a pager longitudinally across the mediastinum to see if its diameter is greater than that of the pager. The differential diagnosis for a widened mediastinum should also include sternal fracture, thoracic vertebral fracture, or ligamentous injury. Other abnormalities that may be encountered with great vessel injury include the apical cap, loss of aortic contour, tracheal/esophageal deviation to the right, depression of the left main stem bronchus, or a left pleural effusion. The accuracy of chest x-ray for screening for aortic/great vessel injury has been called into question since the advent of multi-slice computed tomography (CT). At our own institution, we found that liberal use of chest CT did not disclose an increased incidence of aortic injury in the blunt setting, but in those with high ISS (>27) and other significant other injuries (i.e., pelvic fracture), chest x-ray was inadequate in 13.9% [1]. It is difficult to extrapolate this data to those with penetrating injury. A single center experience with penetrating trauma to upper thorax was able to retrospectively validate the use of clinical exam and chest radiography in accurately excluding great vessel injury in those with negative clinical and radiologic exams [13]. However, if you are suspicious of major vascular injury based upon trajectory (i.e., transmediastinal) or physical examination, then there is no question that additional imaging is necessary in the hemodynamically stable patient [14].

Tracheo-bronchial injuries occur almost twice as commonly in the blunt setting compared to penetrating trauma. Early radiographic findings may include subcutaneous emphysema, pneumothorax, or pneumomediastinum. Classic radiographic signs (albeit rare) associated with tracheo-bronchial injury include the "double wall" sign that occurs secondary to intra-mural gas in the proximal transected airway, and the "fallen lung" sign associated with inferior lung collapse [9]. More commonly encountered findings clinically are: increasing soft tissue emphysema and persisting/enlarging pneumothorax despite adequate tube thoracostomy drainage (often with a large continuous air leak). Occasionally, frank herniation of the endotracheal tube through the tracheal defect may occur.

Esophageal injuries secondary to trauma account for 10–20% of all injuries [15]. An injury tract traversing the mediastinum should make one suspicious for aero-digestive injury. The most common findings on plain films include cervical emphysema, pneumomediastinum, and a left pleural effusion. Contrast esophagography under conventional fluoroscopy is the confirmatory test of choice.

13.4.4 The Asymptomatic Patient

We have presented multiple injury scenarios in the preceding paragraphs, but what about the asymptomatic patient who has just sustained a penetrating injury to the thorax? Up to 60% of civilian penetrating thoracic injuries are asymptomatic and have normal chest x-rays upon presentation [16]. Delayed complications after penetrating chest x-ray such as hemo/pneumothorax are well known and occur in 8–12% of patients [17]. There is general agreement that these asymptomatic patients typically only require observation with repeat chest radiography. A recent prospective trial found that there was no increased incidence of delayed injury when shortening the period of observation and repeat chest x-ray from 12 to 3 h [3]. We agree with and strongly recommend this policy in the asymptomatic patient. This change in management has the potential to reduce crowding in the emergency room, decrease patient radiation exposure, and improve patient compliance.

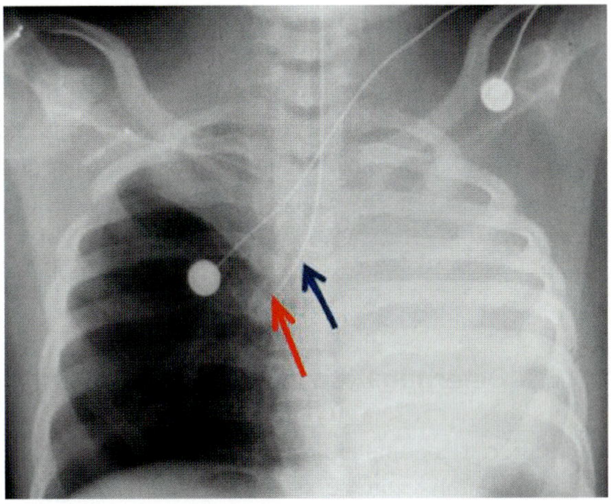

Fig. 13.7 Right mainstem intubation (*blue arrow*) with the tip of the endotracheal tube terminating at the bronchus intermedius (*red arrow*)

13.4.5 Iatrogenesis Imperfecta

One of the greatest utilities of chest radiography is to evaluate therapeutic interventions in a rapid manner. No chest radiograph is completely evaluated unless all tubes and catheters placed into the patient have been accounted for and found to be in the appropriate position. The laundry list includes: endotracheal tubes, nasogastric tubes, thoracostomy tubes, and central venous catheters. The endotracheal tube should terminate approximately 2–3 cm above the carina. When haphazardly placed, it is often in the right main stem bronchus (1–6%) (Fig. 13.7) or an esophageal intubation (4–8%) [9]. Often incorrect positioning of the endotracheal tube is identified on the first chest radiograph after the intervention [18]. These abnormal tube positions must be identified quickly to avoid adverse clinical outcomes. Nasogastric tube position can also be validated on chest x-ray. This is particularly important if there is no return of gastric contents after placement or there is concern over potential airway or pleural placement. Chest tubes are notorious for incorrect placement by inexperienced operators. Common errors include: subcutaneous placement, placement against mediastinal structures, through the lung parenchyma, or through the diaphragm itself. Once erroneous placement is identified, the tube should be repositioned or removed. If there is doubt over whether the tube is intra-parenchymal or trans-diaphragmatic, additional imaging can be of assistance.

13.5 Abdominal Radiography

Though less frequently utilized than chest x-ray, there are select indications in which plain abdominal films may be useful in guiding further diagnostics after penetrating injuries. This is especially true since the acceptance of selective nonoperative management of penetrating abdominal wounds.

13.5.1 Determination of Trajectory

In addition to a complete physical examination, plain abdominal films can be useful in determining the approximate trajectory of a missile. A common practice is to mark the external surface wounds with a radio-opaque marker (i.e., paper-clip or EKG lead) and obtain a two-image series of the abdomen. This will allow one to determine the relative tract of the missile by aligning the surface markers with projectiles. Abdominal films can also be helpful in suspected tangential injuries to the abdominal wall. This should never be assumed as fact since this may represent two separate deep wounds with vastly differing trajectories. Another useful tip to remember is that the sum of surface wounds plus projectiles must equal an even number. If this is not the case, a redirected physical exam paying close attention to evaluation of the axillae, inguinal region, and perineum is advised, as these are areas that are frequently overlooked. If repeat physical examination is unremarkable, the patient may be a "victim" of trauma recidivism or require additional imaging to rule out embolism.

13.5.2 Diaphragmatic Injury

Though penetrating injury to the diaphragm is less frequent than blunt injuries, the radiographic diagnosis is similar. Chest and abdominal radiographs are highly variable in their diagnostic accuracy of diaphragmatic injury (28–70%) [9]. Serial plain film imaging may increase this yield an additional 12% [19]. Findings consistent with injury include: asymmetric elevation of hemi-diaphragm, herniation of abdominal contents into the chest, or opacification of the lower lung field with diaphragm asymmetry (Fig. 13.8). Due to the low yield of plain film imaging, we cannot recommend plain radiographs as a screening test. Patients with penetrating left-sided thoracoabdominal trauma at our institution are initially observed if asymptomatic and offered diagnostic laparoscopy prior to discharge to definitively exclude diaphragmatic injury.

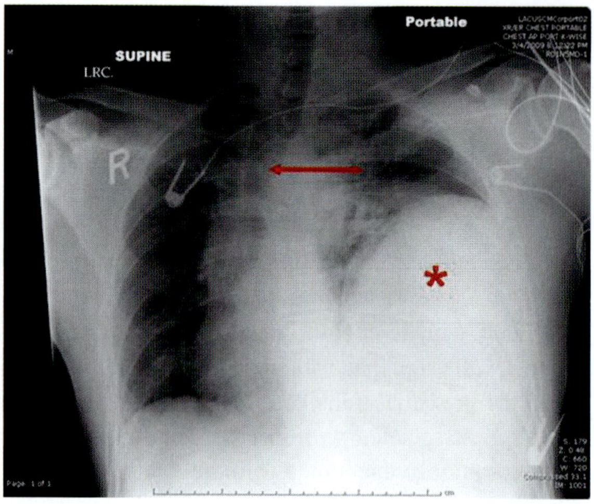

Fig. 13.8 Chest X-ray consistent with diaphragmatic injury. Opacification of the left hemi-thorax with abdominal contents (*red asterisk*) and deviation of mediastinal structures to the right (*red arrow*)

13.6 Missile Embolism

Missile injury is secondary to the kinetic energy released as it passes through the human body. Rarely does a projectile enter the vascular tree and embolize through the body to a site remote from the initial injury. Only 200 cases of missile embolus have been reported in the literature since 1900 [20]. The vast majority of missile embolism cases are from civilian low-caliber weapons [21]. This diagnosis should be considered in patients in whom the sum of surface wounds plus intracavitary foreign bodies is equal to an odd number or in those with missiles in obscure locations. Plain films of the trunk and extremities (Fig. 13.9) can assist in making the diagnosis and result in less radiation exposure than total body fluoroscopy or computed tomography. Once the missile is identified on plain film imaging, additional diagnostic tests can be performed to plan removal as indicated.

Despite the limitations of x-rays, they can provide a wealth of rapid information to those experienced in their interpretation. We have presented several scenarios in

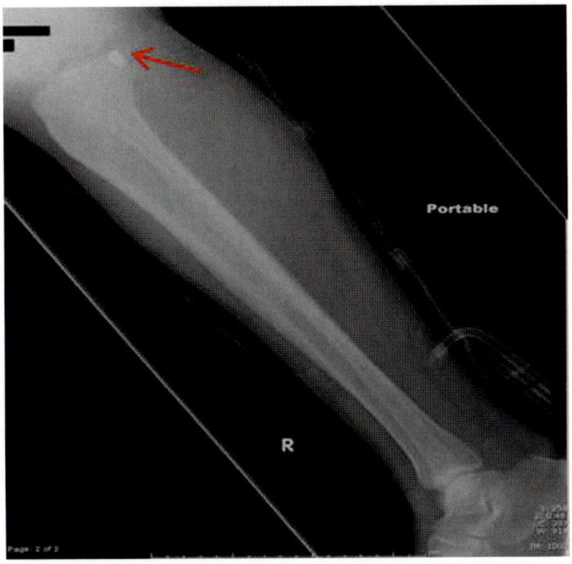

Fig. 13.9 Missile embolism into left popliteal vein (*red arrow*) secondary to a penetrating injury to the inferior vena cava

which plain film imaging can be used for the initial evaluation in the patient sustaining penetrating trauma. In conjunction with physical examination, conventional radiography allows for more judicious use of adjunctive imaging studies, which in turn can reduce health care costs and resource utilization. We hope that this review has enhanced your armamentarium of knowledge for care of the injured patient. After all, you never know when the "scanner" is going to be out-of-service.

Important Points

- Radiographs have their limitations; learn them, because there is no substitute for the quick diagnostic information provided in the unstable patient.
- Subcutaneous Emphysema + Rib Fractures = Pneumothorax (Even if you cannot see it!)
- If you find one injury on a chest X-ray, suspect and look for another.
- Remember to check the subpulmonic and antero-medial recesses on the portable chest film. This is where a pneumothorax may hide.
- The most common cause of pneumomediastinum is a pneumothorax.
- Do not rely on an x-ray to assess drainage of a hemothorax.
- The differential diagnosis for a widened mediastinum is broad, but only one of them can kill your patient.
- Three hours is enough time to wait to repeat a chest film in an asymptomatic patient with penetrating chest trauma.
- Check the position of all tubes and lines that are placed into your patients.
- X-rays are the cheapest and least radioactive way to screen for missile embolism.

References

1. Plurad D et al (2007) The increasing use of chest computed tomography for trauma: is it being overutilized? J Trauma 62(3):631–635
2. Spaite DW (2006) The future of emergency care in the United States: the Institute of Medicine Subcommittee on Prehospital Emergency Medical Services. Ann Emerg Med 48(2):126–130
3. Seamon MJ et al (2008) Follow-up after asymptomatic penetrating thoracic injury: 3 hours is enough. J Trauma 65(3): 549–553
4. Ho ML, Gutierrez FR (2009) Chest radiography in thoracic polytrauma. AJR Am J Roentgenol 192(3):599–612
5. Stapakis JC, Thickman D (1992) Diagnosis of pneumoperitoneum: abdominal CT vs. upright chest film. J Comput Assist Tomogr 16(5):713–716
6. Woodring JH, Heiser MJ (1995) Detection of pneumoperitoneum on chest radiographs: comparison of upright lateral and posteroanterior projections. AJR Am J Roentgenol 165(1):45–47
7. Tocino I, Miller MH (1987) Computed tomography in blunt chest trauma. J Thorac Imaging 2(3):45–59
8. von Oppell UO, Bautz P, De Groot M (2000) Penetrating thoracic injuries: what we have learnt. Thorac Cardiovasc Surg 48(1):55–61
9. Costantino M, Gosselin MV, Primack SL (2006) The ABC's of thoracic trauma imaging. Semin Roentgenol 41(3): 209–225
10. Tocino IM, Miller MH, Fairfax WR (1985) Distribution of pneumothorax in the supine and semirecumbent critically ill adult. AJR Am J Roentgenol 144(5):901–905
11. Velmahos GC et al (1999) Predicting the need for thoracoscopic evacuation of residual traumatic hemothorax: chest radiograph is insufficient. J Trauma 46(1):65–70
12. Shanmuganathan K, Matsumoto J (2006) Imaging of penetrating chest trauma. Radiol Clin North Am 44(2):225–238
13. Gasparri MG et al (2000) Physical examination plus chest radiography in penetrating periclavicular trauma: the appropriate trigger for angiography. J Trauma 49(6):1029–1033
14. Hanpeter DE et al (2000) Helical computed tomographic scan in the evaluation of mediastinal gunshot wounds. J Trauma 49(4):689–695

15. Jones WG II, Ginsberg RJ (1992) Esophageal perforation: a continuing challenge. Ann Thorac Surg 53(3):534–543
16. Kerr TM et al (1989) Prospective trial of the six hour rule in stab wounds of the chest. Surg Gynecol Obstet 169(3): 223–225
17. Shatz DV et al (2001) Efficacy of follow-up evaluation in penetrating thoracic injuries: 3- vs. 6-hour radiographs of the chest. J Emerg Med 20(3):281–284
18. Omert L et al (2001) Role of the emergency medicine physician in airway management of the trauma patient. J Trauma 51(6):1065–1068
19. Rodriguez-Morales G, Rodriguez A, Shatney CH (1986) Acute rupture of the diaphragm in blunt trauma: analysis of 60 patients. J Trauma 26(5):438–444
20. Bertoldo U et al (2004) Retrograde venous bullet embolism: a rare occurrence-case report and literature review. J Trauma 57(1):187–192
21. Michelassi F et al (1990) Bullet emboli to the systemic and venous circulation. Surgery 107(3):239–245

14 Computed Tomography in the Workup of Patients with Penetrating Trauma

Mark E. Hamill

Penetrating trauma presents one area where operative management has long been considered the gold standard of care. When presented with a patent who has been the victim of a penetrating injury, physiologic status often dictates the need for rapid operative exploration with the goal of control of active hemorrhage and contamination from hollow viscus injuries. Certainly no qualified surgeon, when faced with a victim of penetrating trauma who is hemodynamically unstable with active hemorrhage or evidence of peritonitis, would seriously argue to undertake an extensive radiological workup. However, when faced with the stable patient, there is evolving evidence that information obtained from newer generation computed tomography (CT) scanners, augmented with contrast to allow for CT Angiography, can be valuable in guiding further care and limiting nontherapeutic operative exploration. While historically not typically considered an area of major concern, these nontherapeutic explorations can be a significant source of morbidity and mortality as well as dramatically increasing the length of stay and overall cost [1]. This chapter will examine some of the available evidence with regard to various anatomic locations and provide some guidelines for the appropriate use of CT imaging in the workup of the stable patient with penetrating trauma. Specifically we will examine its use in the workup of penetrating injuries to the abdomen, back and flank, thorax, neck, and extremities.

M.E. Hamill
Department of Surgery, State University of New York
Upstate Medical University, 750 East Adams Street,
Syracuse 13210, NY, USA
e-mail: hamillm@mac.com, hamillm@upstate.edu

14.1 Abdomen

When faced with the workup of a patient with penetrating injuries to the abdomen, it is essential to consider all available information and resources available. In the stable patient without evidence of peritonitis, many centers have explored nonoperative management in patients injured with low-energy edged weapons and, more recently, those with higher-energy injuries caused by gunshot wounds. The first consideration, of course, is determining the need for any advanced imaging. In a small series, it was shown that in patients with abdominal stab wounds and confirmed peritoneal penetration by local wound exploration, physical exam, when combined with a variety of diagnostic and imaging modalities, allowed nonoperative management of 79% of patients [2]. Another study examining the use of serial physical examinations in patients with abdominal stab wounds demonstrated successful nonoperative management in 89% of patients without indication for laparotomy at presentation [3]. However, it should be noted that in this group, no attempts were made to determine peritoneal penetration. A variety of imaging modalities including conventional radiography and ultrasound have been examined specifically to determine their usefulness in evaluating patient with penetrating trauma. Overall their roles are likely limited due to their relatively low sensitivity in determining the need for further intervention or laparotomy [4–6].

In penetrating abdominal trauma with both low-energy mechanisms (such as stab wounds) as well as higher-energy mechanisms (gunshot wounds), multiple institutions have evaluated the use of CT scan in the workup of patients without obvious indication for immediate laparotomy. Initially, these studies were

G.C. Velmahos et al. (eds.), *Penetrating Trauma*,
DOI 10.1007/978-3-642-20453-1_14, © Springer-Verlag Berlin Heidelberg 2012

aimed at the determination of peritoneal penetration with subsequent operative exploration if the peritoneum had been violated. Several studies, both retrospective and prospective in nature, have demonstrated a high sensitivity, specificity and negative predictive value for CT imaging to determine peritoneal penetration [7, 8]. While IV contrast was used in all studies, the use of Triple Contrast – IV, oral and rectal – did improve the specificity [8, 9]. However, a recent review of single contrast CT imaging, using IV contrast alone, demonstrated a high sensitivity in predicting the need for laparotomy in penetrating trauma, highest in patients with gunshot wounds [10].

When considering abdominal stab wounds, there is a large amount of data supporting the increasing use of nonoperative management of stable patients. Certainly local wound exploration is an important part of any treatment algorithm. If it can be definitively determined that peritoneal penetration has not occurred, the patient can often be safely discharged directly from the emergency department. However, once peritoneal penetration has been established, the issue is somewhat less clear. Multiple protocols have been suggested including serial abdominal exams, imaging followed by serial abdominal exams, serial abdominal exams and laboratory analysis and selective imaging. Evidence exists that contrast-enhanced CT scans can reliably demonstrate the likely absence of injury requiring laparotomy [11]. A recent US multicenter trial clearly demonstrated that once peritoneal penetration has been established, nonoperative management has a definite role. Abdominal CT scan was used in decision making in half of the patients. Their conclusions support the use of CT imaging, though not as the sole determinant for the need for laparotomy [12].

Abdominal gunshot wounds represent an area of even greater controversy. Given the increased energy involved, the relative risk of significant injury is somewhat higher than with wounds involving edged weapons. However, a subset of patients can clearly tolerate and even benefit from nonoperative management. Initial reports used serial exams primarily, with the adjunctive use of DPL and radiographic imaging [13]. Others have demonstrated that CT imaging can reliably demonstrate the need for laparotomy with a negative predictive value of 95% [14]. Another larger prospective study clearly demonstrated the usefulness of CT scan in the evaluation of patients selected for nonoperative management, with a resulting high sensitivity and specificity [15]. It is important to note that in this study, patients with tangential wounds were completely excluded and only 38% of patients presenting with abdominal gunshot wounds were considered eligible for nonoperative management. CT imaging has been demonstrated to be useful in determining missile trajectory, as well as the likelihood of organ or vascular injury [16]. One important word of caution regarding this approach – if higher power firearms are involved, especially modern military rifles, the possibility of blast effect and resulting hydrostatic pressure causing intraperitoneal injury exists even with a tangential wound and the absence of peritoneal penetration [17].

One subset of patients with penetrating abdominal trauma deserves a special mention – those with isolated solid organ injury identified on abdominal imaging. Looking specifically at penetrating abdominal trauma, both retrospective and prospective data have demonstrated that in the hemodynamically stable patient without peritonitis in whom isolated wounds to solid organs are identified by CT scan, most can be safely managed nonoperatively with observation [18, 19]. An added benefit in nonoperative management was the rapid identification via CT imaging of patients who would benefit for angiographic treatment of solid organ hemorrhage. Additionally, nonoperative management led to an overall decrease in the length of stay, even in the face of more serious injuries.

The issue of penetrating abdominal trauma has recently been addressed by the Eastern Association for the Surgery of Trauma. In the practice management guideline for Selective Nonoperative Management of Penetrating Abdominal Trauma, a recommendation was made that abdominopelvic CT scan be strongly considered as a diagnostic tool to facilitate initial management decisions [20].

A patient presenting with hemodynamic instability or peritonitis after penetrating injury clearly requires emergent operative intervention. However, just as clear is the increasing role for nonoperative management in the stable patient. In the stable patient, with an abdominal stab wound, nonoperative intervention is clearly an option, especially with a CT scan that is suggestive of no injury. One possible exception is a patient with a wound which places them at risk for a diaphragm injury; these patients would probably benefit from diagnostic laparoscopy to exclude this injury. Gunshot wounds are another matter. My personal bias is to have a low threshold for operative intervention for abdominal gunshot wounds given the tremendous energy transfer that can take place and sometimes unpredictable missile path. However, in the completely stable patient with a benign abdominal exam, CT imaging can prove to be an extremely useful adjunct if nonoperative management is being considered.

14.2 Back and Flank

Penetrating injuries to the flank and back present a especially difficult diagnostic challenge. It has been clearly noted that, overall, these mechanisms have a low risk for injury requiring surgical intervention [21]. However, due to the anatomic considerations involved, diagnosis of these rare injuries may be significantly delayed with subsequent increase in morbidity and mortality. Modalities such as diagnostic peritoneal lavage and laparoscopy offer limited usefulness, as the main concern is injury to retroperitoneal structures. Since the 1980s, CT scan, enhanced by the administration of contrast to ensure opacification of the colon and other retroperitoneal structures, has been demonstrated to be a safe, reliable, and effective method to rule out significant injuries due to back or flank stab wounds [22–24]. The use of the "triple contrast CT" allows for rapid identification of those patients with injury, as well more rapid discharge of those without and clinically significant trauma [25–27].

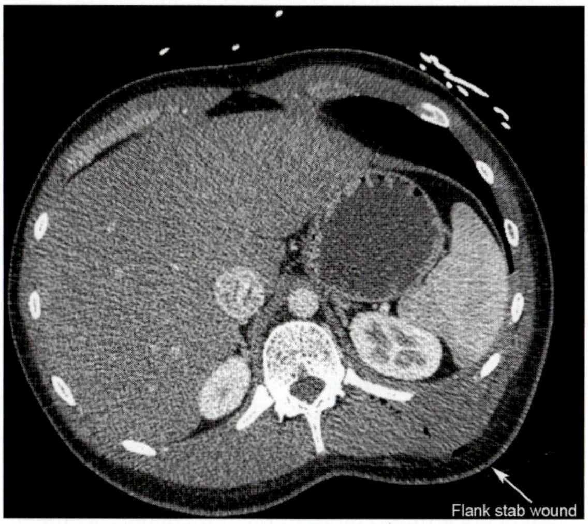

Fig. 14.1 Stab wound to the left back without intraperitoneal or retroperitoneal penetration

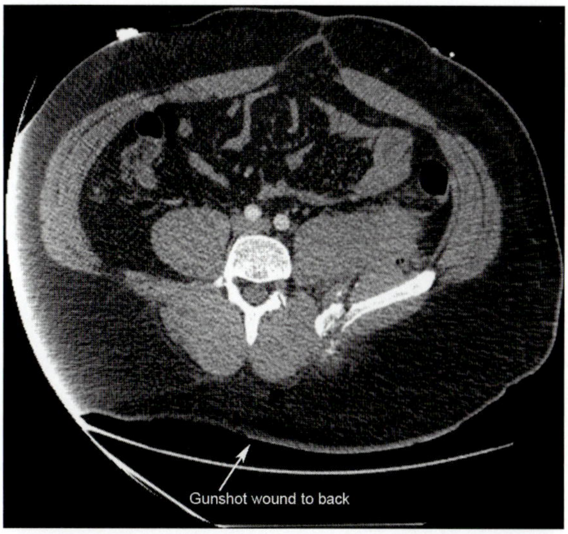

Fig. 14.2 Gunshot wound to back with evidence of intraperitoneal penetration. Patient found to have multiple enterotomies at laparotomy

It should be noted, however, that the same potential issue regarding high-energy firearms exists in penetrating gunshot wounds to the back and flank. A clinician should have a high index of suspicion for occult injury with bowel wall contusion and potential late presentation of injury in cases where the weapon used is of an especially high-energy one, such as a military or large game rifle. In these cases, significant injury can occur even with the absence of direct bowel penetration and with tangential missile paths. With these injuries, it is reasonable that, at the very minimum, the patient be observed for up to 24 h and further investigation be undertaken as dictated by the patient's clinical status [28].

14.3 Thorax

Penetrating injuries to thorax represent a critical diagnostic dilemma. While certain presentations such as massive hemothorax or ongoing bleeding mandate rapid operative exploration, the large majority of injuries can be managed by simple tube thoracostomy or observation alone. In fact, only approximately 15% of patients with penetrating chest trauma require any type of therapeutic operative procedure [29]. However, given the potential for serious morbidity and mortality associated with injury to heart, great vessels, or aerodigestive tract structures, rapid accurate diagnosis is essential.

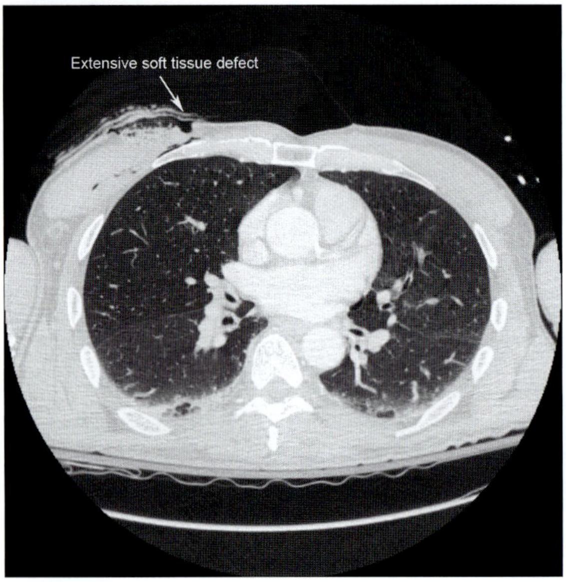

Fig. 14.3 Saw injury to right anterior chest wall without evidence of intrathoracic penetration. Complicated wound care due to extensive tissue defect

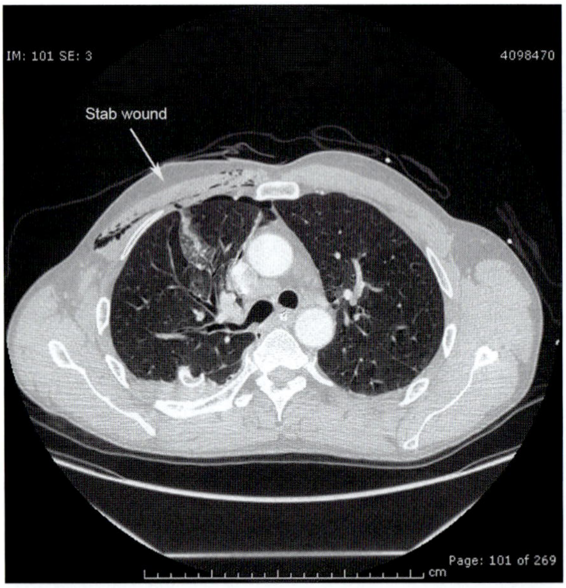

Fig. 14.4 Stab wound to right chest with intrathoracic penetration and lung injury. No evidence of mediastinal or intrathoracic vascular injury. Successfully treated with thoracostomy tube drainage

The use of Chest CT and CT angiography as a tool for triage of stable patients with penetrating chest trauma has been well described in the literature. When combined with echocardiography, chest CT has been

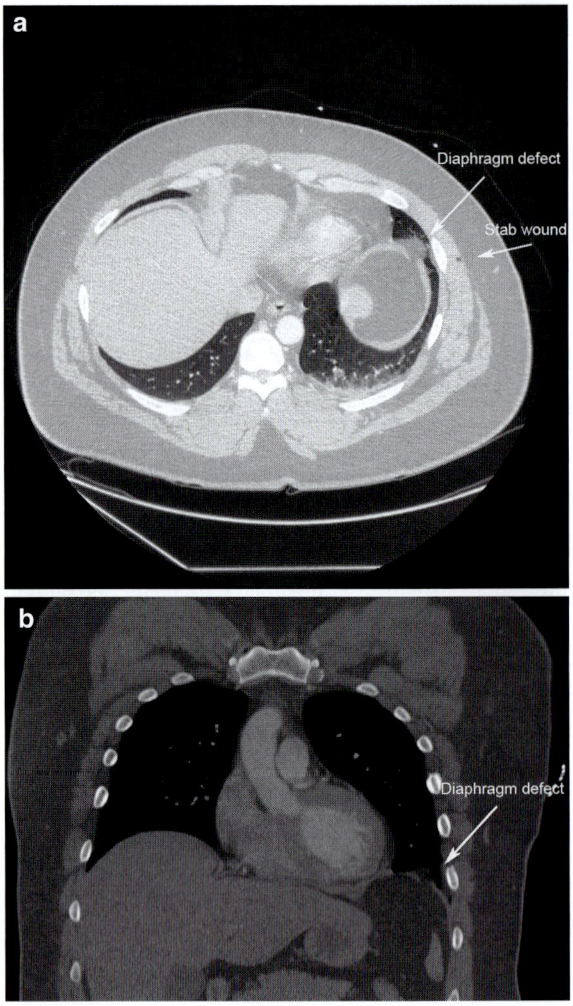

Fig. 14.5 (**a**) Stab wound to left chest with evidence of diaphragm injury adjacent to wound tract. (**b**) AP reconstruction of diaphragm injury showing herniation of abdominal fat through defect

demonstrated as able to exclude injury in approximately 80% of patients [30, 31]. For those patients who have CT findings concerning for significant injury, additional diagnostic procedures such as bronchoscopy or esophagoscopy are useful to further evaluate the areas of concern. Chest CT and CT Angiography have been shown to be a useful screening tool for patients with transmediastinal gunshot wounds [32]. It can be used with good accuracy to evaluate for hemopericardium suggestive of penetrating cardiac injury, especially when echocardiography is not immediately available [33]. High-resolution CT angiography is especially helpful in assessing for subclavian and axillary artery injury [34], and has virtually supplanted conventional angiography at the initial mechanism to screen for thoracic vascular injury [35]. In addition, it has been demonstrated that chest CT was far better than conventional chest radiography at predicting the presence of significant undrained hemothorax needing surgical evacuation [36]. Furthermore, in patients who have injuries identified which require operative intervention, chest CT has been shown to accurately locate the injury, and in some cases provide information leading to a change in the operative approach best suited for the injuries identified [37].

One area where newer generation CT scans have become very useful is the detection of diaphragm injuries. New multidetector CT scanners can now resolve the presence of diaphragm injuries with a sensitivity and specificity of 94% and 95.9% with an overall accuracy of almost 96% [38]. This represents a significant improvement from the older technology scanners which had reported sensitivities of as low as 14%. However, when assessing for diaphragm injuries, a high index of suspicion remains important.

An additional area where chest CT has been reported as extremely useful is in the initial screening of patients with minor penetrating chest trauma. In a recent study comparing the use of serial conventional chest radiographs with CT imaging, it was found that CT scan more accurately depicted the injuries present. In addition, in stable patients, a normal chest CT was shown to obviate the need for admission and follow-up chest imaging, leading to a potential cost savings, decreasing the proportion of patients signing out prior to the completion of their workup and allowing for expedited discharge directly from the emergency department [39].

All said, chest CT and CT angiography provide a rapid means or triage and diagnosis of injuries in stable patients with penetrating chest trauma. When used as a screening tool to allow for rapid discharge of patients without significant injury and to identify those patients either with definitive evidence of injury or for whom further workup is needed, it can provide a wealth of information. While some suggest that it is overutilized [40], it has the ability to rapidly detect life-threatening injuries and provide the information needed for optimal treatment. Conversely, it also provides a means to facilitate rapid discharge of patients without significant injury, freeing scarce resources for the treatment of patients more in need.

14.4 Head and Neck

In the evaluation of penetrating injuries to the neck, the availability of high-resolution CT scan and CT Angiography has had a dramatic impact on the need for surgical neck exploration. In the past, penetrating injures to the neck with violation of the platysma, especially those in Zone II (cricoid cartilage to angle on mandible), were thought to mandate surgical exploration. This resulted, however, in a high rate of negative explorations leading many to suggest the need for more selective exploration based on diagnostic evaluation using modalities such as bronchoscopy and esophagoscopy.

With the advent of newer generation CT scan technology in the late 1990s, several institutions began to question the need for invasive diagnostic procedures in the workup of stable patients with penetrating neck trauma. In two small series done by urban United States level 1 trauma centers, CT scan was evaluated for its usefulness in the diagnosis of significant vascular or aerodigestive tract injuries. Mazolewski et al.

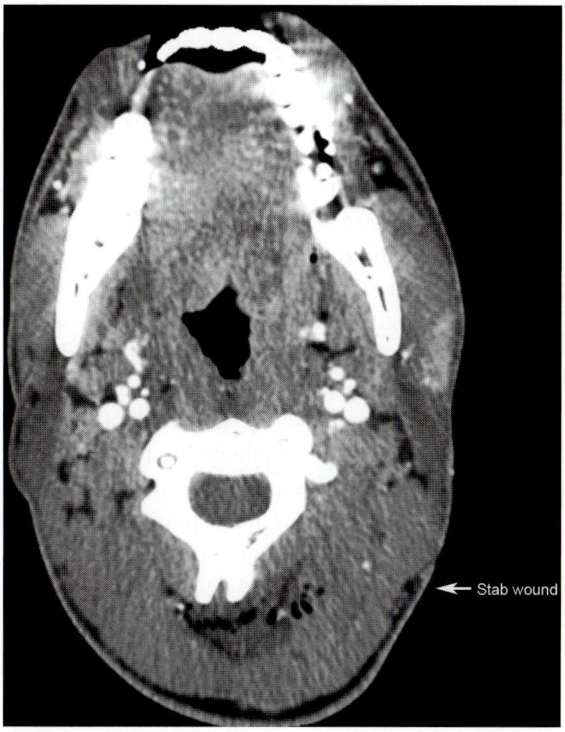

Fig. 14.6 Stab wound to left posterior neck clearly showing wound tract without evidence of proximity to vascular structures

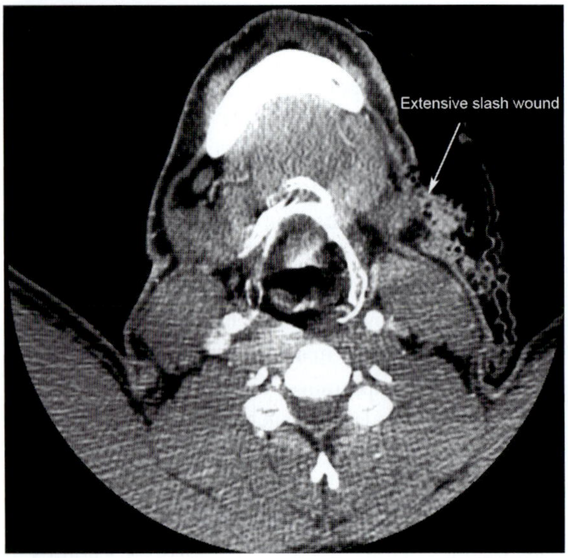

Fig. 14.7 Slash wound to left neck which clearly penetrated platysma on exam. CTA neck demonstrating no evidence of proximity or injury to vascular or aerodigestive tract structures. Treated with wound washout and closure without formal neck exploration

evaluated CT scan results with operative findings and determined that CT had a high sensitivity and specificity (100% and 91% respectively) for detection of significant injuries in penetrating zone II neck trauma [41]. Another study by Gracias et al. used CT scan as the sole initial diagnostic study in stable patients. They found that CT scan effectively ruled out injuries in 56% based on a wound trajectory remote from vital structures [42]. Based on a 3–6-month follow-up, there were no missed injuries. This early enthusiasm was not universal. Another center reported that CT scan had only a 50% sensitivity in detecting aerodigestive tract injury from penetrating neck trauma and contributed only minimally to the results of physical exam [43].

Several large series have been reported looking specifically at the use of CT Angiography to evaluate for vascular injury in penetrating neck trauma. Absent hard signs of vascular injury, it is reported the physical exam alone in the region has an especially poor sensitivity and specificity (57% and 53%) for detection of occult vascular injury [44]. In specifically evaluating CT Angiography, Munera et al. compared the results of CT Angiography with conventional angiograms. They clearly demonstrated a good correlation with conventional angiography as well as a high sensitivity and specificity (90% and 100%) for the detection of vascular injuries diagnosed by [45].

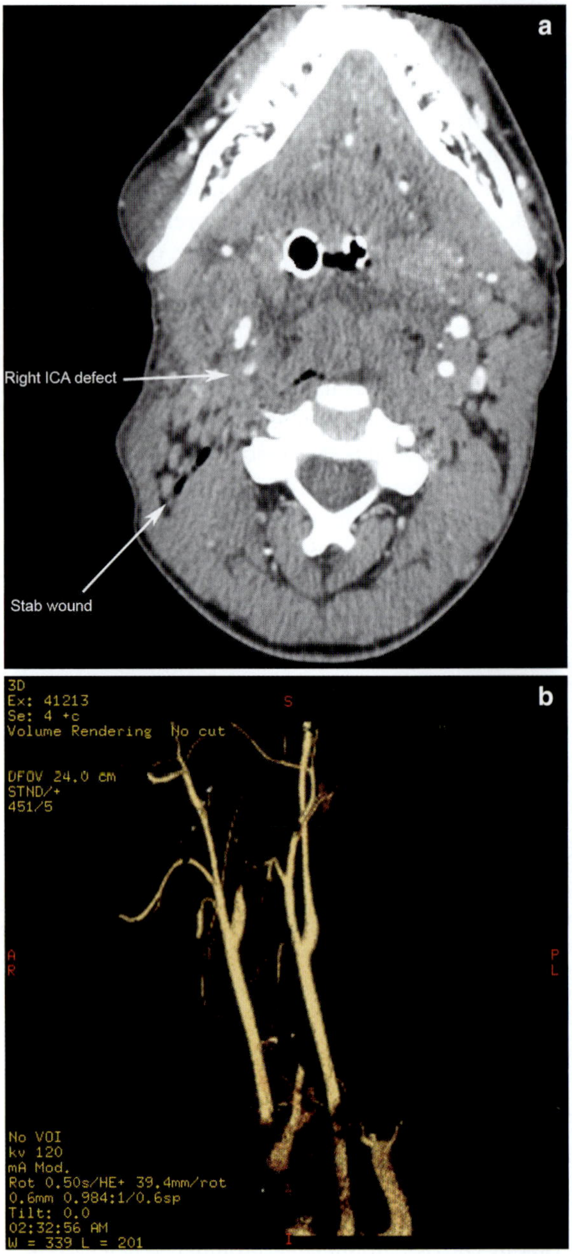

Fig. 14.8 (**a**) Stab wound to right neck with evidence of internal carotid artery injury. Patient with large MCA territory thrombotic stroke successfully treated with neurointerventional extraction of thrombus and coiling of right proximal and distal ICA with excellent functional recovery. (**b**) CTA reconstruction of right ICA injury demonstrating abrupt cutoff of right ICA without distal reconstitution

Another study prospectively examined the usefulness of CT Angiography as the initial screening mechanism in stable patients with neck injuries penetrating the platysma. Inaba, et al. demonstrated a sensitivity of

100% and specificity of 93.5% for detection of vascular and aerodigestive tract injuries [46]. The use of CT Angiography has been shown to decrease the rate of formal surgical neck exploration, as well as the rate of negative neck exploration when used in stable patients not requiring emergent exploration [47].

In 2008, the Eastern Association for the Surgery of Trauma issued a practice management guideline regarding penetrating zone 2 neck trauma. After an exhaustive review of the relevant literature, it was concluded that selective operative management of penetrating zone 2 neck injuries is recommended to minimize unnecessary operations. High-resolution CT angiography was identified as the initial diagnostic study of choice when available [48].

Again, patients with signs of obvious life-threatening injury including massive hemorrhage, expanding hematoma, airway compromise, or extensive subcutaneous emphysema require emergent surgical exploration [49]. However, in the stable patient with a penetrating neck injury accompanied by an unimpressive physical exam, CT and CT Angiography represent excellent tools for diagnosis. Their liberal use, followed by the appropriate use of other diagnostic modalities and selective surgical exploration, is associated with timely intervention for injures, with the prevention of a large number of negative surgical explorations.

14.5 Extremities

When dealing with penetrating extremity trauma, the use of CT and CT Angiography can enhance the clinical picture in the appropriately selected patient. Certainly in a patient with hard signs of vascular injury (including pulsatile bleeding, expanding hematoma, pulselessness, thrill/bruit) and active hemorrhage or limb-threatening ischemia, the primary intervention should be operative, with the use of on-table angiography as dictated by the operative findings. However, in the stable patient with soft signs of vascular injury including decreased pulses or ABI, non-expanding hematoma, history of significant bleeding or concerning proximity of the wound tract to major vascular structures, CT angiography can be of benefit both in confirming the injury as well as determining the character and location of the injury, and potential appropriateness of nonoperative and less invasive interventions such as stenting or angioembolization.

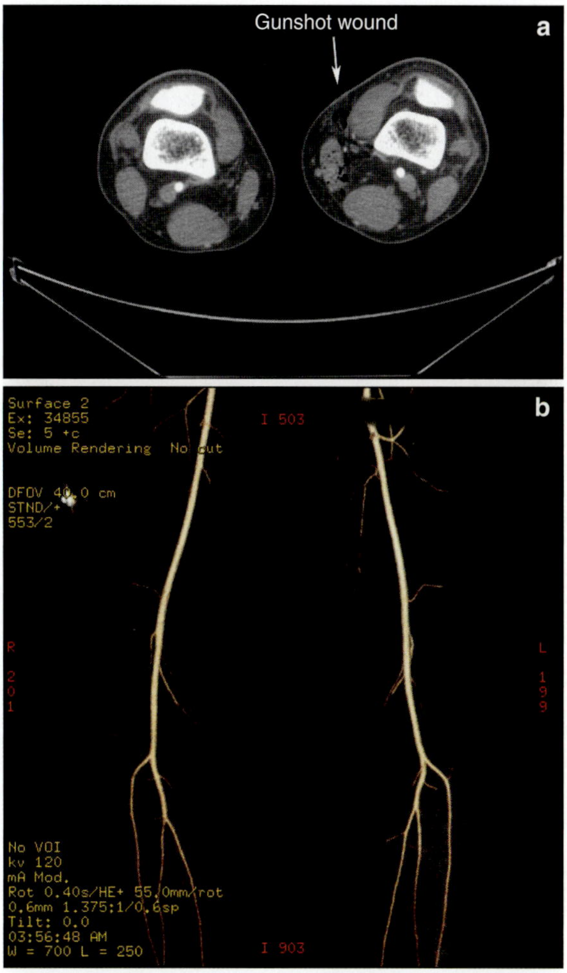

Fig. 14.9 (**a**) Gunshot wound to left lower extremity. No evidence of significant bony or vascular injury. Treated with local wound care. (**b**) CTA reconstruction of lower extremity vasculature demonstrating no evidence of vascular injury

In the radiographic evaluation of extremities for vascular injuries, conventional angiography has long been considered the gold standard. However, over the past several years with the development of multidetector CT scanners, CT Angiography has been shown by several authors to offer both a high sensitivity (95–100%) and specificity (87–100%) for the detection of injuries, without the potential drawbacks of conventional angiography such as access site thrombosis, groin hematoma, distal plaque embolization, or intimal dissection [50]. When the use of CT Angiography was retrospectively evaluated at an urban US level 1 trauma center, Peng et al. found that its use effectively ruled out injuries in 55% of studies and was associated

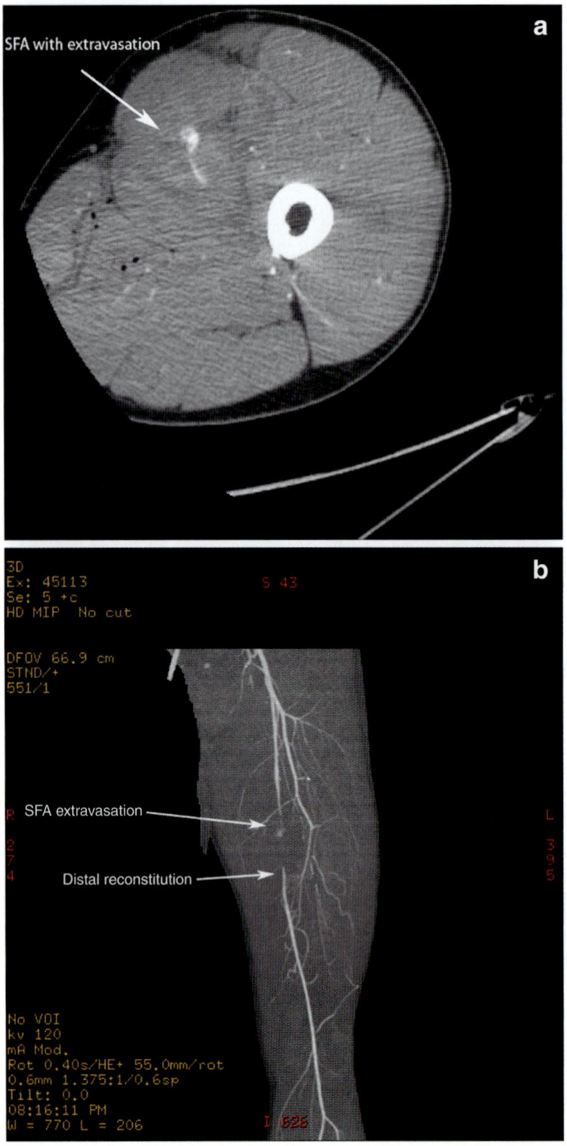

Fig. 14.10 (**a**) Gunshot wound to left lower extremity with evidence of contrast extravasation in territory of superficial femoral artery. Patient required vascular repair using vein graft. (**b**) Vascular reconstruction demonstrating SFA injury with extravasation as well as distal reconstitution of vessel

with zero false-negatives or missed injuries as well as excellent correlation between CT Angiography results and operative findings in patients who had injuries identified and subsequently underwent operative exploration [51]. Furthermore, the authors noted that by the end of their study period, CT Angiography had become the radiographic study of choice in the initial evaluation of extremity vascular trauma at their institution. Another review of the technique by Soto et al. at a Columbian trauma center demonstrated excellent sensitivity and specificity (95% and 98%, respectively) with one false-positive result over 139 patients [52]. The authors did point out that almost 4% of the studies performed were so degraded by scatter artifact from retained metal fragments that they were non-interpretable. Injuries were effectively ruled out by 55% of the interpretable studies.

CT Angiography represents a step forward in the workup of stable patients with extremity injures concerning for vascular injury without hard signs. While it only allows for diagnosis, it does so without many of the potential hazards associated with conventional angiography. With its high sensitivity and specificity and low potential for complications compared to conventional angiography, CT Angiography offers an excellent radiographic tool for the rapid diagnosis of peripheral vascular injuries. Once the presence of CT Angiographic signs of arterial injury, including active extravasation, pseudo-aneurysm formation, abrupt narrowing of a vessel, loss or opacification of an arterial segment or arteriovenous fistula, has been confirmed [53], either operative intervention, interventional radiographic intervention, or appropriate observation can be undertaken as dictated by the injury. It is important to note that the ability to detect injury is potentially related to the resolving power of the scanner. One author notes that the lack of intimal injuries detected over a 3-year period at their institution may have been related to the limited resolution of the four-row multidetector CT scanner used at the time [53]. As more advanced scanners are becoming available, this should become less and less of an issue in the future.

14.6 Conclusion

The use of CT scanning in penetrating trauma has led to a number of important advances in the care that can be provided. Given the rapid and accurate information that it provides, we are now able to more accurately determine which patients will benefit from operative intervention. It has allowed the expansion of selective nonoperative care for penetrating wounds to a variety of regions. In addition, with high-resolution scanners and CT angiography, it allows for screening and diagnosis previously only available through more invasive techniques. With it, we can be better at identifying those patients with significant injury and more rapidly commence appropriate treatment. At the same time, we are able to more rapidly exclude significantly large number of patients, leading to faster discharge and less use of scarce resources. Their use represents a major step forward in the diagnosis and treatment of patients with both blunt and penetrating trauma.

Important Points

- The place for an unstable patient after penetrating trauma is the operating room, not the CT scanner.
- CT scanning is recommended in patients selected to undergo nonoperative management of penetrating injuries to the abdomen.
- CT scanning, augmented by colonic contrast, is the modality of choice in evaluating for injury to retroperitoneal structures in penetrating trauma to the back and flank.
- High-energy mechanisms (e.g., military rifles) can lead to significant injury even with tangential wounds that do not appear to penetrate the peritoneal cavity by CT.
- Chest CT and CTA provide a rapid method of diagnosing significant intrathoracic injury after penetrating trauma.
- Absence of significant injury on CT chest can be used to facilitate rapid discharge.
- Stable patients with penetrating zone 2 neck injuries can be successfully nonoperatively managed; CTA is the recommended diagnostic modality in these cases.
- CT and CTA of the extremity can provide information just about equivalent to conventional angiography when evaluating for lower extremity vascular injury after penetrating trauma to the extremities.
- The place for an unstable patient after penetrating trauma is the operating room, not the CT scanner.

References

1. Hasaniya N, Demetriades D, Stephens A et al (1994) Early morbidity and mortality of non-therapeutic operations for penetrating trauma. Am Surg 60(10):744–747
2. Ertekin C, Yanar H, Taviloglu K et al (2005) Unnecessary laparotomy by using physical examination and different diagnostic modalities for penetrating abdominal trauma. Emerg Med J 22(11):790–794
3. Navsaria PH, Berli JU, Edu S et al (2007) Non-operative management of abdominal stab wounds – an analysis of 186 patients. S Afr J Surg 45(4):128–130
4. Boulanger BR, Kearney PA, Tsuei B et al (2001) The routine use of sonography in penetrating torso injury is beneficial. J Trauma Inj Infect Crit Care 51(2):320–325
5. Soffer D, McKenney MG, Cohn S et al (2004) A prospective evaluation of untrasonography for the diagnosis of penetrating torso injury. J Trauma Inj Infect Crit Care 56(5): 953–957
6. Varin DSE, Ringburg AN, VanLieshout EMM et al (2009) Accuracy of conventional imaging of penetrating torso injuries in the trauma resuscitation room. Eur J Emerg Med 16(6):305–311
7. Ginzburg E, Carrrilllo EH, Kopelman T et al (1998) The role of computed tomography in selective management of gunshot wounds to the abdomen and flank. J Trauma Inj Infect Crit Care 45(6):1005–1009
8. Salim A, Sangthong B, Martin M et al (2006) Use of computed tomography in anterior abdominal stab wounds: the results of a prospective study. Arch Surg 141(8):745–750
9. Shanmuganathan K, Mirvis SE, Chiu WC et al (2004) Penetrating torso trauma: triple contrast helical CT in peritoneal violation and organ injury – a prospective study in 200 patients. Radiology 231(3):775–784
10. Ramirez RM, Cureton EL, Ereso AQ et al (2009) Single contrast computed tomography for the triage of patients with penetrating torso trauma. J Trauma Inj Infect Crit Care 67(3):583–588
11. Soto JA, Morales C, Munera F et al (2001) Penetrating stab wounds to the abdomen: use of serial US and contrast-enhanced CT in stable patients. Radiology 220(2):365–371
12. Biffl WL, Kaups KL, Cothren CC et al (2009) Management of patients with anterior abdominal stab wounds: a Western Trauma Association multicenter trial. J Trauma Inj Infect Crit Care 66(5):1294–1301
13. Chmielewski GW, Nicholas JM, Dulchavsky SA et al (1995) Nonoperative management of gunshot wounds of the abdomen. Am Surg 61(8):665–668
14. Munera F, Morales C, Soto JA et al (2004) Gunshot wounds of abdomen: evaluation of stable patients with triple contrast helical CT. Radiology 231(2):399–405
15. Velmahos GC, Constantinou C, Tillou A et al (2005) Abdominal computed tomographic scan for patients with gunshot wounds to the abdomen selected for nonoperative management. J Trauma Inj Infect Crit Care 59(5):1155–1161
16. Grossman MD, May AK, Schwab CW et al (1998) Determining anatomic injury with computed tomography in selected torso gunshot wounds. J Trauma Inj Infect Crit Care 45(3):446–456
17. Tien HC, van der Hurk TW, Dunlop MP et al (2007) Small bowel injury from a tangential gunshot wound without peritoneal penetration: a case report. J Trauma Inj Infect Crit Care 62(3):762–764
18. Demetriades D, Gomez H, Chahwan S et al (1999) Gunshot injuries to the liver: the role of selective nonoperative management. J Am Coll Surg 188(4):343–348
19. Demetriades D, Hadjizacharia P, Constantinou C et al (2006) Selective nonoperative management of penetrating abdominal solid organ injuries. Ann Surg 244(4):620–628

20. Como JJ, Bokhari F, Chiu W et al (2010) Practice management guideline for selective nonoperative management of penetrating abdominal trauma. J Trauma Inj Infect Crit Care 68(3):721–733
21. Miller FB, Cryner HM, Chilikuri S et al (1989) Negative findings on laparotomy for trauma. South Med J 82(10):1231–1234
22. Meyer DM, Thal ER, Weigelt JA et al (1989) The role of abdominal CT in the evaluation of stab wounds to the back. J Trauma Inj Infect Crit Care 29(9):1226–1230
23. Phillips T, Sclafani SJA, Goldstein A et al (1986) Use of the contrast enhanced CT enema in the management of penetrating trauma to the flank and back. J Trauma Inj Infcct Crit Care 26(7):593–601
24. Plorde JJ, Boyle EM, Mann FA (1997) Triple contrast CT interrogation of the retroperitoneal colon after a stab wound. AJR Am J Roentgenol 169(2):484
25. Albrecht RM, Schermer CR, Demarest GB III et al (1999) Stab wounds to the back/flank in hemodynamically stable patients: evaluation using triple contrast computed tomography. Am Surg 65(7):683–688
26. Hauser CJ, Huprich JE, Bosco P et al (1987) Triple contrast computed tomography in the evaluation of penetrating posterior abdominal injuries. Arch Surg 122(10):1112–1115
27. Kirton OC, Wint D, Thrasher B et al (1997) Stab wounds to the back and flank in the hemodynamically stable patient: a decision algorithm based on contrasted-enhanced computer tomography with colonic opacification. Am J Surg 173(3):189–193
28. Macleod J, Freiberger D, Lewis F et al (2007) What is the optimal observation time for a penetrating wound to the flank? Am Surg 73(1):25–31
29. LeBlang SD, Dolich MO (2000) Imaging of penetrating thoracic trauma. J Thorac Imaging 15(2):128–135
30. Burack JH, Kandil E, Sawas A et al (2007) Triage and outcome of patients with mediastinal penetrating trauma. Ann Thorac Surg 83(2):377–382
31. Ibirogba S, Nicol AJ, Navsaria PH (2007) Screening helical computed tomographic scanning in haemodynamic stable patients with transmediastinal gunshot wounds. Injury 38(1):48–52
32. Stassen NA, Lukan JK, Spain DA et al (2002) Reevaluation of diagnostic procedures for transmediastinal gunshot wounds. J Trauma Inj Infect Crit Care 53(4):635–638
33. Nagy KK, Gilkey SH, Roberts RR et al (1996) Computed tomography screens stable patients at risk for penetrating cardiac injury. Acad Emerg Med 3(11):1024–1027
34. Staller B, Munera F, Sanchez A et al (2005) Helical and multislice CTA following penetrating trauma to the subclavian and axillary arteries. Emerg Radiol 11(6):336–341
35. Mirvis SE (2006) Thoracic vascular injury. Radiol Clin North Am 44(2):181–197
36. Velmahos GC, Demetriades D, Chan L et al (1999) Predicting the need for thoracoscopic evacuation of residual traumatic hemothorax: chest radiograph is insufficient. J Trauma Inj Infect Crit Care 46(1):65–70
37. O'Connor JV, Scalea TM (2010) Penetrating thoracic great vessel injury: impact of admission hemodynamics and preoperative imaging. J Trauma Inj Infect Crit Care 68(4): 834–837
38. Stein DM, York GB, Boswell S et al (2007) Accuracy of computed tomography (CT) scan in the detection of penetrating diaphragm injury. J Trauma Inj Infect Crit Care 63(3):538–543
39. Magnotti LJ, Weinberg JA, Schroeppel TJ et al (2007) Initial chest CT obviates the need for repeat chest radiograph after penetrating thoracic trauma. Am Surg 73(6):569–573
40. Plurad D, Green D, Demetriades D et al (2007) The increasing use of chest computed tomography for trauma: is it being overutilized? J Trauma Inj Infect Crit Care 62(3):631–635
41. Mazolewski PJ, Curry JD, Browder T et al (2001) Computed tomographic scan can be used for surgical decision making in zone II penetrating neck injuries. J Trauma Inj Infect Crit Care 51(2):315–319
42. Gracias VH, Reilly PM, Philpott J et al (2001) Computed tomography in the evaluation of penetrating neck trauma: a preliminary study. Arch Surg 136(11):1231–1235
43. Gonzales RP, Falimirski M, Holevar MR et al (2003) Penetrating zone II neck injury: does dynamic computed tomographic scan contribute to the diagnostic sensitivity or physical exam for surgically significant injury/a prospective blinded study. J Trauma Inj Infect Crit Care 54(1):61–65
44. Mohammed GS, Pillay WR, Barker P et al (2004) The role of clinical examination in excluding vascular injury in haemodynamically stable patients with gunshot wounds to the neck. A prospective study of 59 patients. Eur J Vasc Endovasc Surg 28(4):425–430
45. Munera F, Soto JA, Palacio D et al (2000) Diagnosis of arterial injuries caused by penetrating trauma to the neck: comparison of helical CT angiography and conventional angiography. Radiology 216(2):356–362
46. Inaba K, Munera F, McKenney M et al (2006) Prospective evaluation of screening multislice helical computed tomographic angiography in the initial evaluation of penetrating neck injuries. J Trauma Inj Infect Crit Care 61(1):144–149
47. Osborn TM, Bell RB, Qaisi W et al (2008) Computed tomographic angiography as an aid to clinical decision making in the selective management of penetrating injuries to the neck: a reduction in the need for operative exploration. J Trauma Inj Infect Crit Care 64(6):1466–1471
48. Tisherman SA, Bokhari F, Collier B et al (2008) Clinical practice guideline: penetrating zone 2 neck trauma. J Trauma Inj Infect Crit Care 64(5):1392–1405
49. Bell RB, Osborn T, Dierks EJ et al (2007) Management of penetrating neck injuries: a new paradigm for civilian trauma. J Oral Maxillofac Surg 65(4):691–705
50. Foster BR, Anderson SW, Soto JA (2006) CT angiography of extremity trauma. Tech Vasc Interv Radiol 9(4):156–166
51. Peng PD, Spain DA, Tataria M et al (2008) CT angiography effectively evaluates extremity vascular trauma. Am Surg 74(2):103–107
52. Soto JA, Munera F, Morales C et al (2001) Focal arterial injuries of the proximal extremities: helical CT angiography as the initial method of diagnosis. Radiology 218(1):188–194
53. Miller-Thomas MM, West OC, Cohen AM (2005) Diagnosing traumatic arterial injury in extremities with CT angiography: pearls and pitfalls. Radiographics 25(Suppl 1):S133–S142

Portable Ultrasound as an Adjunct in Penetrating Trauma

15

Jim Connolly

Ultrasound machines are becoming increasingly portable, cheap and robust leading to them becoming increasingly available for use outside of the radiology department, and increasingly out of hospital. All practicing trauma surgeons should consider embracing this modality when they are managing penetrating trauma.

You should think of point-of-care ultrasound as nothing more than a 'Visual Stethoscope' that can add visual images as an adjunct to your examination rather than as a radiological test. Multiple studies attest to the fact that limited training can achieve highly focussed views which can answer highly focused question in time critical situations. Such focussed practice has a sharp learning curve. You should not use point-of-care ultrasound as a replacement for examination, rather as a fundamental part of your examination. Its major value is in adding extra information to your assessment.

15.1 Introduction

Certain attributes are important in a machine. Machines must be easy to use and most modern machines can be defined down to an important set of buttons. They should be quickly ready to use: Machines designed for point-of-care usage should be ready to use within seconds. To achieve this, they often have a preset application set (best settings for each purpose) for ease of use. The machine should meet your needs. For example, if you work in an isolated area with intermittent power supply, the machine needs a good battery life. Reliability, robustness and portability may be important to withstand the environment you are working in.

15.1.1 How Should You Use Point-of-Care Ultrasound?

Point-of-care ultrasound is useful for defining the injury, assessing volume status and managing patients in the initial and recovery phases of their injury.

15.1.2 Defining the Injury

The major value of point-of-care ultrasound is in triaging the body cavity that you need to access first. This allows you to consider your best first incision to approach the injury. If used in the primary survey, it highlights injury much more rapidly than physical examination alone. Point-of-care ultrasound is of value in detecting pericardial bleeding, intra-abdominal bleeding as well as pneumothoraces and haemothoraces. It is not good at detecting which organ is injured or retroperitoneal blood.

J. Connolly
Emergency Dept Royal Victoria Infirmary Newcastle-upon-Tyne, Newcastle General, Westgate Road, Newcastle upon Tyne, NE4 6 BE, UK
e-mail: jim.connolly@nuth.northy.nhs.uk

G.C. Velmahos et al. (eds.), *Penetrating Trauma*,
DOI 10.1007/978-3-642-20453-1_15,

15.2 Focussed Ultrasound Is Good at Triaging Body Cavities

15.2.1 Detecting Abdominal Blood (FAST Scan)

The term ‘FAST’ (Focussed Assessment with Sonography for Trauma) was coined by Grace Rozycki and her team in Washington in the mid-1990s. FAST is a highly sensitive screen for free fluid in trauma. Invariably, it is the right hepatorenal pouch that becomes [1] positive first whatever the area of intra-abdominal injury. The minimum fluid volume is in the order of a few hundred millilitres.

With limited training, you can achieve sensitivities in the order of 85% for all bleeding, but this has been shown to rise to nearer 100% in those with shock In the context of penetrating trauma, particularly gun shot wounds, the presence of fluid is highly indicative of the need for exploration (coeliotomy)

Standard views (Fig. 15.1) are obtained of the six Ps (Pericardial, Perihepatic, Perisplenic, Pelvic, and Pleurae (2)). The probe positions are as shown – you should start with the probe indicator uppermost, and with the dot on the right hand of the screen (as per Fig. 15.2 scans). This standardises the images (head to the left). It is precisely this standardised approach (same picture every time) that will allow you to achieve rapid competence in the technique. All rotations of the probe in FAST should be anticlockwise, so that the patient’s right side comes to lie to the right of the screen. Fluid is black and will collect in one of the areas as depicted below in Fig. 15.2a–c.

You should be aware of the significant pitfalls in performing a FAST scan. Most important of these is

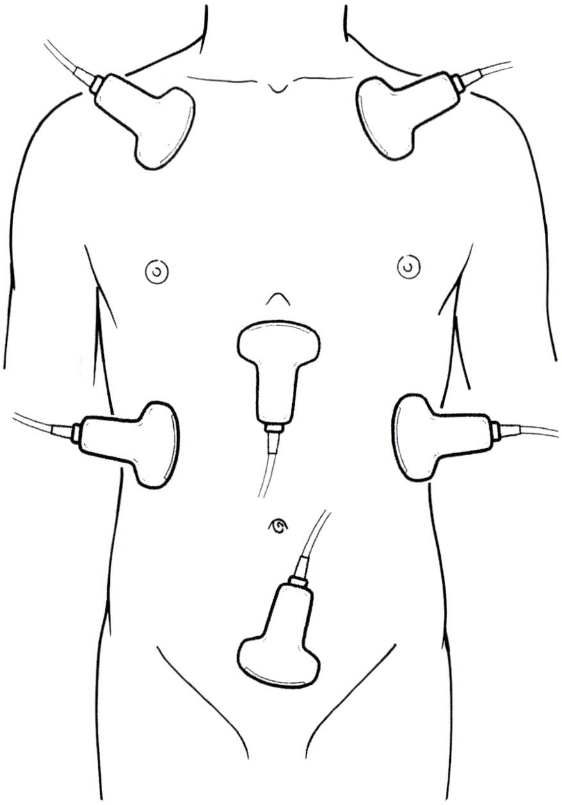

Fig. 15.1 Probe positions for FAST

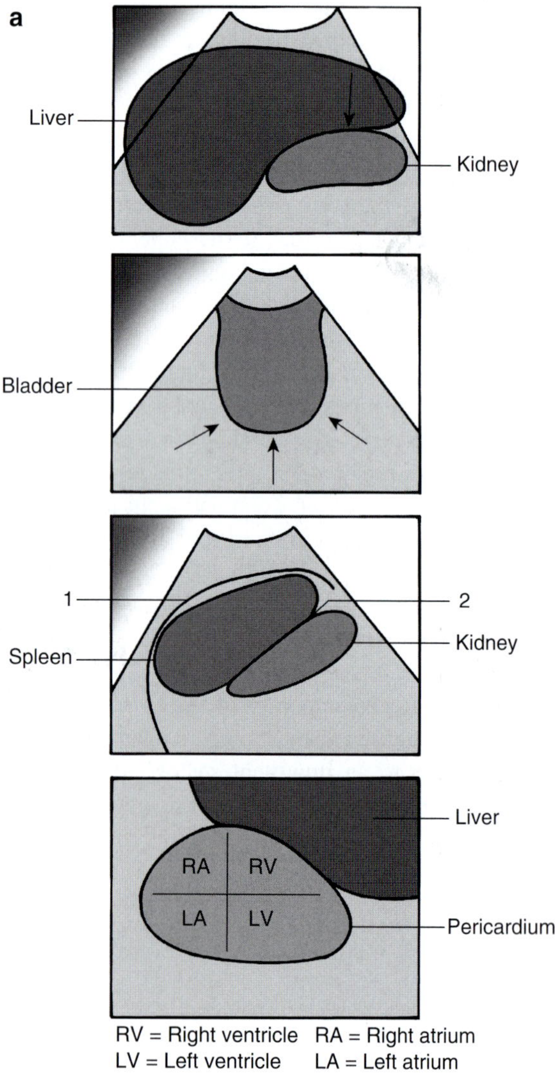

Fig. 15.2 (a) Schematic drawings of scans. (b) Four normal scans. (c) Four abnormal scans

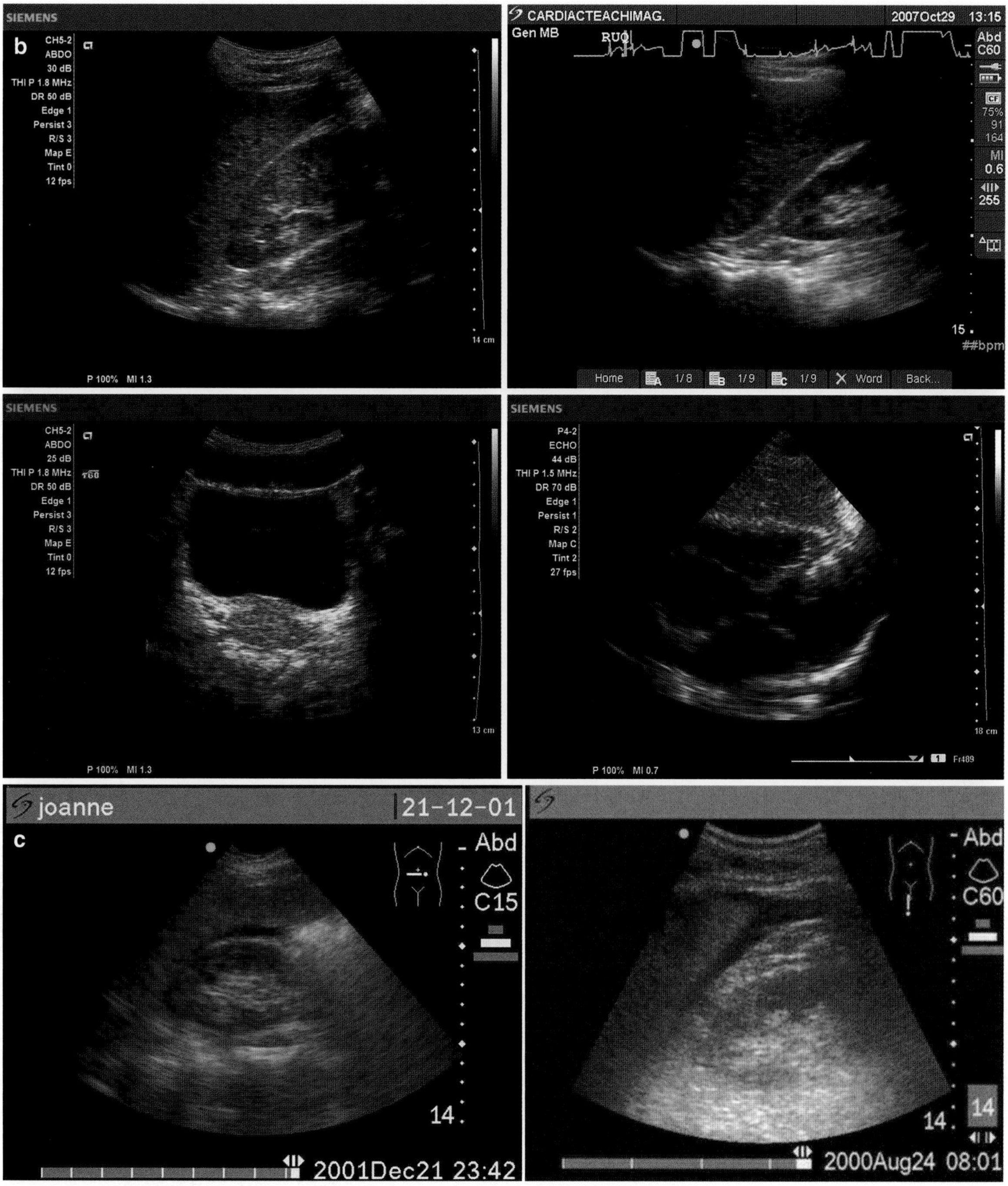

Fig. 15.2 (continued)

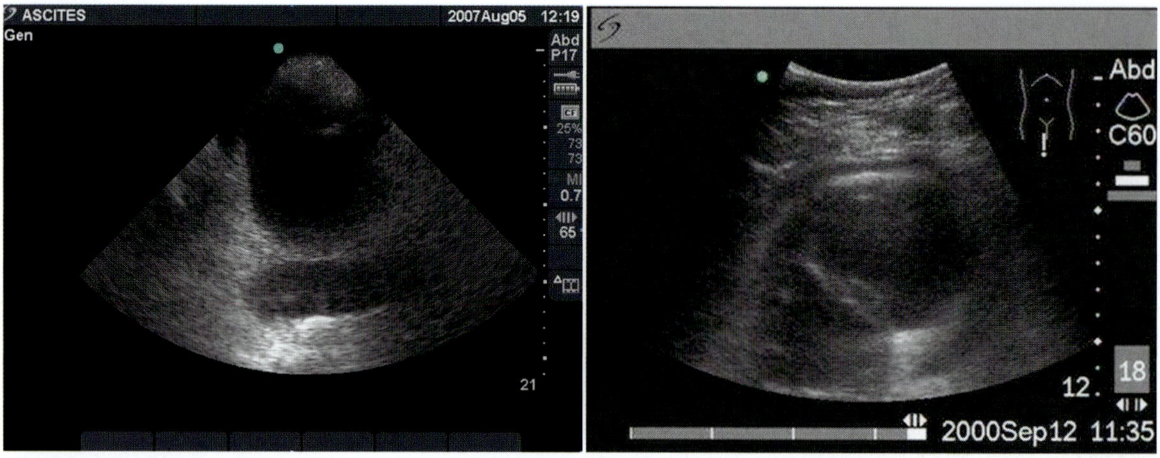

Fig. 15.2 (continued)

the fact that you need blood to bleed (i.e., a polytraumatised patient may have such significant other losses, e.g., external so as to preclude significant intra-abdominal bleeding). Remember in all situations to trust your clinical judgement

15.2.2 You Need Blood to Bleed

The presence of significant surgical emphysema can make an image impossible to interpret (air is the enemy of ultrasound!). As you learn this technique, be wary of false-positives, particularly interpreting the gallbladder and IVC as free fluid in the abdomen. The only way to avoid this is to look for fluid in pre-defined spaces – if you are not getting the views as shown in diagram 2, you should not be interpreting the images!

15.2.3 Pearls

1. Always start with notch (US probe indicator) at the top to orientate your image.
2. Make all rotations anticlockwise.
3. Look at the pericardium first to define fluid as black.
4. Repeat! Repeat! Repeat!
5. And do not forget – you need blood to bleed.

15.3 Pneumothorax

Detection of Pneumothorax is an exciting recent development in point-of-care ultrasound and is in fact more sensitive than chest X-ray in this regard. It also has the value of being fast, portable and repeatable, and in the often-noisy world of trauma, the 'visual stethoscope' has obvious advantages over the auditory stethoscope.

Air is considered the enemy of ultrasound, so in this scanning modality, it is not the detection of air that is the goal, rather the detection of the lack of normal signs. When visualising the interface between the two layers of pleura, certain signs are normal.

1. *Sliding* – you will see this as a sliding motion between the two layers of the pleura; if air interposes between them, then this is lost.
2. *Comet tail artefacts* – these are reverberation or ring-down artefacts caused by fluid in the interstitium of the lung – if the lung cannot be visualised because air has interposed, this artefact may be lost.
3. You can use M Mode to look for motion of the lung – where there is motion of the lung, there is the appearance of a seashore sign (Fig. 15.3a, b).

15.3.1 Pitfalls

1. Right main bronchus intubation will mean only the right lung moves – before you diagnose a

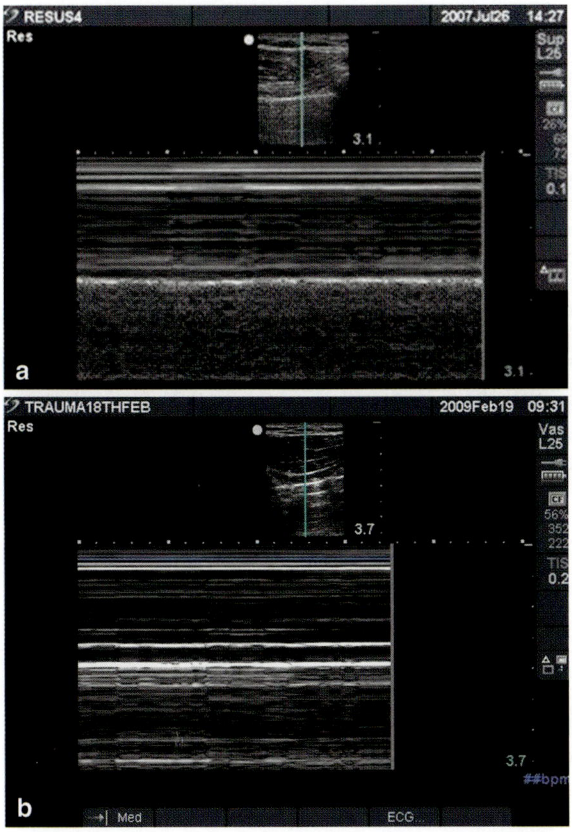

Fig. 15.3 Photo of seashore sign (**a**) M Mode – note the lower part of image has texture like a beach with sea distal – beach – this disappears with a pneumothorax (**b**)

Pneumothorax in the intubated patient, check the tube distance at the teeth and consider pulling the tube back a bit. (You may of course also find this useful as an adjunct in noisy environments for checking the tube position!).

2. Bullae can be confused for Pneumothorax, so you should proceed with caution in patients with chronic lung disease. Surgical emphysema may cause you great difficulty in visualising anything.
3. A one-off anterior probe position in the same site as you would listen for a Pneumothorax will merely alert you to the presence of a Pneumothorax. It is only possible to quantify the size by multiple site sampling or a Chest X-ray. In this context, however, an ill patient with signs of a Pneumothorax gets a drain, a well patient further imaging.

Pneumothorax Detection Is Possible by Looking for the Absence of Normal

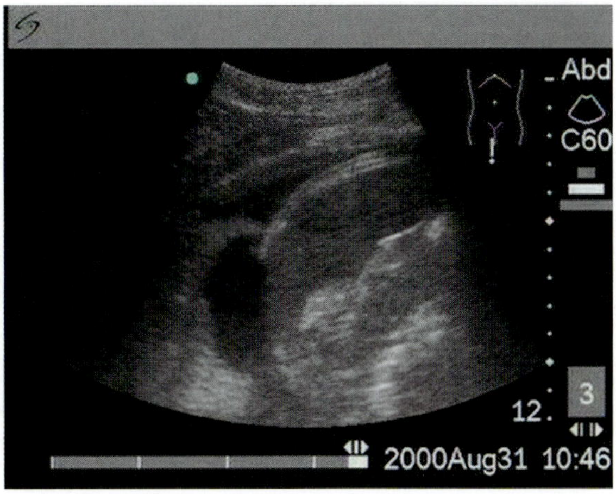

Fig. 15.4 Image of Haemothorax – note black above the diaphragm

15.4 Haemothorax

Ultrasound is very sensitive at visualising the dependent costophrenic angle on both the right and left. In fact, this view is seen on the standard FAST views as demonstrated in Fig. 15.4.

The appearance above the diaphragm is normally made up of a composite of lung and solid organs below the diaphragm being reflected above the diaphragm. (Often producing a mirror image of the liver or spleen above the diaphragm). If fluid is present above the diaphragm, this is lost and the space appears black, indicating fluid in the pleural space. Simple measures of depth can help to quantify the volume.

15.5 Pericardial Tamponade

This is seen well on the subcostal FAST view. In those patients with poor access to this view, alternative views may be needed. A simple transverse scan in the fifth intercostals space will suffice for a rapid view further echo views are beyond the scope of this text but are easily learnt.

15.5.1 Pitfalls

Clotted blood may be grey rather than black, so confuse the beginner. A very small amount of fluid is normal physiologically. If the fluid goes all the way around

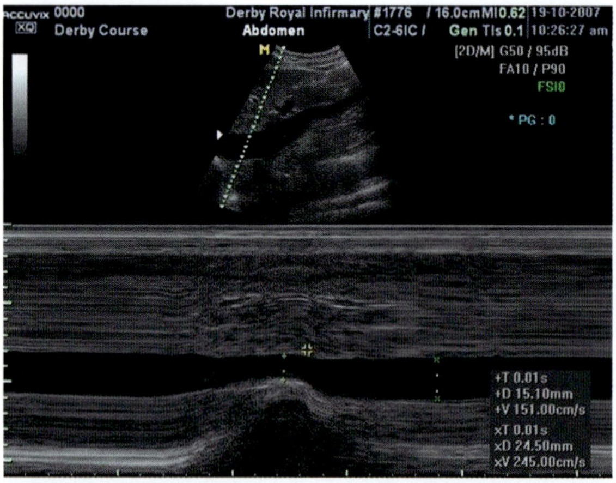

Fig. 15.5 Image of IVC Collapse – black structure is IVC. Note as M Mode is applied how it collapses with inspiration by about 30% (normal)

the heart, it is likely to be significant. Diastolic collapse of the R ventricle and IVC non-collapsibility are good indicators of physiological compromise. However, in the context of a penetrating wound, with haemodynamic compromise, anything but the smallest amount of fluid should be considered significant.

15.6 Assessment of Volumetric Status

A major value for point-of-care ultrasound is its ability during the primary survey and resuscitation stage to add information to the assessment of volume status.

Kissing ventricles: You will recognise an empty heart by the fact that the front wall of the left ventricle touches the back wall in systole, the classic kissing ventricles.

IVC visualisation: Even when you are a relative beginner, direct observation of the IVC will give you a rapid indication of volume status. The IVC is often visualised in the Pericardial FAST view and occasionally at the back of the liver in the Perihepatic views (Fig. 15.5 IVC). Care should be taken not to confuse the IVC with the aorta. Even simply eyeballing the IVC can be of value. In the normovolaemic patient, its diameter is normally 2 cm, a few cm below the diaphragm, and it collapses by between a quarter and a third. In extreme hypovolaemia, the collapse is almost total.

The IVC can be distinguished from the aorta as it is thin walled with a less forceful beat and travels behind the liver into the right atrium. Be aware that IVC collapse may be lost in the intubated positively ventilated patient! Total collapse of the IVC or near-total collapse indicates a very deplete vascular status. Non-collapse may indicate a right-sided pressure problem (Tension/Tamponade/PE)

Direct Visualisation of the IVC Enables a Rapid Assessment of Volumetric Status

15.7 Using Ultrasound to Manage Penetrating Trauma

15.7.1 Vascular Access

You will find ultrasound useful in severe hypovolaemia for both peripheral and central access. Most simply you can use the high-frequency probe to identify patent vessels (patent vessels compress). With more experience, the probe may be used to guide a cannula into the vessel.

For peripheral access, after applying a tourniquet set the machine at the lowest depth Using a high-frequency probe, apply only light pressure (as you will easily compress vessels). Veins are black and if they are patent are compressible. If peripheral access is not possible, you can use the probe to identify the location of central vessels (most commonly femoral/Internal jugular). The purpose of ultrasound is to guide your initial puncture into the vein. Once the needle is in the vein, use a standard access technique. (However, if you are going to dilate the tract or pass a large bore line, it is worth scanning to see if the guide wire is in the appropriate place).

15.7.2 Pericardial and Pleural Drainage

Ultrasound guidance can be used to more accurately visualise the needle to aid in more accurate localisations of fluid. (You can often best achieve this by a more longitudinal approach so that the needle depth is well assessed). As pericardial blood is likely to rapidly reaccumulate, this will likely need conversion to pericardial drainage.

15.8 Postoperative Management

With more training, you will develop increased potential skills in the post-operative period. Even with simple FAST scanning experience, you can start to use ultrasound as a valuable adjunct in the shocked post-operative patient.

In a valuable study by Jones et al. [2] of patients with undifferentiated shock presenting at ED, the use of simple ultrasound questions helped to define the most likely aetiology in 80% (versus 50% of those not scanned) and half the potential differential list. You can look at the following:

Heart function: Is it beating? A simple eyeball of how effective has been shown to correlate well with ejection fractions. Assessment for pericardial fluid and Right Ventricle size, as well as simple valvular colour assessments are easily learnt.

Vascular status: Visualisation of the IVC as above can aid fluid resuscitation.

Lung status: Practitioners like Lichtenstein working in ITU are increasingly using ultrasound to detect lung abnormalities (wet lung, consolidation, Pneumothorax, empyema, pleural effusion, etc.) with reported accuracies better than examination and as good as simple portable chest X-ray [3].

Focussed Ultrasound Is Rapidly Becoming an Important Part of the Assessment of the Critically Ill and Injured

15.9 Summary of Important Pitfalls

15.9.1 Fast Scanning

- You need blood to bleed!!!!
- Do not call a scan positive unless you have one of the standard image!
- Clotted blood in the pericardium looks grey.
- Do not rely on a one-off scan! Repeat! Repeat! Repeat!
- The scan should add to your judgement of the situation, not replace it!!!

15.9.2 Pneumothorax

- In the intubated patient, a right main bronchus intubation will look like a pneumothorax on the left.
- Bullae appear the same as pneumothoraces.
- The scan should add to your judgement of the situation, not replace it!!!

15.9.3 IVC Scanning

- The IVC in an intubated patient does not collapse in inspiration.
- The scan should add to your judgement of the situation, not replace it!!!
- The scan should add to your judgement not replace it!!!

Important Points

- A poor doctor with an ultrasound probe is still a poor doctor.
- You need blood to bleed.
- Pneumothorax detection is possible by looking for the absence of normality.
- Direct visualisation of the IVC enables a rapid assessment of volumetric status.
- Focussed ultrasound is rapidly becoming an important part of the assessment of the critically ill and injured.
- The scan should add to your judgement not replace it!!!

References

1. Rozycki GS, Oschner MG, Schmidt JA (1995) A prospective study of surgeon performed ultrasound as the primary adjunctive modality for injured patient assessment. J Trauma 39: 492–500
2. Jones Vivek et al (2004) RCT of immediate versus delayed Goa; directed ultrasound to identify the aetiology of non traumatic hypotension in ED patients. Acad Emerg Med 11(5):445
3. Lichtenstein D, Goldstein I, Mourgon E (2004) Comparative diagnostic performance of auscultation, chest radiography and lung ultrasonography in ARDS. Anaesthesiology 100(1):1–2

Suggested Reading

Emergency Ultrasound made easy Bowra McLaughlin ISBN-10 0443101507

Ultrasound in Emergency Care Brooks Connolly Chan Blackwell Publishing ISBN 0-7279-1731-5

Manual of Emergency and Critical Care Ultrasound Noble Nelson Cambridge Medical ISBN-13 978–0521688697

Emergency Ultrasound John Ma McGraw-Hill ISBN-10 007147904X

General Ultrasound in the Critically Ill Lichtenstein Springer ISBN-10 3540736239

Laparoscopy and Penetrating Trauma

16

Megan Wolthuis Grunander and Daniel R. Margulies

Laparoscopy and its use in trauma is not a new concept. In the 1920s, laparoscopy was first proposed as a means of identifying hemoperitoneum [1]. In the 1960s, Hesselson performed the first diagnostic laparoscopy [2]. In 1976, Garrzaniga used laparoscopy for evaluation of 37 patients who suffered abdominal trauma [3]. In 1977, Carvevale recommended laparoscopy be used to evaluate patients with anterior abdominal stab wounds and tangential gunshot wounds [4]. Over the past 30 years, laparoscopy has become the standard in diagnosis and treatment of many surgical diseases. As such, the technology and availability of equipment, as well as surgeons' ability have all greatly improved.

Laparoscopy when used as a means of diagnosing peritoneal penetration or intra-abdominal organ injury has become an accepted practice. In so doing, the majority of literature has shown a significant decrease in the number of negative laparotomies being performed. A review of the data when laparoscopy was used as a screening tool prevented 63% of patients from unnecessary laparotomies [5], which subsequently leads to lower hospital costs secondary to a shorter length of stay [5, 6]. Laparotomy patients have an overall higher morbidity and mortality, with a higher incidence of complications such as deep vein thrombosis and pulmonary embolism, pneumonia, wound infection, wound dehiscence, and abscess formation [5]. Although no study has documented long-term follow-up, it could be reasoned that a lower laparotomy rate also leads to fewer long-term complications such as bowel obstructions from adhesions as well as a lower number of ventral hernias subsequently requiring repair. Diagnostic laparoscopy for penetrating trauma has been shown to have a 3% complication rate in comparison to a 22% complication rate associated with negative laparotomies [6, 7].

Nevertheless, the fear of a missed injury still exists. Early studies reported missed injury rates as high as 82%. Multiple studies since that time, however, report a 1% incidence of such [4, 8]. Studies evaluating laparoscopy solely as a diagnostic tool have shown that it was 100% accurate in determining the need for laparotomy [4, 7]. The goal of diagnostic laparoscopy is to prevent unnecessary laparotomies with complete confidence that no injury went unrecognized. Laparotomy must be performed in patients where any doubt of injury remains.

Therapeutic laparoscopy becomes a topic of debate. There are numerous case reports and small series citing laparoscopy as an appropriate means of diagnosis and treatment of penetrating trauma [4, 6, 7, 9]. The use of laparoscopy, not only as a diagnostic tool but also as a means of therapy, is expanding as the skills and comfort level of trauma surgeons improve.

Extreme care must be taken in selecting patients to undergo this management. The ideal patient will have limited penetrating injury to the thoracoabdominal region or abdomen [7]. Contraindications to diagnostic laparoscopy include patients with hemodynamic instability with evidence of shock or active bleeding [8]. Relative contraindications include peritonitis, known intra-abdominal injury, or posterior penetrating trauma with high likelihood of bowel

M.W. Grunander • D.R. Margulies (✉)
Director of Trauma and Surgical Critical Care,
Department of Surgery, Cedars-Sinai Medical Center,
Suite 8215, 8700 Beverly Blvd, 90048 Los Angeles, CA, USA
e-mail: marguliesd@cshs.org

G.C. Velmahos et al. (eds.), *Penetrating Trauma*,
DOI 10.1007/978-3-642-20453-1_16, © Springer-Verlag Berlin Heidelberg 2012

injury, concern for retroperitoneal injury, previous abdominal surgery, and lack of equipment and expertise [7, 8]. The positive predictive value of shock and generalized peritonitis in predicting the presence of abdominal organ injury requiring surgical repair is well over 80% [10]. Laparoscopy holds no advantage over laparotomy in someone suspected of having multiple intra-abdominal injuries that will require attention [6].

The possibility of an intra-operative pneumothorax occurring while obtaining pneumoperitoneum from an undiagnosed diaphragmatic injury exists and must be something that the operating surgeon and anesthesiologist are monitoring for and prepared to handle quickly if the problem should arise [4, 7, 8].

Another consideration in your patient selection includes those with traumatic brain injury (TBI). It has been shown that intracranial pressure rises with the pneumoperitoneum required to perform laparoscopy, and as such, this may not be the best means of diagnosing and treating multi-trauma patients with a component of TBI [4, 7].

16.1 General Techniques of Laparoscopy

Prep and drape the patient in a position that allows for easy conversion to exploratory laparotomy if need be. Secure the patient to the table as to facilitate positioning in Trendelenburg, reverse Trendelenburg, left or right side up as to give you optimal visibility when examining each of the four quadrants. If possible, place a tower at the head and foot of the bed. Insert the Veress needle with standard technique and insufflation obtained to 15 mmHg. If chest tubes were previously placed, position the pleurovac lateral to the bed in a position of visibility to facility monitoring for the presence of a new airleak during insufflation. In the inferior umbilical position, insert a 5-mm trocar for use with 30° camera. If the patient has a known pelvic fracture, however, the trocar should be placed superior to the umbilicus. Prefer blunt trocars to bladed. If you find that visualization is insufficient with a 5-mm camera, you may easily convert your trocar to accommodate a 10-mm scope. Place two additional 5-mm trocars lateral to the umbilicus and rectus, one to the right and the other to the left to facilitate easy manipulation and examination of the entire small bowel

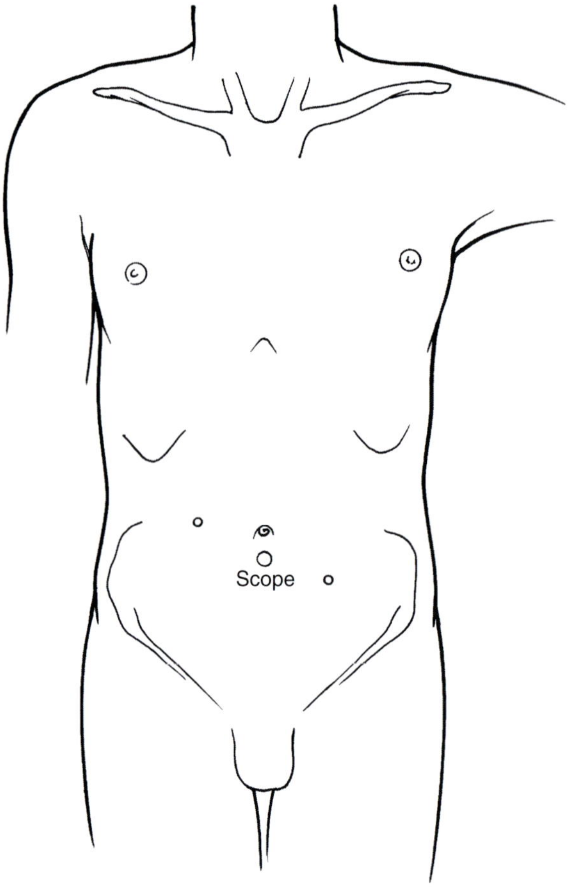

Fig. 16.1 Troikar positions for best overview

(Fig. 16.1). These trocars should be placed in a position distanced from the penetrating wound. Use atraumatic graspers with a hand-over-hand technique in order to examine the small bowel from ligament of Treitz to cecum (Fig. 16.2). Keep the graspers always in view of the camera. Examine the colon along its entire length. The right and left colon are easily mobilized along the white line of Toldt via laparoscopy. This should be done particularly if blood or hematoma is visualized along the colon or its mesentery as the likelihood of retroperitoneal colon injury is increased. If an anterior colon injury is observed, suspect a posterior injury. The lesser sac is also able to be dissected, opened, and examined completely laparoscopically. You can inject methylene blue via a nasogastric tube or intravenously to further assist you in the identification of injuries. Additional 5- or 10-mm trocars may easily be placed as needed if proceeding with therapeutic laparoscopy.

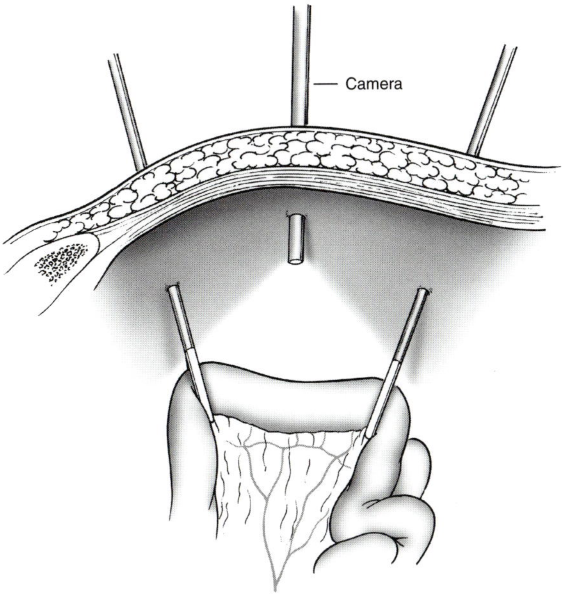

Fig. 16.2 Lift and inspect bowels from both sides from Treitz to rectum

16.2 Technical Considerations

In the obese patient, an Optiview© or similar trocar is recommended to use if available. The trocar should be placed lateral to the umbilicus but still within the rectus. Place the trocar with a 0° scope and then change to a 30° scope.

If hemoperitoneum is seen, evacuate the blood and examine the abdomen completely if the patient remains hemodynamically stable. The blood may be from a small liver or spleen injury or from the abdominal wall, all of which can be managed laparoscopically.

16.3 Laparoscopy and Anterior Abdominal Wall Stab Wounds

Patients with penetrating trauma to the anterior abdominal wall can present a challenge in management as up to 45% of hemodynamically stable patients may not have suffered peritoneal penetration [7]. Diagnostic laparoscopy in this circumstance provides a clear benefit as a minimally invasive means of evaluating for peritoneal penetration.

Local wound exploration with subsequent diagnostic peritoneal lavage (DPL) if peritoneal penetration is found has been used in combination for evaluation of bowel or solid organ injury. However, DPL can have false-positives secondary to blood from insignificant liver or splenic injuries as well as bleeding from the anterior abdominal wall [11]. Selective nonoperative management has been used as a treatment strategy as a means of decreasing the rate of negative exploratory laparotomies [12]. However, concern exists over the delay in diagnosis of an injury as the management is based on subjective physical exam findings [12]. In this circumstance, diagnostic laparoscopy provides abdominal exploration in a minimally invasive fashion as well as information regarding the extent of injury [10]. Hospital length of stay and cost are higher for patients managed nonoperatively verses those who undergo negative diagnostic laparoscopy [10]. If diagnostic laparoscopy is completely negative, considerations for discharge of the patient from the PACU avoid unnecessary hospitalization.

Technical considerations particular to laparoscopy with stab wounds:

If there has been penetration into the peritoneum, air and bubbling may be observed at the injury site while pneumoperitoneum is being obtained. A penetrating towel clip may need to be used at the stab wound entrance in order to maintain pneumoperitoneum. Blood within the abdomen may be from the abdominal wall only and may not mandate a laparotomy.

16.4 Laparoscopy and Gunshot Wounds

It has long been the accepted standard that all abdominal gunshot wounds (GSW) must be evaluated by laparotomy. However, with the use of FAST (Focused Assessment with Sonography for Trauma) scans, as well as improvement in CT imaging and the increasing utilization of diagnostic laparoscopy, this standard is being challenged [11]. Zantut et al. reported that 58% (113 of 194) of stable patients with gunshot wounds who were evaluated with laparoscopy were discharged home with confidence after a brief hospital stay without need for laparotomy [13].

16.5 Laparoscopy and Thoracoabdominal Trauma

The risk of diaphragmatic injury exists with penetrating trauma in the thoracoabdominal region [9]. Several studies have shown that penetration in the

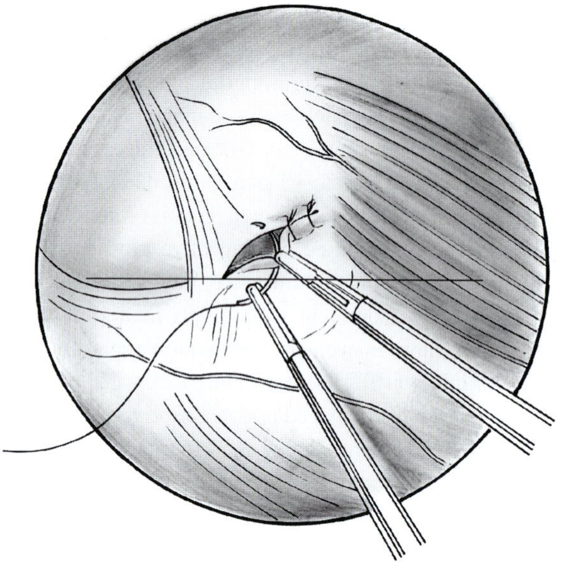

Fig. 16.3 Laparoscopic repair of a diaphragmatic injury is the most commonly reported therapeutic laparoscopic intervention

thoracoabdominal region has an 18–35% incidence of diaphragmatic injury [9, 11]. A stab wound below the nipple, lateral to the xiphoid, and medial to the mid-axillary line that traverses through the ribs has a chance of causing a diaphragmatic injury. Laparoscopy is particularly useful in making this diagnosis [6, 7, 9, 11]. Spann et al. found that 31% of patients with a hemo – or pneumothorax on chest x-ray had a diaphragmatic injury later identified with laparoscopy [14]. Multiple studies have found that laparoscopy is safe and effective not only for diagnosis but also for treatment of such an injury [14]. Laparoscopic repair of a diaphragmatic injury is the most commonly reported therapeutic laparoscopic intervention (Fig. 16.3) [7].

When repairing a diaphragmatic injury laparoscopically, you should use a braided permanent suture. However, large traumatic diaphragmatic injuries adjacent to or including the esophageal hiatus are best approached via laparotomy.

16.6 Laparoscopy and Extraperitoneal Rectal Injury

The current consensus in regards to rectal injuries is that intraperitoneal injuries are repaired primarily. Extraperitoneal injuries are also repaired primarily if minimal dissection is needed or if the injury is exposed during dissection to examine and repair other injuries [15]. The feasibility of laparoscopic fecal diversion as a means of managing an isolated extraperitoneal GSW injury has been documented [7, 15, 16]. With laparoscopy, you are able to rule out other injuries and perform mobilization of the colon, allowing for creation of a loop sigmoid colostomy [7]. Presacral drainage is also able to be established laparoscopically. The urinary tract is also evaluated to exclude injury.

16.7 Laparoscopy and Definitive Repair of Injuries Secondary to Penetrating Trauma

One small series documents 26 of 28 patients undergoing successful repair of intra-abdominal injury following penetrating trauma. Repairs included closure of gastrostomies, repair of liver lacerations, cholecystectomy, and repair of diaphragmatic injuries [16].

One small series of children demonstrates successful repair of bowel injury secondary to trauma [17]. When small bowel injuries are identified, you are able to do all of the following laparoscopically: primary repair, stapled resections with side-to-side anastomosis as done in laparoscopic bariatric surgery [6].

Liver and splenic injuries: Laparoscopy allows for evacuation of blood and establishment of hemostasis with electrocautery, argon beam, and/or hemostatic agents. Drains should only be left in place for large injuries.

Gallbladder: Cholecystectomies may be performed in a standard fashion.

Bladder: Primary repair may be performed with a laparoscopic suturing device. However, the inside of the bladder must be fully examined with the laparoscope or cystoscopy prior to closure.

Important Points

- Laparoscopy as a diagnostic tool in penetrating trauma can reduce the rate of negative laparotomies. Its use as a therapeutic means is also increasing. Limitations to its use for diagnosis and definitive repair include patient stability as well as surgeons' ability.

- If the patient is hemodynamically unstable or multiple injuries are suspected, do not attempt laparoscopy.
- Prep and drape the patient in such a way as to facilitate easy conversion to laparotomy.
- Blood identified with laparoscopy may be from a liver or splenic injury, or from the anterior abdominal wall and is not an indication alone for conversion to laparotomy.
- The entire small bowel can be evaluated with meticulous care via laparoscopy.
- Stab wounds to the left lower chest should be evaluated to rule out diaphragmatic injury. Inspection as well as repair of such injuries can be accomplished laparoscopically.

References

1. Villavicencio RT, Aucar JA (1999) Analysis of laparoscopy in trauma. J Am Coll Surg 189:11
2. Rossi P, Mullins P, Thal E (1993) Role of laparoscopy in evaluation of abdominal trauma. Am J Surg 166:707–711
3. Gazzaniga AB, Stanton WW, Bartlett RH (1976) Laparoscopy in the diagnosis of blunt and penetrating injuries to the abdomen. Am J Surg 131:315–318
4. Chelly JR, Major K, Spivak J, Hui T, Hiatt J, Margulies DR (2003) The value of laparoscopy in management of abdominal trauma. Am Surg 69:957–960
5. Miles EJ, Dunn E, Howard D, Mangram A (2004) The role of laparoscopy in penetrating abdominal trauma. JSLS 8: 304–309
6. Gorecki P, Cottam D, Angus L, George D, Shaftan G (2002) Diagnostic and therapeutic laparoscopy for trauma: a technique of safe and systematic exploration. Surg Laparosc Endosc Percutan Tech 12(3):195–198
7. Goettler C, Bard M, Toschlog E (2004) Laparoscopy in trauma. Curr Surg 61(6):554–559
8. Stefanidis D, Richardson WS, Chang L, Earle DB, Fanelli RD (2009) The role of diagnostic laparoscopy for acute abdominal conditions: an evidence-based review. Surg Endosc 23:16–23
9. Matthews BD, Bui H, Harold KL, Kercher KW, Adrales G, Park A, Sing RF, Heniford BT (2003) Laparoscopic repair of traumatic diaphragmatic injuries. Surg Endosc 17:254–258
10. Leppaniemi A, Haapiainen R (2003) Diagnostic laparoscopy in abdominal stab wounds: a prospective, randomized study. J Trauma 55(4):636–645
11. Simon RJ, Rabin J, Kuhls D (2002) Impact of increased use of laparoscopy on negative laparotomy rates after penetrating trauma. J Trauma 53(2):297–302
12. Saribeyoglu K et al (2007) Laparoscopy offers diagnosis and treatment in abdominal stab injuries. Surg Laparosc Endosc Percutan Tech 17(5):396–401
13. Zanut LF, Ivatury RR, Smith RS et al (1997) Diagnostic and therapeutic laparoscopy for penetrating abdominal trauma: a multicenter experience. J Trauma 42:825
14. Spann JC, Nwariaku FE, Wait M (1995) Evaluation of video-assisted thoracoscopic surgery in the diagnosis of diaphragmatic injuries. Am J Surg 170:628
15. Navsaria PH, Graham R, Nicol A (2001) A new approach to extraperitoneal rectal injuries: laparoscopy and diverting loop sigmoid colostomy. J Trauma 51(3):532–535
16. Hope WW, Christmas AB, Jacobs DG, Sing RF (2009) Definitive laparoscopic repair of penetrating injuries to the colon and small intestine: a case report. J Trauma 66:931–932
17. Streck CJ, Lobe TE, Pietsch JB, Lovvorn HN III (2006) Laparoscopic repair of traumatic bowel injury in children. J Pediatr Surg 41:1864–1869

17 Angiography and Interventional Radiology

Marc Kalinowski

Due to technical innovations over the last decades especially in the field of computed tomography (CT), catheter-based procedures have evolved more and more from a diagnostic modality to a primary treatment option for severely injured trauma patients. Whether remote aortic occlusion is performed to avoid a secondary cavity incision, embolization of bleeding vessels or an endovascular stent is placed to cover a lacerated vessel, all these techniques can minimize the physiologic burden placed on patients who may have very little physiologic reserve. The application of endovascular technology to the management of penetrating and blunt traumatic vascular injuries represents an exciting and significant advance in modern trauma centers. Utilization of these techniques to stabilize a patient in extremis or to serve as a "bridge" to future elective procedures to correct the same problem represents an attractive alternative with potentially lower morbidity and mortality rates than conventional management. It is of utmost importance that these procedures must be carried out by experienced providers in an environment conducive to such repair. A variety of imaging equipment as well as endovascular inventory must be readily available for the successful management of these injuries.

M. Kalinowski
Hanserad-Radiology, Tabea Hospital Kösterbergstrasse 32, 22587 Hamburg, Germany
e-mail: marc.kalinowski@googlemail.com

17.1 General Comments

Due to the growing availability of fast CT scanners, the diagnosis of arterial trauma should be established primarily by using this fast and noninvasively imaging modality even in unstable patients [1]. Modern multislice CT scanners can detect bleeding rates of 0.3 cc of blood/min whereas digital subtraction angiography (DSA) needs a blood loss of approximately 0.5–1 cc/min for detection. Suspicion of arterial injury is usually based on the findings of clinical examination. Careful evaluation can detect abnormalities in patients with major arterial injuries. But it is known that arterial injuries may present with so-called soft signs (stable hematoma, adjacent nerve injury, unexplained hypotension, or proximity of the penetrating wound to the underlying major blood vessels) and may be overlooked. In case of suspected vascular injury, a contrast-enhanced CT scan (presumably a whole body CT) defines on the best way where a patient is bleeding. Contrast extravasation on CT proves a vascular injury resulting in early intervention. Holding unstable patients in the emergency room (ER) to achieve cardiovascular stability is not wise and not needed neither for imaging nor for percutaneous interventions. Usually, patients lose more blood during stabilization possibly resulting in a "bloody vicious cycle" (coagulopathy, acidosis, hypothermia). Therefore, imaging and interventions should be understood as a continuous process even during ongoing resuscitation [1, 2].

There are some basic algorithms in case of suspected bleeding which are useful for suspected vascular trauma even if CT is not available using FAST-Ultrasound. If CT is available, consider the following basic algorithm (Fig. 17.1).

G.C. Velmahos et al. (eds.), *Penetrating Trauma*,
DOI 10.1007/978-3-642-20453-1_17, © Springer-Verlag Berlin Heidelberg 2012

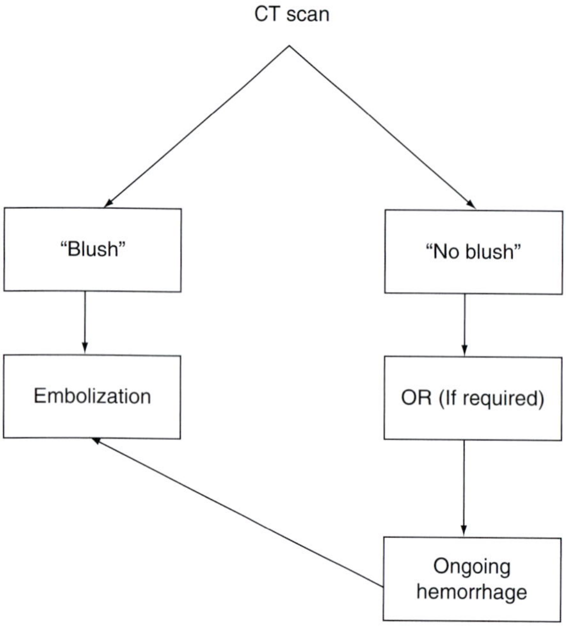

Fig. 17.1 Basic algorithm for endovascular treatment decisions according to identifiable contrast-media extravasation on CT scan

You should always keep in mind that due to the wide range of materials needed for vessel occlusion or covering (coils, plugs, glue, particles, gelatine-based embolics and covered stents), you should be familiar with this "interventional zoo." The complexity of these procedures reaching the bleeding target site by catheter-based procedures adds to this difficulty. So think twice and check your surrounding before you jump. You also need an appropriate facility even in an operating room or an angio-suite. A wide range of different materials must be immediately available and the most crucial point in such situations is that experienced operators are on call on a 24/7 fashion [3].

17.2 Technical Considerations

In case of penetrating trauma, there are only a handful scenarios where percutaneous interventions may provide life-saving bleeding control especially in areas that are difficult to access surgically. These interventions may prevent the need for reoperation in the presence of rebleeding or assist in nonoperative management. This includes head and neck injuries, extremities and pelvic trauma, great vessel, and thoracic and solid abdominal organ injuries.

For all these scenarios, the common femoral artery is the recommended access site. All vascular regions of the body can be reached easily using specific catheters and guidewires. The retrograde puncture site should be located on the lower third of the femoral head seen on fluoroscopy. Avoid an arterial puncture above the inguinal ligament due to an increased chance of retroperitoneal bleeding that of course is not compressible or a puncture site too low because of the same reason. Especially, in case of extensive vascular trauma and the need for aortic stentgrafts, a surgical cut down of the groin should be performed. Percutaneous access for stentgraft placement is also possible, but specific closure devices and techniques are necessary. In shock situations where blood pressure could be extremely low, ultrasound-guided puncture is recommended due to possible collapsed and nonpulsatile arteries. You should use preferential 4 F catheters with a 0.038 in. inner lumen, as you can use these devices as guiding-catheters for ongoing superselective catheterization by microcatheters. Time-consuming exchange of standard 0.035 in. catheters should be avoided. Never lose your guide wire. Use one (or better two) French greater vascular sheaths than the catheters you use because the side port of the sheath can then be used for intra-arterial blood pressure measurements during the intervention by your anesthesiologists. They will appreciate you.

17.3 Basic Imaging Aspects

There are some basic imaging principles which should be kept in mind especially when searching bleeding sites. Four different imaging patterns of injured vessels could be identified during angiography (Fig. 17.2).

- Contrast extravasation "blush"
- Vascular occlusion "arterial stump"
- Pseudoaneurysms
- Arterio-venous fistulas

Considering the following top ten points, you can save much time, and therefore, these tips are recommended for a successful intervention.

1. Perform angiographic series as selective as possible with a contrast-media injector; avoid hand injections. Most of the available microcatheters are designed even for higher injections rates

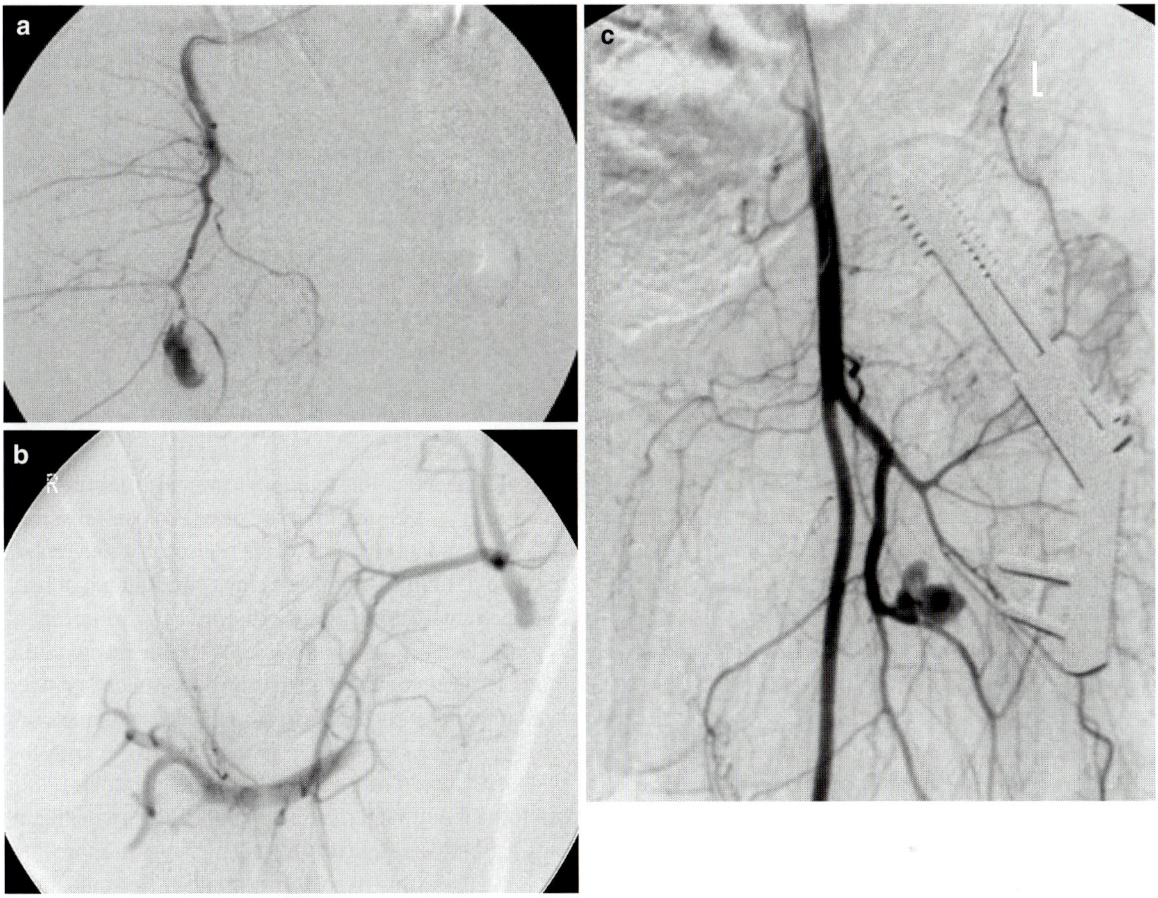

Fig. 17.2 Different imaging patterns of vessel injury presenting at angiographic evaluation. Contrast extravasation (**a**), arterial stump (**b**), pseudoaneurysm (**c**)

resulting in superior visualization of the target vessel region.

2. Perform long series including parenchymal and venous phase for detection of even subtle contrast-media extravasation.
3. Use additional i.v. butylscopolamine in the abdominal region to reduce bowel motion artifacts.
4. When reviewing your angio series, always look on subtracted and unsubtracted images for better differentiation of possible bleeding sites and bowel motion artifacts.
5. Always look for side branch and collateral flow, because according to specific situations, additional vessels have to be embolized for successful bleeding control.
6. The complete target region must be imaged. If the vascular region is greater than your field of view, perform additional series. Especially, in the abdominal and pelvic regions, all visceral arteries must be selectively catheterized including the celiac trunk, both internal iliac and common femoral arteries.
7. Look for "cut offs." Treat visible arterial stumps like an active bleeding. These lacerated or dissected vessels are possibly compressed by surrounding hematoma and could rebleed after hemodynamically stabilization.
8. In case of negative angio, do not use a heparin bolus or other lytics to induce artificial bleeding; this is not recommended.
9. Leave the sheath in place after your intervention because in some cases, additional secondary embolizations must be performed by reopened vessels due to better cardiovascular status of your patient.
10. Avoid time-consuming negative angios and unnecessary interventions.

In an optimal situation, the previous performed CT images guide you to the suspected bleeding area. That means that on the one hand if you do not have suspected signs of arterial bleeding, there is no indication for further time-consuming angiographic evaluation. On the other hand, if bleeding site was identified and the following angio is negative, prophylactic embolization due to possible end-organ failure and concomitant complications should be avoided. Primary goals of interventional procedures are stabilization of the patient and preservation of function of bleeding organs. However, in some cases, a less selective embolization ("shower-embolization") and a surviving patient is better than an interventional "tour de force" and a dead patient.

Common causes for negative angios are local vasospasm, local thrombosis, a venous bleeding, or a wrong catheter position. Therefore, angiographic images must be reviewed extensively in every case.

17.4 Head and Neck Injuries

Cervical blood vessels are the most commonly injured structures following penetrating neck injuries. Their location relative to defined anatomic landmarks dictates the diagnostic workup and therapeutic approaches of these injuries. The neck is divided into three zones. Zone I (from the clavicles to cricoid cartilage), Zone II (between the cricoid cartilage the angle of the mandible), and Zone III (above the angle of the mandible). Regardless of which zone is injured, any hard signs of vascular injury including overt hemorrhage, an expanding hematoma, or ongoing neurologic deficits demand an operative exploration. Endovascular techniques should not be used as a first-line therapy in these cases. Patients who present with soft signs of vascular injury, e.g., stable hematoma are typically hemodynamically stable and you have enough time for detailed evaluation. However, endovascular techniques may assist classical operative approaches like balloon catheter blocking until surgery is done and could potentially avoid the morbidity of median sternotomy, a high thoracic incision, difficult vertebral dissection, or dissections at the base of the skull [4, 5].

17.5 Key Points

- Direct surgical repair remains the gold standard for injuries in all neck zones.
- An occlusion balloon can be used from the groin to provide endoluminal proximal control of the great vessels allowing surgical exposure in a more controlled fashion.
- Endoluminal therapy can be performed under local anesthesia allowing direct assessment of the patient's neurologic status.

17.6 Thoracic and Abdominal Aortic Injuries

Thoracic vascular injuries carry a high mortality rate. Endovascular techniques using stentgrafts are limited to patients presenting hemodynamically stability and are useful in the treatment of delayed manifestations such as pseudoaneurysms, dissections, or arterio-venous fistulas. Usually, trauma patients are often younger than patients treated with stentgrafts for aortic aneurysmal disease. In the first cohort, the mean aortic diameter is approximately 20 mm. The smallest device available today for the thoracic aorta has a diameter of 26 mm. Some interventionalists stated that oversizing up to 40% could be performed without sequelae, but it has to be mentioned that the manufactures recommend only a 10–15% oversize. Oversizing the graft more than 15% can possibly result in secondary complications such as graft compression, graft collapse, endoleak formation, and stentgraft pleating. According to the injury site in some cases, left subclavian artery has to be overstented. Some authors recommend routinely overstenting of the left subclavian artery resulting in an appropriate proximal landing zone. This has proven to be a relative harmless procedure. If secondary symptoms arise, a carotid-to-subclavian artery bypass can be performed.

Vascular injuries in the abdomen remain the leading cause of death after penetrating abdominal aorta and typically require operative exploration to stop hemorrhage because concomitant solid organ and gastrointestinal sites of injuries are common. Nevertheless, endovascular therapies have some advantages in acute and delayed manifestations of abdominal aortic trauma including avoidance of aortic cross clamping and avoidance of opening the retroperitoneum, consecutively placing prosthetic material in possibly contaminated regions if perforated viscus is present and in patients with previous abdominal surgery. Especially, for delayed manifestations, morbidity and mortality rates are dramatically lower compared to open surgical repair.

In the acute setting, aorto-monoilical prosthesis are recommended with contralateral occluders followed by femoro-femoral crossover bypass grafting. If a bifurcated prostheses is used, the patient may bleed to death due to time-consuming catheterization of the contralateral leg [6–11].

17.7 Key Points

- In preinterventional planning scenario for stent-grafting always check iliac diameter. Introducer devices range from 18 to 24 French; therefore, external iliac diameter should not be below 7–8 mm.
- Length of the proximal landing zone should be not less than 10 mm and the stentgraft should be approximately 4 cm longer than the treated segment.
- If the left subclavian artery must be overstented, watch for an occluded right vertebral artery, dominant or indispensable left vertebral artery and patients with left internal mammarian coronary bypass.
- In acute abdominal vascular injuries, aorto-monoiliical prostheses must be on hand because you may get into trouble if catheterization of the contralateral leg joining the main body of bifurcated stent-grafts takes longer than a couple of seconds (this is daily routine even in experienced centers).

17.8 Extremities and Pelvic Injuries

The majority of extremity vascular trauma can be controlled with direct tamponade or tourniquets. Due to the relative long-lasting ischemia tolerance of 4–6 h, there is usually enough time to address other life-threatening injuries and detailed evaluation. Lower as well as upper extremity vascular injuries can be easily approached via femoral access. In case of lower extremity injury, preferentially, use contralateral retrograde access and crossover techniques to avoid deterioration of injury by ipsilateral antegrade access. All kinds of acute or delayed injuries could be treated easily, e.g., pseudoaneurysms, a.v. fistulas, active bleeding, or thrombosis by using embolics, covered stents, or thrombectomy devices. Iliac vessel injuries with expanding pelvic hematomas are among the most challenging to trauma surgeons. The utility of angiographic embolization of bleeding pelvic vessels is well documented and could be reached easily by ipsi- or contralateral femoral approach [12–15].

Important Points

- Assure stable catheter position and be selective as possible to avoid dislodgement of embolics and malperfusion of downstream located regions.
- If embolization of both internal iliacs is necessary, inform patient and/or relatives if possible due to specific complications such as buttock claudication, sexual dysfunction, and gluteal necrosis.
- In case of multiple bleeding sites under these circumstances, proximal "shower-embolization" could be the best and fastest procedure.

References

1. Huber-Wagner S, Levering R, Quick LM et al (2009) Effect of whole-body CT during trauma resuscitation on survival: a retrospective, multicentre study. Lancet 373:1455–1461
2. Sampson MA, Colguhoun KB, Hennessy EL (2006) Computed tomography whole body imaging in multitrauma: 7 years experience. Clin Radiol 61:265–269
3. Arthurs ZM, Sohn VY, Starnes BW (2007) Vascular trauma: endovascular management and techniques. Surg Clin N Am 87:1179–1192
4. Feliciano DV (2001) Management of penetrating injuries to the carotid artery. World J Surg 25:1028–1035
5. Martin MJ, Mullenix PS, Steele SR et al (2005) Functional outcome after blunt and penetrating carotid artery injuries: analysis of the National Trauma Data Bank. J Trauma 59: 860–864
6. Kasirajan K, Heffernan D, Langsfeld M (2003) Acute thoracic trauma: a comparison of endoluminal stentgrafts with open repair and nonoperative management. Ann Vasc Surg 17:589–595
7. White R, Krajcer Z, Johnson M et al (2006) Results of a multicenter trial for the treatment of traumatic vascular injury with a covered stent. J Trauma 60:1189–1195
8. Lin PH, Bush RL, Zhou W et al (2006) Endovascular treatment of traumatic thoracic aortic injury – should this be the new standard of treatment? J Vasc Surg 43:22A–29A
9. Symbas PN, Sherman AJ, Silver JM et al (2002) Traumatic rupture of the aorta: immediate or delayed repair? Ann Surg 235:796–802
10. Hoornweg LL, Dinkelman MK, Goslings JC et al (2006) Endovascular management of traumatic ruptures of the thoracic aorta: a retrospective multicenter analysis of 28 cases in the Netherlands. J Vasc Surg 43:1096–1102

11. Mattison R, Hamilton IN Jr, Ciraulo DL et al (2001) Stent-graft repair of acute traumatic thoracic aortic transection with intentional occlusion of the left subclavian artery: case report. J Trauma 51:326–328
12. Hafez HM, Woolgar J, Robbs JV (2001) Lower extremity arterial injury: results of 550 cases and review of risk factors associated with limb loss. J Vasc Surg 33:1212–1219
13. Busquets AR, Acost JA, Colon E et al (2004) Helical computed tomographic angiography for the diagnosis of traumatic arterial injuries of the extremities. J Trauma 56:625–628
14. Mavili E, Donmez H, Ozcan N (2007) Endovascular treatment of lower limb penetrating arterial traumas. Cardiovasc Intervent Radiol 30:1124–1129
15. Velmahos GC, Toutouzas KG, Vassiliu P et al (2002) A prospective study on the safety and efficacy of angiographic embolization for pelvic and visceral injuries. J Trauma 53:303–308

Imaging of Penetrating Urologic Trauma

18

Beat Schnüriger and Donald J. Green

18.1 Imaging of Penetrating Urologic Trauma

Penetrating injury to the abdomen causes ureteral injury in approximately 2%, kidney injury in up to 8%, and injury to the bladder in up to 20% [1–4]. It is important to keep in mind that microscopic or gross hematuria is unreliable as a diagnostic tool for any urological injury, with a maximal overall sensitivity of 75% [5, 6]. Hematuria may be even absent in cases of complete transection of one ureter [7]. In addition, significant penetrating injuries to the major collecting system may present without hematuria because urine from the injured kidney exits into the retroperitoneum, preventing ureteral conduction.

Maintain a high index of suspicion for urinary tract involvement in all penetrating injuries to the abdomen, flank, pelvis, and perineum. For all gunshot injuries to the trunk, stab wounds to the flank, and cases where the length of the knife may reach the retroperitoneum, you should proceed to further investigations to rule out urinary tract injury.

About half of the patients with injuries to the urinary tract are hypotensive on presentation, indicating the overall severity of trauma and not the urologic injury itself [5]. These patients require immediate laparotomy without delay. Additionally, nearly all gunshot injuries with involvement of the urinary tract are associated with significant concomitant injuries [8]. The decision making regarding diagnostic procedures and treatment of penetrating urologic trauma clearly depends on the hemodynamic status and associated injuries of the patients. As soon as the patient is stable, an evaluation of the urinary tract should follow as part of the secondary survey. The vast majority of urologic injuries are not life threatening. However, failure of diagnosis and delay in treatment may lead to significant patient morbidity [7]. The unique consequence of a penetrating injury to the urinary tract is extravasation of urine with the risk of local and systemic intra- or extra-peritoneal subsequent infection.

Fortunately, the urinary tract has an amazing ability to heal itself. If the flow of urine can be maintained without obstruction, then healing of the injury is likely [7]. To examine the integrity of the urinary tract, a wide spectrum of radiologic investigations is available.

18.2 Computerized Tomography

In hemodynamically stable, clinically evaluable patients without peritoneal signs, perform computerized tomography (CT) scan routinely as part of the secondary survey after penetrating trauma to the trunk. A properly

B. Schnüriger (✉)
Division of Trauma and Critical Care, Department of Surgery, Naval Trauma Training Center, Los Angeles County General Hospital (LAC+USC), University of Southern California, 1200 North State Street, IPT, C5L100, Los Angeles, CA 90033 – 4525, USA

Keck School of Medicine, University of Southern California, Los Angeles, CA, USA
e-mail: beat.schnuriger@gmail.com

D.J. Green
Division of Trauma & Surgical Critical Care, Naval Trauma Training Center, LAC+USC Medical Center, Room 6341 1200N State Street, Los Angeles, CA 90033, USA
e-mail: donaldgr@usc.edu

G.C. Velmahos et al. (eds.), *Penetrating Trauma*,
DOI 10.1007/978-3-642-20453-1_18,

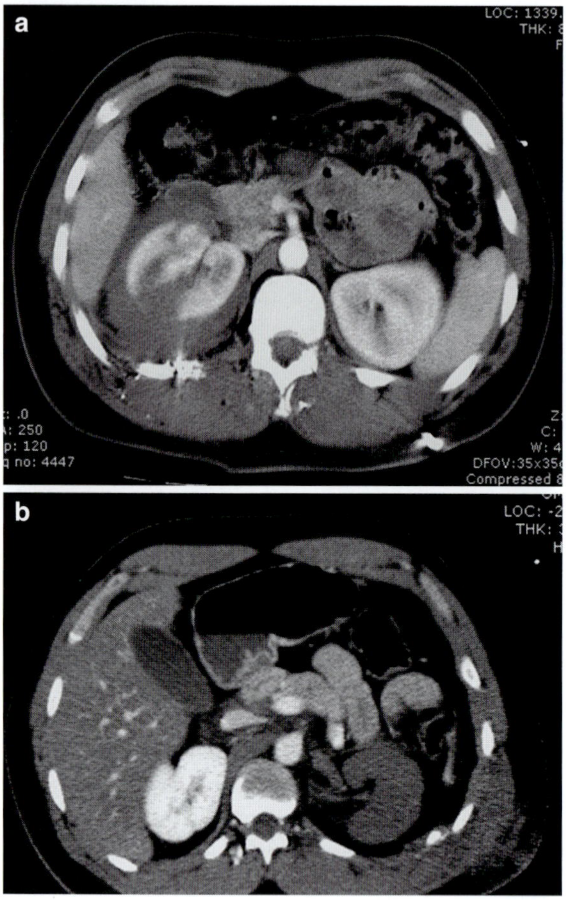

Fig. 18.1 (**a**) Grade IV right kidney injury with retroperitoneal hematoma (zone II) after multiple gunshot injuries to the back. I.V. contrast-enhanced CT scan of the abdomen is highly sensitive in diagnosing parenchymal injuries to the kidneys as well as in detecting active extravasation and associated intra-abdominal injuries. (**b**) Early contrast-enhanced abdominal CT scan after stab wound to the left flank. There is no contrast enhancement of the left kidney due to a renal arterial lesion

performed contrast-enhanced CT scan of the abdomen and pelvis is highly sensitive to detect vascular and parenchymal injuries of the kidneys as well as proximal urine leaks and urinomas (Fig. 18.1) [7]. Acquisition of multiple thin overlapping slices provides excellent 2D and 3D visualization of the entire urinary tract and improves its sensitivity in detecting urinary tract lesions.

Initially, an early phase intravenous contrast CT scan of the abdomen and pelvis is performed. This investigation is highly sensitive in diagnosing parenchymal or vascular injuries to the kidneys as well as in detecting associated injuries (Fig. 18.1). To fully evaluate the collection system, a second CT scan is performed, approximately 10 min after intravenous contrast injection. This technique is known as intravenous CT pyelography (CT-IVP). These delayed-phase images are highly sensitive in diagnosing parenchymal injuries, proximal urine leaks or urinomas, and in confirming bilateral functional renal moieties (Fig. 18.2). However, with a low sensitivity of 37% to detect subtle ureteral injuries, small leaks at this location might be missed [5, 9]. Nevertheless, failure of the distal ureter to opacify on a contrast-enhanced CT scan should raise concern of an injury and should lead to further investigations or intraoperative evaluation of the affected ureter [10].

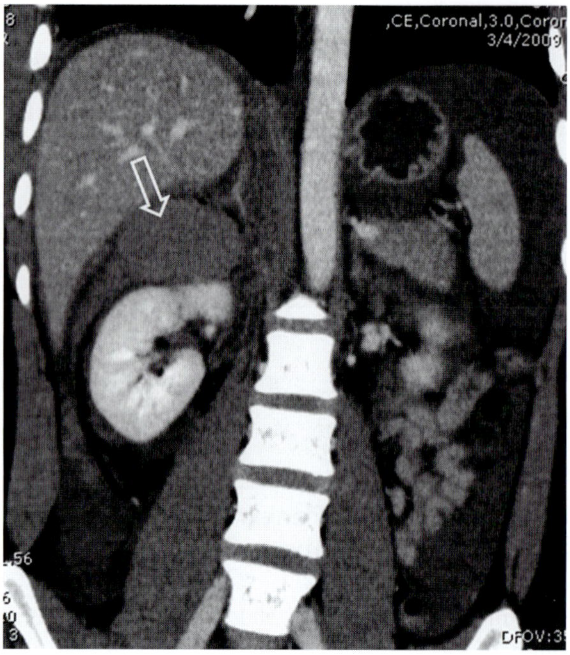

Fig. 18.2 Urinoma (*white arrow*) detected on I.V. contrast-enhanced CT scan after a stab wound to the right upper quadrant. The knife went through the right portion of the liver into the right kidney, where it perforated the major collection system

To further improve the value of the initial CT workup and to save time, a CT cystogram can be easily done simultaneously. CT cystography is equally as sensitive as conventional cystography for the detection of bladder rupture [11]. Immediately before the CT scan, the urinary bladder is gently filled with approximately 350 ml of diluted iodine contrast through the urethral catheter. In the absence of an urethral injury,

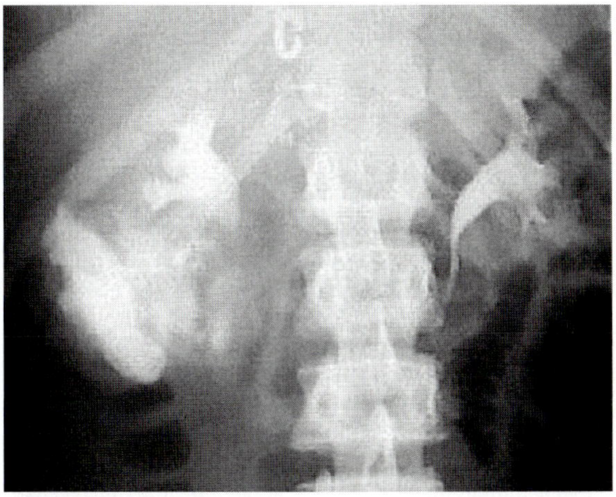

Fig. 18.3 Intraoperative excretory pyelography with complete proximal ureteral disruption. This intraoperative investigation of the urinary tract was made after completion of the damage control procedure

this procedure is safe and provides an accurate visual assessment of the integrity of the bladder. An urethral injury should be suspected in patients with pelvic fractures or penetrating injuries to the perineum. In these cases, you should consider a retrograde uretherogram before placing a urethral catheter [2].

18.3 Pyelography

Pyelography can be performed either as an excretory pyelography or as a retrograde pyelography. With a sensitivity of approximately 30%, *excretory pyelography* is relatively insensitive for the diagnosis of renal injuries and urine leaks [12, 13]. However, in initially unstable patients, excretory pyelography may be useful to investigate the urinary tract intraoperatively after completion of the damage control procedure (Fig. 18.3). In the presence of hematuria or a suspicious penetrating injury tract, a "single shot" excretory IVP is performed intraoperatively. Ten minutes after intravenous injection of 2 cc/kg of contrast, a single abdominal plain film is taken. This investigation has been shown to obviate renal and ureteral exploration in 32% [12].

A *retrograde pyelography* is extremely sensitive in identifying ureteral injuries [14]. However, in the emergency setting of patients sustaining abdominal penetrating injury, its value and practicability is limited. As an adjunct to CT-IVP, or to confirm and further delineate the extent of a ureteral injury postoperatively, it is very helpful. Additionally, this investigation should be considered when planning further secondary surgical management of urinary tract injuries.

18.4 Cystography

All patients with abdominal gunshot wounds or pelvic fractures are at risk of having a ruptured bladder. Gross hematuria is very common in case of a bladder injury, occurring in over 95% of cases [15, 16]. Imaging of the bladder using only excreted contrast material by CT scan or by conventional radiography is not adequate and has been shown to result in false-negative studies [17]. The only definitive study to rule out a ruptured bladder is a retrograde static cystogram [18]. The bladder is gently filled with approximately 350 ml of diluted iodine contrast through a urethral catheter. After that, an extravasation of contrast is captured by conventional plain film or, as described previously, by CT scan. In patients with a suspected urethral injury, a retrograde uretherogram should be considered before placing a urethral catheter. If a urethral rupture is found, the bladder is filled through a suprapubic tube.

18.5 Retrograde Uretherogram

The most common clinical finding in patients with uretheral injuries are gross hematuria or blood at the meatus. Retrograde injection of contrast medium into to urethra is safe and has a high sensitivity for making the diagnosis of urethral rupture (Fig. 18.4) [13]. Multiple techniques have been described in the literature [7, 19]. We have had good results by inserting a 14-Fr Foley catheter at the meatus for about 3–4 cm to the fossa navicularis where the balloon is then gently inflated with 2–3 cc of sterile water. A Toomey syringe is then used to administer 30–40 cc or water-soluble contrast and a plain conventional film is obtained while the last 10 cc is instilled. A large extravasation without filling of the bladder indicates a complete disruption, whereas partial filling of the bladder with some extravasation is indicative of partial disruption of the urethra. If there is no extravasation, the catheter should be advanced into the bladder and a cystogram should be added.

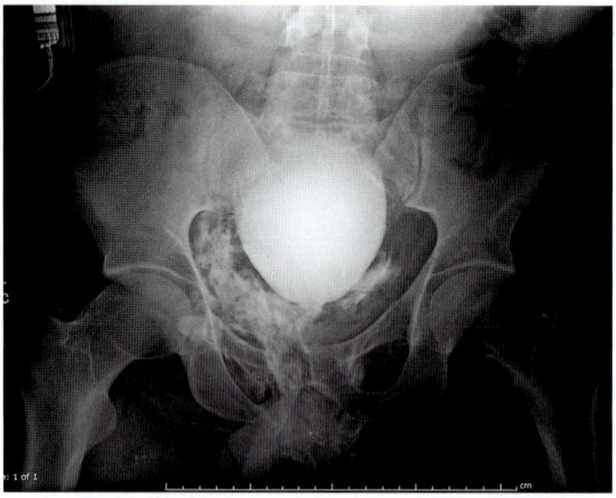

Fig. 18.4 Retrograde uretherography. Large extravasation of contrast into the extraperitoneum including scrotum without filling of the bladder indicates a complete disruption of the urethra. The distended bladder is filled with excreted contrast material from the previous I.V.-enhanced CT scan

Important Points

- Penetrating injuries to the abdomen, flank, pelvis, and perineum involve the urinary tract in up to 20%.
- Hematuria may be absent even in significant upper urinary tract injury.
- The diagnostic procedure and treatment of penetrating urologic trauma clearly depends on the hemodynamic status and associated injuries of the patient.
- In patients with suspected urethral injury, a retrograde uretherogram should be considered before placing a urethral catheter.
- By adding a CT-IVP and a retrograde CT cystogram, the initial CT workup can be improved and accelerated significantly.
- In initially unstable patients, intraoperative excretory pyelography is useful to investigate the urinary tract and may obviate unnecessary renal and ureteral surgical exploration.
- A retrograde pyelography is time consuming but extremely sensit ive in identifying ureteral injuries in the tertiary survey of the patient.

References

1. Cass AS (1984) The multiple injured patient with bladder trauma. J Trauma 24(8):731–734
2. Corriere JN, Sandler CM Jr (1986) Management of the ruptured bladder: seven years of experience with 111 cases. J Trauma 26(9):830–833
3. Pitts JC 3rd, Peterson NE (1981) Penetrating injuries of the ureter. J Trauma 21(11):978–982
4. Presti JC Jr, Carroll PR, McAninch JW (1989) Ureteral and renal pelvic injuries from external trauma: diagnosis and management. J Trauma 29(3):370–374
5. Elliott SP, McAninch JW (2003) Ureteral injuries from external violence: the 25-year experience at San Francisco General Hospital. J Urol 170(4 Pt 1):1213–1216
6. Palmer LS, Rosenbaum RR, Gershbaum MD et al (1999) Penetrating ureteral trauma at an urban trauma center: 10-year experience. Urology 54(1):34–36
7. Jankowski JT, Spirnak JP (2006) Current recommendations for imaging in the management of urologic traumas. Urol Clin North Am 33(3):365–376
8. Coburn M (2008) Genitourinary trauma. In: Feliciano DV, Mattox KL, Moore EE (eds) Trauma, 6th edn. McGraw-Hill, New York
9. Brown SL, Hoffman DM, Spirnak JP (1998) Limitations of routine spiral computerized tomography in the evaluation of blunt renal trauma. J Urol 160(6 Pt 1):1979–1981
10. Townsend M, DeFalco AJ (1995) Absence of ureteral opacification below ureteral disruption: a sentinel CT finding. AJR Am J Roentgenol 164(1):253–254
11. Peng MY, Parisky YR, Cornwell EE 3rd et al (1999) CT cystography versus conventional cystography in evaluation of bladder injury. AJR Am J Roentgenol 173(5):1269–1272
12. Morey AF, McAninch JW, Tiller BK et al (1999) Single shot intraoperative excretory urography for the immediate evaluation of renal trauma. J Urol 161(4):1088–1092
13. Obenauer S, Plothe KD, Ringert RH et al (2006) Imaging of genitourinary trauma. Scand J Urol Nephrol 40(5): 416–422
14. Campbell EW Jr, Filderman PS, Jacobs SC (1992) Ureteral injury due to blunt and penetrating trauma. Urology 40(3): 216–220
15. Corriere JN, Sandler CM Jr (1999) Bladder rupture from external trauma: diagnosis and management. World J Urol 17(2):84–89
16. Morey AF, Iverson AJ, Swan A et al (2001) Bladder rupture after blunt trauma: guidelines for diagnostic imaging. J Trauma 51(4):683–686
17. Haas CA, Brown SL, Spirnak JP (1999) Limitations of routine spiral computerized tomography in the evaluation of bladder trauma. J Urol 162(1):51–52
18. Corriere JN Jr, Sandler CM (2006) Diagnosis and management of bladder injuries. Urol Clin North Am 33(1):67–71
19. Gallentine ML, Morey AF (2002) Imaging of the male urethra for stricture disease. Urol Clin North Am 29(2): 361–372

Video-Assisted Thoracic Surgery in Penetrating Chest Trauma

19

François Pons, Federico Gonzalez, and Jean Philippe Arigon

Video-Assisted Thoracic Surgery (VATS) has gained a place of choice in the surgical management of thoracic injuries since 1991. It is an efficient and safe procedure to assess and manage chest trauma. In specific indications of chest trauma, VATS is associated with decreased morbidity and mortality, and shortened hospital stay [1–6]. Because in trauma patients, VATS is sometimes more challenging than in elective surgery, outcome is strongly related to precise indications and a good thoracoscopic expertise.

19.1 Indications

Hemodynamic instability is an absolute contraindication for VATS. Unstable patients should undergo open surgery: emergency thoracotomy and/or laparotomy in the supine position. Indications for VATS in stable patients are based upon initial findings and the patient evolution. They can be immediate or delayed [3, 7] (Table 19.1).

F. Pons (✉) • F. Gonzalez • J.P. Arigon
Department of Surgery, Ecole du Val de Grâce, Paris, France

Department of Thoracic and General Surgery, Percy Military Hospital, 101 avenue Henri Barbusse, 92140 Clamart, Paris, France
e-mail: fpons@neuf.fr

- Immediate: (immediately or within a couple of hours following the wound):
  - Significant hemothorax (>1 or 1.5 L at chest tube insertion).
  - Continuous bleeding (>300 cc/h within the first 3 h after chest tube insertion).
  - Suspected diaphragmatic injury (quite probable when the entrance wound is inferior to the nipple line) [8].
  - Suspicion of a penetrating heart wound (stable patients with penetrating injuries in cardiac proximity and doubtful pericardial ultrasound examination). The procedure aims at ruling out any pericardium or heart wound which can decompensate at any time [9].
  - Withdrawal of a stab in situ under direct vision [10].
- Delayed (up to several days after the trauma) in case of:
  - Retained or clotted hemothorax [11]. The goals of VATS in the management of these retained collections are (1) evacuation and culture of the collection, (2) release of the trapped lung with decortication, and (3) drainage of the chest cavity and lung reexpansion.
  - Prolonged air leak and/or recurrent pneumothorax [12].
  - Secondary empyema (often secondary to an incompletely drained hemothorax) [13].
  - Chylothorax.
  - Foreign body extraction such as bullets, wires, etc. It should be discussed depending on the proximity of the vascular structures and on the predictable operative difficulties [14].

G.C. Velmahos et al. (eds.), *Penetrating Trauma*,
DOI 10.1007/978-3-642-20453-1_19, © Springer-Verlag Berlin Heidelberg 2012

Table 19.1 Indications for VATS in penetrating chest trauma

Clinical picture (stable)	Interest in penetrating trauma	Time of thoracoscopy	Diagnosis or Treatment	Indication	Position
Significant hemothorax or continuous bleeding	+	Immediate	Diagnosis: source of the bleeding, complete exploration	Discussed, careful	Supine
			Treatment: evacuation of clotted hemothorax, hemostasis		
Residual hemothorax	+	Delayed (third, seventh day)	Treatment	Well admitted	Lateral decubitus
Persistent pneumothorax, air leak	+	Delayed (third day)	Treatment	Well admitted	Lateral decubitus
Suspicion of diaphragmatic injury	++ (wound under the nipple horizontal line)	Immediate	Diagnosis	Well admitted	Supine
			Treatment (sometimes)		
Suspicion of hemopericardium	++ (wound in the "cardiac box")	Immediate	Diagnosis (conversion if hemopericardium)	Discussed, careful	Supine
Post-traumatic empyema	++	Delayed	Treatment	Well admitted	Lateral decubitus
Foreign body	++	Immediate	Treatment	Admitted	Supine or lateral decubitus
		Delayed			
Chylothorax	+	Delayed	Treatment	Admitted, rare	Lateral decubitus

19.2 Technique of Immediate VATS for Penetrating Trauma

The aim of the treatment is twofold: (1) to inspect and accurately diagnose the injuries (hemothorax, chest wall, lung, diaphragm, pericardium), and (2) to proceed accordingly, evacuating an hemothorax, ensuring hemostasis, suturing a diaphragmatic defect, treating a pulmonary lesion etc.… The extent of the lesions and the operator's expertise will decide whether to hold on to VATS or convert to open thoracotomy.

19.2.1 Anesthesia

General anesthesia using a double lumen endotracheal tube is recommended in order to facilitate the ipsilateral lung collapse and optimize the view in the thoracic cavity. When selective endotracheal intubation fails, the exploration is made much more difficult and most of the time you should better convert to an open thoracotomy.

19.3 Positioning of Patient

Penetrating chest injuries may involve various organs, some of them are best dealt with by laparotomy (abdominal viscus), sternotomy, or thoracotomy (heart, contralateral hemithorax, massive bleeding). Patient positioning is therefore paramount in view of a possible thoracic, abdominal extension, and more therapeutic options.

- The lateral decubitus position is the easiest approach to perform VATS, but as laparotomy or sternotomy requires different patient positioning, the surgeon should eliminate diaphragmatic or pericardiac lesions before. In practice, we mainly recommend lateral position for delayed thoracoscopic exploration.
- The supine position (Fig. 19.1) makes the VATS slightly more difficult, but this setting allows accesses in all directions as and when required. Elevate the injured chest with a cushion, the arm folded over the head. If necessary, tilt the operating table up to 30° in order to improve the exposure. Should you need to proceed through a sternotomy or a laparotomy, you just have to remove the cushion and replace the arm in abduction.

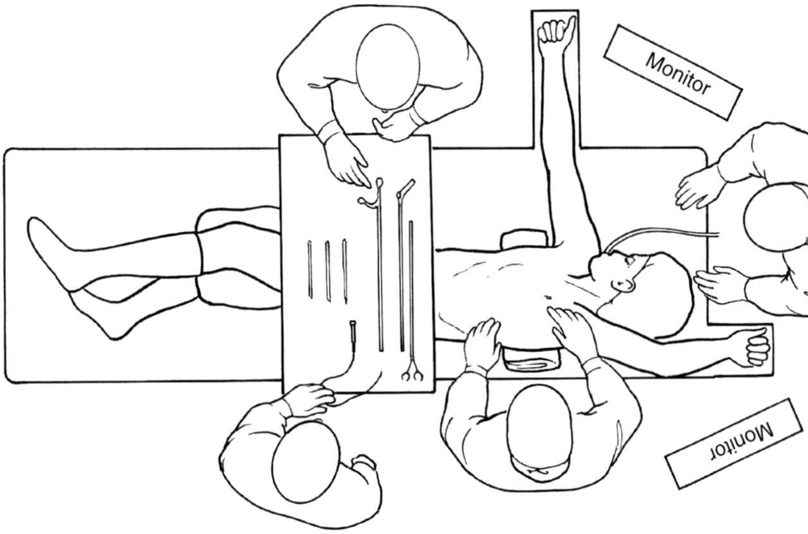

Fig. 19.1 Team allocation and port positions

19.4 Setup and Equipment

The operator stands at the site of the injured chest, his assistant next to him, and the scrub nurse facing him. Formal thoracotomy instruments are prepared and available on an auxiliary table.

The equipment is as follows:

- Two or three trocars (10 mm, sometimes 5 mm), one 10 mm 0° optical (a 30° optical may facilitate the visualization of chest wall lesions), one irrigation-suction cannula, bipolar diathermy forceps, coagulating scissors, lung grasping forceps (Duval type = endoscopic or open surgery forceps), endostaplers Ethicon® or Covidien®, straight or articulated with blue reloads.

19.5 Operative Technique

A large hemothorax should ideally be drained before general anesthesia. The tube is then removed just before the procedure.

19.6 Port Sites

- Use 10-mm ports as it allows you to swap the optical from one site to another.
- Avoid placing the first port in the wound as it may reactivate bleeding.
- The first port site depends on the place of the wound; in most cases, you should place the first port at the level of the inferior angle of the scapula, posterior to the midaxillary line around the fifth intercostal space. It may then be necessary to aspirate blood pouring throughout the port before inserting the optical if the thorax has not been drained before. The inspection immediately focuses on the internal orifice(s) of the chest wound and on adjacent lung lesions. A second port should rapidly follow, either through the seventh or eighth intercostal space, the previous drain orifice, or through the wound itself (Fig. 19.1). Drain the hemothorax under direct vision, swapping instruments if necessary to achieve a systematic and meticulous inspection. A third port disposed in an appropriate triangulation will allow the insertion of a retracture or forceps and careful mobilization of the lung.

19.7 Exploration

This stage may be demanding and stressful. Impaired vision is frequent as the hemothorax absorbs the light and gives the disturbing impression that the patient is still bleeding. You should keep composed and constantly share information with the anesthetist. As long as the patient is stable, you can pursue the thoracic washout, aspirating the blood and clots from the apex to the diaphragmatic cul de sac. To remove large clots,

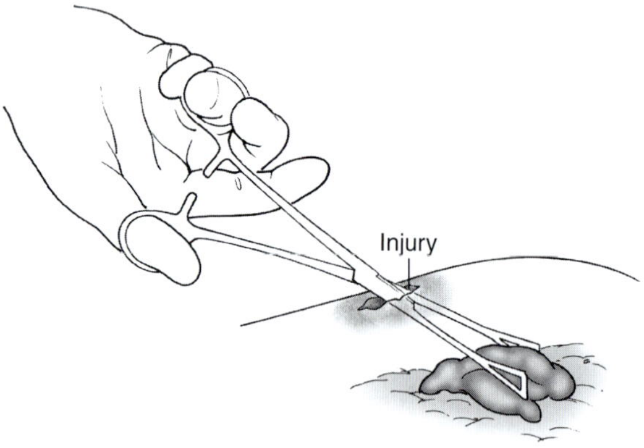

Fig. 19.2 To remove large clots, you can use lung forceps as for open surgery (Kelly or Duval) introduced through the defect without trocar

you can use lung forceps as for open surgery (Kelly or Duval) introduced through the port without trocar (Fig. 19.2). Once evacuation of the hemothorax has been achieved, you should systematically examine the lung, the diaphragm, the pericardium, the internal aspect of the chest, inventory all lesions and decide whether the treatment will remain thoracoscopic or converted into a sternotomy.

19.8 Parietal Lesion Hemostasis

If an intercostal artery bleeds, you can achieve hemostasis with bipolar diathermy, completed if necessary with a hemostatic gauze packed in the orifice. Hemoclips are often unsuccessful. Anterior or lateral wounds may require an enlargement of the wound and a stitch under direct or video-assisted vision. Posterior wound bleeding is more difficult to control through utility incisions; therefore, thoracoscopic hemostatic packing can be an alternative.

19.9 Treatment of Pulmonary Injuries

You should remember that the treatment of a pulmonary injury must be a lung-sparing technique [15]. Inspection determines the site of the wound, its size and depth, the appearance of the adjacent parenchyma, the severity of the bleeding, the air leak, etc.

- A peripheral wound is ideally stapled: Grasp the injured lung and apply one or two series of staples in the adjacent normal parenchyma (Fig. 19.2). The resected lung is then extracted under direct vision through the port.
- In case of a dry deep wound, possibly transfixing: Do not catheterize or manipulate as bleeding may reoccur. Refrain yourself from any deleterious manipulation and prefer a simple lateral stapling or even abstention.
- Pulmonary contusions without breach should just be left well alone.
- Massive bleeding through a deep pulmonary opening is rarely encountered at this stage due to prior hemodynamic instability. In the exceptional case that this occurs, convert into open thoracotomy.
- Some authors reported video-assisted lobectomies in penetrating chest trauma. We share with others the opinion that it should remain the exception to spare as much parenchyma as possible. Most importantly, the patient is hardly ever hemodynamically stable when lobectomy is indicated; therefore VATS is contraindicated [16].
- An insufficient air leak control may be improved with an application of surgical sealant or collagen patch [17].

In conclusion, the main target is to achieve hemostasis. A small residual air leaks may be tolerated as it will dry out with the chest tubes. Keep in mind that massive pulmonary bleeding may lead to thoracotomy and that pulmonary contusions are not as such an indication of resection, as the lung parenchyma has surprising capabilities for recovery.

19.10 Diaphragmatic Injury (DI)

Diaphragmatic injury is suspected when the entrance wound is located below the nipple line. When an associated abdominal injury is present, based upon the abdominal entry wound site, the peritonitic signs, the intraabdominal viscus lesions on ultrasound or CT scan, you should prefer an abdominal approach. When there is only a thoracic wound (especially for a posterior or lateral stab wound), VATS is recommended to rule out a diaphragmatic injury.

Carefully examine the area facing the wound entry into the thoracic cavity and push down the hemidiaphragm to visualize the posterior cul de sac where a small wound can be missed. If you find diaphragmatic injury, a laparotomy should be considered

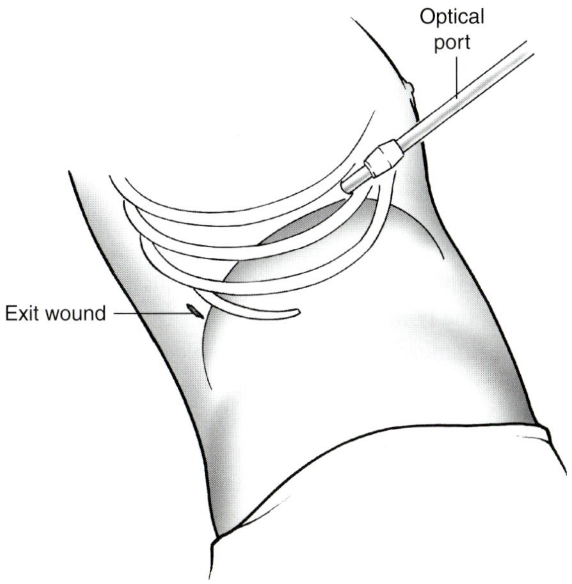

Fig. 19.3 Thoracoscopic visualization of a defect in the diaphragm

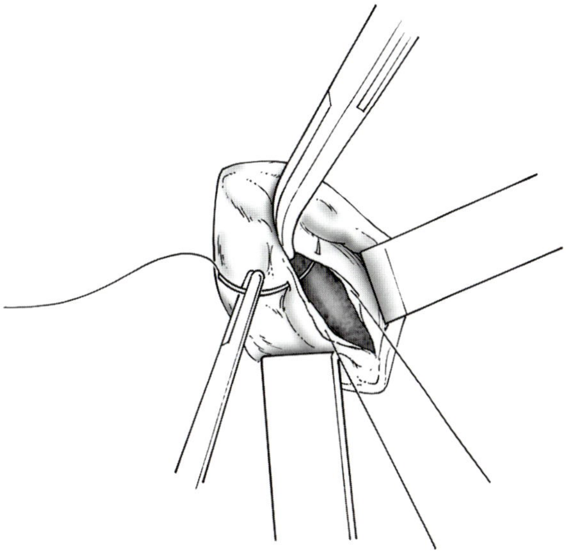

Fig. 19.4 Direct suture through a small utility thoracotomy suture

to diagnose and treat associated intraabdominal injury. Thoracic approach is easier than abdominal to repair posterior DI particularly if you consider laparoscopy. As a result, you may choose the thoracic approach if you are familiar with this access or if laparotomy is not indicated. You can repair the diaphragm either under thoracoscopic vision, or through an utility thoracotomy.

Video-assisted repair of a DI: Interrupted sutures, or a running suture of nonabsorbable material is applied using two ports (one for the forceps, one for the needle holder). Endothoracic knotting may be difficult and time consuming specifically for posterior lesions.

Repair through a utility thoracic incision (Figs. 19.3 and 19.4): The diaphragmatic breach can be exposed, then grasped and sutured through a limited thoracotomy centered on the DI or through the enlarged thoracic wound.

19.11 Pericardial Effusion

Inspect the pericardium systematically. A wound may directly be visible or an effusion may be seen through a stretched pericardium. In this case, be careful and inform the anesthetist of a probable heart wound leading to immediate sternotomy or anterolateral thoracotomy. When pericardial effusion is not obvious, perform a pericardial window to rule out hemopericardium. Identify the phrenic nerve and grasp the pericardium (most of the time posteriorly to it on the left and anteriorly on the right) (Fig. 19.5). Endoscopic forceps may not be as effective as expected to hold the pericardiac sac, in which case use formal forceps (Bengolea or Roberts) directly inserted in an intercostal space will be of great help. A 1–2-cm incision in the pericardium is sufficient to diagnose a hemopericardium. Some authors recommend abstention when minimal bleeding is met. We do not share the same view and strongly advocate immediate conversion to thoracotomy or sternotomy. When pericardiac effusion is eliminated, then the pericardial window should be left open.

19.12 End of Procedure

Insert at least one chest tube through the inferior port under direct vision. The lung is then progressively reinflated showing possible air leaks. Close the remaining incisions.

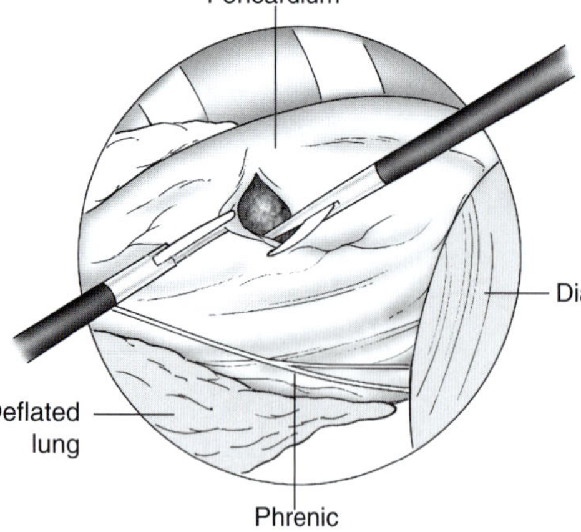

Fig. 19.5 Pericardiotomy after identification of the phrenic nerve. Note that a horizontal incision may be safe especially when the nerve cannot be seen

- Foreign body extraction: It needs first to be precisely localized on CT scans to discuss the feasibility of a VATS extraction and above all anticipate the risks of bleeding. When it is in close proximity to a main vessel, then thoracotomy will probably be the way forward.
- Posttraumatic chylothorax: This is a rare complication that may require surgery when the medical treatment is unsuccessful. VATS will aim at identifying the lymphatic vessel and ensure lymphostasis with diathermy, endoclips, or biologic glues.

Provided that the surgeon sticks to some basic principles, VATS in a stable patient with penetrating trauma of the chest allows a comprehensive exploration of the thoracic cavity and the performance of simple procedures, which will ensure a better outcome in terms of morbidity, mortality, and duration of hospital stay.

19.13 Technique of Delayed VATS for Penetrating Trauma

These procedures are performed 3 or 4 days (or later) after the trauma. They are consequently carried out as elective procedures. We will just emphasize on the main steps.

Anesthesia: A double lumen endotracheal tube is also necessary.

Patient setting: Likewise to elective thoracic surgery, the lateral decubitus position is the position of choice.

Trocar positioning: The optical trocar is placed in the fifth intercostal space slightly posterior to the scapular angle. One or two additional ports will then be positioned depending on the procedure.

The main steps are: (1) exploration; (2) evacuation of a clotted hemothorax (sometimes old clots will need to be fragmented and extracted bit by bit, a gentle dissection and peeling with sponge sticks and ring forceps usually allows the rind to be removed from the visceral and parietal pleuras, thus completely releasing the trapped lung); and (3) reexpansion of the lung to identify air leaks that will be treated as described above with stapler, sealant, collagen patches.

Important Points

- Hemodynamic instability is an absolute contraindication for VATS.
- Double lumen endotracheal intubation is strongly recommended.
- Think of abdominal or thoracic extension: Prefer the supine position for immediate VATS.
- Do not use the wound for the first trocar.
- You can use the wound or a tube incision for the other trocars.
- The treatment of pulmonary injuries must be a lung-sparing technique.
- Repair of a diaphragmatic injury is often easier through a small utility thoracotomy.

References

1. Lieber A, Pons F, Düsel W, Glapa M, Machemehl T, Röhm B, Doll D (2006) The value of thoracoscopy in thorax trauma. Chirurg 77(11):1014–1021
2. Lang-Lazdunski L, Mouroux J, Pons F, Grosdidier G, Martinod E, Elkaim D, Azorin J, Jancovici R (1997) Role of videothoracoscopy in chest trauma. Ann Thorac Surg 67:327–333
3. Ahmed N, Jones D (2004) Video-assisted thoracic surgery: state of the art in trauma care. Int J Care Injured 35:479–489

4. Ben-Nun A, Orlovsky M, Best LA (2007) Video-assisted thoracoscopic surgery in the treatment of chest trauma: long-term benefit. Ann Thorac Surg 83(2):383–387
5. Paci M, Ferrari G, Annessi V, de Franco S, Guasti G, Sgarbi G (2006) The role of diagnostic VATS in penetrating thoracic injuries. World J Emerg Surg 1:30
6. Degiannis E, Bowley D, Smith M (2004) Minimally invasive surgery in trauma: technology looking for an application. Int J Care Injured 35:474–478
7. Divisi D, Battaglia C, De Berardis B, Vaccarili M, Di Francescantonio W, Salvemini S, Crisci R (2004) Video-assisted thoracoscopy in thoracic injury: early or delayed indication? Acta Biomed 75(3):158–163
8. Freeman RK, Al-Dossari G, Hutcheson KA, Huber L, Jessen ME, Meyer DM, Wait MA, DiMaio JM (2001) Indications for using video-assisted thoracoscopic surgery to diagnose diaphragmatic injuries after penetrating chest trauma. Ann Thorac Surg 72(2):342–347
9. Pons F, Lang-Lazdunski L, de Kerangal X, Chapuis O, Bonnet PM, Jancovici R (2002) The role of videothoracoscopy in management of precordial thoracic penetrating injuries. Eur J Cardiothorac Surg 22:7–12
10. Hanvesakul R, Momin A, Gee MJ, Marrinan MT (2005) A role for video assisted thoracoscopy in stable penetrating chest trauma. Emerg Med J 22:386–387
11. Navsaria PH, Vogel RJ, Nicol AJ (2004) Thoracoscopic evacuation of retained posttraumatic hemothorax. Ann Thorac Surg 78:282–285
12. Schermer CR, Matteson BD, Demarest GB III, Albrecht RM, Davis VH (1999) A prospective evaluation of video-assisted thoracic surgery for persistent air leak due to trauma. Am J Surg 177(6):480–484
13. Landreneau RJ, Keenan RJ, Hazelrigg SR, Mack MJ (1996) Thoracoscopy for empyema and hemothorax. Chest 109(1): 18–24
14. Barish H, Edil MD, Aaron L, Trachte MD, Christopher Knott-Craig MD, Roxie M, Albrecht MD (2007) Video-assisted thoracoscopic retrieval of an intrapleural foreign body after penetrating chest trauma. J Trauma 63:E5–E6
15. Petrone P, Asensio JA (2009) Surgical management of penetrating pulmonary injuries. Scand J Trauma Resusc Emerg Med 17(1):8
16. Kaseda S, Aoki T, Hangai N, Yamamoto S, Kitano M, Yajima Y (1997) A case of deep laceration of the lung treated with video-assisted thoracic surgical lobectomy: case report. J Trauma 43(5):856–858
17. Carrillo EH, Kozloff M, Saridakis A, Bragg S, Levy J (2006) Thoracoscopic application of a topical sealant for the management of persistent posttraumatic pneumothorax. J Trauma 60(1):111–114

Diagnostic Peritoneal Lavage (DPL) Unplugged

20

Terence O'Keeffe

The original technique for performing a Diagnostic Peritoneal Lavage was described by Root et al. in 1965 [1]. At one time, it was the diagnostic test of choice to detect the presence of blood in the abdominal cavity. With the advent of the CT scan and later the FAST exam, it now enjoys a more limited use. However, as described in the new eighth edition of the ATLS manual, DPL can be performed rapidly, is 98% sensitive, can detect bowel injury, and is still taught as a skills station during the ATLS course [2].

In the real world, a note of caution must be expressed regarding the speed with which it can be performed; because of the limited use of DPL, it may be difficult to find the necessary equipment and the lack of technical familiarity may extend the time it takes to get a definitive result. The increasing obesity of trauma patients also makes the placement of the catheter challenging, while the infusion of saline is not always rapid, and the laboratory will often take up to 30 min to report the results.

Notwithstanding the above, the safe and rapid performance of a DPL should remain part of the diagnostic skillset of the trauma surgeon. It retains its usefulness especially in the hemodynamically abnormal patient with a negative or equivocal FAST exam.

T. O'Keeffe
Division of Trauma/Critical Care and Emergency Surgery, University of Arizona, 1501 N Campbell Avenue, Rm 5411, P.O. Box 245063, Tucson, AZ 85724-5063, USA
e-mail: tokeeffe@surgery.arizona.edu

20.1 Open or Closed?

The technique as originally described consisted of placing a catheter through the abdominal wall into the peritoneal cavity, and aspirating for gross blood or bile, with subsequent infusion of a liter of saline into the abdomen, followed by removal and analysis of the effluent [1].

Both an open and a percutaneous technique have been described, the choice generally being operator preference, with the closed technique generally being quicker; however, the open technique may at times be safer [3–5]. Both procedures use the infraumbilical approach, which should be altered only for atypical circumstances such as a pelvic fracture or pregnancy (to prevent decompression of pelvic hematomas or avoid the gravid uterus respectively).

Prior to performing a DPL, you should always place a nasogastric tube and Foley catheter to decompress the stomach and bladder. Relative, but not absolute, contraindications to the performance of a DPL include prior surgery, advanced cirrhosis, coagulopathy, and morbid obesity.

20.1.1 Percutaneous Technique

Otherwise known as a closed DPL, this method employs the Seldinger technique i.e., passing a catheter over a wire placed into the abdomen through a needle inserted through the fascia. The initial preparation of the patient is the same in both methods; you need to sterilely prepare the area around the umbilicus with Betadine or chlorhexidine, and drape widely to ensure a sterile field. In the hemodynamically normal

G.C. Velmahos et al. (eds.), *Penetrating Trauma*,
DOI 10.1007/978-3-642-20453-1_20, © Springer-Verlag Berlin Heidelberg 2012

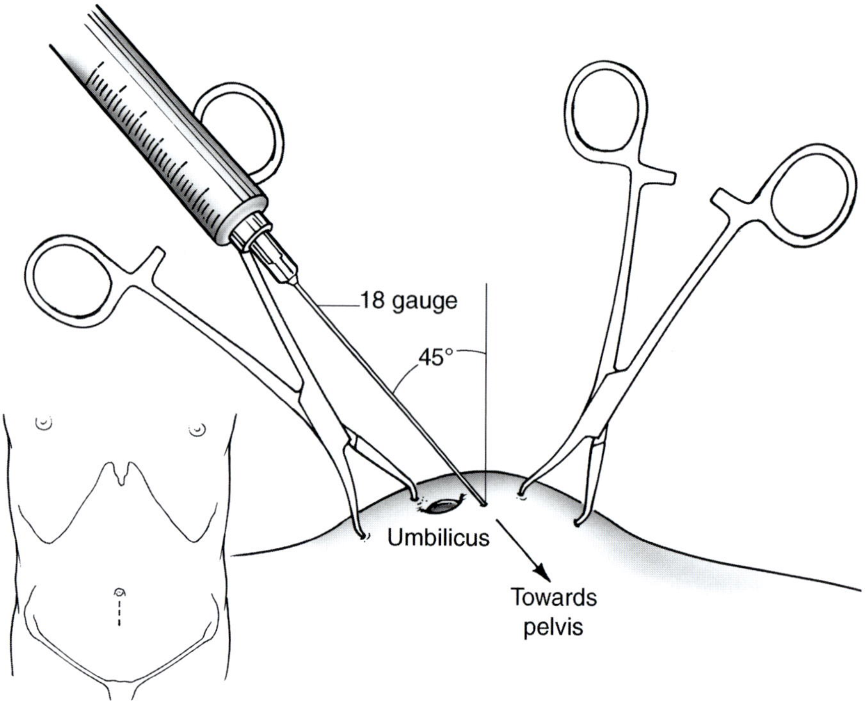

Fig. 20.1 Grasp the abdominal wall with towel clips and inject saline

and awake patient, infiltration with local anesthesia will help to ensure the procedure is comfortable for the patient. Conscious sedation is rarely, but sometimes, necessary. A vertical stab incision is sufficient for the percutaneous method, and you should then securely grasp the abdominal wall (usually with towel clips) to allow good counter-traction. Then attach the needle from the DPL kit to a syringe containing a few ccs of saline and place it percutaneously through the fascia (Fig. 20.1). You will feel two distinct changes in the tension on the needle (two "pops") as you penetrate the fascia and enter the peritoneal cavity.

You should confirm that you are in the peritoneal cavity by watching saline flow easily from the needle into the abdomen; double-check this by disconnecting the syringe and watching the saline flow freely down the needle. Then place the wire through the needle, which you subsequently withdraw leaving only the wire in place. Some DPL kits come with a dilator, which you should use at this point to make the placement of the catheter easier. Next, you insert the DPL catheter over the wire and into the abdomen (Fig. 20.2). If you hold the catheter close to its point of insertion and rotate it continually as it is inserted, this helps it pass through the abdominal wall more easily. Angle the needle and subsequent catheter insertion toward the pelvis, as the whole purpose of the DPL is to identify fluid in the dependent portions of the abdomen.

Once the catheter is in place, you should aspirate it gently, looking for the presence of >10 ccs of blood or enteric contents such as bile or vegetable matter. If none of these are present, infuse a liter of warmed saline into the patient's abdominal cavity. As some DPL kits have relatively small catheters, you will normally find it necessary to squeeze the fluid in at this point, or place it on a pressure bag. A very rapid infusion can be accomplished using the Level One infuser to infuse the saline into the patient.

It is important to retain a small amount of saline in the bag at the end of the procedure, and not to allow air to enter the tubing; otherwise the capillary effect will be lost. After about 970–980 ccs have been instilled, you should lower the bag below the level of the patient and the capillary effect will draw back the fluid that has been instilled (Fig. 20.3). You can help this by gentle pressure and agitation on the patient's abdomen, and also with some careful rotation and movement of the catheter, while being vigilant not to withdraw it and allow air to enter the tubing. It is important to try and get out as much fluid as possible, as this can influence the results of the

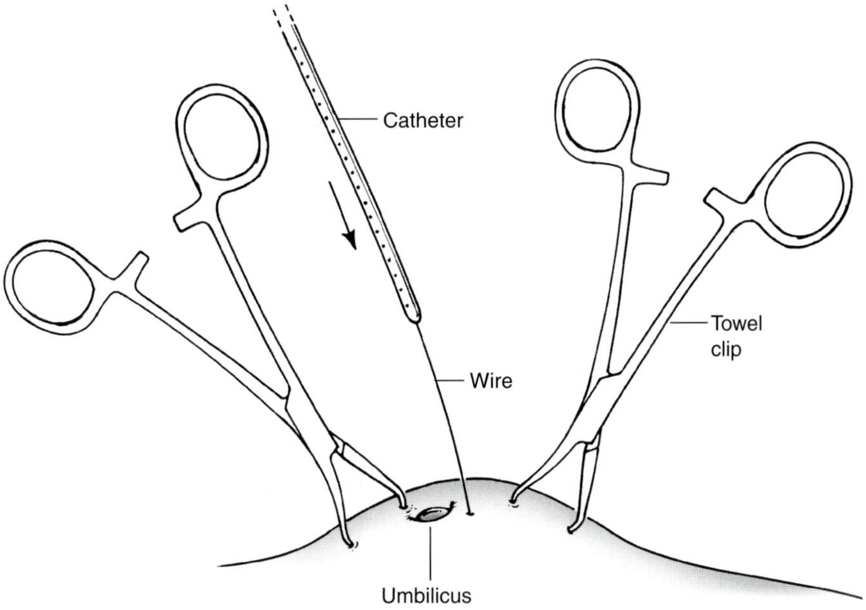

Fig. 20.2 Insert the DPL catheter over the wire and into the abdomen

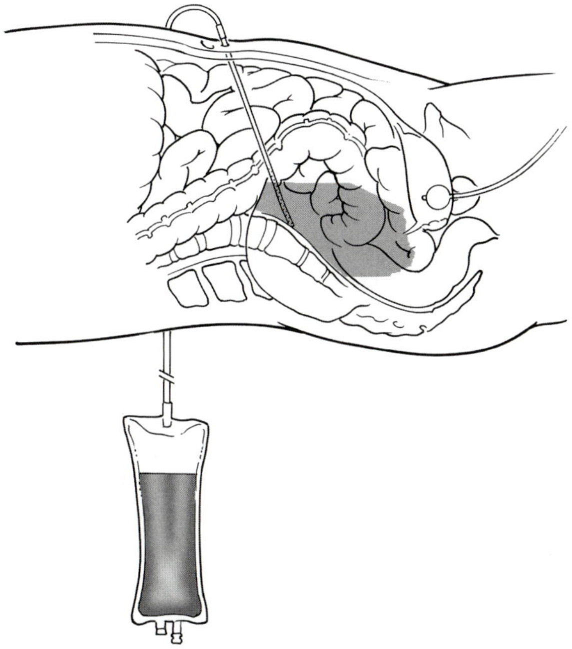

Fig. 20.3 Lower the bag below the level of the patient, and the capillary effect will draw back the fluid that has been instilled

cell count [6]. Although prior studies have shown that a negative DPL can be obtained with as little as 100 ccs of fluid, you should wait until at least 400 ccs have been collected, before sending the effluent for analysis [7].

20.1.2 Open Technique

The open technique does not differ in its initial steps, but instead of a vertical stab, a 2–5-cm vertical incision is usually necessary, with the exact size depending on the thickness of the abdominal wall and the operator's skill. Again you should make this just above or below the umbilicus depending on the presence or absence of pelvic fractures or a gravid uterus. Next, dissect down to the level of the fascia, taking care to minimize bleeding from the subcutaneous tissues and fat, which could potentially interfere with the result. Although having an electrocautery device is useful, if it is not available, using Lidocaine with epinephrine can help to reduce any bleeding. Once you visualize the linea alba, make a small incision in the fascia (Fig. 20.4). Then grasp the peritoneum with two fine hemostats and under gentle upward tension make a small nick to safely enter the peritoneal cavity. Place the DPL catheter under direct vision into the peritoneal cavity and aspirate using a 10-cc syringe (Fig. 20.5). If it is not grossly positive, infuse a liter of warmed saline into the patient as per the closed technique.

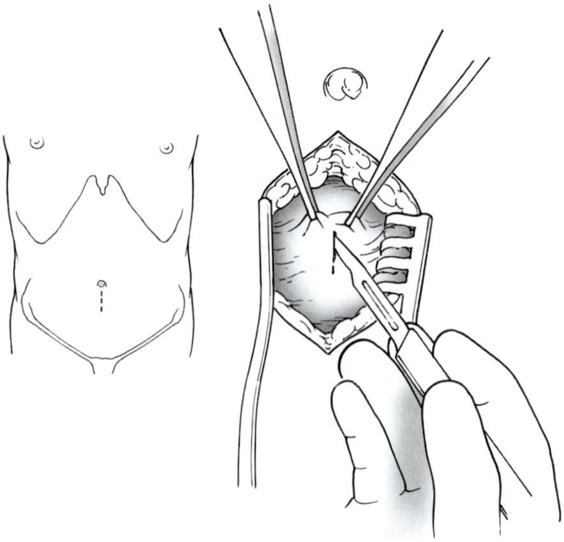

Fig. 20.4 Make a small incision in the fascia

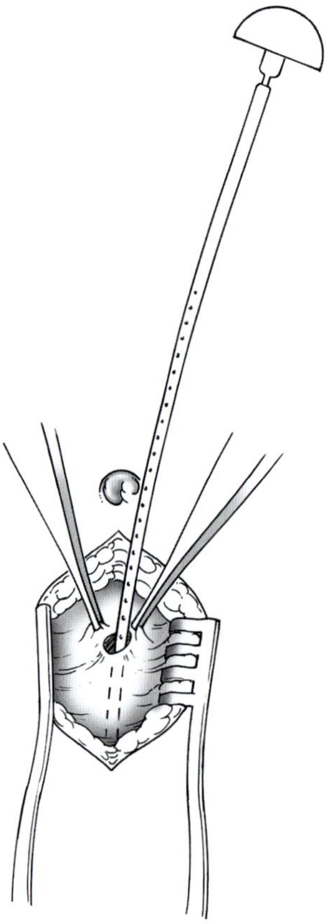

Fig. 20.5 Place the DPL catheter under direct vision into the peritoneal cavity and aspirate using a 10-cc syringe

20.2 Interpretation

If after placing the catheter into the abdominal cavity, your initial aspiration yields greater than 10 ccs of blood or if bile or vegetable matter is present, then this is considered a positive test and the patient should be taken directly to the operating room. While there is general agreement of what constitutes a positive test for blunt trauma patients (>100,000 RBCs/mm^3, >500 WBCs/mm^3, bile, food fibers, or amylase higher than the serum amylase), the same is not true for patients sustaining penetrating trauma.

If a red cell count of 100,000/mm^3 is used, there is a low risk of a nontherapeutic procedure, but some authors feel there is a greater risk of a missed injury (false-negative) of 9–11% [8, 9]. The converse is also true; if the cell count is lowered to 10,000 RBCs/mm^3, there is a false-positive rate of between 12% and 14%. One must weight the risk/benefit of a missed injury vs. a nontherapeutic celiotomy. Recent data would suggest that if the same criteria are used (RBCs, WBCs, bile, food fibers and amylase) for penetrating trauma as recommended above for blunt trauma, there will be no greater risk of a missed injury [8]. It is our preference to use 100,000/mm^3 as a positive cell count, but observe the patient closely for 23 h even if negative to prevent missed injuries. If there is a suspicion for a diaphragm injury, then diagnostic laparoscopy is preferred, as DPL has a low sensitivity for this injury. The old adage of "inability to read newsprint through the saline bag" as an indication of a positive DPL has been scientifically disproven and should be abandoned [10].

The white cell count, although also controversial, is helpful in identifying bowel injuries if the DPL is performed at least 3 h after injury. The accuracy of enzyme assays from lavage fluid has unfortunately been shown to be of limited value [11].

Although rarely used in the pediatric population, there are some variances that need to be considered. The amount of fluid infused should be 10–15 ccs/kg and the cell counts must be adjusted for the smaller amount of fluid infused. The values used for adult patients are then adjusted on the basis of a 1-L dilution. If only 500 ccs are infused, a positive red cell count would be greater than 200,000.

Table 20.1 Summary of DPL versus other diagnostic modalities

	DPL	Fast	CT scan
Time	20–30 min	1–2 min	Variable
Repeatability	Possible, but rarely performed	Easy	Repeatable
Safety	Low risk (<2%)	No risk	Unknown risk (Long-term radiation)
Reliability	Not organ specific	Operator dependent	Obesity, movement
	Not indicated for retroperitoneal injuries	Not organ specific	Misses some injuries
Sensitivity	High	Medium	High
Specificity	Low	High	High
Advantages	Can be performed anywhere	Can perform anywhere can take machine	Noninvasive Highly accurate
	Inexpensive	Noninvasive	
	May detect bowel injury	Rapidly performed	
		Inexpensive	
Disadvantages	Invasive	Hampered by	Requires transport
		• Subcutaneous air	
		• Intraabdominal air	
		• Obesity	
		• Pelvic fractures	
		• Only detects presence of fluid	
	Misses injuries	Initial outlay for ultrasound machine	Misses injuries
	• Retroperitoneum		• Diaphragm
			• Small bowel
	• Diaphragm		• Pancreas
			Expensive
			Radiation exposure

20.3 Current Status of DPL

As paradigms shift, so does the management of patients. With the advent of nonoperative management of many trauma patients and the introduction of newer studies such as the FAST, and newer high-speed CT scans, diagnostic peritoneal lavage has assumed far less of a role than in years past. Because of its limited use, it has been abandoned in some centers and newer trainees now have little or no experience with its use [12, 13]. In spite of the popularity of the FAST, one must take into account that it is operator dependent and there are technical limitations. Likewise, a CT scan can be time consuming, expensive, and exposes the patient to considerable radiation exposure. Table 20.1 summarizes the advantages and disadvantages for the various investigative modalities.

Therefore, where does DPL come into the picture? The ideal time to use DPL is in the hemodynamically abnormal (shock) patient with multiple injuries secondary to blunt trauma. It is imperative to rapidly localize the bleeding or the cause of hypotension. If the FAST is equivocal, negative, or unavailable, a DPL that is positive can quickly make that determination and allow one to proceed to the operating room without delay. If on the other hand, the DPL is negative, one can rule out the abdomen as the source of bleeding with reasonable confidence and avoid an unnecessary abdominal procedure. Recent data has shown the validity of this approach, with DPL 100% accurate in the hemodynamically unstable patient (where the FAST was only positive in 45% of the time) [14].

The most important current application for DPL in penetrating trauma remains in the investigation of anterior abdominal stab wounds. With the abandonment

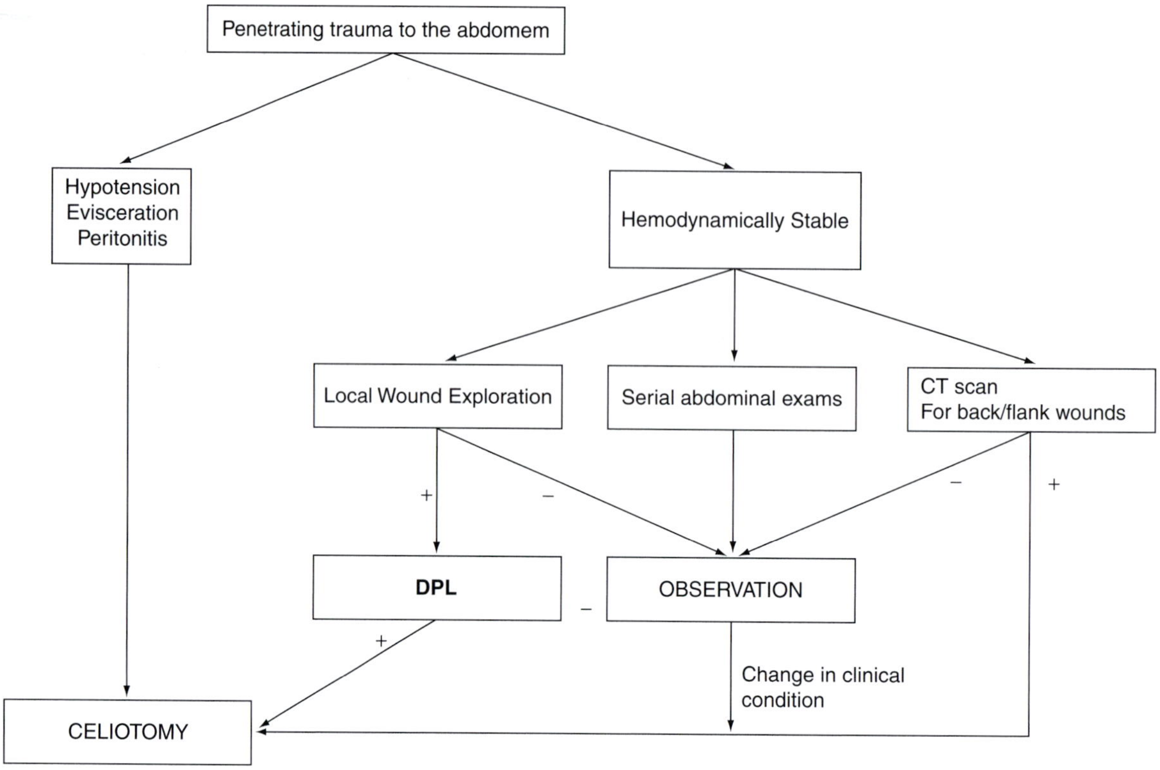

Fig. 20.6 Schema for the investigation of the patient with penetrating trauma to the abdomen, including the use of DPL where appropriate

of mandatory operative intervention for abdominal stab wounds, most centers today rely on close observation and serial examinations for patients who do not have clear-cut indications for surgery. In situations where there are limited personnel resources, the DPL can afford a quick answer in patients with these stab wounds. There may also be a limited role in patients with lower anterior chest wounds, although laparoscopy is a better choice in these cases, as the DPL will miss many diaphragmatic injuries.

In those hospitals that utilize local wound exploration, there is another role for DPL. If the wound exploration (performed under local anesthesia and sterile technique, with extension of the wound and direct visualization of the depth of penetration) is either inconclusive and/or positive (fascial penetration) and the patient remains asymptomatic, DPL can assist in the decision as to whether or not the patient needs an operation. If it is negative, the length of stay in the hospital can be considerably shortened. It must be emphasized that its greatest utility is in patients with anterior and perhaps selected flank wounds and it should not be used to rule out retroperitoneal injuries, as it is highly likely it will miss injuries to the kidneys, pancreas, or retroperitoneal colon.

Although reports are beginning to appear regarding the use of DPL in gunshot wounds, this should not be adopted at this time. Missiles do not travel in straight lines and there is no guarantee that the tract can be accurately determined. DPL cannot address the issue of blast injury, which may not be manifest for several hours or even days. As stated above, the DPL has no role in the assessment of retroperitoneal injuries.

There has been a renewed interest in diagnostic peritoneal aspiration (DPA) [15]. The technique is similar to the DPL; however the fluid is not infused. This approach is most useful to determine quickly if the cause of hypotension in a patient is due to an intra-abdominal source, if FAST is not available or is unreliable. There may be an advantage to this technique if the patient needs a CT scan, as there will be less confusion if the abdomen is not filled with lavage fluid. If the aspirate is positive, it is extremely accurate, but the false-negative rate is significantly higher than a full DPL with lavage, and a negative result should be interpreted with caution.

Figure 20.6 proposes a schema for the investigation of the patient with penetrating trauma to the abdomen, including the use of DPL where appropriate.

There may also be a need for DPL in those institutions that do not possess capabilities in ultrasonography or CT scanning. This may be because the hospital itself does not have the resources, or the practitioners caring for the patient do not have the technical expertise. Although DPL is invasive, it is associated with a low complication rate (<2%) and can be easily and quickly taught to non-surgeons. In an austere environment, DPL may be a more useful examination, as other imaging or investigative modalities may not be available. As a DPL kit currently costs approximately $35 in the USA, compared to a $30,000 ultrasound machine or million-dollar CT scanner, this is much more in the budget of a smaller and less well-equipped hospitals, such as may be found in less industrialized nations.

Despite its introduction over 40 years ago, this simple test is still the subject of controversy in terms of indications, technique, and interpretation, particularly since the development of the FAST exam and the advent of CT scanning. There remains a group of selected patients in which it may be helpful and its simplicity, ease of performance, and acceptable sensitivity and accuracy warrant its continued use. Perhaps, since the procedure has been put on the back shelf in many institutions, it may be time to dust it off and teach our new trainees how to perform it.

Important Points

- Know where the DPL kit is in your ED.
- Make a point of teaching DPL to your residents/staff.
- Always use the IV tubing that comes in the kit (normal IV tubing has a one-way valve).
- A Level One introducer can infuse the fluid VERY rapidly.
- NEVER put in all 1,000 ccs – leave 20–30 ccs in the bag.
- Remember the Foley and nasogastric tube.
- Consider Lidocaine with Epinephrine if doing open DPL.
- In pediatric patients, use 10–15 ccs/kg of saline.

References

1. Root HD, Hauser CW, McKinley CR, Lafave JW, Mendiola RP Jr (1965) Diagnostic peritoneal lavage. Surgery 57: 633–637
2. American College of Surgeons (2008) Abdominal trauma. In: Advanced trauma life support for doctors, 8th edn. American College of Surgeons, Chicago, pp 111–129
3. Velmahos GC, Demetriades D, Stewart M et al (1998) Open versus closed diagnostic peritoneal lavage: a comparison on safety, rapidity, efficacy. J R Coll Surg Edinb 43:235–238
4. Hodgson NF, Stewart TC, Girotti MJ (2000) Open or closed diagnostic peritoneal lavage for abdominal trauma? A meta-analysis. J Trauma 48:1091–1095
5. Whitehouse JS, Weigelt JA (2009) Diagnostic peritoneal lavage: a review of indications, technique, and interpretation. Scand J Trauma Resusc Emerg Med 17:13
6. Sullivan KR, Nelson MJ, Tandberg D (1997) Incremental analysis of diagnostic peritoneal lavage fluid in adult abdominal trauma. Am J Emerg Med 15:277–279
7. Sweeney JF, Albrink MH, Bischof E, McAllister EW, Rosemurgy AS (1994) Diagnostic peritoneal lavage: volume of lavage effluent needed for accurate determination of a negative lavage. Injury 25:659–661
8. Thacker LK, Parks J, Thal ER (2007) Diagnostic peritoneal lavage: is 100,000 RBCs a valid figure for penetrating abdominal trauma? J Trauma 62:853–857
9. Merlotti GJ, Marcet E, Sheaff CM, Dunn R, Barrett JA (1985) Use of peritoneal lavage to evaluate abdominal penetration. J Trauma 25:228–231
10. Bellows CF, Salomone JP, Nakamura SK, Choe EU, Flint LM, Ferrara JJ (1998) What's black and white and red (read) all over? The bedside interpretation of diagnostic peritoneal lavage fluid. Am Surg 64:112–118
11. McAnena OJ, Marx JA, Moore EE (1991) Peritoneal lavage enzyme determinations following blunt and penetrating abdominal trauma. J Trauma 31:1161–1164
12. Fakhry SM, Watts DD, Michetti C, Hunt JP (2003) The resident experience on trauma: declining surgical opportunities and career incentives? Analysis of data from a large multi-institutional study. J Trauma 54:1–7; discussion 7–8
13. Bhan C, Forshaw MJ, Bew DP, Kapadia YK (2007) Diagnostic peritoneal lavage and ultrasonography for blunt abdominal trauma: attitudes and training of current general surgical trainees. Eur J Emerg Med 14:212–215
14. Cha JY, Kashuk JL, Sarin EL et al (2009) Diagnostic peritoneal lavage remains a valuable adjunct to modern imaging technique. J Trauma 67:330–334; discussion 4–6
15. Kuncir EJ, Velmahos GC (2007) Diagnostic peritoneal aspiration–the foster child of DPL: a prospective observational study. Int J Surg 5:167–171

Mass Casualties and Triage

21

James M. Ryan and Dietrich Doll

In considering the topic of mass casualties and triage, there is an immediate problem on agreed definition. In the context of war and conflict, the term 'mass casualties' has an exact definition – NATO defines a mass casualty incident as follows: 'A mass casualty situation is one in which an overwhelming number of seriously injured or otherwise incapacitated individuals, within a limited area or multiple areas and a brief period of time are placed upon locally available medical facilities quite unable to supply medical care for them. This definition, carefully worded, implies an overwhelming of medical facilities and implies that the aim of military medical services in the area must be to assume care to the greatest benefit of the largest number. More recently, NATO has refined their approach to Mass Casualties and now uses the term 'MASCAL'. In a later section on Triage, this will be discussed further.

J.M. Ryan (✉)
Centre for Trauma, Conflict & Catastrophes,
St. George's Hospital Medical School, University of London,
London, UK
e-mail: jryan@sgul.ac.uk

D. Doll
University of the Witwatersrand Medical School,
Chris Hani Baragwanath Academic Hospital,
Trauma Directorate, 7 York Road, Parktown,
2193 Johannesburg, South Africa (RSA)

Department of Visceral, Vascular and Thoracic Surgery,
Phillips-University of Marburg,
Baldingerstraße, D-35043 Marburg, Germany
e-mail: ddoll@gmx.de

While this definition may be appropriate to total war and some catastrophic natural disasters, it requires revisiting in the context of civilian needs and experience.

> **Take Home Point**
>
> Mass Casualty Triage in the military and civilian environments is fundamentally different.

21.1 Multiple Casualties and Mass Casualties

The immediate problem here is the lack of international civilian agreement on appropriate definition. In the United States and Israel, the term '*Mass Casualty Incident (MCI)*' is in common usage and is defined as: 'A mass casualty incident is an incident where the emergency medical personnel and equipment at the scene are overwhelmed by the number and severity of casualties at that incident'. In the United Kingdom for the purposes of mass casualty planning, the Department of Health divides major incidents resulting in casualties into [1]:

- Major Incidents resulting in casualties – casualty numbers in multiples of 10 – the receiving hospital is able to cope within existing resources.
- Mass Casualty Incidents – casualty number in hundreds requiring multiple local hospital facilities.
- Catastrophic Casualty Incidents – more than 1,000 casualties. Response exceeds the capacity of local facilities and demands a regional or national response.

G.C. Velmahos et al. (eds.), *Penetrating Trauma*,
DOI 10.1007/978-3-642-20453-1_21, © Springer-Verlag Berlin Heidelberg 2012

In the midst of this confusion and lack of consensus it falls to the authors of this chapter to suggest a way forward. The authors suggest for clarity that one term is used for casualty numbers which exceed the existing resources of a medical facility – *Mass Casualties*.

The following definition is suggested: 'A Mass Casualty event is a disastrous single or simultaneous event (s) or other circumstances where the normal major incident response of one or several health organisations must be augmented by extraordinary measures in order to maintain an efficient, suitable and sustainable response.'

By definition, such events have the potential to overwhelm or threaten to exceed the local capacity to respond even with implementation of local major incident planning.

Mass casualty incidents are usually associated with victims of trauma. However, this is not always the case. An incident resulting in mass casualties can be sudden, such as a transport disaster or a series of smaller incidents, which stretch a health facility in a short space of time. Equally, an incident can also creep up gradually, such as a developing infectious disease outbreak or a capacity or staffing crisis such as pandemic flu. Extreme weather conditions can cause a surge in admissions to hospitals and capacity in specialist areas is particularly vulnerable such as intensive care, paediatrics and burns care. In total, there are six ways of categorising these incidents. They are:

1. Big bang – Sudden incident, train crash, bomb
2. Rising tide – Slow onset, epidemic, winter bed crisis
3. Cloud on the horizon – Protracted, war, catastrophic incident overseas
4. Headline news – Media-driven public alarm, scan scares
5. Internal incidents – Internal workings affected, power cut, flooding
6. Deliberate release of chemical, biological or nuclear materials – the sarin attack in Tokyo 1995

So – in summary, so far, there is a need to separate incidents which result in large numbers of ill or injured patients presenting to a medical facility in need of medical care – Multiple Casualty Incidents (called major incidents in the UK) or Mass Casualty Incidents. In this work, the authors are concerned with Mass Casualties which require novel or unusual solutions. Underpinning an effective response is the concept of Triage, and this is the major topic of concern here.

21.2 Triage

What is Triage? In short, it is an attempt to impose order during chaos and make an initially overwhelming situation manageable. Its aim is to get the right patient to the right place at the right time. In US parlance, it is '*to do the most for the most when faced with multiple or mass casualties*'. Triage is now a widely used (and misused) term. It has its origins in military medical practice on the battlefield. The word Triage is derived from the old French verb *trier* and was used during the Napoleonic Wars and American Civil War, meaning to sift or to sort [2]. It is still used in coffee markets in Paris to grade coffee beans using sieves into different qualities or sizes. If a system for sorting casualties is not used, many of the injured who are salvageable may die unnecessarily. A commonly used definition is: The sorting of casualties and assignment of treatment and transfer priorities to the wounded at each level of medical care [3].

21.3 Triage Systems

Before turning to Triage for Mass casualties, it is necessary to examine Triage in general. It is heartening to note that there are moves towards a common understanding and agreement on definition across the European Union. However, marked differences exist between Europe and North America. Here the authors will confine themselves to an evolving European understanding.

Historically, military and civilian teaching across European nations, especially those within NATO, encouraged the use of two parallel systems – one for use for multiple casualties, the other for Mass Casualties. These were respectively the 'P' or Priority system and the 'T' or Treatment system. Hodgetts [4] has rightly commented that the parallel use of two systems has fundamentally undermined the need for simplicity and all should adhere to one system, namely, the T or Treatment system. His advice remains to be heeded, at least within the civilian community.

Within Europe, a variety of descriptive terminologies were (and still are) used incorporating labels, colour codes and descriptors. Table 21.1 summarises these.

P or Priority System – this has historically been used within United Kingdom major incident planning where casualty number associated with IRA bombings

Table 21.1 Triage systems in common use in the UK [5]

Priority	Colour	Label
Immediate	Red	P1 or T1
Urgent	Yellow	P2 or T2
Delayed	Green	P3 or T3
Expectant	Blue/black	T4
Dead	Black/white	T0

has been small, resulting in what an experienced London-based surgeon has described as a 'sweaty morning' in the emergency room. In these situations, the relatively small numbers of injured were managed within existing resources with little impact on the day-to-day working of the affected hospitals. Three patient groups were defined:

P1: Immediate – cannot wait – patients needing immediate resuscitation/surgery

P2: Urgent – can tolerate short delay >30 min

P3: Delayed – can tolerate long or indefinite delay

Plainly, this system works well with small numbers being cared for in a major European general hospital but will not cope with overwhelming numbers. In these situations, the T or Treatment system was suggested. Four or five categories are defined.

T1: Immediate – but not patients with such severe injury that good outcome is unlikely or where care would overburden resources in terms of time and material

T2: As P2 above

T3: As P3 above

T4: Expectant group which includes patients with severe, multi-system injury where prognosis is poor and care unduly time consuming and demands scarce resources

It is interesting to observe that one of the drivers for change from conventional Triage to Mass Casualty Triage has been the recent threats of international terrorist attacks. There is now a growing trend to move towards the T system but also incorporating a coloured label and a description as outlined in Table 21.1 above. This recognises the need to conform to one system in all events and makes training easier, particularly across national boundaries. Sensibly, there remains a degree of flexibility. In the UK, for example, while the T system is agreed where casualty numbers are small (in the 10 s) after a transport accident, the T4 or expectant category is not invoked. However, when managing hundreds of patients, the T4/expectant category may be invoked, at least for a time.

In summary, a sensible suggestion for future use is summarised below:

T1 – Red label – Immediate: These cannot wait. Treatment needed as soon a possible.

T2 – Yellow label – Urgent: Casualties with serious injury. Treatment needed after a limited delay.

T3 – Green label – Delayed: Indefinite delay, while not desirable can be tolerated.

T4 – Blue or Black label – Expectant: Likely not to survive but optimism maintained and will be treated if and when conditions improve.

T5 – Black or White label – Dead: Should not enter the clinical arena but may do so.

Take Home Point

When faced with overwhelming casualties, the P or priority system will fail resulting in unnecessary morbidity and mortality.

Take Home Point

Civilian Triage systems maintain an optimistic outlook in the face of Mass Casualties. In our modern cities, it is hard to visualise a total overwhelming of resources.

21.4 Methodology

We have suggested a system to sort casualties in the event of mass casualties. The next question is how to apply the system. Historically, Triage was performed by the most senior doctor present – usually a senior surgeon – and decisions were based on observed anatomical injury. This is now recognised to be a poor method and results on both overtriage and undertriage. In brief, this approach is flawed for a number of reasons:

- Anatomical triage requires a fully exposed patient which is rarely possible in the chaos of Mass Casualty incident.
- Considerable experience is required and will rarely be available.
- Even in experienced hands, full anatomical examination will fail to detect significant bleeding in the chest and abdomen in over 40% of cases.

Fig. 21.1 Major incident triage sieve flow diagram

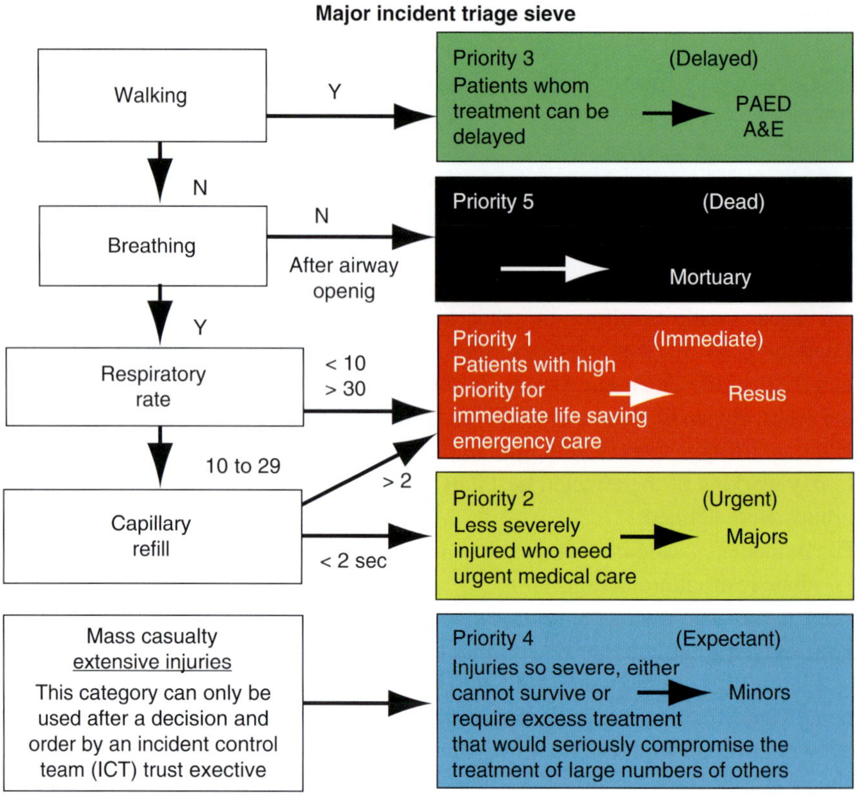

This realisation has resulted in a move towards a more discriminating approach – namely measurement of physiological parameters. A two-part physiological system has evolved referred to a sieve-sort methodology [6].

21.5 The Sieve-Sort Approach to Mass Casualties

This is a two-part approach when applying Mass Casualty Triage to injured patients.

Triage Sieve – The first part – the Sieve is an algorithm and is illustrated at Fig. 21.1. This figure is from the author's hospital major incident policy. While the word 'priority' is used to describe the patient categories, the method uses the Mass Casualty T System and an expectant group is included.

The sieve is a physiologically based method using the ABC approach advocated by the ATLS programme of the American College of Surgeons [7]. It is ideally suited to pre-hospital sorting by trained but not necessarily medically qualified first responders but is also used by Emergency Room medical teams working at a hospital entrance selecting patients for admission to resuscitation room bays in receiving hospitals. Figure 21.2 shows triage sieve in operation during a major incident exercise at a London hospital.

Triage Sort – This component is a hospital (resuscitation room) based method requiring a more time-consuming and accurate assessment. Its aim is to iron out undertriage or overtriage. It is typically performed by a trained triage officer and needs skill and equipment to perform accurately. The method uses the physiological findings outlined in Table 21.2 and yields a score or coded value for each of three physiological measurables. The sum of the three scores gives the Triage Revised Trauma Score (TRTS). Table 21.3 shows the relationship between the TRTS and Triage priority.

This is not a one-off method. It may be repeated over time and allows a refining of priorities following therapeutic interventions. Figure 21.3 below shows a summary of Triage Sort included in a major

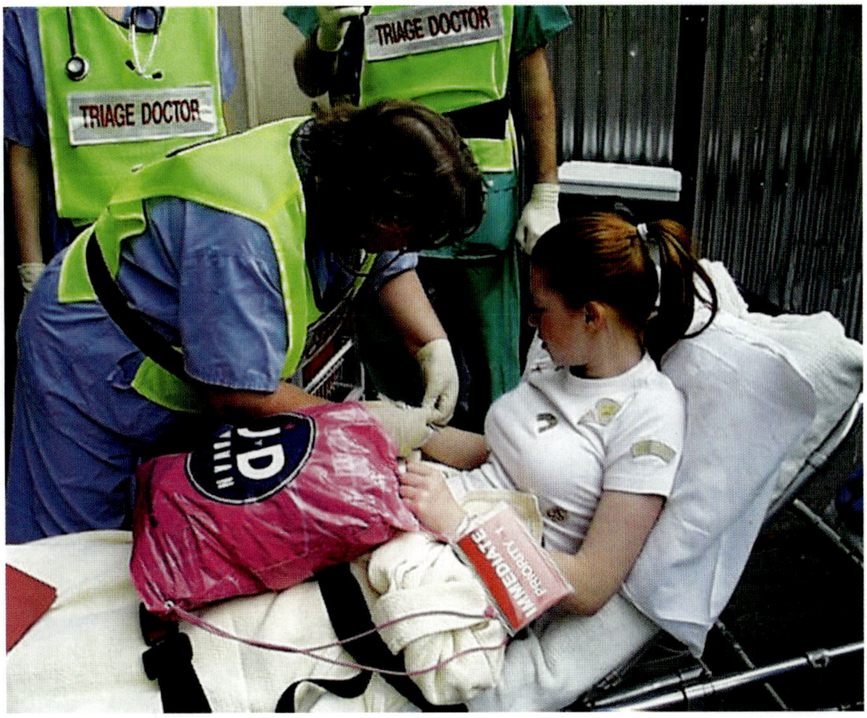

Fig. 21.2 A London hospital triage training exercise in 2006. Note the field triage label using both red colour code and 'immediate' description

Table 21.2 Triage sort based on revised trauma score

Score	Respiratory rate	Systolic BP	Glasgow coma score
0	0	0	3
1	1–5	1–49	4–5
2	6–9	50–74	6–8
3	>29	75–90	9–12
4	10–29	>90	13–15

Table 21.3 Scores converted to triage priorities

Triage revised trauma score	Triage group or priority
4–10	T1
11	T2
12	T3
1–3 (hospital only)	T4
0	Dead

Source for all tables used: Ministry of Defence [8] publication – with permission

London hospital's major incident policy. Note the comment that a decision to invoke Mass Casualties is a high-level political decision by medical and management senior staff working in concert. Note too that it utilises the newly agreed T – Treatment approach.

21.6 Effect-Related Triage

In an attempt to add a scientific basis to the application triage and of therapy, following triage Lennquist has described *Effect-related triage* [9]. This approach to triage is based on which effect a decision or therapy will have for a given injury in a given situation. For example, in considering a 40% burn, if intravenous fluid therapy is instituted as early as possible, average mortality is between 5% and 10%. If therapy is delayed for up to 24 h because of a poor triage decision, then average mortality is >90%. Effect-related triage forces triage raters to consider available resources and to set priorities in an effect-related way. Lennquist clearly shows that failure to do so results in increased mortality. This approach lends itself to wider application and has relevance for facial injuries with threatened airway,

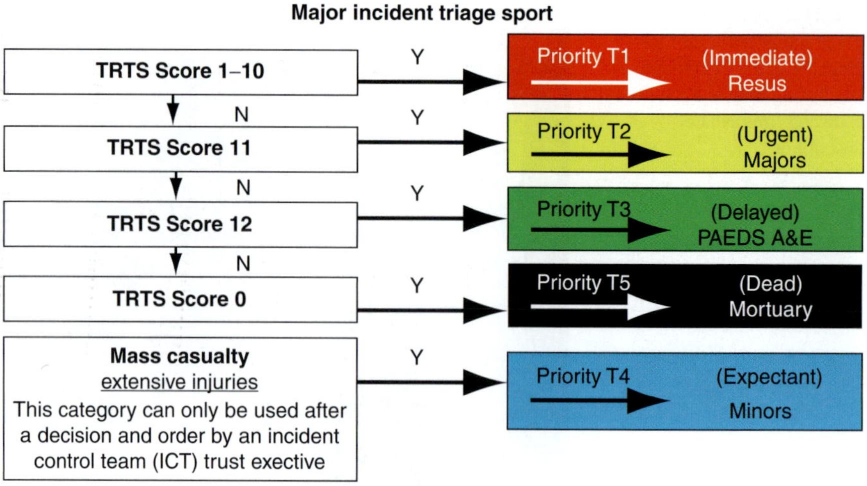

Triage revised trauma scoring system		
Physiological variable	Measured value	Score
Respiratory rate	10–29	4
	>29	3
	6–9	2
	1–5	1
	0	0
Systolic blood pressure	>90	4
	76–89	3
	50–75	2
	1–49	1
	0	0
Glasgow coma scale	13–15	4
	9–12	3
	6–8	2
	4–5	1
	3	0

Fig. 21.3 Major incident triage sort flow diagram

life-threatening thoracic injuries, intra-abdominal injuries and major injuries to the musculoskeletal system. Application of effect-related triage requires knowledge and training. It is particularly suited to hospital triage where a more scientifically based approach is mandated.

21.7 Triage in Austerity

Triage was born of need on the battlefields of Europe and North America. It later spread to the civilian arena. War and disaster provide the most extreme and testing environments for the application of triage. Triage here is influenced by matters not encountered in the civilian setting even when faced with terrorist outrages. In war and following natural catastrophes such as earthquakes, unique influences impact upon decision making. These include casualty numbers, availability of transport, hostile terrain, distance and danger. Figures 21.4 and 21.5 are illustrative. Decisions here can be agonising – evacuating badly injured patients to a partially destroyed and non-functioning hospital may not be possible and a correct Triage decision may be to hold casualties in a functioning pre-hospital medical facility who may die but not in the back of an ambulance or in the waiting area of a hospital quite unable to care for them.

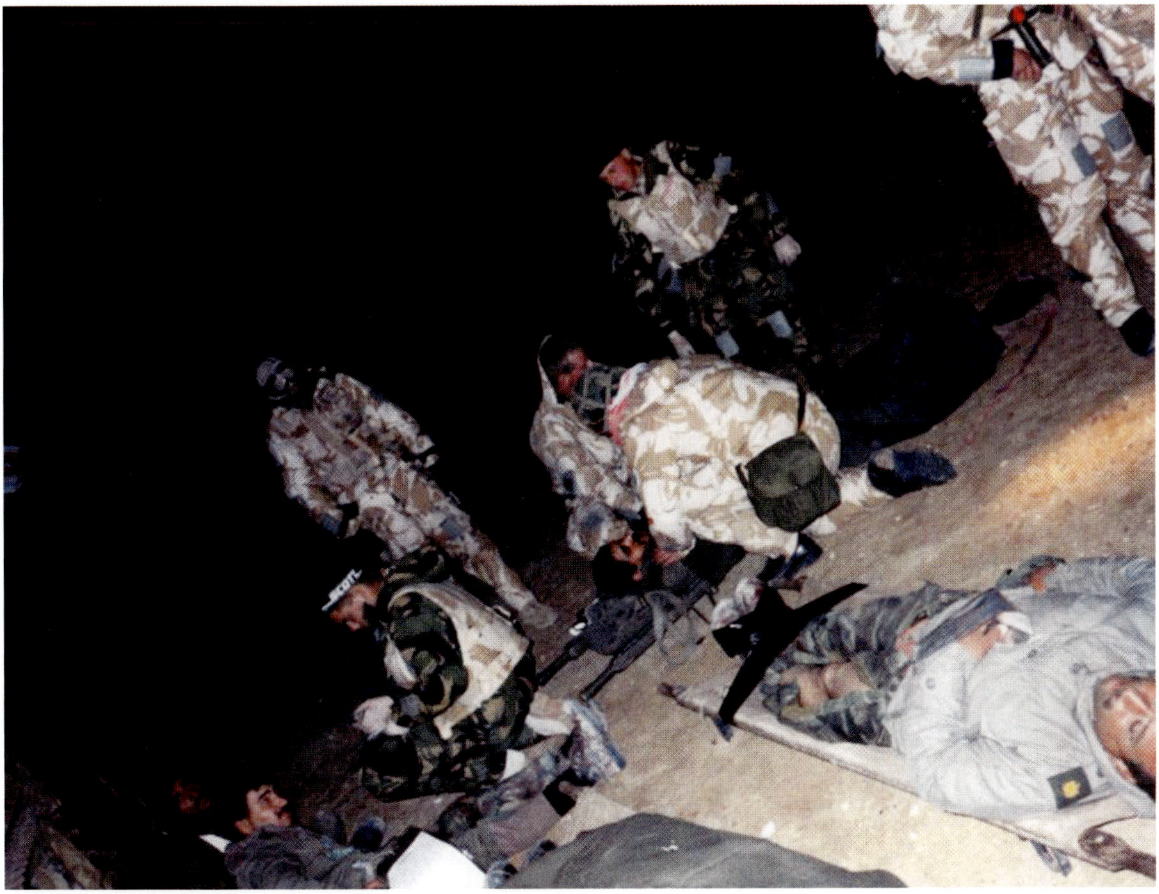

Fig. 21.4 An infantry regiment's triage location in desert at night

21.8 Training

Triage is a medical skill and requires knowledge, training and appropriate temperament. It can be taught and many organisations provide such training. Proof of the need is provided by Frykberg who has shown a clear correlation between overtriage or undertriage and avoidable morbidity and mortality [10]. Lennquist has shown that the most effective way to avoid such tragedies is training and regular exercising [11] (Figs. 21.6 and 21.7).

21.9 Conclusions

Mass Casualty situations have historically been regarded as the lot of military medical personnel during conventional war. With the rise in the incidence of international terrorism and catastrophic natural disasters, Mass Casualty management is now the lot of civilian health care professional and will be for the foreseeable future. Appropriate systems and methods are required and are out there in the public domain. All working in health care have an obligation to be informed.

Important Points

- You must understand the fundamental difference between multiple and mass casualties – the management approaches are very different.

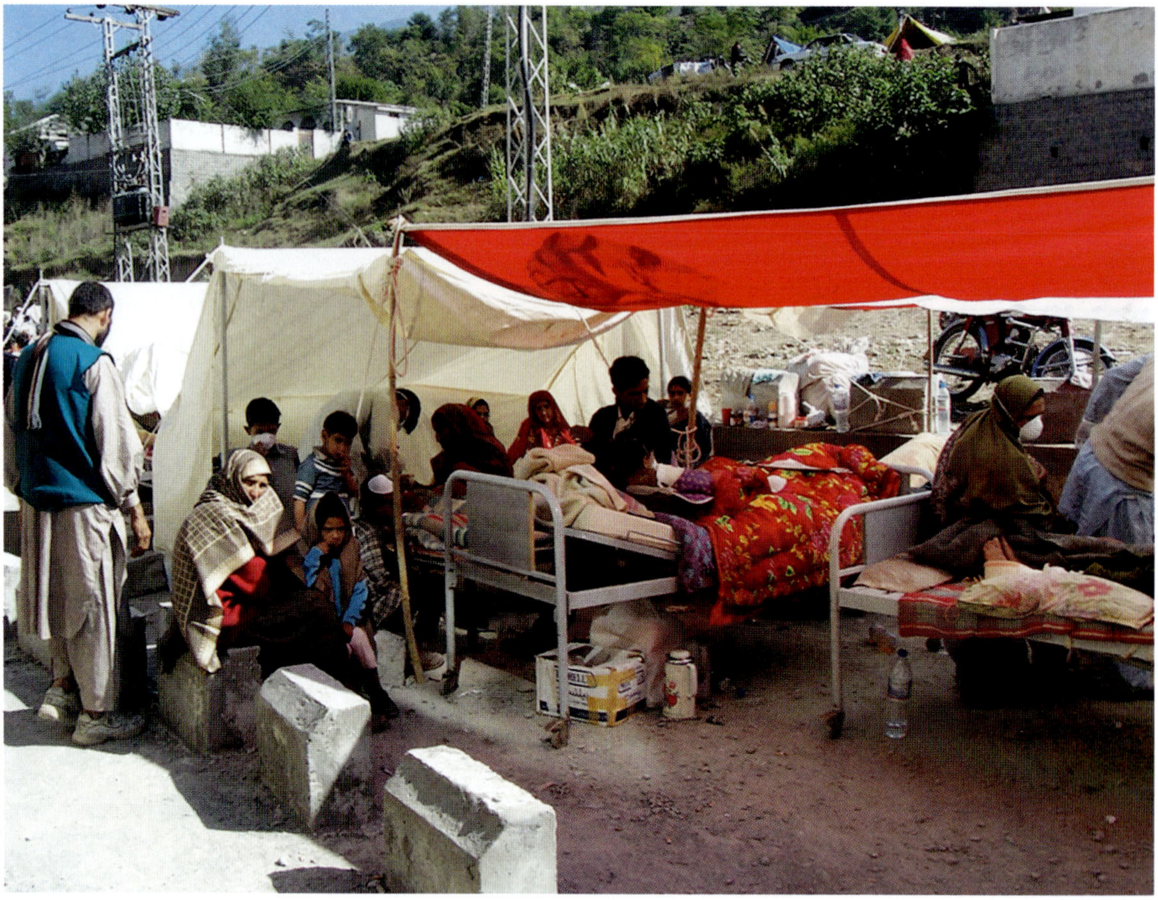

Fig. 21.5 Ill and injured patients evacuated from a partially destroyed hospital and awaiting re-triage in a new hospital location – following the earthquake in Pakistan (Photograph by one of the authors (JMR))

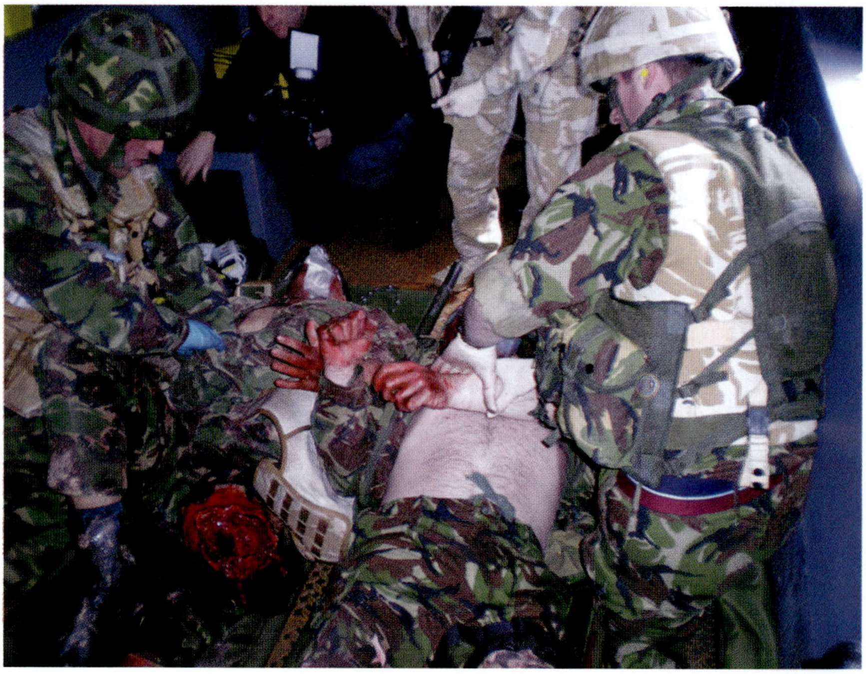

Fig. 21.6 Realistic pre-deployment triage training by British combat medical personnel (Photo by one of the authors (JMR))

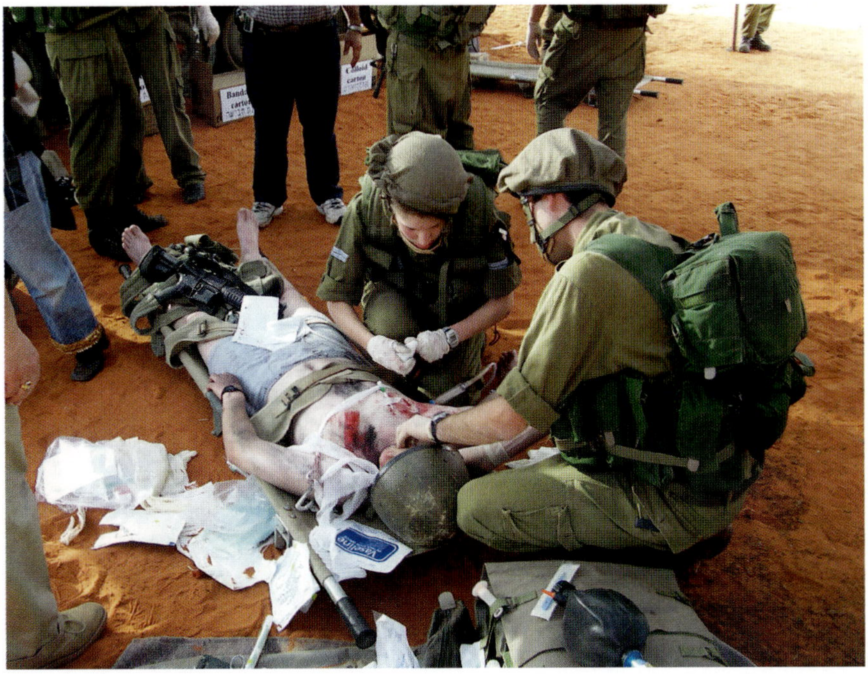

Fig. 21.7 Effective triage training in the desert by Israeli Defence Forces (IDF) combat medical personnel (Photograph by one of the authors (JMR))

- Please do not assume that military triage will work in the civil pre-hospital or hospital setting – it will not!
- The above does not mean we cannot work together or learn from each other – we can.
- Experience of managing a handful of patients following an autobahn/motorway pile up does not prepare you for handling mass casualties.
- Please know that while we are making progress, we have not yet reached full consensus on either definition or management strategies – we will get there.
- Triage requires a knowledge base, realistic training and constant practice – not everyone is temperamentally suited.
- Triage is a dynamic process applicable across the entire patient journey – many hand and many people are involved – separated in time and place – a common language and understanding are critical.
- Triage in austerity, whether a civilian calamity or in a war zone have issues wider than clinical.
- Finally, management of mass casualties and application of effective and accurate triage are team based, multi-disciplinary activities.

References

1. Department of Health Emergency Planning Division (2007) Mass casualty incidents – A framework for planning. http://www.dh.gov.uk. Accessed 10 Oct 2009
2. Hodgetts TJ (2006) Triage. J R Army Med Corps 152: 151–162
3. Roberts P (ed) (2004). Triage. In: The British military surgical pocket book. Ministry of Defence Publication, London, pp 107–113
4. Hodgetts TJ, Porter C (2002) Major incident management systems. BMJ Publishing, London
5. Ryan JM (2008) Triage: principles and pressures. Eur J Trauma Surg 5:427–432
6. Bond Alison (2007) Major incident and mass casualty trust wide policy and plans. University College London Hospitals NHS Foundation Trust Publication, London
7. American College of Surgeons Committee on Trauma (2009) Advanced trauma life support for doctors, 8th edn. ACS, Chicago
8. Ministry of Defence (2005) Battlefield advanced trauma life support (BATLS) manual, 1st edn. Ministry of Defence, London
9. Lennquist S (2007) Management of major accidents and disasters: an important responsibility for the trauma surgeon. J Trauma 62:1321–1329
10. Frykberg ER (2005) Triage and practice. Scand J Surg 94: 272–278
11. Lennquist S (2005) Education and training in disaster medicine. Scand J Surg 94:300–310

Part II

Surgical Strategies in Penetrating Trauma to Head, Face, and Neck

22 Surgical Strategies in Trauma

Hasan B. Alam

The surgical management of significantly injured trauma patients has undergone a major change over the last decade. The basic principles of the contemporary approach include an emphasis on:

1. Damage control operations
2. Damage control resuscitation
3. Appropriate utilization of adjunctive hemorrhage control strategies

22.1 Damage Control Operations

Damage control operations are widely performed today in severely injured patient [1]. Rotondo [2] borrowed this term for the trauma literature from naval vocabulary where it refers to the ability of a ship to absorb damage while maintaining mission integrity. In the context of severely injured patients, damage control approach has three phases. The goal of the first phase is to perform an abbreviated operation focusing on controlling the hemorrhage and contamination. Time is of critical importance, and you must select surgical maneuvers that rapidly achieve the goals of the operation, including packing, vessel ligation, temporary shunting, bowel resection without anastomosis, and placement of drains. Time should also not be wasted on closing body cavities at the time of the initial operation, relying instead on various methods of temporary closure (e.g., plastic sheet/negative pressure sponge closure of the abdominal wall). Leaving the cavities open not only saves time, but it also avoids potential problems with tight compartments during the postoperative period that can predispose to various types of compartment syndromes. As the trauma surgeon, you must accept the fact that definitive repair of all the injuries at the time of the first operation is not in the best interest of the patient. This initial life-saving operation is followed by a period of resuscitation in the intensive care unit to correct acidosis, hypothermia, and coagulopathy [3, 4]. Once normal physiology has been restored, the third phase starts where the patient is taken back to the operating room for definitive repair of the injuries. During this phase, vascular and bowel continuity is restored, injured organs are repaired or removed, packs are taken out, and body cavities are properly closed. It may require multiple operations to achieve all these goals.

The principles of damage control have been applied to almost all types of major injuries, in nearly all parts of the body. As a concept, it is equally valid even for procedures that are not typically considered trauma operations, such as angiographic embolization, splinting and application of external fixation devices, control of external bleeding with tourniquets or advanced hemostatic dressings.

1. *Patient selection*: Damage control approach is clearly not benign as it commits the patient to multiple operations, prolonged sedation and mechanical ventilation, and repeated administration of general anesthesia. It also increases the risks related to leaving the body cavities open, including infections, fluid and heat loss, excessive metabolic demands, loss of domain (e.g., large hernia), and organ injury (e.g., enteric fistulae). Thus, it must be

H.B. Alam
Harvard Medical School,
Division of Trauma, Emergency Surgery, and Surgical Critical Care, Massachusetts General Hospital, 165 Cambridge Street, Suite 810, Boston, MA 02114, USA
e-mail: hbalam@partners.org

G.C. Velmahos et al. (eds.), *Penetrating Trauma*,
DOI 10.1007/978-3-642-20453-1_22, © Springer-Verlag Berlin Heidelberg 2012

applied in a group of patients where the risk-benefit ratio justifies this approach. Equally important is to make the decision early in the course of the operation. Choosing to apply damage control strategies too late in the operation is equally harmful. You must identify the presence of hypothermia, acidosis, and coagulopathy early in the course. Often labeled as the "lethal triad," these factors perpetuate each other creating a vicious cycle that is difficult to interrupt [5]. Late coagulopathy often reflects dilution of platelets, hemoglobin, and clotting factors, but early coagulopathy is a well-recognized marker of injury severity, and its presence is associated with significantly greater mortality. Similarly, hypothermia is not only due to loss of body heat and drop in temperature due to infusion of cold fluids, but more importantly, it reflects presence of significant tissue ischemia. Maintaining normal body temperature is an energy-dependent process that patients in shock are unable to maintain. Acidosis reflects the presence of shock, which in turns further perpetuates coagulopathy and hypothermia. Thus, the surgeon must actively monitor the patient for the development of these markers, and use their presence as a trigger to switch into a damage control mode. There are no universally agreed-upon criteria, but a reasonable list would include: core temperature <35°C, a base deficit >10 mmol/L, requirement for vasoactive agents to maintain a systolic blood pressure >90 mmHg, a pH less than 7.20, transfusion of >10 units of packed red blood cells, and clinical evidence of coagulopathy/diffuse oozing. Experienced trauma surgeons know that it is better to avoid development of the lethal triad rather than to reverse it, because by the time all these signs become obvious, it may already be too late. If you are not sure, it is better to err on the side of being too cautious and opt for a damage control approach. Remember that you can always come back to fight another day, if the patient survives today.

2. *Basic goals*: The major aim during the initial operation is to control the bleeding as soon as possible to minimize the blood loss and the limit the duration of shock. As time is of critical importance, the quickest exposure should always be selected. Thus, laparoscopic or minimally invasive approach is not appropriate for patients where every minute counts. Once in the body cavity, tools that can expedite controlling the source of bleeding should be liberally used. For example, a stapler fired through a tract of a bullet (tractotomy) is a fast way to open the track and expose the bleeding vessels in the lung. When the source of bleeding is exposed, consider ligation if it can be done without excessive morbidity (e.g., most veins, and many arteries can be safely ligated). If ligating the blood vessel is likely to result in significant tissue loss, select a temporary shunt instead of a formal anastomosis/graft, which should be delayed for a later stage. When unable to get quick exposure of the blood vessel, which is not uncommon in the head and neck region, consider tight packing with or without balloon tamponade (e.g., Foley catheter) of the tract as a damage control strategy. Similarly, for nonvascular injuries (e.g., solid organs, pelvic fractures, mangled extremities) packing combined with rapid inflow control could be life saving. Always remember that saving life takes priority over saving organs or limbs, and doing a quick, focused operation is better than doing a perfect operation that takes too long. The second goal (after controlling hemorrhage) is to control contamination, mostly from bowel but also from other sources such as bile, pancreatic juices, saliva, and urine. In these seriously injured patients, dividing the bowel proximal and distal to the injury with a stapler rapidly controls the spillage. There is no need to restore continuity of the bowel if the patient's physiology is critically deranged. Simply, drop the stapled ends of the bowel back in the abdomen and take care of the anastomosis during the next operation. When unable to fix the source of contamination, try to get a controlled leak. Drainage catheter and tubes can be rapidly placed to achieve this goal.

22.2 Damage Control Resuscitation

The concept of damage control has been extended to resuscitation methods as well. The aim is to select strategies that can decrease bleeding, avoid development of coagulopathy, minimize cellular damage, and can maintain cellular viability, while keep hemostatic parameters within the normal range. As this is a rapidly evolving and controversial area, some background information is provided to justify the recommendations.

1. *Futility of current methods/adverse effects of aggressive resuscitation*: Although it is widely believed that early aggressive fluid resuscitation is beneficial, clinical and basic science literature fails to provide conclusive supporting evidence [6–9]. As a matter of fact, the basic rationale for administering intravenous fluids in patients with ongoing bleeding has been challenged repeatedly for almost a century [10]. Theoretically, fluid resuscitation in the absence of (or prior to) hemorrhage control can exacerbate bleeding due to the disruption of early soft thrombus, coagulopathy, and hemodilution [11–14]. A systematic review of 52 animal trials concluded that fluid resuscitation appeared to decrease the risk of death in models of severe hemorrhage (RR = 0.48), but increased the risk of death in those with less severe hemorrhage (RR = 1.86) [15]. Furthermore, hypotensive resuscitation, whenever tested, reduced the risk of death (RR = 0.37). Similarly, a critical review of the literature failed to find any evidence that prehospital advanced life support improved outcomes in trauma patients [16]. In a study that has generated vigorous debate since its publication in 1994 [17], hypotensive patients with penetrating torso injury were randomized to routine fluid resuscitation, or resuscitation was delayed until bleeding had been surgically controlled. The results of this study demonstrated a survival advantage in the delayed resuscitation group (70% vs. 62%, $p = 0.04$). Despite all the controversy, the most impressive finding remains that withholding fluid resuscitation until hemorrhage control did not increase the mortality. The issue of timing and volume of fluid resuscitation in bleeding patients has also been addressed by The Cochrane Database of Systematic Reviews [18]. Only six randomized clinical trials met the inclusion criteria, and a careful review failed to provide any evidence in support of (or against) *early* or *large volume* intravenous fluid administration in uncontrolled hemorrhage. In addition to the impact of resuscitation on bleeding, resuscitation fluids have profound cellular effects. It is now widely recognized that resuscitation fluids are not completely innocuous, and they may actually potentate the cellular injury caused by hemorrhagic shock [19]. Therefore, in addition to the immediate side effects (worsening of hemorrhage), delayed complications of fluid resuscitation such as systemic inflammatory response, fluid overload (leading to compartment syndromes, pulmonary edema, etc.), anemia, thrombocytopenia, electrolyte/acid-base abnormalities, and cardiac and pulmonary complications must also be kept in mind [20]. Excessive fluid resuscitation increases the chances of developing abdominal compartment syndrome in critically ill surgical/trauma, burn, and medical patients [21–23]. Similarly, in a multicenter study of burn patients, administration of excessive fluids (in excess of 25% of predicted) increased the odds of ARDS (OR 1.7), pneumonia (OR 5.7), multiple organ failure (OR 1.6), blood stream infections (OR 2.9), and death (OR 5.3) [24]. Based upon all this information, it is reasonable to conclude that fluid resuscitation is not a substitute for early hemorrhage control. You should consider low volume, careful resuscitation, especially when trying to control bleeding in a dying patient. However, early aggressive fluid resuscitation, in the absence to hemorrhage control, should be avoided.
2. *New developments*: Despite a paucity of good randomized controlled trials (RCT) in this arena, clinical practices are rapidly changing. In general, large volume aggressive fluid resuscitation is becoming increasingly rare, and low volume, carefully guided resuscitation is more common. Controlled mild hypotension in appropriate patients (e.g., in young victims of penetrating trauma) prior to hemorrhage control is fairly routine practice in large trauma centers. Blunt trauma patients with associated head injury should still be resuscitated to a higher blood pressure, in an attempt to maintain adequate cerebral perfusion, but early use of blood products and vasopressors is replacing large volume crystalloid infusion. Prompted by the recommendations of some consensus conferences [25, 26], and due to the unique logistical challenges of the battlefield, the resuscitation strategies being utilized by the US military have changed dramatically: Resuscitation is selective, emphasizing low volume and practical endpoints, and the use of fluids with logistical advantages (e.g., hetastarch) is preferred. The concept of "hemostatic or damage control resuscitation" has also gained prominence [27]. Trauma patients are often coagulopathic due to shock and tissue injury, and this coagulopathy is worsened by resuscitation with crystalloids and packed red blood cells (PRBC), as both are deficient in clotting

factors. Observational data from civilian trauma centers and the battlefield seem to suggest that early administration of component therapy (fresh frozen plasma and platelets) may be beneficial [28, 29]. A recent retrospective analysis of mixed trauma patients requiring surgery and massive transfusion compared FFP:PRBC ratios of 1:1 and 1:4, and showed that only 26% of patients treated with the former ratio died while 87.5% of patients treated with the latter ratio died ($p<0.0001$). In this high-risk group with an overall mortality of 55.5%, a 1:4 ratio of FFP:PRBC increased the relative risk of dying by 18.9 ($p<0.001$) when controlling for all other patient variables [30]. Holcomb's study of trauma patients at 16 trauma centers who required massive transfusion found that an FFP:PRBC ratio of 1:2 or higher ($N=252$) compared to lower ratios ($N=214$) was associated with improved 30-day survival (59.6% with high ratio vs. 40.4% with low ratio, $p<0.01$) [31]. These conclusions have recently been questioned by a study that suggests that the observed survival differences between patients receiving high and low ratios in the first 24 h may simply be due to the fact that survivors live long enough to receive component therapy (survivor bias) [32]. The US Army has instituted a policy of using a 1:1:1 ratio of PRBC:FFP:platelets in the battlefield for those that meet the criteria for massive resuscitation (expected to receive >10 units PRBC). Our policy is to start FFP infusion as early as possible in massively bleeding patients, using a PRBC:FFP ratio of 2:1, and administer 6 units of platelets for every 10 units of PRBC.

The basic guidelines include: (1) Accept low blood pressure in young patients as long as they have adequate tissue perfusion as evidenced by mental status, (2) delay the full resuscitation until the source of hemorrhage has been controlled, (3) prioritize hemorrhage control, (4) use limited volume of crystalloids, (5) switch to blood products early during the initial resuscitation (after the first liter of crystalloids), and (6) transfuse plasma and platelets early and in a high ratio along with red cells in massively bleeding patients. And most importantly, remember that resuscitation is not a substitute for early hemorrhage control. Patients hardly ever die because you run out of resuscitation fluids/blood products, they die due to a delay in the hemorrhage control.

22.3 Appropriate Utilization of Adjunctive Hemorrhage Control Strategies

A major change over the last decade has been a dramatic improvement in medical technology, especially in the fields of diagnostic and interventional radiology. Angiographic embolization has become an indispensable method for controlling bleeding in various areas. In most hospitals, bleeding in the head/face region as well as the pelvis is preferentially controlled using this approach. It should be emphasized that embolization and surgical control are not mutually exclusive. Often the critically bleeding patients are taken to the operating room for packing of major bleeding such as liver or pelvis, which is followed by angioembolization to consolidate the hemorrhage control, allowing for early and safe removal of the packs. These adjunctive angiographic procedures should be performed in the operating room if logistically possible to avoid transporting critically ill patients. The second important point is that urgent embolization (a life-saving intervention) is fundamentally different from procedures that are performed in stable patients, and it should follow the principles of damage control. A classic example is the control of retroperitoneal bleeding following pelvic fractures. The radiologist must appreciate that the goal is to rapidly, and temporarily, control the source of blood loss, without wasting time in doing sub-selective coil embolization of the precise bleeding points. Following this concept, pelvic embolization should routinely involve injection of gelatin sponge slurry into both of the internal iliac arteries. This can be done within minutes, and it decreases the pelvic perfusion, which slows down the bleeding and allows clotting to occur. Usually, there is still sufficient blood supply to insure organ viability and significant ischemic complications are extremely rare. The sponge particles are reabsorbed within the next few days resulting in restoration of normal perfusion. But most importantly, damage control embolization is a quick procedure that can be performed in most of the institutions without a need for very advanced equipments. Embolization of other organs, such as the liver or kidney, requires a higher degree of selectivity and is usually performed by placing coils in the bleeding branch. Splenic hemorrhage can also be controlled by embolizing the main splenic artery. However, this should be avoided in unstable patients as it goes against the principles of damage control. A prompt splenectomy is a much better option for the vast majority of unstable patients with splenic hemorrhage.

References

1. Lee JC, Peitzman AB (2006) Damage-control laparotomy. Curr Opin Crit Care 12:346–350
2. Rotondo M, Schwab CW, Mullins RJ et al (1993) Damage control: an approach for improved survival in exsanguinating penetrating abdominal injury. J Trauma 35:375–383
3. Maegele M, Lefering R, Yucel N et al (2007) Early coagulopathy in multiple injury: an analysis from the German Trauma Registry on 8724 patients. Injury 38:298–304
4. Niles SE, McLaughlin DF, Perkins JG et al (2008) Increased mortality associated with the early coagulopathy of trauma in combat casualties. J Trauma 64:1459–1465
5. Dirkmann D, Hanke AA, Görlinger K, Peters J (2008) Hypothermia and acidosis synergistically impair coagulation in human whole blood. Anesth Analg 106(6):1627–1632
6. Turner J, Nicholl J, Webber L et al (2000) A randomized controlled trial of prehospital intravenous fluid replacement therapy in serious trauma. Health Technol Assess 4(31):1–57
7. Greaves MW, Hussein SH (2002) Fluid resuscitation in prehospital trauma care: a consensus view. J R Coll Surg Edinb 47(2):451–457
8. Dula DJ, Wood GC, Rejmer AR, Starr M, Leicht M (2002) Use of prehospital fluids in hypotensive blunt trauma patients. Prehosp Emerg Care 6(4):417–420
9. Dutton RP, Mackenzie CF, Scalea TM (2002) Hypotensive resuscitation during active hemorrhage: impact on in-hospital mortality. J Trauma 52:1141–1146
10. Cannon WB, Faser J, Collew EM (1918) The preventive treatment of wound shock. JAMA 47:618
11. Stern SA, Dronen SC, Birrer P, Wang X (1993) Effect of blood pressure on hemorrhage volume and survival in a near-fatal hemorrhage model incorporating a vascular injury. Ann Emerg Med 22:155–163
12. Selby JB, Mathis JE, Berry CF, Hagedorn FN, Illner HP, Shires GT (1996) Effects of isotonic saline solution resuscitation on blood coagulation in uncontrolled hemorrhage. Surgery 119:528–533
13. Sondeen JL, Coppes VG, Holcomb JB (2003) Blood pressure at which rebleeding occurs after resuscitation in swine with aortic injury. J Trauma 54(suppl):S100–S107
14. Rotondo MF, Schwab CW, McGonigal MD, Phillips GR III, Fruchterman TM, Kauder DR et al (1993) "Damage Control": an approach for improved survival in exsanguinating penetrating abdominal trauma. J Trauma 35:375–383
15. Mapstone J, Roberts I, Evans P (2003) Fluid resuscitation strategies: a systematic review of animal trials. J Trauma 55:571–589
16. Liberman M, Mulder D, Sampalis J (2000) Advanced or basic life support for trauma: meta-analysis and critical review of the literature. J Trauma 49:584–599
17. Bickel WH, Wall MJ, Pepe PE, Martin RR, Ginger VF, Allen MK et al (1994) Immediate versus delayed fluid resuscitation for hypotensive patients with penetrating torso injuries. N Engl J Med 331:1105–1109
18. Kwan I, Bunn F, Roberts I (2003) WHO Pre-Hospital Trauma Care Steering Committee: timing and volume of fluid administration for patients with bleeding following trauma. Cochrane Database Syst Rev (3):CD002245
19. Alam HB (2006) An update on fluid resuscitation. Scand J Surg 95:136–145
20. Cotton BA, Guy JS, Morris JA, Abumrad NN (2006) The cellular, metabolic, and systemic consequences of aggressive fluid resuscitation strategies. Shock 26:115–121
21. Daugherty EL, Hongyan L, Taichman D et al (2007) Abdominal compartment syndrome is common in medical intensive care unit patients receiving large volume resuscitation. J Intensive Care Med 22:294–299
22. O'Mara MS, Slater H, Goldfarb IW, Caushaj PF (2005) A prospective, randomized evaluation of intra-abdominal pressures with crystalloids and colloid resuscitation in burn patients. J Trauma 58:1011–1018
23. Balogh Z, Moore FA, Moore EE, Biffl WL (2007) Secondary abdominal compartment syndrome: a potential threat for all trauma clinicians. Injury 38:272–279
24. Klein MB, Hayden D, Elson C et al (2007) The association between fluid administration and outcome following major burn. A multicenter study. Ann Surg 245:622–628
25. Champion HR (2003) Combat fluid resuscitation: introduction and overview of conferences. J Trauma 54(supp):7–12
26. Rhee P, Koustova E, Alam HB (2003) Searching for the optimal resuscitation method: recommendations for the initial fluid resuscitation of combat casualties. J Trauma 54(supp):52–62
27. Holcomb JB, Jenkins D, Rhee P et al (2007) Damage control resuscitation: directly addressing the early coagulopathy of trauma. J Trauma 62:307–310
28. Gonzales EA, Moore FA, Holcomb JB et al (2007) Fresh frozen plasma should be given earlier to patients receiving massive transfusion. J Trauma 62:112–119
29. Borgman MA, Spinella PC, Perkins JG et al (2007) The ratio of blood products transfused affects mortality in patients receiving massive transfusions at a combat support hospital. J Trauma 63:805–813
30. Duchesne JC, Hunt JP, Wahl G, Marr AB, Wang YZ, Weintraub SE, Wright MJ, McSwain NE Jr (2008) Review of current blood transfusions strategies in a mature level i trauma center: were we wrong for the last 60 years? J Trauma 65:272–276; discussion 6–8
31. Holcomb JB, Wade CE, Michalek JE, Chisholm GB, Zarzabal LA, Schreiber MA, Gonzalez EA, Pomper GJ, Perkins JG, Spinella PC et al (2008) Increased plasma and platelet to red blood cell ratios improves outcome in 466 massively transfused civilian trauma patients. Ann Surg 248:447–458
32. Snyder CW, Weinberg JA, McGwin G Jr, Melton SM, George RL, Reiff DA, Cross JM, Hubbard-Brown J, Rue LW III, Kerby JD (2009) The relationship of blood product ratio to mortality: survival benefit or survival bias? J Trauma 66:358–362; discussion 62–64

Surgical Strategies in Trauma to the Head, Face and Neck

23

Heather L. Evans and Eileen Bulger

23.1 Initial Evaluation

23.1.1 Airway and Breathing

The initial evaluation begins, as always, with an assessment of the patient's airway [1]. Direct penetrating injury to the larynx or trachea can cause airway obstruction or disruption, making endotracheal intubation difficult or impossible. When penetrating injury to the airway is suspected, regardless of the presenting symptoms, it should be assumed that the patient has a difficult airway and appropriate intubation adjuncts such as an indirect laryngoscope (e.g., GlideScope), fiberoptic bronchoscope or laryngeal mask airway should be on hand. As increasing number of intubation attempts is associated with poorer outcomes, the most experienced person available should attempt the initial intubation and the surgeon should be prepared for immediate cricothyrotomy if intubation fails [2]. In some cases, the patient may require a surgical airway during pre-hospital management. It is essential to confirm the patency of the surgical airway upon arrival in the Emergency Department and to assess the need for emergent revision due to malpositioning, associated airway injury, or for hemorrhage control. In the setting of a large anterior neck wound, if the defect to the trachea can be identified, the distal trachea may be directly intubated through the wound.

H.L. Evans (✉) • E. Bulger
Department of Surgery,
University of Washington, Seattle, WA, USA
e-mail: hlevans@uw.edu; ebulger@u.washington.edu

Alternatively, if the patient is able to oxygenate and ventilate during the primary survey, but airway injury is evident from physical examination, the safest airway management involves immediate transport to the operating room for awake fiberoptic intubation or awake tracheostomy with local anesthesia under optimal operative conditions. This is particularly important when the larynx is injured, as the usual anatomic landmarks may be absent. When the trachea is penetrated, but not transected, use of fiberoptic bronchoscopy facilitates localization and characterization of the extent of the airway injury, as well as the ability to confirm that the endotracheal tube balloon has been placed distal to the injury enabling positive pressure ventilation. In general, blind nasotracheal intubation and retrograde intubation techniques are not recommended due to the potential for exacerbation of injury or nasopharyngeal hemorrhage complicating air exchange. In extreme situations, such as complete transection of the trachea, ventilation through rigid bronchoscopy may be required to facilitate control of the distal airway until definitive control is achieved through thoracotomy and intubation of the distal trachea on the operative field.

Compromise of the airway may also occur without direct trauma to the airway itself. Aspiration of blood, teeth or soft tissue from intraoral or pharyngeal trauma may precipitate lobar collapse and severely impact gas exchange. Loss of consciousness from direct trauma to the cranium and its contents may cause asphyxia due to airway obstruction or loss of respiratory drive. Vascular injury to the neck may evolve to expanding hematoma and associated airway inflammation or obstruction. These cases are particularly challenging

G.C. Velmahos et al. (eds.), *Penetrating Trauma*,
DOI 10.1007/978-3-642-20453-1_23,

endotracheal intubations and impending airway loss should be avoided by pre-emptive airway control when signs and symptoms of cervical penetrating trauma are present. The importance of re-evaluation of the airway throughout the initial evaluation cannot be understated, as progression of hemorrhage or airway injury can quickly transform an initially patent airway to a life-threatening airway obstruction.

Following establishment of the airway, and confirmation by capnometry and oximetry, physical examination of breathing should proceed to rule out distal airway injury and associated life-threatening conditions such as tension pneumothorax, massive hemothorax or open chest wound. Due to the relative rarity and high acuity of airway injuries, there is a risk that providers will be distracted from the appropriate full evaluation of the trauma patient and life-threatening injuries may be overlooked. Furthermore, deviation of the trachea, one of the key findings in tension pneumothorax, may be obscured by direct cervical trauma. When the patient is hypotensive or hypoxic, thoracostomy should be performed when pneumothorax is suspected even without prior confirmation on chest radiograph.

23.1.2 Hemorrhage Identification and Temporary Control

While definitive airway management always takes precedence, in reality, the team caring for the patient with penetrating head, face or neck trauma must simultaneously begin physiologic monitoring, evaluate for all sources of hemorrhage and attempt preliminary hemorrhage control. Penetrating trauma may be localized or multiple, and can be coincident with blunt injury as well. For this reason, it is imperative that the initial evaluation of the patient includes a thorough survey of the entire body so that significant wounds are not overlooked.

Providers should adhere to a systematic evaluation of the common causes of life-threatening bleeding including an assessment of the external blood loss. Although rare when considering all patients with life-threatening trauma, isolated hemorrhage from head and face can cause hemorrhagic shock, and delayed recognition of this source of acute blood loss can be fatal [3]. Lacerations to the scalp should be expeditiously irrigated then sutured (or stapled) to avoid occult blood loss; posterior lacerations are most often missed due to supine positioning. Compression and packing of facial lacerations are preferred over blind clamping to prevent possible nerve injury. Penetrating neck wounds may require manual direct control of hemorrhage until emergent exploration is possible in the controlled setting of the operating room. Anterior nasal hemorrhage may be controlled with direct pressure, but persistent nasopharyngeal hemorrhage may require posterior packing with 1:10,000 epinephrine or even embolization or ligation of the internal maxillary or external carotid arteries. Furthermore, profuse nasopharyngeal hemorrhage is an indication for intubation for airway protection. Nasopharyngeal bleeding due to direct trauma should be distinguished from that seen with coagulopathy which is common in patients with head injury and multi-system involvement, the latter better addressed with administration of coagulation factors rather than direct hemorrhage control.

23.2 Identification of Injury and Prioritization of Treatment

This section will address the scope of penetrating injuries by anatomic location. Common injury patterns, key physical examination findings, diagnostic adjuncts to the secondary survey and basic tenets of therapy will be discussed.

23.2.1 Penetrating Brain Trauma

Civilian penetrating head injuries are most commonly the result of low-velocity gunshot wounds and are frequently due to suicide attempts. In the United States, firearms are the leading mechanism of traumatic brain injury mortality, particularly among young persons, but even in the elderly, death from self-inflicted TBI ranks third after that due to TBI from motor vehicle crashes and falls [4]. The predominant injury from projectiles is facilitated through the velocity of the object, as the energy conveyed to the tissue is proportional to the square of velocity. Injury occurs via three different mechanisms. The direct disruption of the missile tract lacerates parenchyma and blood vessels. Shock waves produce pressure gradients that impact neural tissue and function beyond the path of the missile tract. Cavitation facilitates further direct tissue damage and increased intracranial pressure (ICP). For this reason, military injuries from high-velocity

Table 23.1 Predictors of mortality in penetrating brain injury (Adapted from J Trauma, 2001;51:S44–S86)

Category	Predictor	Class of evidence
Demographics	Increasing age	III
Epidemiology	Perforating (through and through) injury	III
	Suicide	II
Systemic measures	Hypotension	III
	Coagulopathy	III
	Respiratory distress (<10 breaths/min)	III
Neurologic measures	Fixed and dilated pupils	III
	Increased intracranial pressure	II
	Low glasgow coma score	I (civilian), III (military)
Neuroimaging features	Missile track	
	Bihemispheric involvement	II
	Ventricular involvement	III
	Cisternal effacement	I
	Subarachnoid hemorrhage	I
	Intraventricular hemorrhage	I

projectiles are usually associated with a higher rate of death that caused by civilian weapons [5]. It has been observed that the majority of soldiers that present for medical attention with penetrating head injuries sustain low-velocity shrapnel or shell wounds [6].

Because of the potential for secondary brain injury due to hypotension and hypoxia, any initial management of penetrating head injury must begin with efforts to restore homeostasis. The airway must be secured, adequate oxygenation and ventilation confirmed, and an attempt made to improve circulation before the patient is transported for brain imaging or operative intervention. The secondary survey begins with evaluation of neurologic disability, including pupillary examination, determination of spontaneous respirations, and motor-sensory evaluation. With penetrating wounds due to sharp objects, such as nails fired from pneumatic nail guns, the entrance wounds may be deceivingly small and initial neurologic assessments benign, particularly in injuries to the anterior temporal and frontal regions [7]. A normal mental status may mask evolving intracranial hemorrhage, and neurologic deterioration can be rapid. Alternatively, penetrating head trauma can be associated with massive blood loss and direct pressure may be inadequate to achieve more than transient hemostasis, such as that from the nasopharynx. Combination injuries to the face, neck and cranium may require the early involvement of multiple surgical specialists to coordinate control of the airway and bleeding sources.

Computed tomographic (CT) scans of the brain and cervical spine facilitate evaluation of the tract of the penetrating object, missile debris, and the secondary effects of the projectiles including cerebral edema, hemorrhage and bone fragmentation. Computed tomographic angiography (CTA) has largely supplanted cerebral angiography and should be employed liberally to evaluate for carotid and vertebral arterial injury when injuries involve the sphenoid and temporal bones and posterior fossa. Early and rapid identification of vascular injury by screening CTA can allow planning for angiographic embolization or stenting of pseudoaneurysms. The limitations of CTA, with a sensitivity as low as 80% in some studies due to shrapnel artifact, should be recognized and targeted evaluation of potential injuries supplemented with subsequent duplex ultrasound or angiography [8].

The prognosis of penetrating head injury is extremely poor; the overall mortality rate is 88%, significantly higher than that of blunt head injury. Table 23.1 summarizes a number of factors identified by various investigators as predictors of mortality [6, 9]. Of note, midline effacement, presence of brain matter in open wounds and caliber of weapon have not been demonstrated to influence a fatal outcome.

Although increased ICP is associated with higher mortality in PBI patients, there is little published data on the use of ICP monitoring in this patient population, primarily focused on the directed evacuation of hematoma or relief of intractable cerebral swelling [10]. In the absence of guidelines, it is generally accepted that ICP monitors may be employed to follow ICPs for evidence of deterioration when neurologic examination is not possible, as is the practice in blunt head injury [11].

Harvey Cushing's experience during World War I established the standard for early and meticulous debridement of penetrating head wounds [12]. The subsequent military experience of World War II and the Vietnam War largely supported the aggressive operative management of high-velocity weapon injuries, but the evidence seems to support a less invasive management strategy in low to moderate velocity missile injuries, even in the context of military conflicts [13, 14]. In general, the practice in low-velocity penetrating injury is one of minimal intervention to prevent subsequent intracranial infection, and there is some evidence that cerebrospinal fluid leak and air sinus involvement are independent predictors of infection. Broad-spectrum antibiotic prophylaxis is recommended, based on the extrapolation of data from clean craniectomy antibiotic prophylaxis studies, although there is no evidence from the penetrating head injury population [15]. Local debridement of the wound, removal of immediately accessible foreign bodies and watertight closure of the dura are favored over extensive craniectomies to remove all devitalized brain tissue. Several authors suggest that the only indication for craniectomy is mass effect due to hematoma; there are no prospective clinical trials of hematoma evacuation in this patient population, so this remains a class III recommendation [14].

23.2.2 Penetrating Facial Trauma

Although detailed evaluation of the extent of facial trauma is usually delayed until the secondary survey, 25–35% of patients with penetrating injuries to the face will require an emergent airway [16–18]. Oral intubation is always preferred over nasal intubation in the setting of midface instability, cerebrospinal fluid leak and basilar skull fracture in order to avoid cranial intubation [19]. Success rates of 85% have been reported in large series of patients sustaining penetrating facial trauma [20]. As mentioned in the introduction to this chapter, early elective intubation should be considered if the potential for deterioration of airway patency is high such as in intraoral bleeding and edema, gunshot wounds to the mandible, and close-range shotgun wounds. Additionally, brisk hemorrhage from lacerations to the face, scalp and underlying structures should be identified and controlled with direct pressure during the initial evaluation.

There is no universal approach to the diagnosis and classification of penetrating facial trauma, but several authors have described schema to identify the location of the external wound and predict underlying structures at risk. The original designation of three zones of the face included everything below the hairline to the superior orbital rim (Area 1), the midface from the superior orbital rim to the upper lip extending laterally to the preauricular area (Area 2), and the lower face from the upper lip to the hyoid bone (Area 3) [21]. Use of this system directed further diagnosis and management of injuries based on the identifiable injuries on screening physical examination [22]. Additionally, particular attention was paid to the injuries posterior to the angle of the mandible, as this location was associated with a higher incidence of vascular injury due to the proximity of the carotid artery and jugular vein, but these are really Zone III neck injuries (see *Penetrating Neck Trauma*). This approach has been generally supplanted by a more simple two area designation of midface and mandible; this is largely due to the fact that significant Area I injuries are intracranial and not truly facial injuries, as well as to avoid the confusion due to the nomenclature and overlap with the previously named three zones of the neck. In the newer designation, the midface includes the area from the supraorbital rim superiorly to the oral commissure inferiorly to the external auditory meatus laterally, and the mandible designates the area below the oral commissure, but not including Zone III of the neck [16, 17].

Although useful for description of findings during the secondary survey, these anatomic schemas do not reliably distinguish between the extent or severity of injury, as the path of projectiles is largely unpredictable. External and intraoral examinations are often insufficient to identify the trajectory and extent of penetrating injury, particularly if concomitant neck or head injury is suspected, and additional diagnostic modalities must be employed. Plain radiographs are of little use today, as CT with reconstructed multidimensional views facilitates a detailed analysis of the path of the projectile and the scope of the tissue damage, including possible intracranial and cervical spine involvement. Three-dimensional bony reconstructions of the face are regarded by many surgeons as essential tools for planning operative reconstruction of facial fractures. Associated vascular injury can be quickly identified using CT angiography, including evaluation of the cerebral circulation, and may assist in planning angiographic intervention of vessels notoriously difficult to expose surgically.

The mechanism of injury also bears importance in the evaluation. In general, the degree of soft tissue loss and overall structural disruption is greater in ballistic injuries than that seen in stabbings, and knife lacerations to vascular structures or nerves may be amenable to primary repair. Gunshot and close-range shotgun blasts are commonly associated with fractures and tissue loss due to their substantial kinetic energy and may leave behind significant shrapnel and bony fragmentation. Shotgun injuries are more commonly spread across multiple areas and have a high incidence of globe injury. Although low-velocity, objects such as knives have unpredictable depth of penetration. If the stab wound implement is still present in the wound at the time of evaluation, it should remain in situ until after any diagnostic studies are performed and the patient is in the operating room. Vascular control can be temporarily obtained endovascularly either before or in conjunction with the operative exposure.

Damage to specialized organs of the face requires evaluation by surgical subspecialists. Ocular and intracranial penetration necessitates early ophthalmological and neurosurgical consultation. Particularly with fractures to the facial bones and involvement of the sinuses, multidisciplinary evaluation and coordinated treatment by craniofacial reconstructive specialists is recommended to obtain the best long-term cosmetic and functional outcomes. Special attention should be paid to meticulous realignment of the eyelids, nasal alar rims, auricular helical rims and oral stoma. Patients who present with obvious facial paralysis should be assumed to have sustained direct injury to one or more branches of the facial nerve. If the wound is posterior to the lateral canthus, a local exploration with primary nerve repair is considered the treatment of choice. In cases of blast trauma, the nerve is debrided beyond the visible injury and nerve grafting should be strongly considered. Delayed onset of paralysis suggests post-injury nerve edema that may resolve without intervention. The parotid duct is commonly injured in association with buccal branch of the facial nerve injuries due to the proximity of these structures. Additional signs of parotid injury include clear fluid draining from a cheek wound or sialocele formation. As the parotid duct rarely heals or recanalizes without intervention, repair over a stent is recommended.

After establishing that the airway is not at risk, maxillofacial bony trauma does not generally pose an immediate threat to life. As such, delayed reconstruction up to 2 weeks after injury is an acceptable approach. At that time, post-injury edema has largely resolved and the reconstructive effort may be more straightforward. In cases of severe wound contamination or tissue loss, multiple staged debridements and serial dressing changes may be required to prepare the recipient bed for grafting or implantation of prosthetic material. Prophylactic antibiotics with activity against oropharyngeal flora are commonly employed, especially when there is communication to the sinuses for fear of development of meningitis. Interestingly, several reports of patients with facial fractures and cerebrospinal fluid leak do not support this practice [23, 24]. Perioperative antibiotics at the time of facial fracture fixation are associated with a significant reduction in the incidence of surgical site infection. [25] However, prolonged administration beyond 24 h does not confer additional protection in contaminated head and neck surgery and may be associated with higher incidence of infectious complications [26]. The only evidence to support administering prophylactic antibiotics from the time of fracture until fixation is from a single retrospective series of complex mandibular fractures [27]. As foreign bodies and necrotic, contaminated tissue serve as a nidus for infection, early debridement and extraction of bullets, shrapnel and debris is indicated. This is especially true for bullets as projectiles carry clothing and other debris along the projectile track. While knives and other sharp implements tend to breach clothing rather than drag it into the wound, irrigation and debridement of devascularized tissue is just as important in these wounds. Removal of fragments may not be possible due to the risk of damage to adjacent structures, or the inaccessibility of the approach. There is no consensus as to the duration or appropriateness of antibiotic therapy in these circumstances, and delayed removal of debris may be required if infection develops. Timing of bony reconstruction is controversial, but earlier definitive treatment, including grafting and fixation, is possible in some patients and may result in fewer infectious complications [24].

23.2.3 Penetrating Neck Trauma

The neck is anatomically unique. No other area of the body contains a focused collection of vital structures from the cardiovascular, respiratory, digestive, endocrine and nervous systems. As such, the proper evaluation of penetrating trauma to the neck is crucial due to the consequences of missed injury that vary depending upon the structures affected. The zones of the neck are defined by anatomic features readily identified on physical examination. The caudal most zone is Zone I, spanning the area from the clavicle to the cricoid cartilage. Zone II is defined between the cricoid cartilage to the angle of the mandible. Above this, Zone III extends to the skull base. Reference to these zones provides a means to describe the location of penetrating injury, and further implies the degree of difficulty of operative exposure required for adequate proximal and distal vascular control due to bony structures such as the clavicle, the angle of the mandible, and the skull base. Table 23.2 lists the major structures at risk for injury by zone. Interestingly, Monson and Saletta, who first described the zones of the neck, defined Zone II as the area from the angle of the mandible all the way to the clavicle, relegating Zone III to the infraclavicular location and making it's distinction from thoracic trauma curiously indistinct [28].

Table 23.2 Anatomic structures at risk in penetrating neck trauma characterized by zone

Location	Structure at risk
Zone III	Pharynx
	Distal carotid artery
	Distal vertebral artery
	Parotid gland
	Cranial nerves
Zone II	Carotid artery
	Vertebral artery
	Jugular vein
	Larynx
	Esophagus
	Trachea
	Vagus nerve
	Recurrent laryngeal nerve
Zone I	Proximal carotid artery
	Subclavian artery
	Vertebral artery
	Upper lung
	Esophagus
	Trachea

Evaluation of the patient with suspected penetrating neck trauma begins, as always, with the airway. About 10% of patients will present with a compromised airway; both direct and indirect airway obstruction must be considered. Any significant penetrating injury to the aerodigestive tract may compromise the airway due to fistula, obstruction or more commonly, hemorrhage into the trachea; these are indicators for mandatory neck exploration (Table 23.3). Alternatively, adjacent injury may progressively occlude the airway. Two main fascial layers, the superficial and deep cervical, envelope the contents of the neck, often limiting bleeding to the compartments defined by the fascia. While this generally prevents exsanguination from most penetrating wounds, the real danger is often airway compromise due to compression by expanding hematoma. Pre-emptive definitive airway control to prevent impending airway loss should be the rule, as an expanding hematoma can rapidly change a stable situation into a frantic struggle to obtain a patent airway (see previous section on *Airway and Breathing*). If the patient's airway has already been secured by prehospital providers, information about the appearance of the airway on direct laryngoscopy should be obtained, particularly noting any physical findings present at the time and any changes that had occurred in the interim. Fiberoptic bronchoscopy may be employed to examine the proximal trachea by carefully withdrawing the endotracheal tube over the scope, but airway edema due to direct trauma or hematoma compression may demand tracheostomy prior to attempting this. CT of the neck is probably the best test in the intubated patient for detecting fractures of the larynx and to determine which patients should be managed operatively. If the airway is patent on arrival, but a direct injury to the larynx is suspected, formal evaluation of the airway via direct or flexible fiberoptic laryngoscopy, flexible or rigid bronchoscopy may be undertaken in the operating room, where tracheostomy may be performed if indicated.

Along with definitive airway management, the initial management of penetrating neck injury includes an assessment of the overall stability of the patient, and consideration for any other major life-threatening injuries. Chest and lateral cervical spine x-rays are helpful to rule out adjacent intra-thoracic hemorrhage and spinal cord injury as alternative causes of hypotension. Active hemorrhage is controlled with direct pressure.

Table 23.3 Hard and soft signs of vascular, airway or pharyngoesophageal penetrating injury on initial physical examination. In general, hard signs call for operative intervention, while soft signs demand further diagnostic evaluation

Injury	Hard signs	Soft signs
Vascular	Shock Expanding hematoma Active ongoing bleeding	History of pulsatile bleeding Small, stable hematoma Cranial nerve injury Unexplained neurologic deficit Proximity injury without other signs
Aerodigestive	Airway obstruction Air escaping from neck wound Major hemoptysis	Dyspnea Hoarseness Subcutaneous emphysema Odynophagia Rare hemoptysis

Hemorrhaging or hemodynamically unstable patients with Zone II injuries should undergo immediate operative exploration for repair of presumed major vascular injury. Due to the extreme difficulty of obtaining vascular exposure in Zone I or III, unstable patients with injuries to these locations should undergo angiography prior to (or in conjunction with) surgical exploration, if feasible. If the patient is not in shock, and has no other "hard signs" of either vascular or aerodigestive injury, further evaluation of the location and severity of the neck injury can proceed (Table 23.3).

The same principles of injury categorized by weapon as described in facial penetrating injury apply to the neck. In general, ballistic injuries are associated with significantly more collateral damage, retained foreign material and a significantly higher rate of infection than those caused by sharp implements, but the extent of sharp penetrating injury may be initially deceiving due to unpredictable trajectory and depth. The history is sometimes helpful to understand the path of the projectile, but should be confirmed with methods such as plain radiographs or CT to assist in planning further diagnostic or therapeutic intervention. The first determination to be made is whether or not the injury has violated the platysma muscle; superficial wounds need no further workup and may be closed primarily. Removal of a retained penetrating implement is best performed after pre-emptive vascular control is attained, usually by means of operative exposure, but potentially via angiography if the location of the injury is outside of Zone II. Blind exploration of penetrating injuries that violate the platysma is not advised due to potential for reactivation of bleeding from a stable hematoma, but not all of these injuries will require operative exploration.

Few topics in surgery have generated more controversy than the operative exploration of the neck following penetrating trauma. Mandatory exploration of all penetrating neck injuries, including those without hemodynamic compromise or obvious signs of vascular or airway violation, was once the rule out of concern for occult esophageal injury [29]. However, as high rates of negative neck explorations were published in multiple case series, a more selective management approach was developed whereby screening angiography, laryngoscopy, esophagoscopy and bronchoscopy were employed to rule out arterial, laryngeal, esophageal and tracheal injury, respectively. In a landmark review assessing the mandatory versus selective exploration of zone II injuries, Asensio and colleagues failed to conclude that one approach was favored over the other, primarily due to the heterogeneity and retrospective nature of previously reported studies [30]. Since that publication, increasingly accurate and expeditious non-invasive computed tomographic angiography has become commonplace and has largely replaced standard angiography in the initial evaluation of stable Zone II penetrating neck trauma [31–33]. CT has the added benefit of being a single diagnostic modality that may characterize associated hematoma, laryngeal disruption, as well as both arterial and venous injury. However, definitive exclusion of pharyngeal and esophageal injury requires additional diagnostic challenges.

The pharygoesophagus includes the hypopharynx, bounded by the tip of the epiglottis superiorly and the cricopharyngeus inferiorly, and the cervical esophagus. This area is the most protected in the neck and estimates of rates of injury in penetrating trauma range from 1% to 8% [34]. While vascular injuries comprise the predominant cause of early mortality (whether due to exsanguination or airway occlusion), pharyngoesophageal injuries are responsible for the majority of the late deaths seen in penetrating neck trauma. Delay in repair of esophageal injury has been described as an independent risk factor for death [35]. Therefore, the screening test performed should not only have a high sensitivity for detecting injury, it should also be performed and interpreted in a timely manner to facilitate expeditious repair.

Injuries in the pharynx can be reliably diagnosed in the awake patient using flexible fiberoptic laryngoscopy. To definitively rule out esophageal injury, Weigelt and colleagues recommended that patients with negative esophagography also undergo rigid esophagoscopy, citing a sensitivity of 100% [36]. Others suggest that truly asymptomatic patients can be monitored for development of clinical signs, as pharyngoesophageal injury is so uncommon in these patients [34]. However, in a newer review of the use of CTA in cervical penetrating trauma, it is proposed that esophagoscopy could be employed on the basis of high risk injury trajectory determined on CT [33]. For patients undergoing emergent neck exploration, intra-operative rigid esophagoscopy is recommended, as its sensitivity is reportedly higher than flexible esophagoscopy [37]. In practice, the availability of equipment and the expertise to employ it may favor the use of flexible endoscopy. If an injury to the pharynx is discovered and it is <2 cm and does not involve the piriform sinuses below the arytenoids cartilages, the patient may be treated non-operative observation with intravenous prophylactic antibiotics and without anything by mouth. All other hypopharyngeal and all esophageal injuries should be repaired in two layers after necrotic tissue is debrided. Muscle flaps and closed suction drainage are advocated to encourage sealing of the repair and salivary diversion, particularly in the setting of adjacent vascular repair. It may be necessary to mobilize the pharynx from the hyoid bone to achieve greater length and a tension-free repair. If extensive tissue loss is encountered, more commonly experienced in gunshot wounds to the esophagus, a diverting esophagostomy and delayed repair should be performed.

For patients in whom vascular injury is discovered, repair or ligation/embolization of the vessel depends on the nature of the injury, the vessel injured, and the preoperative examination. The vertebral artery is generally very well-protected within the spinal column, with the exception of the portion in Zone I, where it arises from the subclavian artery. As such, the incidence of these injuries is relatively low, and most are asymptomatic, discovered on angiography or CTA [30]. Control may be achieved via angiographic embolization or with proximal and distal direct ligation. Embolization is also recommended in vertebral arteriovenous malformation and pseudoaneurysm. All significant penetrating carotid artery lesions should be repaired when technically feasible, either primarily or with patch angioplasty. If a significant segment of artery is lost, interposition graft or internal to external carotid artery transposition may be performed. Injuries to the distal internal carotid are especially challenging. Options include ligation, extracranial-intracranial bypass, or angiographic stenting [38]. Controversy surrounds the population of injuries with preoperative coma, as initially it was thought that revascularization was associated with a higher incidence of hemorrhagic conversion of ischemic infarction [39]. More recent series suggest that because most deficits remain unchanged or improve after repair, carotid repair should be carried out regardless of preoperative neurologic status, if technically possible [40, 41].

References

1. American College of Surgeons Committee on Trauma (2008) ATLS: Advanced trauma life support for doctors (Student Course Manual), 8th Edition. Amer College of Surgeons
2. Mort TC (2004) Emergency tracheal intubation: complications associated with repeated laryngoscopic attempts. Anesth Analg 99:607–613, table of contents
3. Tung TC et al (2000) Acute life-threatening injuries in facial fracture patients: a review of 1,025 patients. J Trauma 49: 420–424
4. Bruns J, Hauser WA (2003) The epidemiology of traumatic brain injury: a review. Epilepsia 44(Suppl 10):2–10
5. Rosenwasser RH, Andrews DW, Jimenez DF (1991) Penetrating craniocerebral trauma. Surg Clin North Am 71: 305–316
6. (2001) Part 2: prognosis in penetrating brain injury. J Trauma 51:S44–S86
7. Litvack ZN et al (2006) Self-inflicted nail-gun injury with 12 cranial penetrations and associated cerebral trauma. Case report and review of the literature. J Neurosurg 104:828–834
8. Cox MW et al (2007) Traumatic pseudoaneurysms of the head and neck: early endovascular intervention. J Vasc Surg 46:1227–1233
9. Murano T et al (2005) Civilian craniocerebral gunshot wounds: an update in predicting outcomes. Am Surg 71:1009–1014
10. Sarnaik AP et al (1989) Role of aggressive intracranial pressure control in management of pediatric craniocerebral gunshot wounds with unfavorable features. J Trauma 29:1434–1437

11. (2001) Intracranial pressure monitoring in the management of penetrating brain injury. J Trauma 51:S12–S15
12. Cushing H (1917) A study of a series of wounds involving the brain and its enveloping structures. Br J Surg 5:558–684
13. Amirjamshidi A, Abbassioun K, Rahmat H (2003) Minimal debridement or simple wound closure as the only surgical treatment in war victims with low-velocity penetrating head injuries. Indications and management protocol based upon more than 8 years follow-up of 99 cases from Iran-Iraq conflict. Surg Neurol 60:105–110; discussion 110–111
14. (2001) Surgical management of penetrating brain injury. J Trauma 51:S16–S25
15. (2001) Antibiotic prophylaxis for penetrating brain injury. J Trauma 51:S34–S40
16. Chen AY, Stewart MG, Raup G (1996) Penetrating injuries of the face. Otolaryngol Head Neck Surg 115:464–470
17. Cole RD, Browne JD, Phipps CD (1994) Gunshot wounds to the mandible and midface: evaluation, treatment, and avoidance of complications. Otolaryngol Head Neck Surg 111:739–745
18. Dolin J et al (1992) The management of gunshot wounds to the face. J Trauma 33:508–514; discussion 514–515
19. Schade K, Borzotta A, Michaels A (2000) Intracranial malposition of nasopharyngeal airway. J Trauma 49:967–968
20. Demetriades D et al (1998) Initial evaluation and management of gunshot wounds to the face. J Trauma 45:39–41
21. Gant TD, Epstein LI (1979) Low-velocity gunshot wounds to the maxillofacial complex. J Trauma 19:674–677
22. Gussack GS, Jurkovich GJ (1988) Penetrating facial trauma: a management plan. South Med J 81:297–302
23. Choi D, Spann R (1996) Traumatic cerebrospinal fluid leakage: risk factors and the use of prophylactic antibiotics. Br J Neurosurg 10:571–575
24. Clemenza JW, Kaltman SI, Diamond DL (1995) Craniofacial trauma and cerebrospinal fluid leakage: a retrospective clinical study. J Oral Maxillofac Surg 53:1004–1007
25. Chole RA, Yee J (1987) Antibiotic prophylaxis for facial fractures. A prospective, randomized clinical trial. Arch Otolaryngol Head Neck Surg 113:1055–1057
26. Johnson JT et al (1986) Antibiotic prophylaxis in high-risk head and neck surgery: one-day vs. five-day therapy. Otolaryngol Head Neck Surg 95:554–557
27. Zallen RD, Curry JT (1975) A study of antibiotic usage in compound mandibular fractures. J Oral Surg (Am Dent Assoc: 1965) 33:431–434
28. Monson DO, Saletta JD, Freeark RJ (1969) Carotid vertebral trauma. J Trauma 9:987–999
29. Fogelman MJ, Stewart RD (1956) Penetrating wounds of the neck. Am J Surg 91:581–593; discussion, 593–596
30. Asensio JA et al (1991) Management of penetrating neck injuries. The controversy surrounding zone II injuries. Surg Clin North Am 71:267–296
31. Múnera F et al (2000) Diagnosis of arterial injuries caused by penetrating trauma to the neck: comparison of helical CT angiography and conventional angiography. Radiology 216:356–362
32. Múnera F et al (2002) Penetrating neck injuries: helical CT angiography for initial evaluation. Radiology 224: 366–372
33. Osborn TM et al (2008) Computed tomographic angiography as an aid to clinical decision making in the selective management of penetrating injuries to the neck: a reduction in the need for operative exploration. J Trauma 64: 1466–1471
34. Vassiliu P et al (2001) Aerodigestive injuries of the neck. Am Surg 67:75–79
35. Asensio JA et al (1997) Penetrating esophageal injuries: time interval of safety for preoperative evaluation–how long is safe? J Trauma 43:319–324
36. Weigelt JA et al (1987) Diagnosis of penetrating cervical esophageal injuries. Am J Surg 154:619–622
37. Armstrong WB, Detar TR, Stanley RB (1994) Diagnosis and management of external penetrating cervical esophageal injuries. Ann Otol Rhinol Laryngol 103:863–871
38. Maras D et al (2006) Covered stent-graft treatment of traumatic internal carotid artery pseudoaneurysms: a review. Cardiovasc Intervent Radiol 29:958–968
39. Bradley EL (1973) Management of penetrating carotid injuries: an alternative approach. J Trauma 13:248–255
40. du Toit DF et al (2003) Neurologic outcome after penetrating extracranial arterial trauma. J Vasc Surg 38:257–262
41. Unger SW et al (1980) Carotid arterial trauma. Surgery 87: 477–487

Gunshot Injuries to the Head

24

Ekkehard M. Kasper, Markus M. Luedi,
and Burkhard S. Kasper

Traumatic brain injury (TBI) remains a major cause of death and disability worldwide, and missile-induced TBI remains the most deadly of all traumas since first reported and has always been associated with high mortality and morbidity [1]. The prevalence of TBI secondary to gunshots is strikingly variable and reflects the global scenery of violence. Injuries from gunshot wounds (GSW) to the head place an extreme economic burden on the public while disabling the victims in the zenith of their life and imposing enormous medical, legal, and emotional costs [2–5]. Since every gun/projectile combination is associated with a typical pattern of injury [6, 7], war injuries differ significantly from others. We will focus here on predominantly penetrating civilian gunshot wounds with low muzzle velocity (<1,000 f/s) as they occur in the setting of homicide and suicide attempts or during accidents. Many surgeons did take patients to the OR over the last 30 years, and they have achieved a remarkable reduction in morbidity from well above 50% to less than 25% in patients admitted with severe brain injury [8]. However, in the setting of increasingly limited resources, recent research focus has shifted toward more precise prediction of survival as well as on better functional outcome.

E.M. Kasper (✉) • M.M. Luedi
Department of Surgery, Division of Neurosurgery, Beth Israel Deaconess Medical Center, Harvard Medical School, 110 Francis Street, Boston, MA 02215, USA
e-mail: ekasper@bidmc.harvard.edu

B.S. Kasper
Department of Neurology, University of Erlangen, Schwabachanlage 6, 91054 Erlangen F.R.G., Germany

Among firearm injuries, gunshot wounds to the head and brain are nightmares for all involved. Pre-hospital mortality remains >50% and the in-hospital mortality for civilians with penetrating neurocranial injury is around 50–95% depending on the study and the proportion of suicide victims in the series [9]. Of note is the observation that female victims seem to have worse outcome based on a different causative injury pattern [10]. It is clear from all studies that "time is brain," – so we must act swiftly on all patients brought to a trauma center and ensure protocol-guided resuscitation. You must obtain an accurate qualified exam upon arrival, since this is the most relevant determinant and reports of any GSC from the scene are often established pre-resuscitation and hence grossly inaccurate (e.g., secondary to intoxication, hypotension or hypoxia/hypothermia). "Time is brain," so initiate ATLS-guided treatment (pressors, mannitol, hyperventilation) even prior to completing the imaging. To prevent secondary damage perioperatively, always ensure sufficient cerebral perfusion (goal >70 mm Hg) by keeping intracranial pressure below 25 mm Hg and arterial blood pressure above 90 mm Hg and use ICP monitoring, broad-spectrum antibiotics, and anticonvulsants.

Most studies support intervention for patients with a post-resuscitation GCS of greater than 5, but there are exceptions to the rule, and despite a first impression of devastation some will have good outcome "against all odds." So our credo is to treat any not clearly hopeless case as fast and aggressively as possible.

In managing gunshot-injured brain-patients, you should be well aware that **only a part of the neurological harm arises at the moment of impact.** The prognostically relevant damage most frequently evolves

G.C. Velmahos et al. (eds.), *Penetrating Trauma*,
DOI 10.1007/978-3-642-20453-1_24, © Springer-Verlag Berlin Heidelberg 2012

in the time span after the incident and any achieved outcome correlates to the time between injury and the time of intervention [4] and postoperative management. By managing and preventing secondary problems aggressively, you justify swift surgical treatment and improve your outcome.

If the patient is comatose with a GCS of 3–5, we do **initiate intracranial pressure (ICP) treatment already in the trauma bay even prior to the acquisition of imaging**. However, as soon as the patient is systemically stabilized, it is mandatory to immediately obtain a standardized CT scan (5-mm cuts parallel to the skull base in **brain/home/bone windows with reformats in coronal and sagittal planes**) in ALL patients with GSW to the head to make a decision on operative intervention; **CT** scanning does not differ from other trauma patient workup, but we scan the patient **head first** during the trauma protocol workup to get a better idea about the prognosis, the urgency of the situation, and the chance to plan a more precise setup for the OR. Work up and handling of patients with stab injuries to the brain does also not differ significantly from those with gunshot wounds, but injury might be more localized since the impact transforms less energy than that of a projectile.

The acquisition of **CT scans must NOT be postponed** ever because of a good presenting GCS, since approximately 10% of patients with non-penetrating injury (without breach of the neurocranium) may still suffer a significant intracranial injury and will require life-saving neurosurgical intervention ([11, 12]; see also patient illustrated in Fig. 24.2). The reverse is also true: even in the setting of a GSC as low as 3–5, a young patient deserves surgical intervention if a defined space-occupying lesion (e.g., hematoma) is identified on admission CT [5].

Initial patient management should be according to ATLS protocols or equivalent algorithms. Isotonic volume resuscitation, normotonia, normorhythmia, and normothermia should be ensured. Traumatic GSW brain injury is classified as critical in any patients presenting with a GCS score below eight and an abnormal CT scan, e.g., showing a skull fracture or deformation, hematoma, contusion, swelling, or other signs of local or global mass effect possibly causing incipient herniation. Remember that patients with GCS scores >8 and/or a supratentorial single lobe lesion have the best chance to show good outcome after aggressive surgical treatment [5, 9, 12–15].

See web link **www.crash2.lshtm.ac.uk** for a head injury prognosis model calculator

Fig. 24.1 Head injury prognosis model, see www.crash2.lshtm.ac.uk [22]

Recent literature [22] offers also some outcome prediction models (see Fig. 24.1) for head-injured patients using a number of parameters including age, GCS score, pupil reactivity, and the presence of extracranial injuries. Further adjustments are made by including findings on CT scanning. As expected, outcome is also defined by the locally available treatment resources and hence reflects the socioeconomic status of the country. Based on our experience in an urban trauma level 1 center, we strongly suggest aggressive surgical treatment in all not clearly hopeless cases.

24.1 Some Rules for Workup Leading to Operative Management

The most important rule to memorize at the very beginning is: **"Time is brain."**

As profane as it may sound: Clear thinking and a high speed of **coordinated action is crucial** and it requires a well pre-instructed and well-drilled team.

What we really mean here is: Swiftly coordinated actions are vital in the true sense of the word and will define the outcome for such challenging endeavors and are an absolute requirement if you want to succeed. This applies to all parts of the care-provider chain: from Advanced Life Support trained EMTs, who pick up and transport the patient, their management en route, to the presentation upon arrival in the ER. Admission exam and timely work up is critical and potentially life-saving (with its bedside decisions) until a possible intervention in the OR can be performed. The latter can only be successful with a premeditated and very well carriedout surgical plan.

Here are my (EMK) rules:

No. 1: **DO NOT PANIC!** In many ways, it is a case like many others; therefore RUN YOUR

ROUTINE. Do all the workup and related decision like a tree and according to a protocol.

No. 2: **DO NOT WASTE TIME** – and save it where you can do it safely. This means: When the hospital is notified about the arrival of such a GSW patient, GET READY BEFORE THEY ARRIVE. Call the OR upfront to get a room setup. Announce the most likely scenario (e.g., 20-year-old male; R crani/supine or suboccipital crani/prone, etc.). Ask to assemble a team for the OR that you already know/can work with, not newcomers (Fig. 24.3).

No. 3: **GO TO THE ER AND WAIT IN THE TRAUMA BAY FOR THE PATIENT TO ARRIVE.** If you are out of the hospital, start

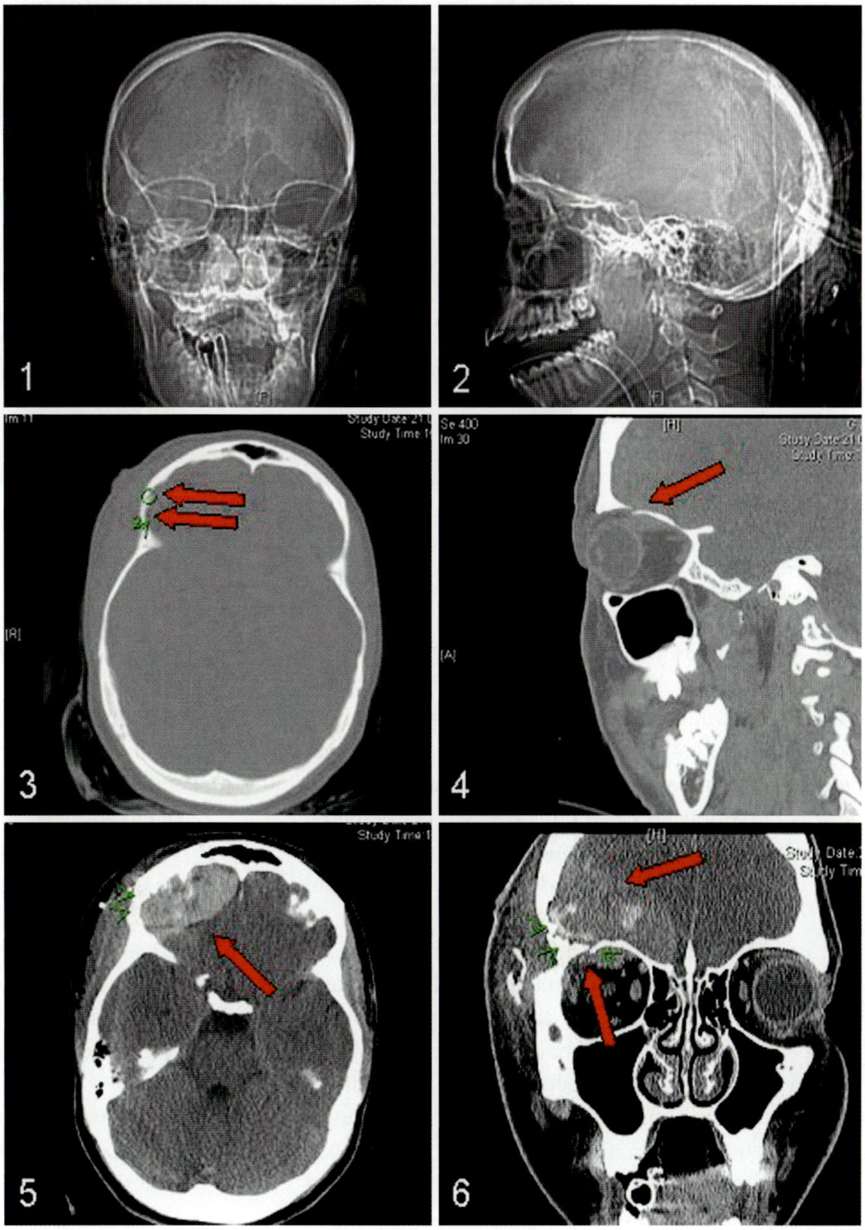

Fig. 24.2 Patient No. 1: 22-year-old female crime victim, who sustained multiple GSW with a single non-penetrating GSW to the head. Entry wound at R cheek, exit wound on R supraorbital forefront. *Plates 1 and 2*: Scout images A/P and lateral without evidence of bullet. *Plate 3 and 4*: preoperative images (bone windows) demonstrating R frontal skull fracture with pneumocephalus and orbital roof fracture. *Plates 5 and 6*: axial and coronal views of large R epidural hematoma and intraorbital hematoma. *Plates 7 and 8*: axial views of postoperative results status post evacuation of hematoma and autologous cranioplasty. *Plates 9 and 10*: reconstructed orbital roof status post transfrontal evacuation of retroorbital hematoma

Fig. 24.2 (continued)

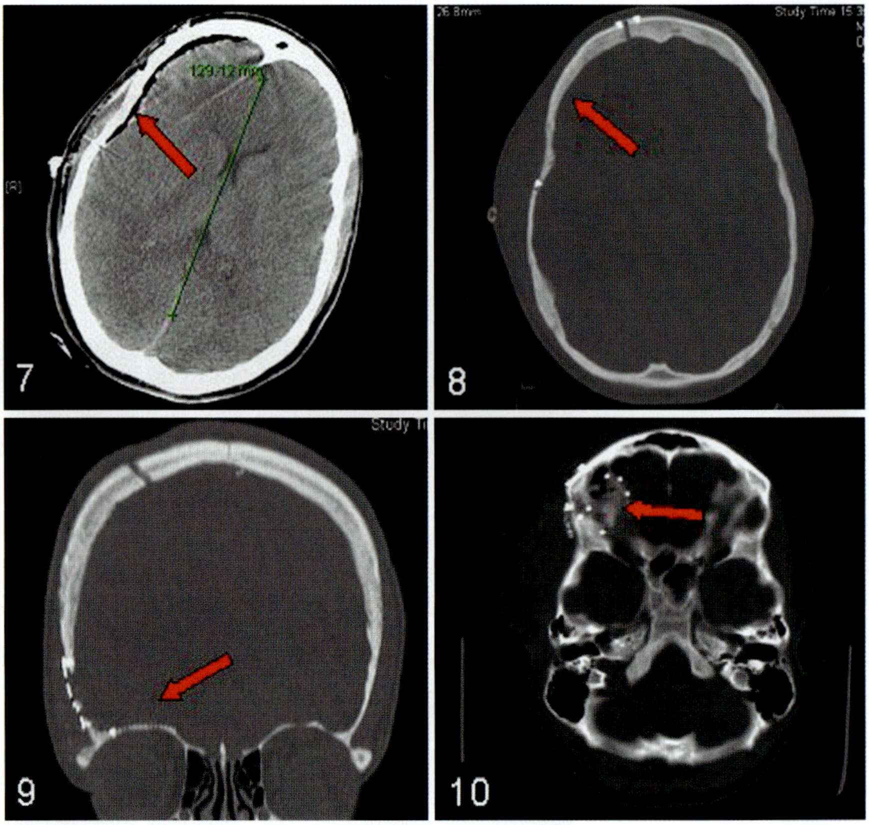

driving in NOW. Meanwhile organize things by phone on your way. These are most valuable minutes that you can save for later (Fig. 24.4).

No. 4: **Touch base with the ER attending**. In an experienced setting, the ER will get prepared early and have identification labels/numbers and a trauma team assigned prior to arrival (Fig. 24.5).

No. 5: Make sure they **notify the blood bank** for possible need of products with "emergent release." Make sure they have pressors and Mannitol/Lasix IV ready, a respiratory therapist to initiate hyperventilation. Remember the rule of 30s: height of bed 30°, hyperventilation with $f=30$ for a goal $pCO_2<30$.

No. 6: Get **the trauma team ready in the bay and assign tasks** by talking to the senior/attending running the case. **THIS IS NOT THE PATIENT TO PRACTICE ON**. Newcomers can stand by and watch, but should stay at a distance and out of the way! Try to pass all preliminary information around as it can be gathered from the EMT-call-in from the scene or en route (ask about patient age, single wound or systemic injury, patient awake or with loss of consciousness (LOC)/comatose; patient intubated, patient stable; blood loss at the scene; other issues).

No. 7: **Call the CT scanner** upfront that you will bring a critically ill patient ASAP so they keep the scanner **FREE for your case!**

No. 8: Listen well to what the transport team has to say upon presenting the case, they sometimes know important details (downtime, seizures at the scene, difficulties with the airway, etc.).

No. 9: **WATCH** if there is any sign of life upon arrival. Get a good glimpse at the patient (I recommend you stand behind the chief running the case at the head end of the patient) and once the primary survey is done.

No. 10: You should **get a 10–30-s neuroexam yourself**.

NOW MAKE THE RUN AGAINST THE CLOCK!

24.2 Preoperative and Intraoperative Management

For most TBI strategies, you will find very little class 1 or 2 recommendations. To get a good grip on how to run these scenarios and treat your patient well, watch as many cases as you can during training. Take home the pivotal steps of decision making from seasoned staff. You can often not randomize patients in critically

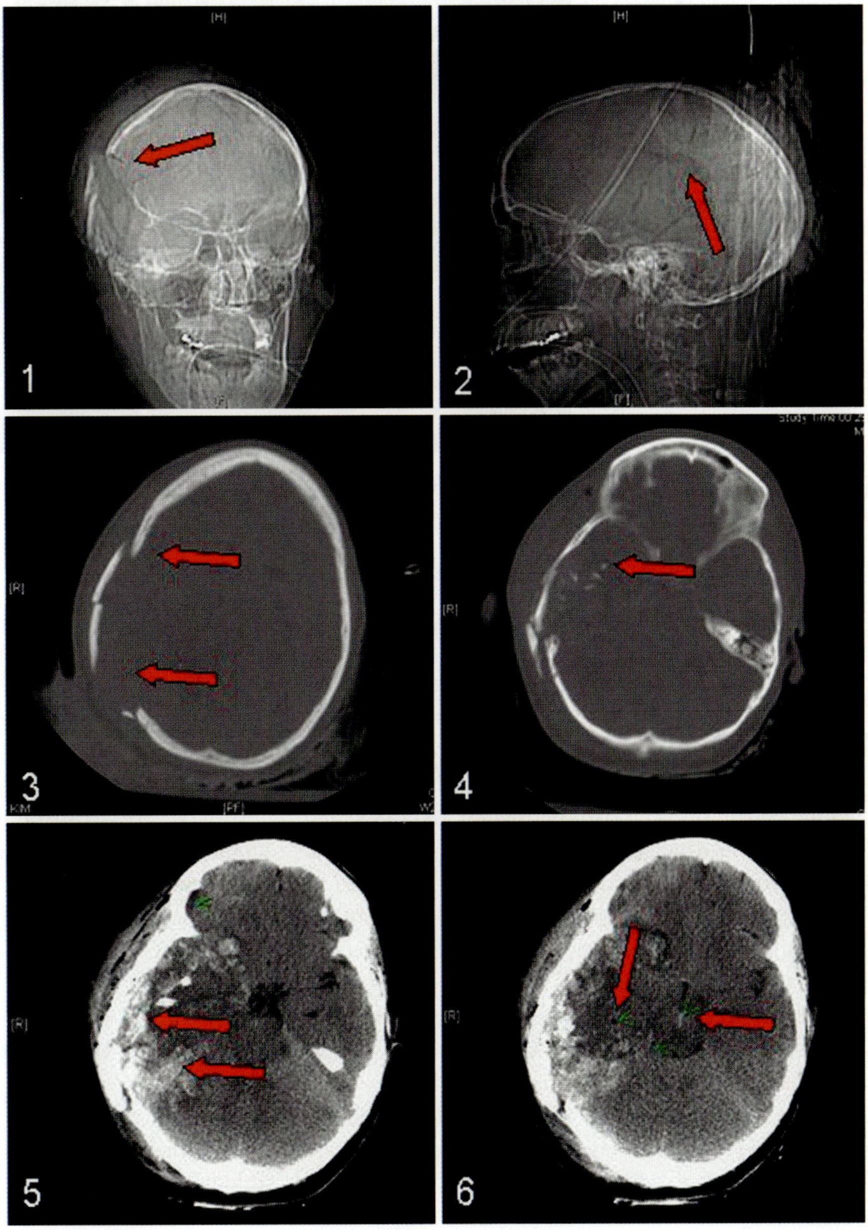

Fig. 24.3 Patient No. 2: 23-year-old female, who sustained a solitary GSW to the head from close range. Entry wound on the R cheek, exit wound R parietal. *Plates 1 and 2*: Scout images A/P and lateral without evidence of bullet but large R sided skull fracture. *Plate 3 and 4*: preoperative images (bone windows) demonstrating R fronto-parieto-temporal blowout skull fracture and skull base fracture from middle cranial fossa entry point. *Plates 5 and 6*: axial views of large R SAH, epidural and intraparenchymal hematoma and contusions with pneumocephalus. *Plates 7 and 8*: axial views of postoperative results status post hemicraniectomy for evacuation of hematoma. *Plates 9 and 10*: final results of reconstructed R allograft cranioplasty with Porex® and encephalomalacia along the bullet tract

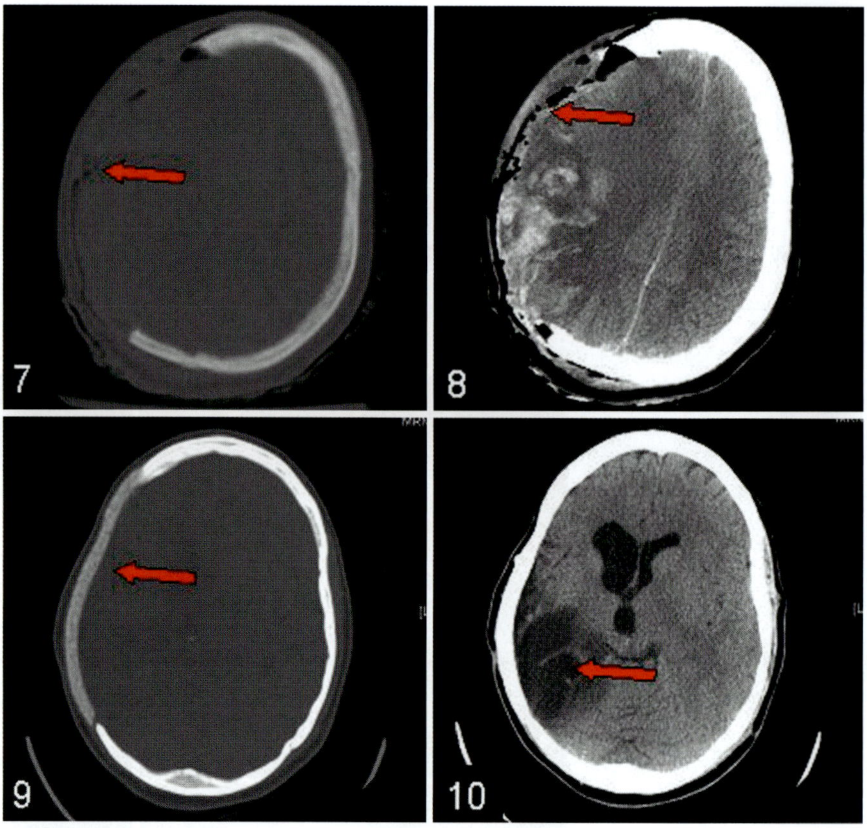

Fig. 24.3 (continued)

ill settings since it often poses an ethical dilemma; therefore, remember the following points to increase the possibility of a satisfying discharge-status of a patient injured by gunshot or a stab wound:

In all trauma patients, let the trauma team perform *systematic reviews* in the bay and stanch blood ASAP; get the patient lined up (two peripheral 16 G IVs) and treat abnormal vital signs (e.g., hypotension, hypoxia/hypothermia!) before you move to the radiological examinations and consider any surgical intervention. The minutes spent here are WELL SPENT and make your part SAVE. No one wants to rush the GSW patient to the scanner and see them crashing there. And remember: NO GSW TO THE HEAD goes to the OR without films EVER!

Have one team member assigned as liaison to the relatives if you do not have the time to communicate during the need of swift action. They will be extremely grateful and less anxious. Once you have obtained your scans, make a swift decision: Patients with a GCS of 3–5 AND a devastating scan (bilateral global injury with transventricular bullet trajectory, massive blood or swelling with near complete herniation, tramtrack signs) may not be salvageable and warrant conservative treatment alone with ICP-bolt placement and medical management only. Other patients with either improved post-resuscitation GCS > 5 and limited supratentorial injury and a vector that does not show involvement of the fatal zone [4] should be considered for surgery.

NOW TO THE POINTS THAT MATTER:

24.3 Operative Management

Always ask yourself
"How can I do the best intervention the fastest possible way"?

Here are the 15 most important points on the road to success:

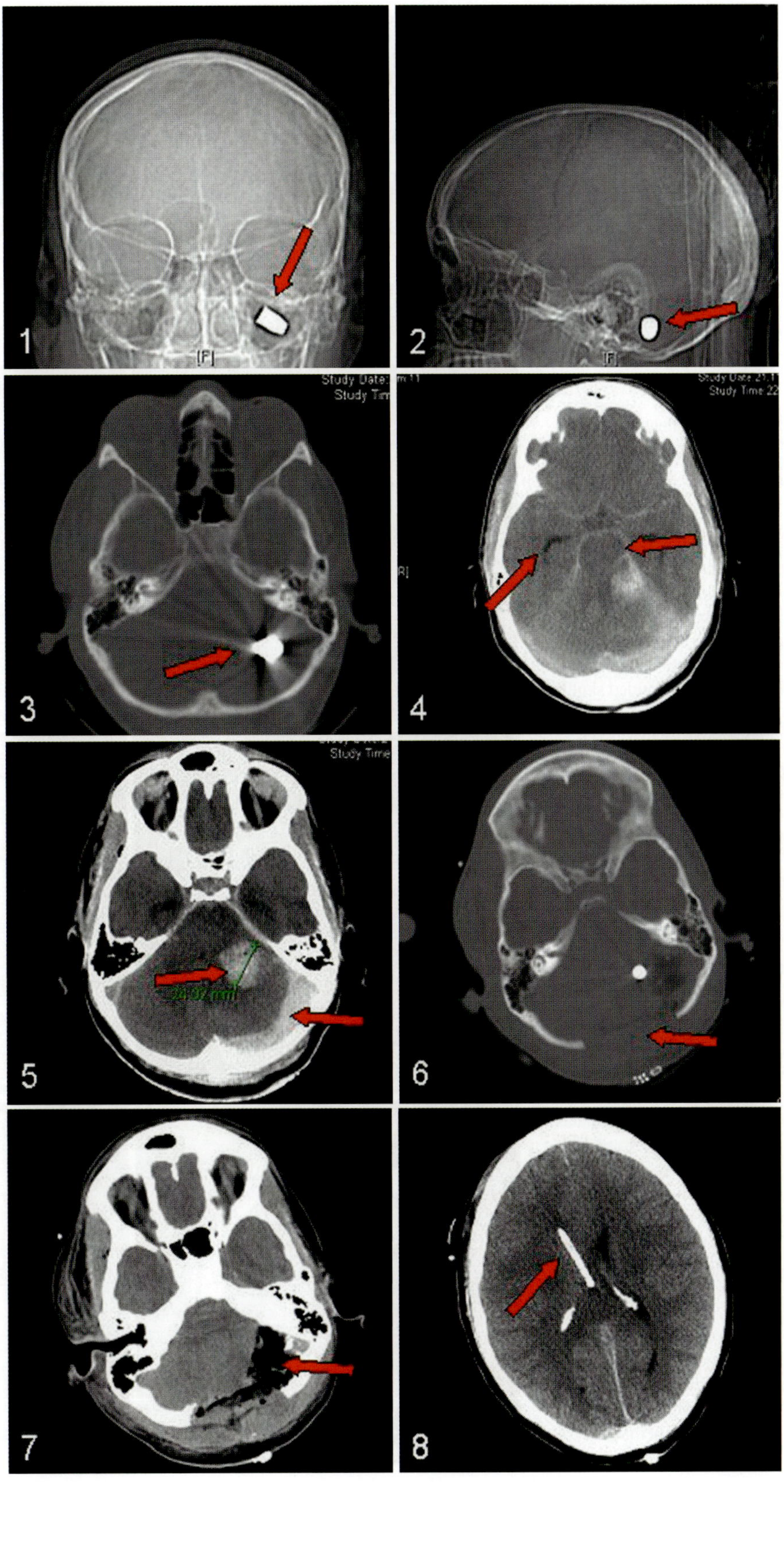

Fig. 24.4 Patient No. 3: 30-year-old female, who sustained a solitary GSW to the back of her head from close range. Entry wound on the occiput and no exit wound. *Plates 1 and 2*: Scout images A/P and lateral with evidence of a lodged bullet in the L cerebellum behind the L mastoid. *Plate 3*: preoperative image (bone window) demonstrating L p-fossa bullet. *Plates 4 and 5*: axial views of significant SAH, L infratentorial epidural hematoma and CPA-intraparenchymal hematoma with pneumocephalus. *Plates 6 and 7*: axial views of postoperative results status post suboccipital craniectomy for decompression and evacuation of hematoma with some residual air in the operative bed. *Plate 8*: supratentorial placement of an R EVD for CSF diversion

1. Transport the patient yourself from the CT scanner straight to the OR.
2. Position the patient by transferring him from the stretcher onto the OR bed (which has been pre-placed correctly in the room since you called from the CT scanner).
3. Apply only the utmost necessary padding to save time (this is not the time to search for pneumo-boots or gelrolls).
4. Pin the patient in a Mayfield headrest at straight angles! (either supine or fully lateral). This helps to keep your orientation once you are deep inside.
5. Shave the entire hemiconvexity (be generous!).
6. Scratch the skin to keep your landmarks and pay attention to especially the midline!
7. Use a quick prep-solution: e.g., soaking beta-iodine sponges followed by Prevail®; this is not the time to go through six sponges of your three soap elective crani routine.
8. Do not waste the time to wait for using local anesthesia/epinephrine for better hemostasis.

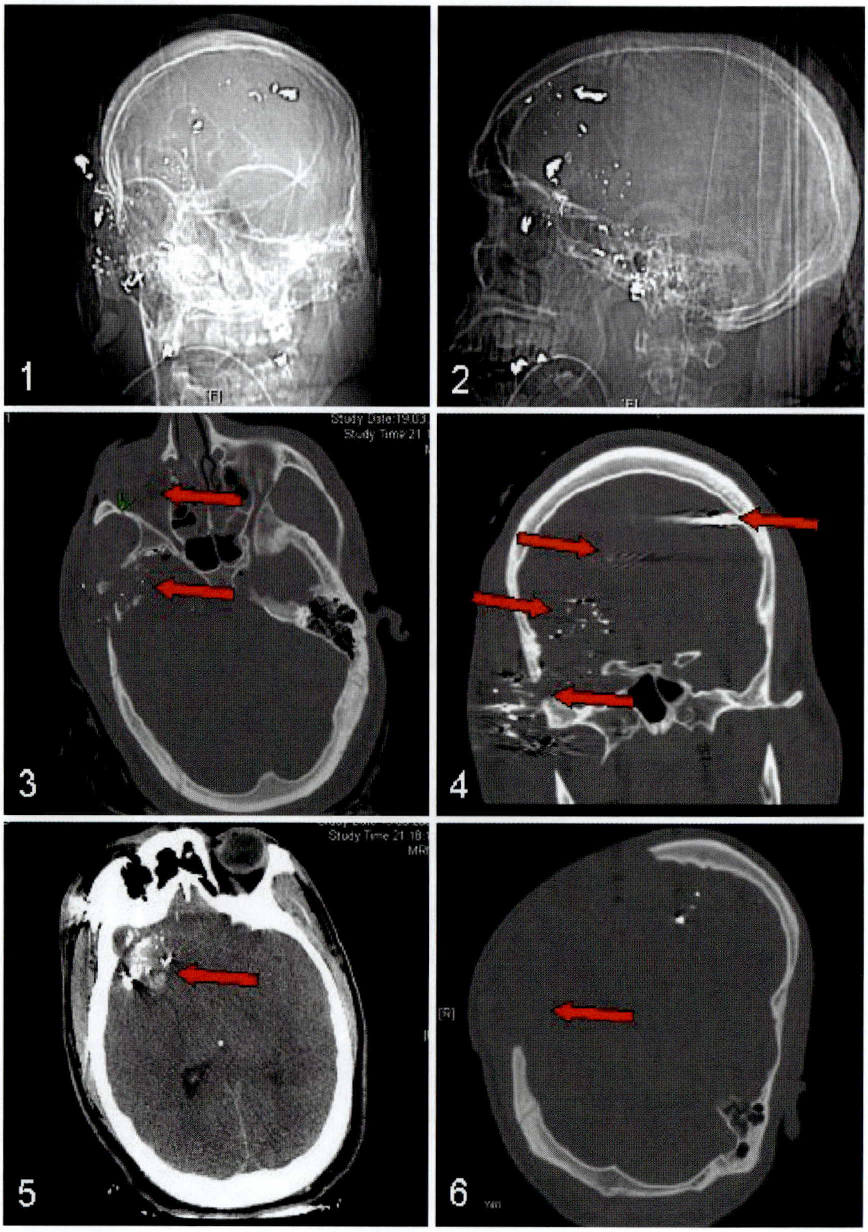

Fig. 24.5 Patient No. 4: 26-year-old male, who sustained a solitary GSW to the head from distant range. Entry wound at the R ear canal, no exit wound. *Plates 1 and 2*: Scout images A/P and lateral with evidence of multiple bullet fragments on the R extra-cranially and bilaterally intra-cranially. Note the large R sided skull fracture. *Plates 3 and 4*: preoperative images (axial and coronal bone windows) demonstrating R infero-temporal blowout skull fracture and skull base fracture from middle cranial fossa entry point and steep trajectory with bullet remnants in the L frontal area. *Plate 5*: axial view of R SAH and temporal intraparenchymal hematoma, contusions, and artifacts from bullet fragments with pneumocephalus. *Plates 6 and 7*: axial and coronal views of postoperative results status post R hemicraniectomy for evacuation of hematoma and status post clipping of R sided MCA branches from avulsion injury. *Plate 8*: postoperative CTA with adequate perfusion to the superior branches of the MCA, 2 aneurysm clips at the MCA, and artifact from bullet fragments. *Plates 9 and 10*: supratentorial views status post hemicraniectomy and small L frontal hematoma along the bullet tract

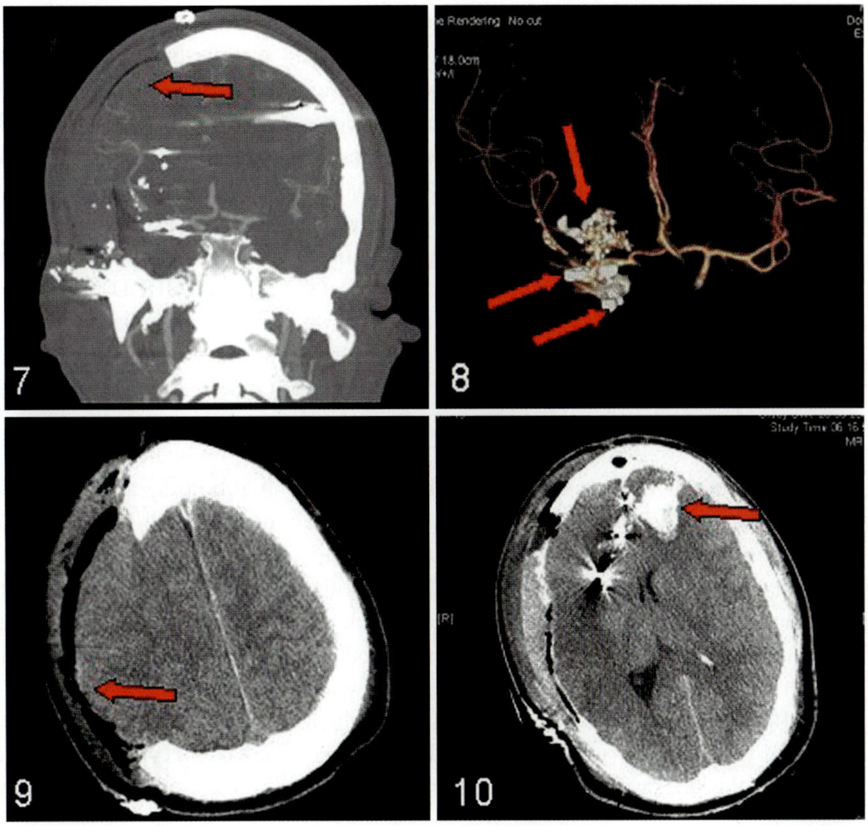

Fig. 24.5 (continued)

9. Incise with the goal of creating a generous flap to allow for post-OP swelling.
10. Perform a really good sized hemicraniectomy for optimal decompression and do not forget to prepare in all p-fossa lesions a **Frazier bur-hole** so you can place an external ventricular drain (EVD) any time.
11. Save the bone flap on the back-table to be used in a freezer-storage protocol and do not waste time on a second (abdominal) incision! You want to get out of the OR ASAP.
12. Always irrigate copiously with antibiotic solution: e.g., bacitracin®.
13. Perform your **wide durotomy BEFORE you place any dural tenting stitches** since this decompresses the brain earlier and you save the brain some more vital minutes.
14. Close the dura provisionally, e.g., with an **onlay dural allograft** (e.g., duragen®) to prevent adhesion-scarring from the brain surface to the undersurface of the muscle flap. A subgaleal CSFoma is of no concern here, since you will be back for a regular cranioplasty.
15. Close the muscle flap in three layers only to save some time: (1) muscle+fascia, (2) galea, (3) skin.

Do not forget to talk to "your team" at all times during the case and announce you next moves clearly and loud. These are fast and stressful cases and performed not for pretty but effective surgery; describe technical details that make a difference (Anesthesia needs to know when you open the dura to anticipate a change in ICP and SBP response).

24.4 Perioperative Management

24.4.1 Cerebral Perfusion Threshold

An adequate cerebral perfusion pressure (CPP) is instrumental to keep brain tissue alive. More is better here. The goal value is the result of subtracting the ICP from the mean arterial pressure (MAP). You may guess via the SBP if your monitor does not calculate and display MAPs.

The critical cerebral perfusion pressure (CPP) threshold for ischemia lies around 50_60 mm Hg [16]; do not overresuscitate with IV fluids and DO NOT USE fluids with concentrations of half normal saline (0.45%), which act as hyposomolar volume expanders and may create significant brain edema. Remember: There is poor outcome in patients with systemic hypotension [17] but there is risk of adult respiratory distress syndrome with too ambitious use of fluids too. So keep ICP low and MAP high enough with mannitol (e.g., 1–1.5 g/kg body **weight is about 100 g I/V** for an average sized person of 70 kg) and do not hesitate to use pressors early (e.g., Neosynephrine) and do NOT bring down systolic blood pressure (SBP) if a patient comes in at 165 before you have a CT scan; he may need that pressure for good perfusion!.

Always monitor blood pressure (BP) frequently (q2–5 min) and avoid **systolic drops of BP < 90 mm Hg** [18]. Now a personal hint: **Do NOT waste time placing an A-line before CT scanning**. In a hemodynamically stable patient, you are better off seeing the intracranial damage early and go to the OR quicker rather than waiting 5 min for line placement before you can make an informed decision. The OR can work more efficiently with teams acting in parallel which saves you vital minutes (needless to say: In the unstable patient, this does not hold true).

24.5 Intracranial Pressure Monitoring

Aim to always maintain adequate cerebral perfusion to prevent secondary damage! So monitor ICP in all necessary settings of severe traumatic brain injury with GCS < 8 to define the need of intervention (level II evidence). But what does that mean here? You are not able to manage CPP correctly without measuring ICP and MAP! However, if the patient goes to the OR anyway, do not waste time placing an ICP-bolt monitor or external ventricular drain upfront. It is more suitable for the post-OP setting [23].

Especially in smaller institutions, the threshold for invasive monitoring remains too high. Here we advocate a low threshold for transferring the patient to an experienced center and correct placement in an ICU setting. CT scans are not appropriate for "guessing" ICP, but good enough pre-OP to make a decision. If the patients scan supports nonoperative management, the patient needs an ICP-bolt placed ASAP.

By the way, if a CT does not present any abnormalities to explain a low admission GCS, then measure ICP when two or more of the following features are noted: negative tox screen, patients above 40 years of age, systolic BP < 90 mmHg, or the patient shows sign of posturing (uni- or bilateral) (level III, see [17, 18]).

Do *not* treat potential high ICP for any prolonged period of time prophylactically without correct monitoring in the ICU setting. (This is NOT true for a sudden change in mental status in a critically ill TBI patient; if you notice a rapid decline in neuroexam, you SHOULD initiate therapy immediately with hyperventilation/HOB30/mannitol and then go to the scanner ASAP to explore the intracranial situation!). Once again, time is brain and less ICP for several minutes can save a lot of tissue if used in the correct setting. Whether you use a parenchymal or ventricular ICP-bolt-device is more a question of preference than of evidence. However, the latter is known for lower costs and offers the chance to also treat by draining off excess cerebrospinal fluid (CSF). Start treatment if ICP is sustained >20 mm Hg (level II) and follow respective clinical and radiological findings.

24.6 Hyperosmolar Therapy and Barbiturates

Mannitol or hypertonic saline lowers ICP and may thereby increase CPP, thus improving neurological outcome. As a rule of thumb, use mannitol at 1 g/kg body weight as a loading dose (level II). Equimolar doses of NaCl may be given according to institutional protocols. Then maintain the dosing but divide it into equal fractions (e.g., 25 g mannitol q6 h) [18]. Do NOT forget to also order holding parameters (e.g., hold next dose for Osm > 320 or Na > 150) to prevent drying the patient out. Also be aware that you might cause transient arterial hypotension! Mannitol outweighs barbiturates in improving ICP, but bears a higher risk of hypotension. Prophylactic administration without evidence of increased ICP is not recommended [19]. Only use barbiturates if ICP cannot be decreased by any other measure to prophylactically slow metabolism. (It also makes brain death determination really difficult.)

24.7 Hyperventilation and Steroids

Hyperventilation can reduce ICP. The mechanism most likely comes from intravasal volume reduction secondary to vasoconstriction. The method works well for 6 h (giving you a good time window to initiate further treatments) but can turn detrimental thereafter. So do not use it without careful consideration and limits! Avoid to excessive a protocol and do not hyperventilate to a $PaCO_2 < 25$ mmHg during the first 24 h after TBI when cerebral blood flow (CBF) is often critically reduced (level II) [17, 18]. Mind you that the day after a significant injury CBF is reduced to less 50% of normal individuals; this means that you risk decreasing CBF even further with aggressive hyperventilation and a subsequent reduction in CBF and you actually worsen the situation to the point that the patient may become ischemic or stroke.

Do NOT apply steroids. Currently, there is no proven benefit for the use of steroids in traumatic closed head /brain injury. Earlier data had reported some benefit but at an increased risk for overall morbidity especially in the population of elderly.

24.8 Infection Prophylaxis

Most general guidelines (level II) suggest periprocedural administration of antibiotics to reduce the incidence of pneumonia after intubation [18] in the patients with significantly decreased mental status. Although gunshots are often considered to be sterile in themselves, we support the notion [20, 21] of a 48–72-h period of broad-spectrum antibiotic prophylaxis for prevention of meningitis secondary to a CSF leak. Vancomycin 1 g Q12 h; Gentamycin 80 mg Q 8 h; and Flagyl 500 mg Q6 will suffice. Since most CSF leaks close spontaneously within 48 h, or will be taken care of during surgery, we do not maintain this regimen beyond day 3, unless there is a significant amount of bony debris translocated into the parenchyma. If that is the case, 7–10 days of antibiotic coverage seems reasonable.

24.9 Prophylactic Hypothermia

Even though preliminary data had shown a possible increase of survival when induced hypothermia is maintained for more than 48 h in TBI patients, we currently do not use prolonged hypothermia on patients with GSW. Pooled data (level III) indicated no improvement in overall mortality [18] and are hinting at increased coagulopathies – hence, we are awaiting further studies to this end.

24.10 Antiseizure Prophylaxis

We strongly recommend the use of antiepileptic medications for a minimum of the first 7 days of injury for subarachnoidal hemorrhage (SAH). If significant parenchymal damage incurred, we keep it on until the first follow-up appointment.

Phenytoin is the drug of choice and clearly decreases the incidence of early posttraumatic seizures (PTS) and associated morbidity. Penetrating trauma to the head is an established risk factor for the development of PTS, but you can relax: These early PTS are not worsening long-term outcome. Since precautionary administration of valproate or phenytoin has not shown to prevent (level II) late posttraumatic seizures, most centers do not use them for anything else but perioperative [18].

24.11 Postoperative Consideration

Excessive postoperative strategies are not topic of this book. All basic postoperative prophylactic strategies apply for GSW trauma victims too. A brief reminder follows and your care protocols should include the following:

- Most patients have a rough course during the first 3–7 days, since swelling seems to peak around POD 3–4 and you have to watch out for it and treat any trends of increase in ICP early and aggressively.
- Wean all patients from the ventilator ASAP; an extubated patient gives you the best scenario for a proper assessment and neurological examination which can be followed once the GCS > 8. If the patient does not regain consciousness soon, opt for an early trachestomy and PEG in anticipation of a long postoperative course.
- Ensure full caloric intake by day 7 post-injury to support wound healing. To achieve best results, begin feeding not later than72 h after injury.
- Combine mechanical DVT prophylaxis via compression stockings or intermittent pneumatic compression stockings with low molecular weight heparin or low-dose unfractionated heparin as early as POD 2
- Provide a decent bowel regimen (including acid blocker and a stool softener to help the slowed guts) and for prevention of stress-induced ICU gastritis.
- Supply adequate pain medications as these patients will not ask for any.

- Support the patient with anxiolytics and sedation in the setting of ICU care.
- Meticulous decubitus prophylaxis must be applied.
- Mobilize the patient early (PT/OT/out of bed to chair).

24.12 Special Circumstances

If you ever face a situation in which you have multiple GSW victims (such as a terror attack or a mass casualty), you have to make a stern decision: Who is going to be treated first, or who is not going to be treated at all. It seems to be acceptable to make that decision based on your available resources and based on the available data reflecting the different prognosis for patients; I recommend to perform the workup in each patient just as outlined above. Based on the clinical information (presenting GCS score) and the CT scan, I feel strongly that a patient with a higher GCS and limited damage on scan (e.g., unilobar right-sided injury) has the best chances for good functional outcome and hence should go to surgery first. However, we acknowledge the ethical dilemma in this scenario and accept differing decisions based on momentary rationale or experience of the treating team.

References

1. Pabuscu Y, Bulakbasi N, Kocaoglu M, Ustunsoz B, Tayfun C (2003) A different approach to missile induced head injuries. Comput Med Imaging Graph 27:397–409
2. Cook PJ, Lawrence BA, Ludwig J, Miller TR (1999) The medical cost of gunshot injuries in the United States. JAMA 282:447–454
3. Denton JS, Segovia A, Filkins JA (2006) Practical pathology of gunshot wounds. Arch Pathol Lab Med 130:1283–1289
4. Kim KA, Wang MY, McNatt SA, Pinsky G, Liu CY, Gianotta SL, Appuzzo MLJ (2005) Vector analysis correlating bullet trajectory to outcome after civilian through and through gunshot wounds to the head: using imaging cues to predict fatal outcome. Neurosurgery 57(4):737–747
5. Kim TW, Lee JK, Moon KS, Kwak HJ, Jpp SP, Kim JH, Kim SH (2007) Penetrating gunshot injuries to the brain. J Trauma 62(6):1446–1451
6. Jandial R, Reichwage B, Levy M, Duenas C, Sturdivan L (2008) Ballistics for the neurosurgeon. Neurosurgery 62(2):472–480
7. Stuehmer C, Blum KS, Kokemueller H, Tavassol F, Bormann KH, Gellrich NC, Rücker M (2009) Influence of different types of guns, projectiles, and propellants on patterns of injury to the viscerocranium. J Oral Maxillofac Surg 67:775–781
8. Lu J, Marmarou A, Choi S et al (2005) Mortality from traumatic brain injury. Acta Neurochir Suppl 95:281–285
9. Rosenfeld JV (2002) Gunshot injury to the head and spine. J Clin Neurosci 9(1):9–16
10. Finlay-Morreale HE, Tsuei BJ, Fisher BS, Davis K, Johannigman JA (2009) Close is dead: determinants of firearm injury lethality in women. J Trauma 66(4):1207–1211
11. Glapa M, Zorio M, Snycker FD, Bowley DM, Yilmaz TH, Doll D, Degiannis E (2009) Gunshot wounds to the head in a civilian practice. Am Surg 75(3):223–226
12. Semple PL, Domingo Z (2001) Craniocerebral gunshot injuries in South Africa – a suggested management strategy. S Afr Med J 91(2):141–145
13. Levy ML (2000) Outcome prediction following penetrating craniocerebral injury in a civilian population: aggressive surgical management in patients with admission GCS scores of 6–15. Neurosurg Focus 8(1):e2
14. Martins RS, Siqueira MG, Santos MT, Zanon-Collange MOJ (2003) Prognostic factors and treatment of penetrating gunshot wounds to the head. Surg Neurol 60(2):98–104
15. Tsuei YS, Sun MH, Lee HD, Chiang MZ, Leu CH, Cheng WY, Shen CC (2005) Civilian gunshot wounds to the brain. J Chin Med Assoc 68(3):126–132
16. Cliffton GL, Miller ER, Sc C et al (2002) Fluid thresholds and outcome from severe brain injury. Crit Care Med 30:739–745
17. Bullock R, Chestnut RM, Clifton G et al (2000) Guidelines for the management of severe head injury. J Neurotrauma 17:451–553
18. Bratton SL, Chestnut RM, Ghajar J et al (2007) Guidelines for the management of severe traumatic brain injury. J Neurotrauma 24(suppl 1):1–106
19. Roberts I (2000) Barbiturates for acute traumatic brain injury. Cochrane Database Syst. Rev. (2): CD000033
20. Bayston R, de Louvois J, Brown EM et al (2000) Use of antibiotics in penetrating craniocerebral injuries. Lancet 355:1813–1817
21. Lozier AP, Sciacca RR, Romagnoli MF et al (2008) Ventriculostomy-related infections: a critical review of the literature. Neurosurgery 62(Suppl 2):688–700
22. MRC CRASH Trial Collaborators, Perel P, Arango M, Clayton T et al (2008) Predicting outcome after traumatic brain injury: practical prognostic models based on large cohort of international patients. BMJ 336:425–429
23. Patel HC, Menon DK, Tebbs S, Hawker R, Hutchinson PJ, Kirkpatrick PJ (2002) Specialist neurocritical care and outcome from head injury. Intensive Care Med. 2002, 28(5): 547–553

Penetrating Injuries of the Face

25

Rizan Nashef and Thomas B. Dodson

The reported frequencies of penetrating maxillofacial injuries in the English literature range from 14% to 52% [1, 2]. The wide range in reported frequencies is a function of the institution's location and referral patterns. Level 1 emergency departments (EDs) located in an urban environment and military units are more likely to see a large volume of penetrating injuries compared to lower level EDs or those located distant from urban environments [2, 3].

25.1 Type and Characteristics of Injuries

Penetrating injuries occur when objects, e.g., a missile or knife, violate skin or mucosal barriers and enter the body and are classified as high energy (missile such as a bullet or shrapnel) or low energy (knife). High-energy penetrating injuries produce avulsive injuries associated with loss of both soft and hard tissue, producing a composite defect (Fig. 25.1a, b). Composite defect wounds are complex wounds to manage acutely and commonly require secondary reconstruction. Internal fixation devices to stabilize bony segments or replace missing bony structures, prudent preservation of soft tissue, and use of advancement flaps can produce excellent anatomic restoration of form.

Low-energy penetrating injuries, such as a knife, machete, or other sharp objects, result in isolated damage to the soft tissue or combination of damage to the soft tissue and facial fractures, generally with preservation of soft and hard tissue mass (Fig. 25.2a, b).

25.2 Structures at Risk for Injury

Maxillofacial injuries, while not generally life threatening, present challenging problems to trauma surgeons because of the concentration of complex, vital anatomic structures with their associated functions. These structures include the brain with its 12 cranial nerves, 4 of the 5 senses, the airway, an intricate bone configuration, the cervical spine, major blood vessels, salivary glands, and the centers for speech and deglutition. In addition, the face has an important esthetic component that affects patients' self-worth and psychological well-being.

25.3 Goals of Management

Maxillofacial penetrating injuries do not usually create major resuscitation challenges [3]. As such, immediate attention needs to be directed toward evaluating and managing the airway and bleeding. After the patient is stabilized, the long-term treatment objectives are to restore facial form and function (Fig. 25.1c, d) while

R. Nashef (✉)
Department of Oral and Maxillofacial Surgery, Hadassah Medical Organization, Kiryat Hadassah, P.O.Box. 12000, Jerusalem 91120, Israel
e-mail: rnashef@hadassah.org.il

T.B. Dodson
Harvard School of Dental Medicine, Harvard University, Boston, MA, USA

Center for Applied Clinical Investigation, Department of Oral and Maxillofacial Surgery, Massachusetts General Hospital, 55 Fruit Street, Warren Building – Suite 1201, Boston, MA 02114, USA
e-mail: tbdodson@partners.org

G.C. Velmahos et al. (eds.), *Penetrating Trauma*,
DOI 10.1007/978-3-642-20453-1_25, © Springer-Verlag Berlin Heidelberg 2012

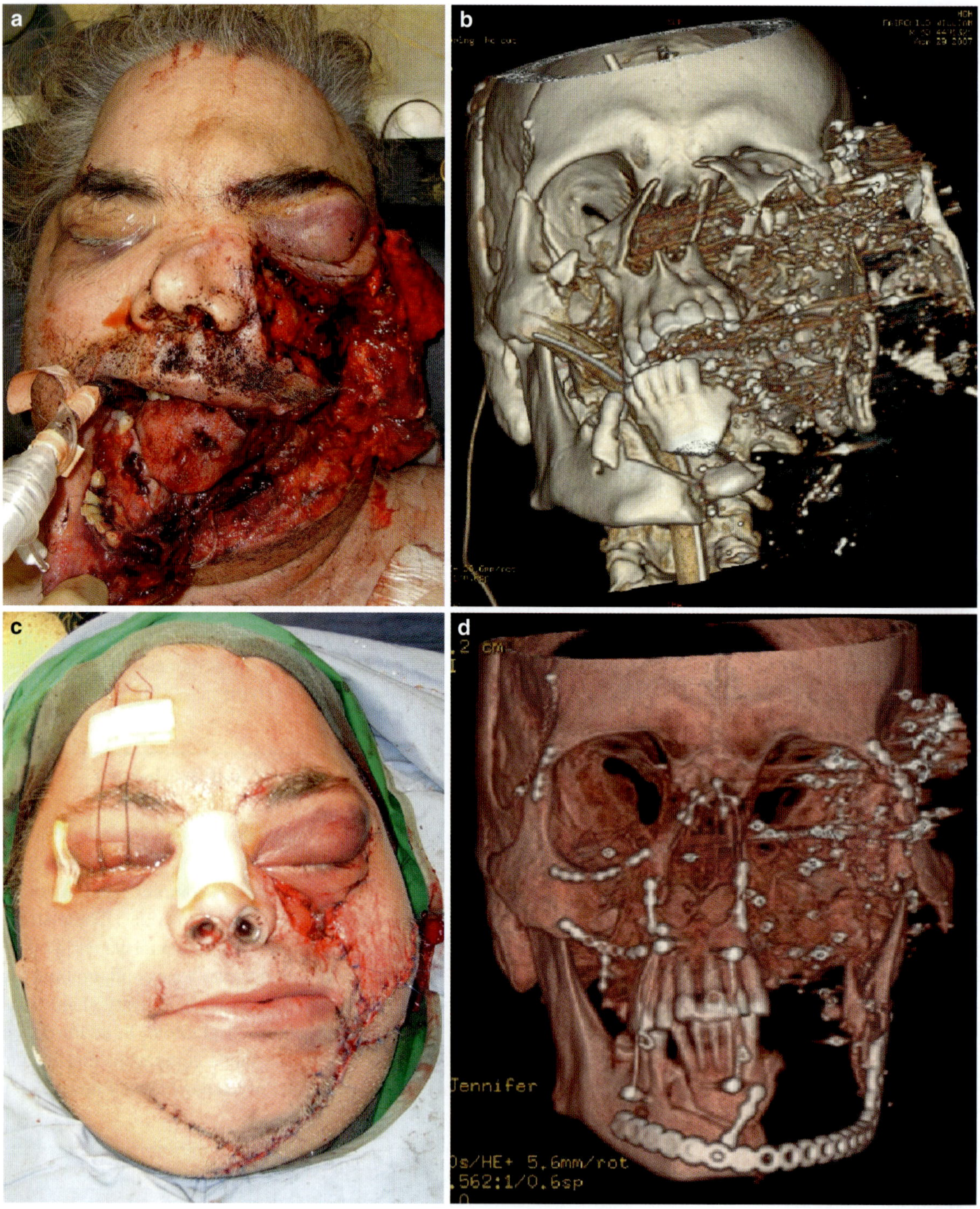

Fig. 25.1 (**a**) Clinical picture of a high-energy penetrating injury. Notice the avulsive injury producing a composite defect characterized by loss of both soft and hard tissue. (**b**) CT demonstrating the hard tissue damage caused by high-velocity penetrating injury. (**c**) Clinical picture of the same patient after treatment which includes restoring facial form. (**d**) CT scan demonstrating reduction and fixation of facial fractures with restoration of facial form

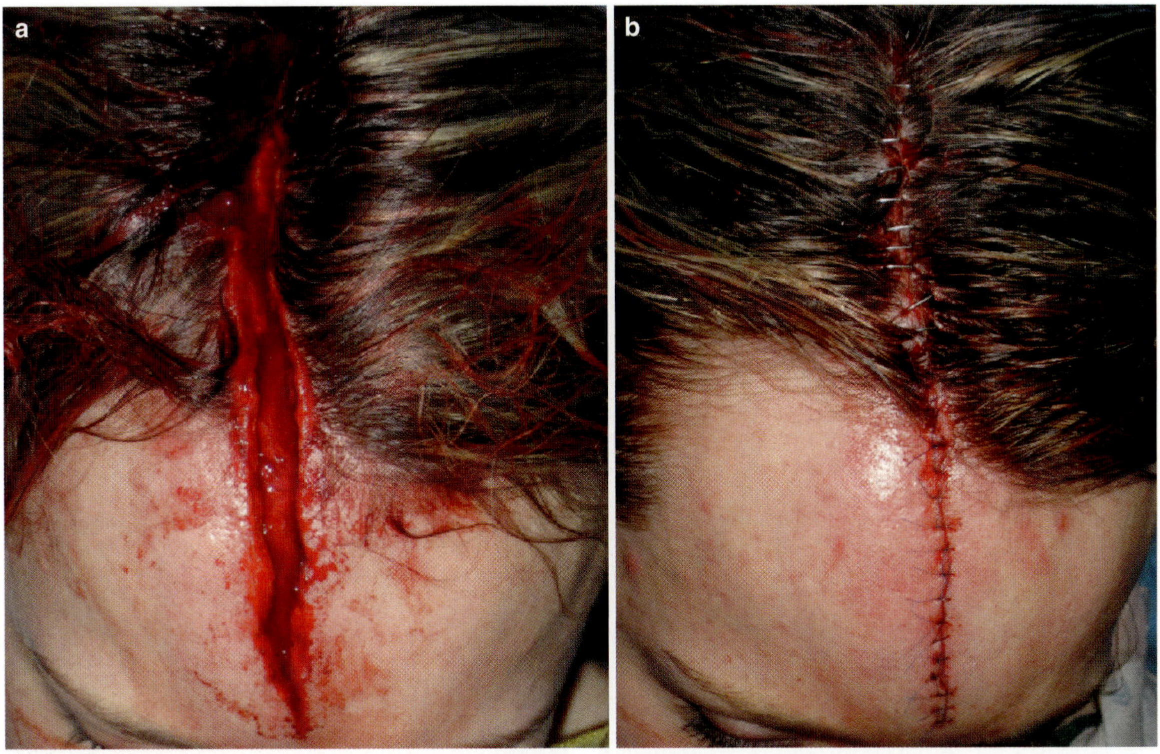

Fig. 25.2 (**a**) Low-energy penetrating injury results in isolated damage to the soft tissue. (**b**) Notice the preservation of soft tissue mass after repair

preventing or minimizing complications, e.g., infection, inadvertent damage to facial nerve, or discarding valuable soft or hard tissue structures.

The purpose of this chapter is to highlight the principles of evaluation and management of patients with penetrating maxillofacial injuries focusing on the acute management skills required by the trauma surgeon and the latter management issues addressed by the specialty service.

25.4 Acute Management

25.4.1 Patient Evaluation

Most maxillofacial injuries are not life threatening and are usually evaluated as a component of the secondary trauma survey. Airway and bleeding, however, require immediate evaluation and control. Simultaneously, the clinician must avoid unnecessary manipulation of the neck pending cervical spine clearance. Ten percent of facial penetrating injuries associate with a motor vehicle collision (MVC) or fall from height have associated cervical spine injuries [4].

Other potential complications initiated during the initial evaluation and management are due to inappropriate management of the maxillofacial soft and hard tissues. For example, careless vessel clamping and legation while trying to obtain homeostasis may result in facial nerve damage. Direct pressure often provides adequate homeostasis. Discarding nearly avulsed tissues, especially those involving the eyelid, may result in soft tissue defects that are challenging to correct. Discarding fracture segments could impair subsequent early or late treatment (Fig. 25.3).

25.5 Airway Management

Airway control is a priority. Obstruction may be due to foreign bodies, e.g., dentures, teeth, fluids (blood or vomit), soft tissue (tongue or loss of tongue support due to a mandible fracture), or direct laryngeal injury. While assessing the airway, bleeding from maxillofacial injuries can be managed acutely with pressure and local haemostatic measures.

Primary airway management is a core competency of the trauma surgeon and addressed in detail elsewhere

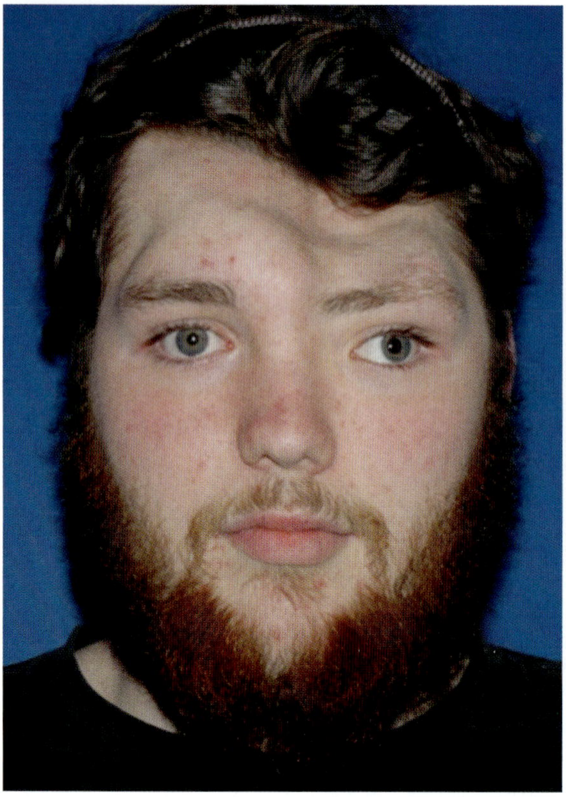

Fig. 25.3 Frontal repose view of frontal bone deformity as a result of discarded hard tissue at the time of neurosurgical treatment

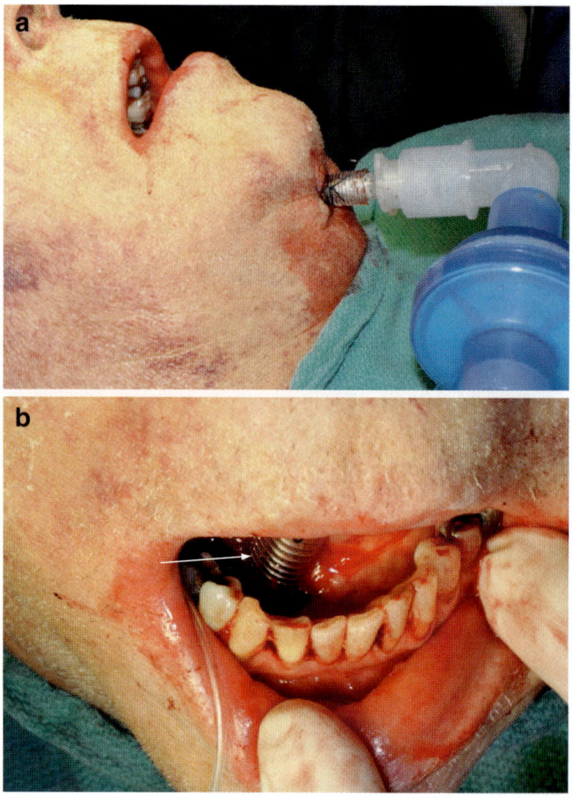

Fig. 25.4 (**a**) Extraoral and (**b**) intraoral view of submental intubation. *Arrow* points to endotracheal tube as it enters the floor of the mouth

in text. There are a few considerations worth noting when managing the airway of patients with maxillofacial injuries. Usually, the initial airway control is by endotracheal intubation or performance of a surgical airway. With few exceptions, at a later stage and depending on oral endotracheal tube needs to be converted to the maxillofacial operative procedure, the orotracheal intubation is changed to nasotracheal or converted to tracheostomy. Occasionally, maxillofacial surgeons can work around an oral airway or may elect to perform submental intubation (Fig. 25.4a, b) [5].

25.6 Evaluation and Management of Maxillofacial Bleeding

Penetrating injuries of the face may bleed profusely due to the highly vascular nature of this region. The corollary of this is that injuries to hard or soft tissues are more likely to survive and be resistant to infection. Many times, because of the copious blood supply and relatively small wounds, maxillofacial injuries appear serious. As such, it is critical to clean the wounds to establish the nature and severity of the injuries and to identify and control bleeding sources. Magnification (loupes) and illumination (headlights) are invaluable to assist in identifying and controlling bleeding. Direct pressure is effective for controlling bleeding from facial injuries. The wounds can be cleaned efficiently with sponges soaked in saline or dilute hydrogen peroxide.

Nasal injuries with associated bleeding are common and can be challenging to manage. Injury of Kiesselbach's plexus accounts for nasal bleeding in 90% of the cases. Nasal bleeding can be caused by laceration of the nasal mucosa, and any of the nasal vessels can be the source of the bleeding. Since the branches of the internal maxillary artery and the anterior and posterior ethmoidal arteries are located in the posterior aspect of the nose, most likely that these vessels will cause posterior bleeding toward the pharynx

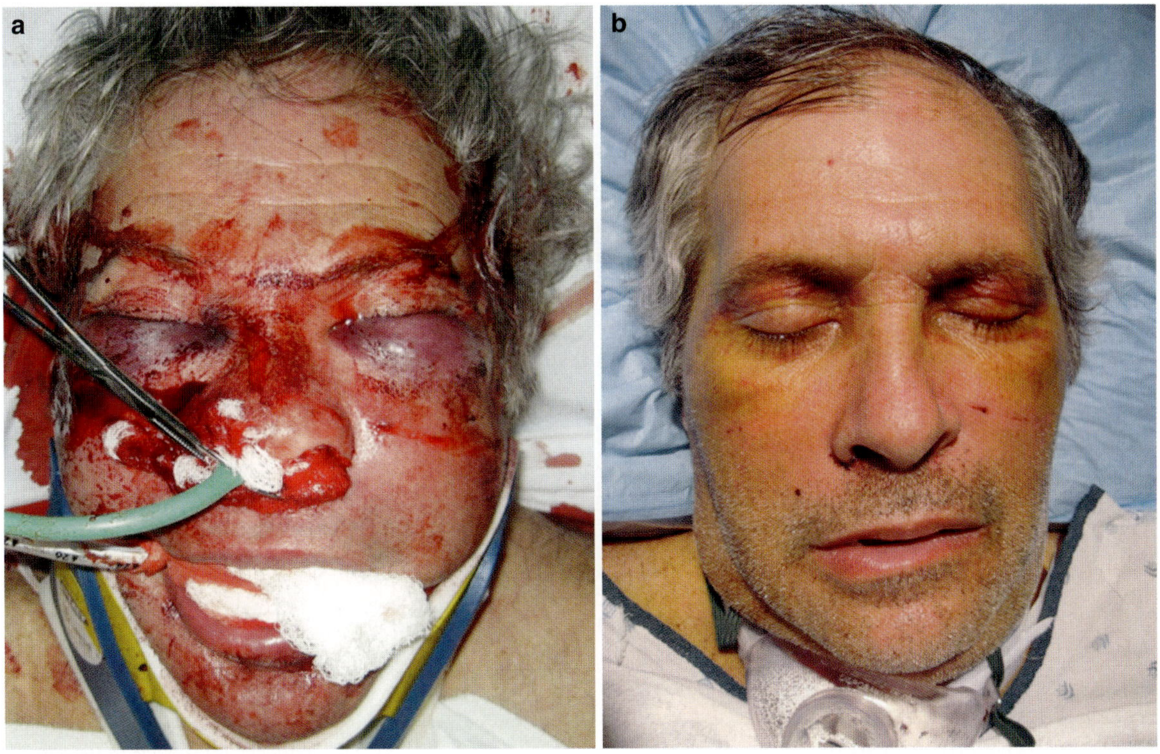

Fig. 25.5 (**a**) Typical blunt midface injury demonstrating stabilization of the neck with a cervical collar, oral intubation, facial edema, periorbital eccymoses, and a posterior nasal pack (Foley catheter) and anterior nasal packing to control nasal bleeding. Marked facial edema develops within a few hours of injury making the physical examination more difficult. (**b**) Same patient few days later. Notice the decreased swelling allows better delineation of the deformity and facilitates operative repair of the injuries

and anterior packing of the nose or packing of the oral cavity is ineffective. As such, posterior nasal packing is indicated. Posterior packing consists of placing a Foley catheter into the far posterior portion of the nasal cavity and then inserting an anterior nasal pack in front of the balloon. The posterior pack is maintained for 1–3 days (Fig. 25.5a).

Nasal septal hematomas are associated with septal fractures. Septal hematomas need to be diagnosed and managed efficiently. Left untreated, a septal hematoma may produce necrosis of the underlying cartilage producing a nasal deformity characterized by collapse of the nasal dorsum and may be very difficult to correct.

Management of the maxillofacial bleeding can be achieved by any one or combination of the following options:

1. Direct pressure:
   Bleeding from maxillofacial injuries responds well to direct pressure. Use dry sponges and abdominal swabs and press on the bleeding site to produce pressure hemostasis (Fig. 25.6).
2. Ligation:
   Ligating vessels is done in the usual manner; however, avoid blind clamping of tissues to prevent iatrogenic injury to vital structures such as the facial nerve.
3. Hemostatic agents:
   Incremental measures to obtain homeostasis include packing with hemostatic agents, e.g., oxidized cellulose, microfibrillar collagen, and chitosan-based hemostatic dressing.
4. Interventional radiology:
   Occasionally, bleeding from the nose, infratemporal fossa, or indeterminate, profuse maxillofacial bleeding cannot be controlled with usual methods. Under these circumstances, consider consultation with interventional radiology for diagnostic angiography and embolization.

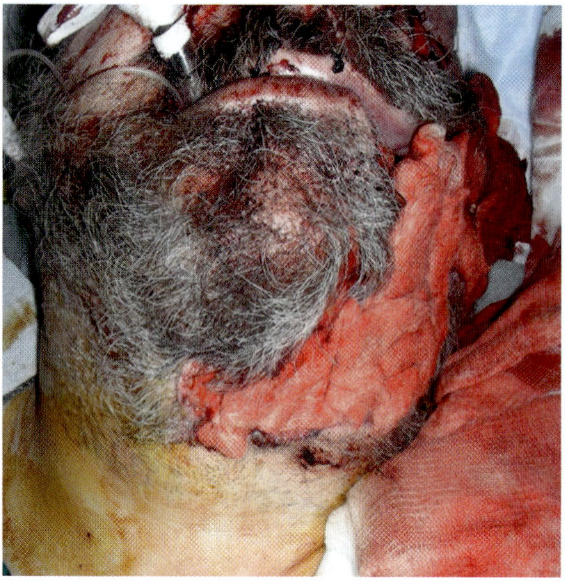

Fig. 25.6 Hemostasis obtained by packing the wound with sponges

25.7 History and Physical Examination of Maxillofacial Injuries

In most cases, evaluating maxillofacial injuries is a component of the secondary trauma survey. Historical information regarding the mechanism of injury, timing, and location of injury can be valuable. Unless the patient is awake and oriented, these data are best collected from witnesses of the incident. Medical history may be important, and family members are helpful with an unconscious or intubated patient. The simplest way to ascertain quickly if there is a fracture of the maxilla or mandible is to ask patients if their bite is altered. If the answer is yes, there is a high likelihood of a fracture. If the answer is no, there is a low likelihood of fracture. The following paragraphs outline a method for completing the initial examination for maxillofacial injuries.

25.8 External Examination

The goal of the examination is to determine quickly and efficiently the presence or absence of maxillofacial injuries. Edema develops within a few hours after injury, masking underlying injuries, making physical identification of injuries more difficult (Fig. 25.5a).

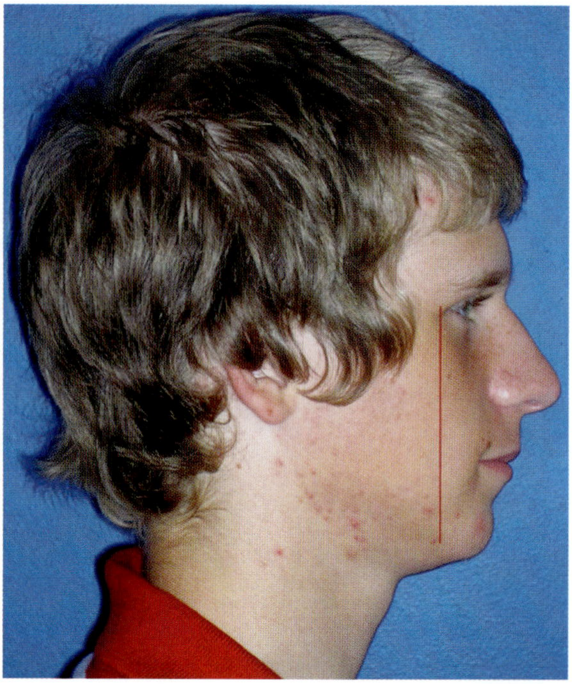

Fig. 25.7 Lacerations located posterior to the line dropped perpendicular to the horizontal at the lateral canthus of the eye are associated with an increased risk for a facial nerve or salivary duct injury

Inspect the scalp and face for obvious lacerations or deformities. Probe the laceration to determine if it communicates with the underling bony structures. Assess facial nerve function by asking patients to raise their eyebrows, squeeze their eyes shut, smile, pucker their lips, and grimace. Lacerations posterior to a line dropped perpendicular to the horizontal at the lateral canthus of the eye increase the risk for a facial nerve or salivary duct injury (Fig. 25.7).

Gently stroke the forehead, infraorbital region, and lower lip to assess trigeminal nerve sensory function. Abnormal sensation suggests a facial bone fracture due to injury to a trigeminal nerve branch.

Palpate the supra-, lateral, and infraorbital rims to identify periorbital or zygomatic fractures as evidenced by bony steps or pain. Examine the nasal bridge and look for deviation of the nose or deformity. Place your non-dominant hand on the patient's forehead to stabilize the head and using your dominant hand, place your index and the thumb fingers over the nasal bride and assess stability by trying to move it side to side (Fig. 25.8). Using a headlight and a nasal speculum, perform an intranasal examination. Inspect the nasal

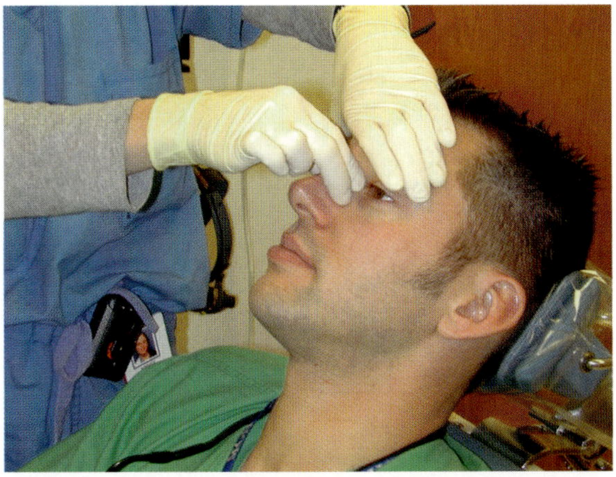

Fig. 25.8 Bimanual palpation to ascertain stability of the nasal bones

septum for evidence of deformity or deviation of the septum and a septal hematoma.

To identify maxillary factures, stabilize the head with your non-dominant hand; hold the premaxilla with the index and thumb fingers on the dominant hand, and try to mobilize the midface. Do not hold the teeth as they may be mobile. Mobility of the inferior maxilla separate from the upper midface indicates a Le Fort I fracture (Fig. 25.9a, b). If the nose and maxilla move as a unit, the injury may be a Le Fort II fracture (Fig. 25.10a, b). If the maxilla, nose, and the lateral orbital rims move as a unit, a Le Fort III fracture is suspected (Fig. 25.11a, b).

Le Fort fractures predispose patients to cerebral spinal fluid (CSF) leaks with rhinorrhea. Clear or yellow

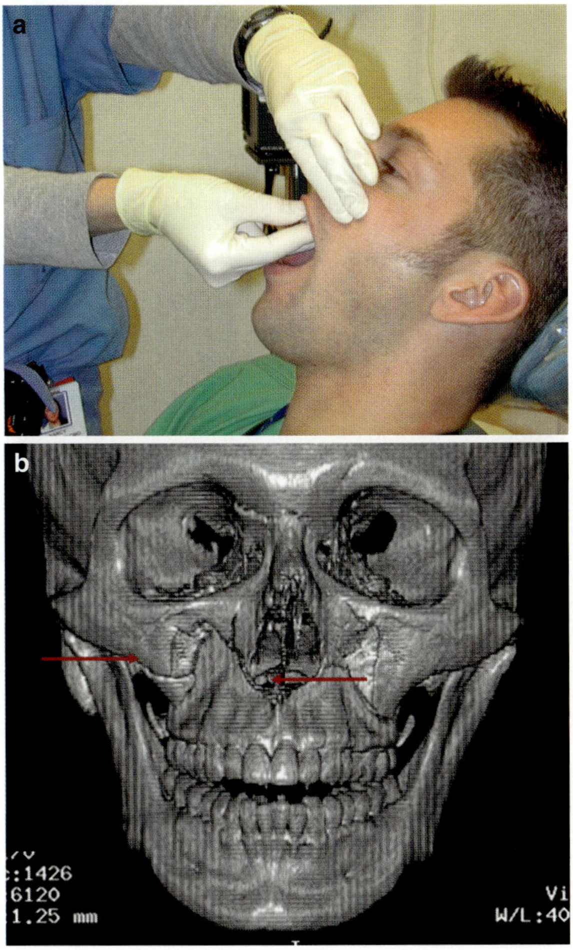

Fig. 25.9 (**a**) Clinical examination and (**b**) three-dimensional CT of Le Fort I fracture. Notice the correlation between the fracture line on CT (*arrows*) and the area being palpated for mobility on the clinical picture

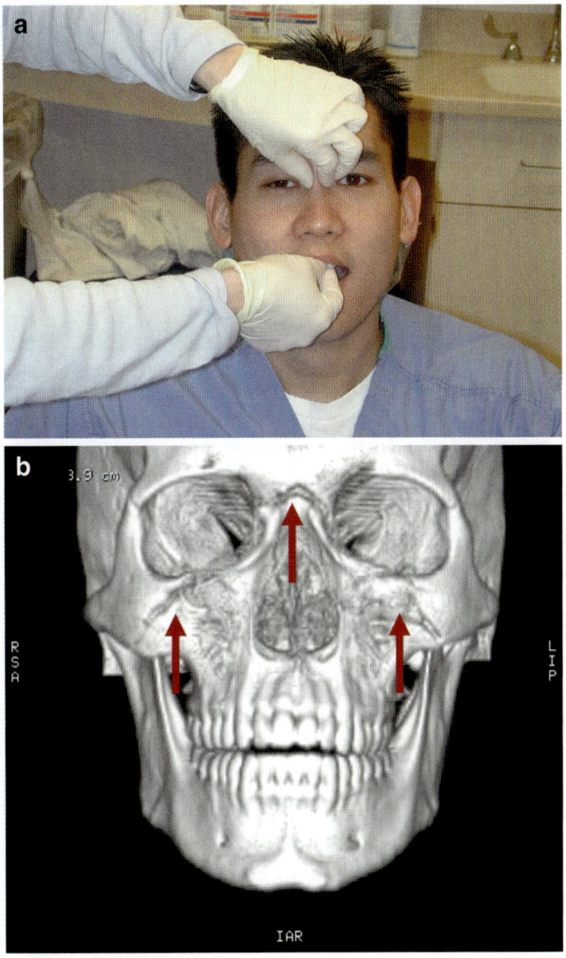

Fig. 25.10 (**a**) Clinical examination and (**b**) three-dimensional CT of Le Fort II fracture. Notice the correlation between the fracture line (*arrows*) on CT and the area being palpated for mobility on the clinical picture

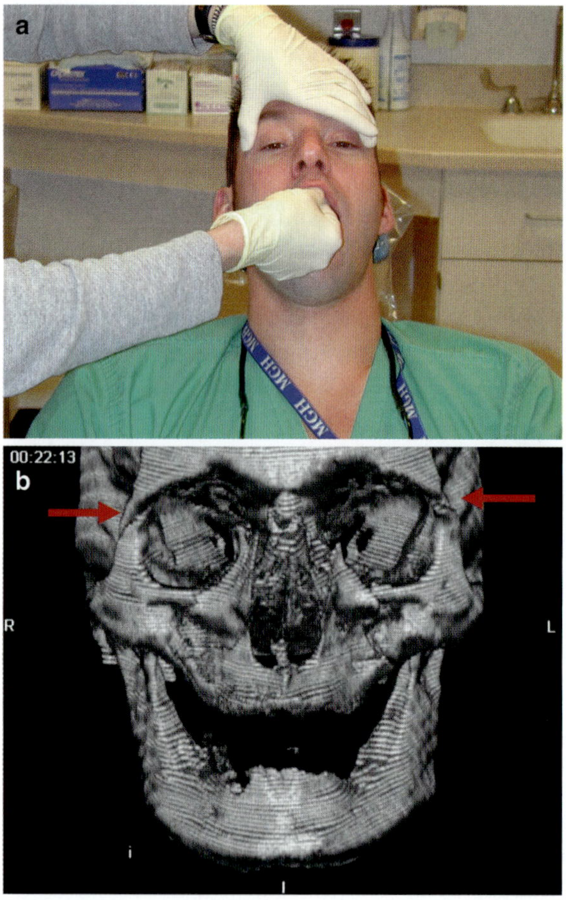

Fig. 25.11 (**a**) Clinical examination and (**b**) three-dimensional CT of Le Fort III fracture. Notice the correlation between the fracture line on CT (*arrows*) and the area being palpated for mobility on the clinical picture

rhinorrhea in patients with midface fractures suggest a CSF leak. The fluid should be accumulated and sent for beta-2 transferrin test.

Use your index fingers and palpate the zygomatic arches bilaterally. Compare the level of the index fingers on both sides from a posterior view. Asymmetry due to depression of the zygomatic arch may suggest an arch fracture.

Palpate the preauricular area and ask awake patients to open fully their mouths while palpating the preauricular area to assess temporomandibular joint function. Normal mandibular opening is 35–55 mm without deviation. Limited range of mandibular motion or deviation with opening suggests injury to the temporomandibular joint, mandible, or muscles of mastication. Palpate the inferior border of the mandible to identify steps or painful areas suggestive of a fracture. Findings from this examination in the intubated patient are compromised.

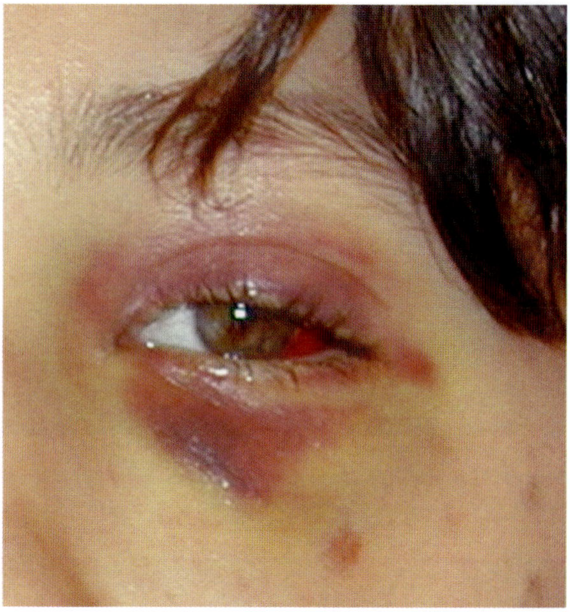

Fig. 25.12 Subconjunctival hematoma, a possible sign for midface fracture

The ocular examination is crucial because 15–20% of patients with major facial trauma suffer from significant ocular injuries [6]. An initial ocular examination should be performed immediately to ascertain visual status, pupillary appearance and function, and extraocular muscle function. When feasible, the ocular examination should be complemented by an ophthalmologist when the eye is at risk for injury, e.g., direct globe injuries or midface injuries.

The ocular examination includes the following elements:

1. External examination:
   Gross inspection of the eye and ocular adnexa can reveal lacerations and abrasions. Eyelid lacerations may be full thickness with underlying globe injury. Examine the conjunctiva and look for subconjunctival hemorrhage (Fig. 25.12). Subconjunctival hemorrhage is associated with midface fractures. In the awake patient, assess extraocular muscle function by asking the patient to follow your moving index finger with his eyes through the major visual fields to confirm that the globe moves freely in all directions while looking for limitation of motion or diplopia. In the intubated patient, evidence of extraocular muscle entrapment can be assessed

using the forced duction technique. With forceps, grasp the insertion of the inferior rectus muscle and rotate the globe. There should be free, passive movement. Restricted movement suggests entrapment of the inferior rectus in an orbital fracture.

2. Optic nerve function:
   Assess grossly whether the patient can perceive light or movement. If light perception or movement is absent, an urgent ophthalmology consultation is indicated. In the cooperative patient, one of the best tests to evaluate the optic nerve function is the subjective red color saturation [6]. A red object is presented to one eye at a time; in case of significant optic nerve injury; ipsilateral color perception will be altered.
3. Pupil evaluation:
   In the nonverbal or uncooperative patient, the pupil examination may be the only measure of ocular function and can provide insights into neurologic function. Inspecting the pupils includes three parts:

(a) Size and shape:
Changes in size might indicate injury in the CN III and V while changes in shape might indicate a damage or trauma to the globe.

(b) Reactivity to bright light:
Each pupil should be viewed independently, followed by swinging the light from one eye to the other and back to determine whether there is a relative afferent papillary defect.

(c) Pupillary accommodation:
This examination assesses miosis during near synkinesis [6]. This test may be of little value when evaluating eye trauma, especially if the remainder of the pupil examination is normal.

Determination of sight, extraocular muscle function, and pupillary status should be completed by the trauma surgeon for every patient with trauma to the periorbital region. More specific and complicated inspection and tests, including visual field determination, penlight examination, and intraocular pressure measurement, should be done by the ophthalmologist when the patient can tolerate these exams or as needed, in the ED.

25.9 Intraoral Examination

Rapidly identify lacerations or other soft tissues injuries, and palpate the wounds for retained foreign bodies such as teeth, parts of teeth, or shrapnel. Sweep your gloved finger to remove loose foreign bodies, e.g., removable dental prostheses, fractured teeth. If an avulsed tooth is intact, do not discard it. Place it into saline, milk, or reinsert it into the socket. Note the presence or absence of teeth. Intraoral lacerations may involve the salivary ducts. This is not an emergency, but should be noted and managed secondarily. Ecchymosis in the floor of the mouth (Fig. 25.13) or in the maxillary buccal vestibule suggests mandibular or midface fractures.

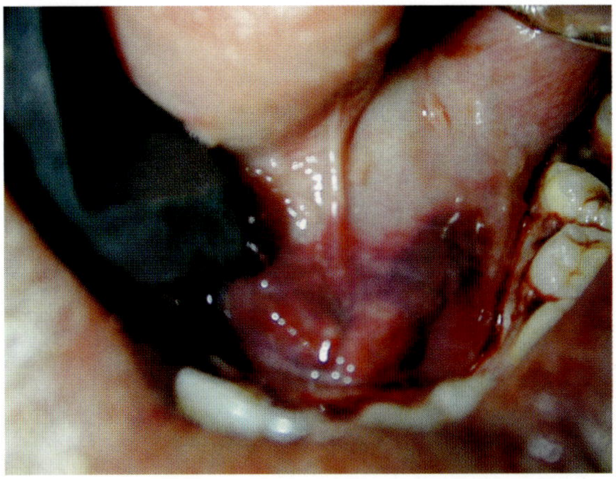

Fig. 25.13 Ecchymosis in the floor of the mouth, a sign of a mandible fracture, is due to disruption of the lingual cortex of the mandible with bleeding into the adjacent soft tissues

Examine the dentition for evidence of fractured or avulsed teeth. Patient complaint of an altered bite, steps or spacing between the teeth, or an inability to interdigitate the teeth suggest a fracture. Check the stability of the mandible by holding it with both hands and try to mobilize (Fig. 25.14). Sublingual ecchymosis suggests a mandibular symphysis fracture. Other finding include gingival lacerations or a biplanar occlusion (Fig. 25.15).

Use your index finger to palpate the zygomatic buttresses, bilaterally; this region could be reached on the deepest point between the buccal mucosa of the cheek and the maxilla. Step-offs on this region indicate a zygomatic fracture.

Most neurosensory injuries are managed as a secondary procedure. Suspected facial nerve injuries should evaluated immediately and managed as soon as the patient is stable enough for operative intervention. Facial nerve exploration and repair is commonly done in conjunction with repair of associated facial lacerations.

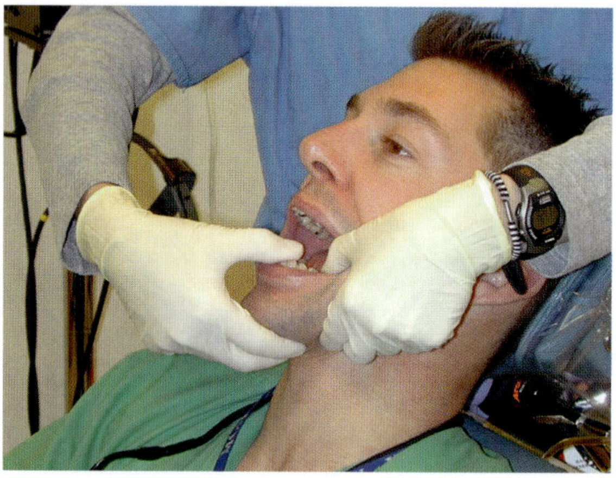

Fig. 25.14 Bimanual palpation of the mandible to assess for stability of the lower jaw

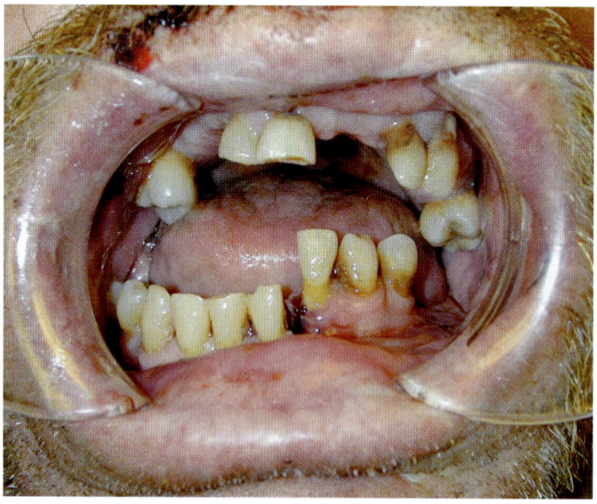

Fig. 25.15 Biplanar occlusion due to mandibular fracture. Notice the laceration of the mandibular gingiva at the fracture

25.10 Imaging

Advances in imaging technique have made it critical component of evaluating maxillofacial injuries. Maxillofacial imaging is usually not an emergent procedure and may be delayed until the patient is stable or completed in conjunction with imaging of the cervical spine or head.

Computed tomography (CT) with three-dimensional reformatting is the current standard (Fig. 25.16). Imaging orders should include axial cuts (1-mm thick) with sagittal, coronal, and three-dimensional reformatting. Contrast is usually not needed unless the injury is old, and there is concern about a secondary inflammatory

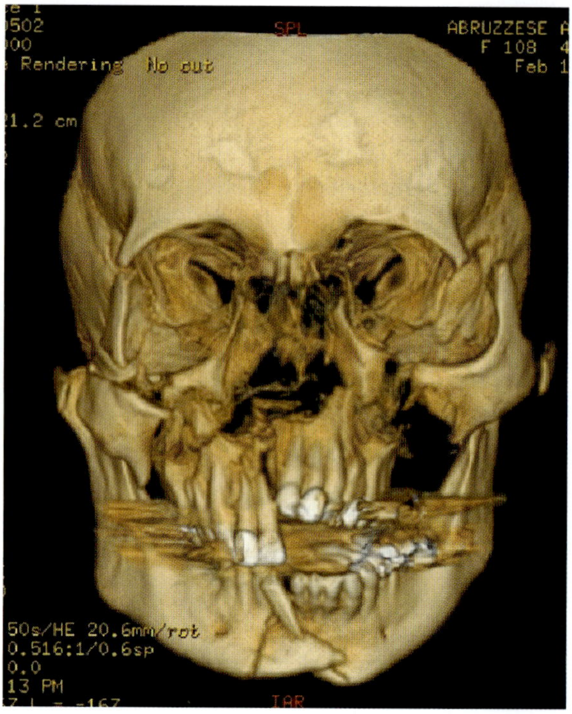

Fig. 25.16 3D CT demonstrating a complex, panfacial fracture

process. Absent CT imaging, alternative imaging choices include panoramic radiographic technique to demonstrate mandibular and dental injuries and a mandibular series, Waters and Caldwell views, and a submental vertex.

25.11 Initial Treatment

25.11.1 Indications for Immediate Treatment in the ED

Many soft or hard tissues in maxillofacial injuries can be managed in the ED as long as treatment time is short, e.g., <60 min, and the patient is conscious, stable, and can tolerate procedures involving the use of local anesthesia. Lacerations that do not involve vital structures such as the facial nerve or parotid duct can be repaired in ED setting. Dentoalveolar, nasal, and some mandibular or zygoma fractures can be reduced and stabilized in the ED. If there is a delay in treating unstable mandibular fracture, these fractures can be temporarily reduced and stabilized by placing a 24-gauge stainless steel wire around teeth on either side of the fractures.

For most maxillofacial injuries, broad-spectrum antibiotics decrease the risk for secondary wound infection [7]. Penicillin, first-generation cephalosporins, or clindamycin are excellent choices for empiric therapy. For intraoral wounds, adding an antibacterial mouth rinse such as 0.12% chlorhexidene is useful.

25.12 Definitive Treatment

25.12.1 Early Versus Late Management

For maxillofacial injuries requiring more extensive treatment, there exists a debate between early (<24 h) and late (>24 h) treatment. Proponents of early treatment claim superior esthetic and functional outcomes, whereas those of the delayed approach claim fewer complications due to infection [8]. In most cases, however, maxillofacial injuries do not require immediate operative treatment. Delaying treatment for a few days after injury allows completion of all diagnostic workups, development of an operative plan, and decreased swelling aids in delineating the degree of deformity and facilitates operative treatment, especially with midface fractures (Fig. 25.5b). When a multidisciplinary approach is indicated for a particularly challenging injury, delayed treatment permits the opportunity to organize treatment resources and develop and implement a rationale treatment plan.

For patients with high-energy penetrating injuries, the treatment plan usually is divided to three stages:

1. Debridement, fracture stabilization, and primary closure – Superficial wounds should be meticulously cleaned and freed from debris and foreign bodies, primary closure of the wound should be attempted, and most maxillofacial injuries can be closed primarily. If the wound cannot be closed primarily, consider packing and dressing changes. This component of the treatment plan may be implemented early or late. At this time, a comprehensive physical examination can also be completed in a well-illuminated controlled setting.
   Fractures can be reduced in a closed manner and stabilized with maxillomandibular fixation (MMF) or treated with open reduction with rigid internal fixation (OR-RIF). Preserve the soft tissue attachments to the bone segments as possible to prevent necrosis of free bony segments. In patients without severe comminuted fractures or infection, using reconstruction plate may be indicated and performed concomitantly with debridement and primary closure. Application of arch bars for penetrating injuries in the jaws has proved invaluable in reestablishing arch form, occlusion and stabilizing of dento-alveolar fragments.
   Reconstruction of soft tissue defects could be done at the same early intervention stage, and it prevents extensive scarring of facial tissues associated with healing by secondary intention [7–9]. In case of large soft tissue defects, absent adequate local tissue, delayed treatment is preferred and the wound edges should be approximated.
2. Reconstruction of the hard tissue defects – Management of bony defects is usually delayed weeks to months and part of the second stage of reconstruction. The goal of delaying bony reconstruction is to allow for soft tissue healing to avoid inadvertent entry into the mouth at the time of bone grafting. Generally, 3 months is adequate if nonvascularized grafting is indicated. If vascularized grafts are being used, the treatment time can be accelerated.
   Delayed treatment is indicated for the following reasons:
   - Early intervention may increase the risk of necrosis due to detachment of bony fragments from the soft tissue surrounding it.
   - MMF may produce a superior functional and esthetic outcome.
   - Late intervention decreases the risk of postoperative infection and increases the success frequency of bony reconstruction or augmentation.
3. Rehabilitation of the oral cavity, including the oral vestibule, alveolar ridge, and secondary correction of residual deformities – This final reconstructive stage restores the jaw and dental function and commonly requires multiple staged procedures with care delivered months after the initial injury.

25.13 Conclusion

Trauma surgeons involved in the early management of penetrating maxillofacial injuries play a key role in determining the ultimate esthetic and functional outcome associated with operative management of these injuries. Establishing an airway, obtaining initial control of bleeding, rapidly assessing the injuries, and requesting efficient imaging of maxillofacial injuries are marks of a well-trained trauma surgeon.

Important Points

- Obtain cervical clearance or inspect your patient with a collar until the c-spine injury is cleared.
- Secure the airway and assure homeostasis prior to initial inspection and treatment of the facial injury.
- Be aware of inappropriate management of the maxillofacial soft and hard tissues. Do not discard broken bones and avoid careless vessel clamping and legation while trying to obtain homeostasis.
- While there are a few exceptions, to manage most maxillofacial injuries involving the dentition, an oral endotracheal intubation needs to be converted to nasoendotracheal intubation or a surgical airway.
- Indications for use of a surgical airway include: complicated injuries such that the nasoendotracheal tube impedes the operative approach, respiratory hygiene, or planned prolonged intubation.
- Most maxillofacial bleeding can be controlled using direct pressure and local hemostatic measures. Occasionally, interventional radiology may need to be consulted.
- Inspection of the maxillofacial injury starts from an external approach and it includes the forehead, orbits, nose, midface, joints, and lower face, based on the later order.
- Intraoral inspection includes soft and hard tissue. Be aware of the following signs, which indicate jaw fracture: ecchymosis in the floor of the mouth, step-offs, and biplanar occlusion on the same jaw.
- The 3D CT is used as the standard for facial trauma imaging. In case CT is not available, plain x-rays can be used instead though with less accuracy.
- Immediate treatment in the ED is indicated for simple lacerations, dento-alveolar trauma, and some of the mandibular and zygomatic fractures.
- For more complicated fractures (high energy), the sequence of treatment is: debridement, reconstruction, and rehabilitation.

References

1. Cunnigham L, Haug R, Ford J (2003) Firearm injuries to the maxillofacial region: an overview of current thoughts regarding demographics, pathophysiology and management. J Oral Maxillofac Surg 61:932–942
2. Ueeck B (2007) Penetrating injuries to the face: delay versus primary treatment – considerations for delay treatment. J Oral Maxillofac Surg 65:1209–1214
3. Glapa M, Kourie J, Doll D et al (2007) Early management of gunshot injuries to the face in civilian practice. World J Surg 31:2104–2110
4. Ward Booth P (2006) Maxillofacial trauma. In: Ward Booth P, Schendel S, Hausamen JE (eds) Maxillofacial surgery, Churchill Livingston, 2nd edn. pp 2–300
5. Schütz P, Hamed HH (2008) Submental intubation versus tracheostomy in maxillofacial trauma patients. J Oral Maxillofac Surg 66:1404–1409
6. Soparkar CN, Patrinely JR (2007) The eye examination in facial trauma for the plastic surgeon. Plast Reconstr Surg 120(Suppl 2):49S–56S
7. Hochberg J, Ardenghy M, Toledo S et al (2001) Soft tissue injuries to face and neck; early assessment and repair. World J Surg 25:1023–1027
8. Motamedi M (2003) Primary management of maxillofacial hard and soft tissue gunshot and shrapnel injuries. J Oral Maxillofac Surg 61:1390–1398
9. Motamedi M (2007) Primary treatment of penetrating injuries to the face. J Oral Maxillofac Surg 65:1215–1218

Operative Strategies in Penetrating Trauma to the Neck

26

Marc de Moya

The neck is a region crowded by vital structures. As such, careful assessment and treatment can significantly affect morbidity and mortality. Penetrating neck injuries, defined as penetration of the platysma, account for approximately 5–10% of all penetrating injuries [1]. How these injuries are assessed and treated has dramatically changed over the last four decades. This chapter will focus on some of the "tricks of the trade" and damage control options for operating on the trauma neck.

In 1969, Cook County investigators divided the neck into three zones [2]. Roon and Christensen recapitulated this classification in 1979 [3] in an effort to standardize therapy and research efforts. Zone I refers to the area from the clavicles to the cricoid cartilage. Zone II refers to the area from the cricoid cartilage to the angle of the mandible, and Zone III refers to the area from the angle of the mandible to the base of the skull. However, since the first description of these zones, much has changed in how we approach, image, and treat patients with neck trauma.

Mandatory exploration of the neck was the standard of care soon after WWII. However, mandatory exploration produced a negative exploratory rate of approximately 50–60% [4–6]. In the 1960s, routine operative explorations were challenged, not just in the abdomen, by Dr. Carter Nance and I. Cohn Jr. [7], but also in the neck by Drs. Shirkey, Beall, and Debakey [8]. This initial push for nonoperative management eventually led to a more careful selection of operative candidates. Over the last decade, larger prospective observational trials have demonstrated success with a more selective approach. Biffl et al. [9] demonstrated in a series of 128 asymptomatic patients by physical exam that only one patient had a missed injury. This injury was from an ice pick. He went on to describe that only 15% of the patients required adjuvant tests. Sriussadaporn et al. [10] observed 17 asymptomatic patients. Only 2 of 40 patients who underwent exploration did not need the operation despite having a "deep" wound. Nason et al. [11] found that 67% of those mandatorily explored had a negative exploration and all zone II injuries were symptomatic. Velmahos et al. [12], described in a large retrospective series, 3% of explorations were unnecessary and in the monitored group, 9% had missed injuries; however, interpretation of the high missed injury rate was difficult. The only randomized clinical trial comparing mandatory exploration to selective observation was Golueke et al. [13] where there was no difference in hospital stay, morbidity, or mortality in 160 patients.

Clinicians began to use the hard signs of injury, i.e., active bleeding, expanding hematoma, a bruit or thrill over the wound, pulse deficit, and a central neurologic deficit to possibly detect a significant vascular injury. Bubbling from wound, massive subcutaneous emphysema, or hemoptysis would be considered hard signs of an airway injury. Some consider crepitance/dysphagia/hematemesis as soft signs of digestive tract injuries. Hard signs of digestive tract injuries usually do not manifest themselves immediately but will lead to neck cellulitis/sepsis. Atteberry et al. in 1994 studied 28 patients with penetrating zone II neck injuries [14].

M. de Moya
Division of Trauma, Emergency Surgery and Surgical Critical Care, Massachusetts General Hospital, Harvard Medical School, 165 Cambridge Street, Suite 810, Boston, MA 02114, USA
e-mail: mdemoya@partners.org

G.C. Velmahos et al. (eds.), *Penetrating Trauma*,
DOI 10.1007/978-3-642-20453-1_26, © Springer-Verlag Berlin Heidelberg 2012

They compared the physical exam to angiographic, operative, and ultrasonic findings. There were no missed injuries albeit a short follow-up period. The same group performed a follow-up study with a larger series in 2000 after having instituted strict physical exam–driven protocols for neck trauma [15]. This follow-up study with 145 patients over an 8-year period confirmed their earlier study. Again the false-negative rate was approximately 0.3% which was quoted to be equivalent to false-negative rates of angiograms. The false-positive rate was 10%. In 1997, Demetriades et al. [16] reviewed their experience of 223 patients and claim that the negative predictive value of physical exam was 100%.

Once the decision to operate is made in either an emergent or urgent manner, there are few guidelines to assist the surgeon. As in other trauma scenarios, bold yet directed/accurate moves are needed to minimize ongoing blood loss and maximize patient outcomes. However, in the neck, the density of vital structures should heighten the surgeon's sensitivity.

26.1 Positioning

A lift (either a roll, thyroid pillow, etc.) is placed posterior to the scapula. This raises the shoulders off the bed causing the neck to passively hyperextend. This hyperextended position is complemented by rotating the head away from the side of interest. Keep in mind that you should be able to rotate the head in the middle of the case if it becomes necessary to explore the opposite side. When the missile or the knife crosses the midline, thought must be given to accessing both sides of the neck. The right arm of the patient can be tucked to allow easier access to the head/neck of the bed by the surgeons. The left arm should be left outstretched to allow for access of the chest for proximal control of the left-sided vessels. Both arms should be left outstretched if the patient sustained multiple stab or GSW in order to maximize options. The patient should be routinely prepped from the base of the skull to the groin.

26.2 Incision/Approach

The most commonly used approach is via an oblique incision just anterior to the sternocleidomastoid (SCM) muscle. Extend this incision from the level 1 cm below the angle of the mandible to the sternal notch to gain easy

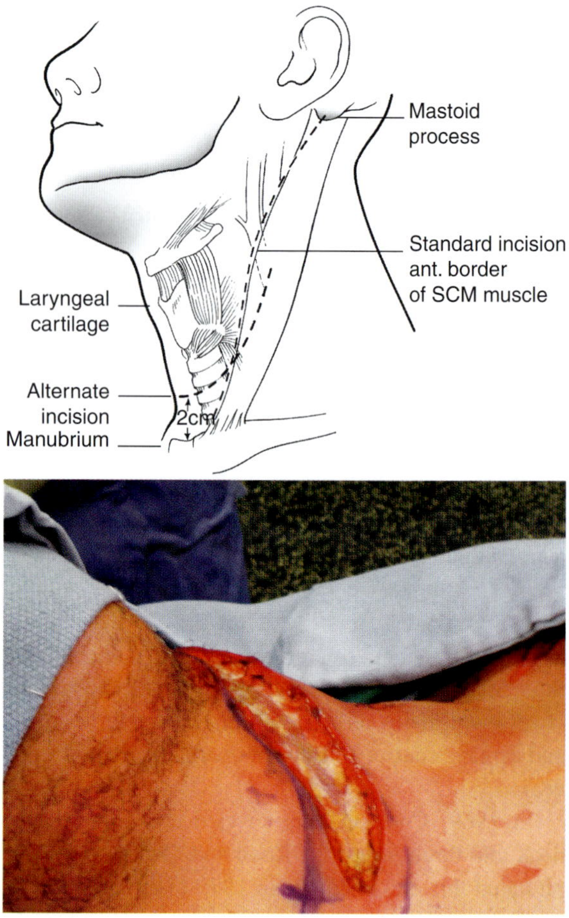

Fig. 26.1 Neck incision through the platysmal layer; then retract the SCM muscle laterally

and wide access to the neck structures. Of particular concern initially is the vascular control. Naturally, the key concept in any vascular repair is proximal and distal control. However, in the neck, this may not always be accessed prior to opening the hematoma given the small area. Carry the incision through the platysmal layer and retract the SCM muscle laterally (Fig. 26.1). Even if the hematoma is centered lateral to the SCM, staying medial provides easier access to the vital structures.

Trick: *Always approach a neck hematoma medial to the SCM*

Once you divide the platysma and retract the SCM laterally, your next objective is to identify the internal jugular vein (IJ) and retract it laterally with a self-retraining blunt retractor. The facial vein usually needs to be ligated and divided to allow the IJ to retract laterally. Often there is a pseudoaneurysm/hematoma encountered at this point; however, if the hematoma

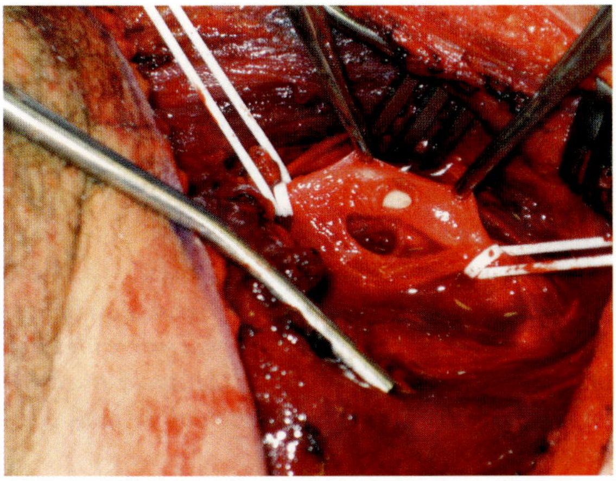

Fig. 26.2 Carotid injury

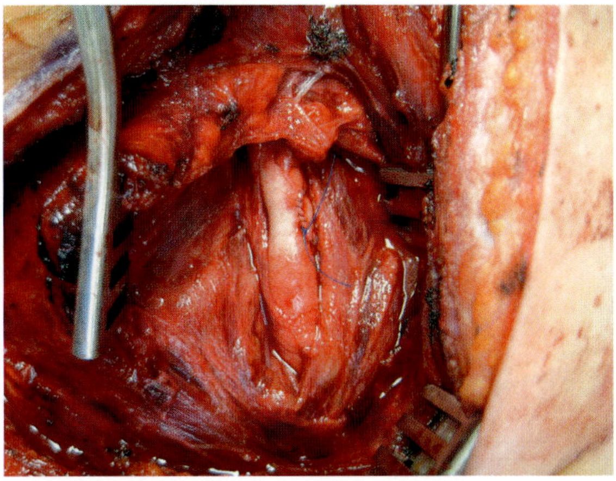

Fig. 26.3 Gunshot wound to the common carotid injury repaired with a bovine pericardial patch

remains intact, it is helpful to dissect alongside the hematoma in order to gain control of either proximal or distal vessels. Depending upon the position of the hematoma, you may only be able to obtain control of one or the other prior to invading the pseudoaneurysm. It is unlikely that you will be able to do both prior to opening the hematoma but if possible certainly gaining both proximal and distal control is ideal. I prefer to gain control with vessel loops vs. vascular clamps in the neck, as the vessel loops are less traumatic to a soft, healthy carotid artery (Fig. 26.2).

Trick: *If the pseudoaneurysm is contained in the neck, dissect either proximally or distally to gain vascular control in more virgin territory.*

Once the most proximal or distal control is obtained, then continuing your dissection to the center of the problem is the next step. You will need to apply digital pressure as the pseudoaneurysm is entered to allow you to evacuate clot and gain better proximal and distal control.

There is no need to heparinize the patient and carotid shunts are only occasionally used if there is an internal carotid artery injury. If you find that the back bleeding from the internal carotid artery is poor, then nothing is lost by placing a shunt. The wound edges then need to be debrided and a decision made about how to repair the defect. This should not be a concern when operating on the common carotid artery as the internal carotid artery has additional inflow from the external carotid artery.

On occasion, a zone I injury will require more proximal control via a median sternotomy. A median sternotomy will facilitate control of both sides, although it is near impossible to gain control of the left common carotid artery at its takeoff given the posterior position on the arch of the aorta. However, usually the neck injuries only require control a few centimeters below the level of the clavicle/sternum, which a sternotomy can afford you. Disarticulation of the sternoclavicular junction can be helpful in this regard. The utility of the highly morbid trap door is minimal and rarely, if ever, necessary.

Trick: *If you enter a pseudoaneurysm and you are unable to control it more proximally, try replacing your finger with a Foley catheter and inflate the balloon. This will often tampanode the bleeding in a GSW track while you perform your sternotomy.*

26.3 Vascular Repair

There are four options for vascular injuries: (1) ligation, (2) primary repair, (3) patch repair, (4) replacement. All internal or common carotid injuries should be repaired. The external carotid artery can be ligated. The most common vascular injury in the neck is the IJ. A unilateral internal jugular vein can be ligated but repair if feasible is preferred.

Caution: *Bilateral IJ ligation has a high mortality associated with it.*

Stab wounds are more likely repaired primarily given the lack of associated tissue loss or blast effect. All GSW wounds need to be debrided prior to repair and are unlikely to allow primary repair (as seen in Fig. 26.3) without tension. Patch repair can be performed with a synthetic patch or a biologic patch (e.g., Bovine pericardium, saphenous vein graft). The

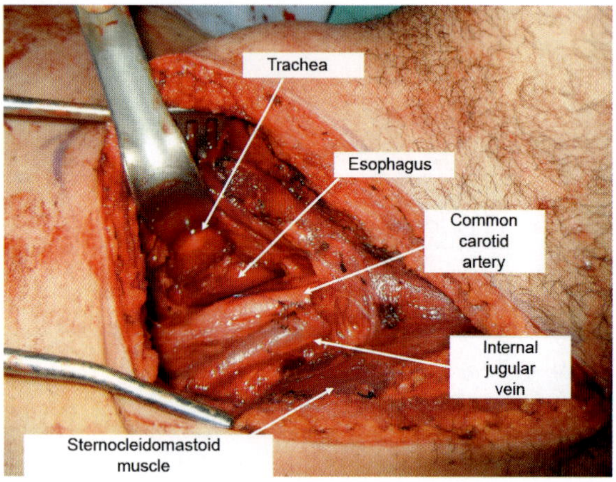

Fig. 26.4 Once the bleeding is controlled, the rest of the neck structures and the tract of the missile/knife can be inspected

biologic or synthetic patches may be quicker than saphenous vein graft with no major downside. Interposition synthetic grafts (PTFE or Dacron 6 mm) are also easy to use and have excellent patency rates.

26.3.1 Damage Control

1. It is OK to ligate common carotid artery, external carotid artery, unilateral IJ, but remember ligation of internal carotid artery is associated with >75% stroke rate.
2. If necessary can place a shunt in the carotid artery if there are other severe injuries requiring control.

Once the bleeding is controlled, then the rest of the neck structures and the tract of the missile/knife can be inspected (Fig. 26.4). Following the tract of the wound may raise or lower your index of suspicion for specific injuries. The trachea/esophagus/vascular structures need to be inspected, and if a bilateral neck exploration is needed, the first incision is then carried in a U fashion from the sternal notch to the angle of the mandible on the opposite side.

26.4 Tracheal Injuries

Tracheal wounds can be approached via either a midline or transverse neck incision. However, if other injuries to the esophagus or vascular structures are suspected, the approach described above for vascular injuries is appropriate. Primary repairs of the trachea are performed using an absorbable suture in a full thickness fashion. If there is significant laryngotracheal damage, an initial life-saving tracheostomy may be necessary. Mathisen and Grillo outlined a few key principles in tracheal repair:

Tricks: *(1) Evaluate associated injuries, (2) Avoid searching for the recurrent laryngeal nerves, (3) Separation of tracheal and esophageal suture lines, (4) Conservation of viable trachea, (5) Avoid tracheostomy through the repair, (6) Flexion of the neck postoperatively to reduce tension.*

The repair should be buttressed with viable muscle, either SCM or strap muscle. This should also be done to separate the tracheal and the associated esophageal repairs.

26.4.1 Damage Control

1. Advance the endotracheal tube beyond the defect and plan a staged repair.

26.5 Esophageal Injuries

Esophageal injuries are approached via either a right or left oblique incision as described for the vascular injuries. It is a little easier to approach from the left given the to-the-left of the midline tract of the cervical esophagus. The identification of a small hole in the esophagus can be challenging. If there is no gaping hole the associated hematoma can be used as a guide. Combining a flexible esophagoscopy with the open approach can help the surgeon rule out any small esophageal injury by insufflating the esophagus under saline looking for bubbles in addition to the intraluminal inspection.

If a hole is discovered, debriding the tissue is necessary and a single or double layer closure is acceptable. The mucosa of the esophagus will retract, and therefore the surgeon must ensure that the entire edge is identified and repaired. In addition, mobilizing a tongue of either strap muscle or SCM to reinforce the repair will provide additional blood supply to the area and separate the esophageal suture line from other repairs. The most common suture line to leak in the neck is the esophagus, and the secretions/ infection may cause the failure of neighboring suture lines.

Trick: *Buttress the esophageal repair with a tongue of viable strap or SCM muscle.*

Always place a drain in the neck following an esophageal repair. If in 72 h, there is no amylase present in the drain, it is OK to remove in order to avoid erosion into the repair or other structures. It is always better to have a controlled fistula with an esophageal leak rather than mediastinitis/death.

26.5.1 Damage Control

1. Create a fistula with a drain, which will close with time.
2. May consider diversion with a cervical esophagostomy with massive destruction of the esophagus.

26.6 Bone Bleeding

An uncommon but distressing problem could be bleeding from a hole in the vertebrae. Usually this type of bleeding in the neck arises from an injured vertebral artery. The treatment is to either stuff bone wax into the hole, a Foley catheter, or pack and perform an angio/embolization.

26.7 Conclusion

These are general guidelines and a few tricks of the trade for surgeons to consider when performing these repairs. This is by no means an exhaustive list of tricks. The surgeon's approach to penetrating neck trauma needs to be considered in the context of the institutional resources. At times for a tracheal injury, airway control with an endotracheal tube with the cuff below the injury and transfer to a higher level of care is necessary. If imaging modalities are limited and follow-up is limited, more liberal exploration of necks may be necessary. This only serves to provide some guidance when you are confronted with a real neck injury and you find yourself in the operating room.

Important Points

- Trick: Always approach a neck hematoma medial to the SCM.
- Trick: If the pseudoaneurysm is contained in the neck, dissect either proximally or distally to gain vascular control in more virgin territory.
- Trick: If you enter a pseudoaneurysm and you are unable to control it more proximally, try replacing your finger with a Foley catheter and inflate the balloon. This will often tampanode the bleeding in a GSW track while you perform your sternotomy.
- Caution: Bilateral IJ ligation has a high mortality associated with it.
- Tricks: (1) Evaluate associated injuries. (2) Avoid searching for the recurrent laryngeal nerves. (3) Separation of tracheal and esophageal suture lines. (4) Conservation of viable trachea. (5) Avoid tracheostomy through the repair. (6) Flexion of the neck postoperatively to reduce tension.
- Trick: Buttress the esophageal repair with a tongue of viable strap or SCM muscle.

References

1. Demetriades D, Asensio JA, Velmahos G et al (1996) Complex problems in penetrating neck trauma. Surg Clin North Am 6:661–683
2. Monson DO, Saletta JD, Freeark RJ (1969) Carotid vertebral trauma. J Trauma 9:987–999
3. Roon AJ, Christensen N (1979) Evaluation and treatment of penetrating cervical injuries. J Trauma 19:391–397
4. Saletta JD, Lowe RJ, Lim LT et al (1976) Penetrating trauma of the neck. J Trauma 16:579–587
5. Elerding SC, Manart FD, Moore EE (1980) A reappraisal of penetrating neck injury management. J Trauma 20: 695–697
6. Bishara RA, Pasch AR, Douglas DD et al (1986) The necessity of mandatory exploration of penetrating zone II neck injuries. Surgery 100:655–660
7. Nance FC, Cohn I Jr (1969) Surgical judgement in the management of stab wounds of the abdomen: a retrospective and prospective analysis based on a study of 600 stabbed patients. Ann Surg 170:569–645

8. Shirkey AL, Beall AC Jr, Debakey ME (1963) Surgical management of penetrating wounds of the neck. Arch Surg 86:955–963
9. Biffl WL, Moore EE, Rehse DH et al (1997) Selective management of penetrating neck trauma based on cervical level of injury. Am J Surg 174:678–682
10. Sriussadaporn S, Pak-Art R, Tharavej C et al (2001) Selective management of penetrating neck injuries based on clinical presentations is safe and practical. Int Surg 86:90–93
11. Nason RW, Assuras GN, Gray PR et al (2001) Penetrating neck injuries: analysis of experience from a Canadian trauma centre. Can J Surg 44:122–126
12. Velmahos GC, Souter I, Degiannis E et al (1994) Selective surgical management in penetrating neck injuries. Can J Surg 37:487–491
13. Golueke PF, Goldstein AS, Sclafani SJ et al (1984) Routine versus selective exploration of penetrating neck injuries: a randomized prospective study. J Trauma 24:1010–1014
14. Atteberry LR, Dennis JW, Menawat SS, Frykberg ER (1994) Physical examination alone is safe and accurate for evaluation of vascular injuries in penetrating zone II neck trauma. J Am Coll Surg 179:657–662
15. Sekharan J, Dennis JW, Veldenz HC, Miranda F, Frykberg ER (2000) Continued experience with physical examination alone for evaluation and management of penetrating zone 2 neck injuries: results of 145 cases. J Vasc Surg 32(3):483–489
16. Demetriades D, Theodorou D, Cornwell E III, Berne TV, Asensio J, Belzberg H, Velmahos G, Weaver F, Yellin A (1997) Evaluation of penetrating injuries of the neck: prospective study of 223 patients. World J Surg 21:41–48

Access to the Neck in Penetrating Trauma

27

Jeffrey Ustin

The neck is an incredibly anatomically complex region of the body containing vital aerodigestive and neurovascular structures. Despite this density of structures, you can access the entire neck by knowing three basic exposures.

Deciding among the incisions requires some knowledge or assumptions about the trajectory of the wound. Ultimately, you are trying to decide which zone or zones (Fig. 27.1) have been injured and if the wound is unilateral or transcervical. It is here that your assessment is critical. What have you learned about the mechanism of injury? Are there any signs or symptoms that indicate which structures have been injured such as the classic "hard signs?" Are there any indications that the trajectory crossed the midline and affected the bilateral necks? Is there a pneumothorax, hemothorax, pericardial effusion, or abnormal brachio-brachial index (BBI) indicating a trajectory into the thoracic cavity as well as the neck? Do you have any imaging studies to guide your decision? It is usually feasible to obtain a quick chest radiograph and thoracic ultrasound.

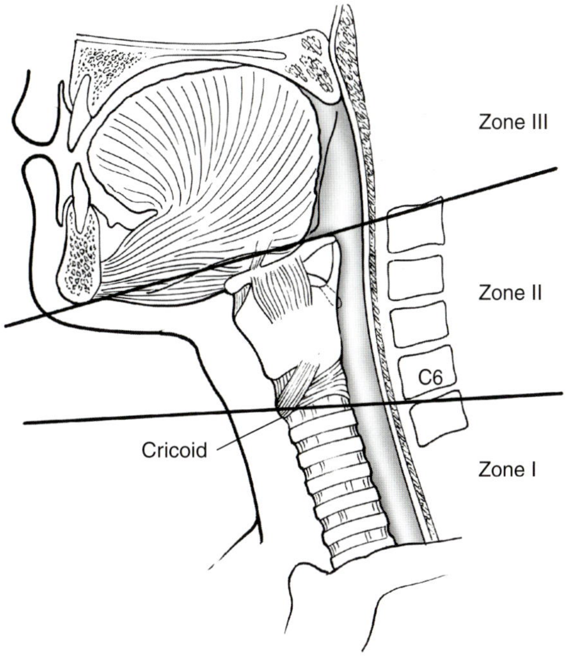

Fig. 27.1 Zones of the neck

Some situations require a definitive maneuver prior to formal exploration. Tracheal injuries require definitive airway control. Laryngoscopic or fiber-optic endotracheal intubation is often possible and worth attempting. Large injuries allow direct intubation through the wound which is an acceptable temporary airway. Otherwise, emergency cricothyroidotomy is the quickest approach and may be left as a definitive airway without conversion to tracheostomy.

Bleeding is usually controllable with digital pressure. Subclavian injuries can be difficult to compress. Place a Foley catheter into the wound, inflate it, and pull against the clavicle for tamponade.

Several steps can help optimize surgical approach. Obviously, the cervical collar is removed. It is unnecessary to follow cervical spine precautions in penetrating neck trauma since the probability of an unstable cervical spine with a penetrating mechanism is exceedingly

J. Ustin
Division of Trauma, Emergency Surgery & Surgical Critical Care, Massachusetts General Hospital, Harvard Medical School, 165 Cambridge Street, Suite 810, Boston, MA 02114, USA
e-mail: justin@partners.org

G.C. Velmahos et al. (eds.), *Penetrating Trauma*,
DOI 10.1007/978-3-642-20453-1_27, © Springer-Verlag Berlin Heidelberg 2012

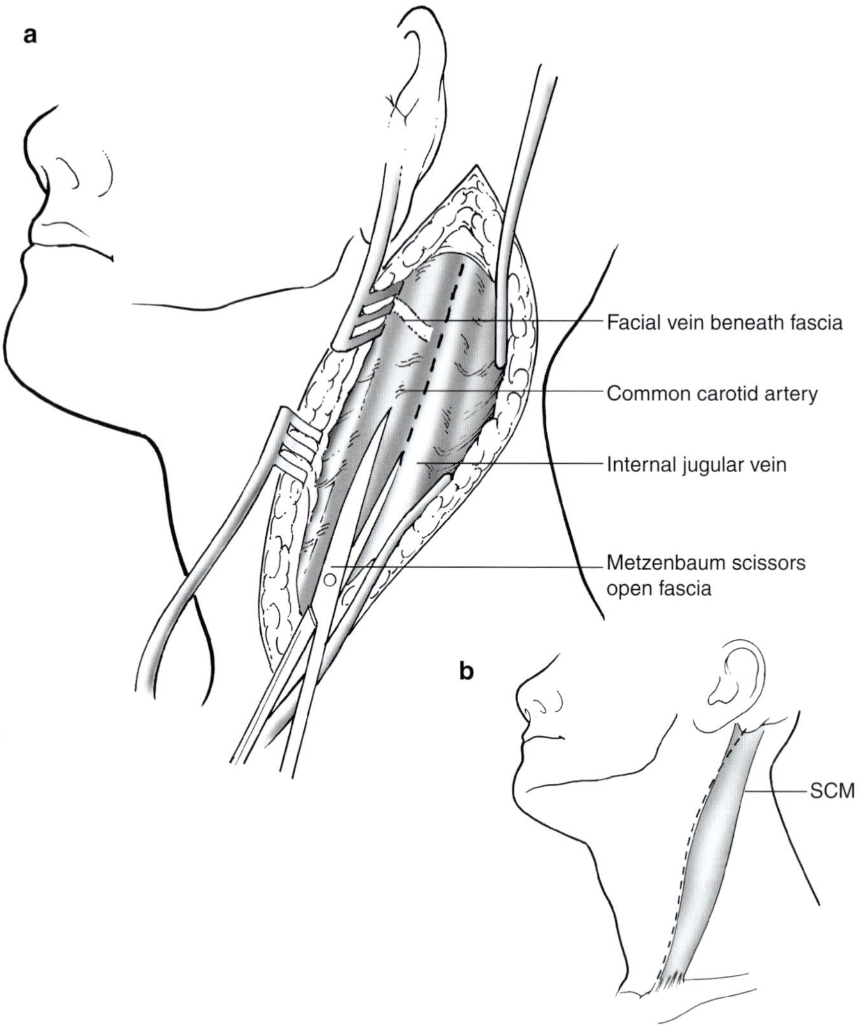

Fig. 27.2 (**a**, **b**) Easiest and most safe access is via the anterior sternocleidomastoid incision

small and suboptimal positioning can seriously impair the ease of access to the neck. Place a transversely oriented shoulder roll to obtain some neck extension. Turn the patient's head away from the side of initial exploration. Prep both sides of the neck starting at the mastoid processed. Leave the tips of the pinnae and angles of the mandible exposed. Prep the sternum into the field for possible extension of the neck incision into a sternotomy. Prep one leg for possible vein graft. Finally, if you are uncertain about the exact trajectory of a missile, consider prepping in the abdomen as well. Make sure to ask to have the following equipment immediately available: vascular suture such as 5-0 prolene, vascular clamps, vascular grafts and patches, a variety of balloon embolectomy catheters, and a sternal saw and sternal retractor. Request the anesthesiologist to place a large bore nasogastric tube.

The workhorse access is the anterior sternocleidomastoid (SCM) incision (Fig. 27.2). Make a generous incision along the anterior border of the sternocleidomastoid. At the angle of the mandible, curve the incision slightly posteriorly to remain at least 2 cm from the mandible and thus avoid injury to the marginal mandibular branch of the facial nerve. The platysma is divided and the dissection is continued anterior to the SCM. Look for the internal jugular vein. The facial vein crosses the wound and empties into the IJ. Divide the facial vein or veins. It is also acceptable to

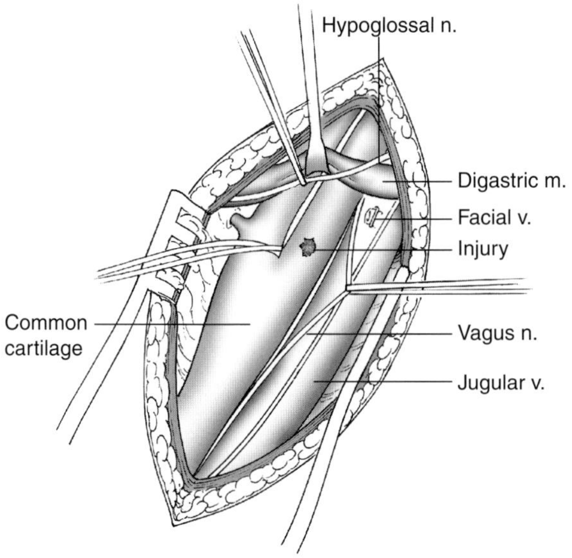

Fig. 27.3 Stay in the adventitial plane of top of the carotid

divide the IJ as well, if there are other injuries, the patient is doing poorly, or the vessel is badly injured.

A large hematoma will often distort the planes as you continue your dissection, advancing the self-retaining retractors deeper into the wound. Prior to entering a large hematoma, gain proximal control. This may require extending the incision caudally toward the sternal notch or even performing a median sternotomy. The omohyoid crosses the wound low in the neck and may need to be divided. Stay in the adventitial plane of top of the carotid (Fig. 27.3). As you pass a vessel loop or clamp around the carotid and IJ, recall the position of the vagus nerve and protect it. Sometimes this requires surrounding it with a vessel loop and gently retracting it laterally.

Distal control can be challenging. The incision may need to be extended toward the mastoid. The hypoglossal nerve crossed the carotid at approximately the level of the bifurcation and often very near the posterior belly of the digastric muscle. Protect the hypoglossal and divide the digastric if needed. By remaining anterior to the SCM, you should not encounter the spinal accessory nerve until you are within several centimeters of the skull base. High carotid injuries are very hard to reach. Dislocating the jaw is possible, but requires special expertise. Use a handheld retractor on the mandible itself in these situations. Often times it is easier to obtain distal control by entering the hematoma and applying distal pressure, vascular clamps, or a balloon embolectomy catheter directly to the open end of the vessel.

To access the trachea, divide the omohyoid or other strap muscles as needed. If needed, mobilize the thyroid by dividing the middle thyroid vein and inferior thyroid artery. Be mindful of the recurrent laryngeal nerve, although frequently, it is not readily identifiable in the trauma situation.

To access the esophagus, mobilize the omohyoid, middle thyroid vein, and inferior thyroid artery. Retract the carotid sheath posterolaterally. Do not hesitate to open the contralateral neck to fully examine the esophagus when needed. The previously placed NG tube helps with the esophageal mobilization.

Bleeding from deep within the posterior neck is coming from a vertebra or vertebral artery. This is best controlled with a hemostatic agent and pressure. You can also try placing bone wax (reference) to control hemorrhage. Avoid exploring these injuries as they are very difficult to directly control.

As discussed above, it is sometimes necessary to perform a sternotomy to gain proximal control of the carotid. This is further described in the chapter on thoracic trauma. Briefly, incise the skin over the sternum from the sternal notch to several centimeters below the xiphoid. Pass a finger deep to the sternum at both ends of the incision to separate the deep surface of the sternum from the underlying soft tissues (Fig. 27.4a). Ask the anesthesiologists to hold respirations and divide the sternum using the saw. Try to remain in the middle of the sternum. Apply gentle traction on the saw toward the ceiling keeping the saw guide against the deep surface of the sternum. Place the sternal retractor and divide the thymus between clamps if needed. Retract the innominate vein to expose the ascending aorta and great vessels. You can divide the left innominate vein to achieve better exposure if retraction alone is insufficient (Fig. 27.4b). The right-sided vessels are easily accessible. The left side is more difficult since the arch extends posteriorly. Identify the vagus and recurrent laryngeal nerves prior to clamping.

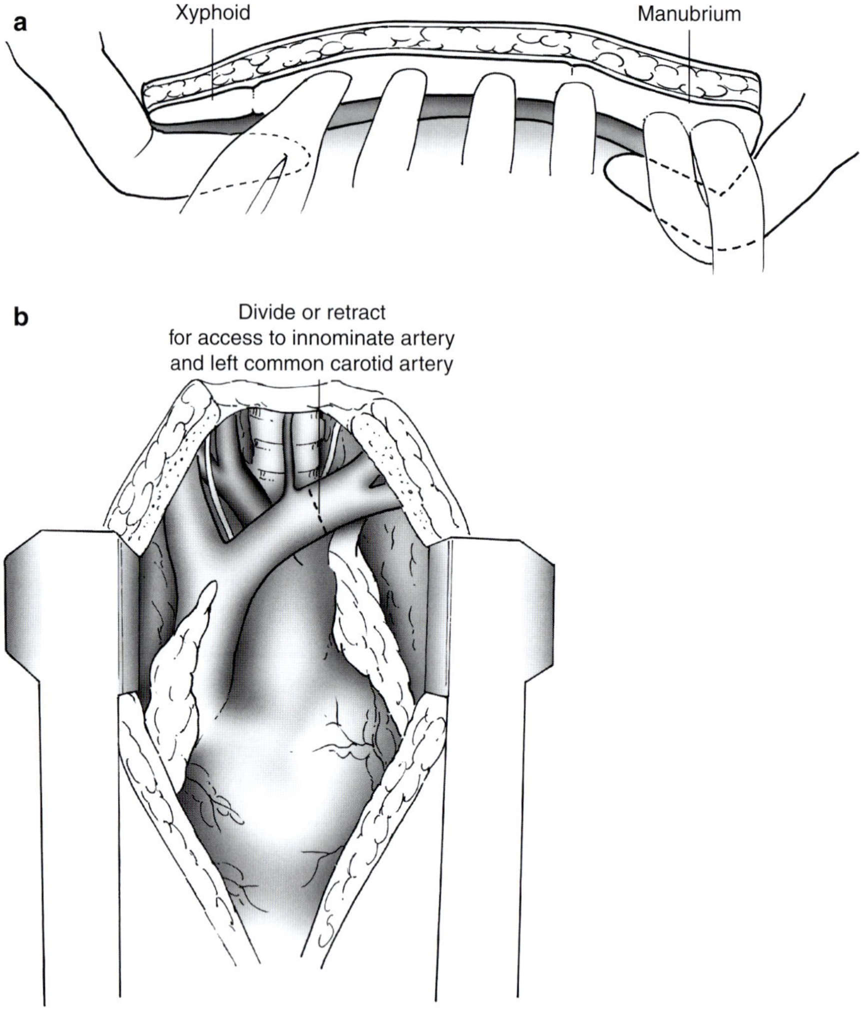

Fig. 27.4 (**a**) Pass a finger deep to the sternum at both ends of the incision to separate the deep surface of the sternum from the underlying soft tissues. (**b**)You can divide the left innominate vein to achieve better exposure if retraction alone is insufficient

For transcervical injuries, perform a "U" incision (Fig. 27.5). Start by making an anterior sternocleidomastoid incision as described above. At approximately 2 cm above the sternal notch, curve the incision toward the contralateral side and continue by incising the skin along the anterior border of the other sternocleidomastoid. Incise the platysma, grasp it with several Allis clamps, and raise a superior flap. Continue to identify the IJ veins, divide the facial veins, and access the carotid sheaths as described above.

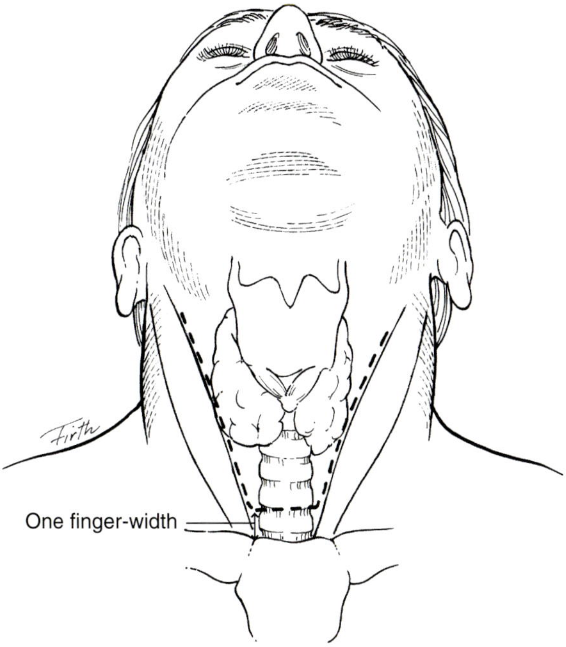

Fig. 27.5 For transcervical injuries, perform a "U" incision to enable bilateral exploration

Penetrating Trauma to the Larynx and the Cervical Trachea

28

Alicia Kieninger and Elliott R. Haut

The management of penetrating neck trauma has evolved over recent years. Historically, penetrating neck injuries have been managed with consideration of injury location and accessibility of surgical exploration. With this in mind, Zone 2 injuries (between the cricoid cartilage and angle of the mandible) that penetrate the platysma have historically all been managed with mandatory neck exploration and direct repair of any injured structures. With advances in radiographic imaging, such as multiplanar computed tomography (CT) and CT angiography (CTA), selective operative management is now the norm. Specifically, some patients with penetrating laryngotracheal trauma may now be managed nonoperatively.

Cervical airway trauma is an uncommon, but not rare occurrence at busy trauma centers. In a review of 1,560 trauma patients with neck injuries, 4.9% of patients suffered from some type of aerodigestive injury. The incidence is higher with penetrating trauma. Specifically, gunshot wounds were associated with a rate of 10% and stab wounds 5%, versus 1% for blunt trauma [1]. As many as 10% of patients have combined aerodigestive injuries due to the close proximity of structures (Fig. 28.1). It is important to keep this in mind when you evaluate a patient with a potential penetrating airway injury. The final approach to penetrating airway trauma should be dependent on the resources and experience of the given institution. However, in all cases, airway control and avoidance of potential airway complications are the most important aspects of initial care.

A. Kieninger
St. Joseph Mercy Oakland Director, Surgical Critical Care Services Associate Director, Trauma Services 44555 Woodward Ave. Suite 501, Pontiac, MI 48341, USA
e-mail: kieninga@trinity-health.org

E.R. Haut (✉)
Division of Acute Care Surgery, Department of Surgery, The Johns Hopkins Hospital, The Johns Hopkins University School of Medicine, 625 Osler, 600 N. Wolfe St, Baltimore, MD 21287, USA
e-mail: ehaut1@jhmi.edu

28.1 Airway Management

Patients who are alert and spontaneously breathing without difficulty likely do not require urgent control of their airway. In a review of 57 patients with penetrating laryngotracheal injuries, 44% required preoperative airway control [2]. However, it is important to know that swelling and hematoma formation can quickly cause deterioration of what would have otherwise been an easily managed airway. Thinking ahead is the key to maintaining control of any airway situation. Consideration of the cervical spine is also essential in all trauma patients. Maintenance of in-line cervical spine immobilization is essential for all blunt trauma patients, until an evaluation of the cervical spine can be completed. Cervical gunshot and stab wounds can cause cervical spine fractures with or without associated neurologic deficit. However, in general, it is safe to remove the collar in the majority of patients [3]. Cervical collars have been suggested to impede airway control and should be removed quickly from patients with penetrating trauma to avoid obscuring wounds [4].

G.C. Velmahos et al. (eds.), *Penetrating Trauma*,
DOI 10.1007/978-3-642-20453-1_28, © Springer-Verlag Berlin Heidelberg 2012

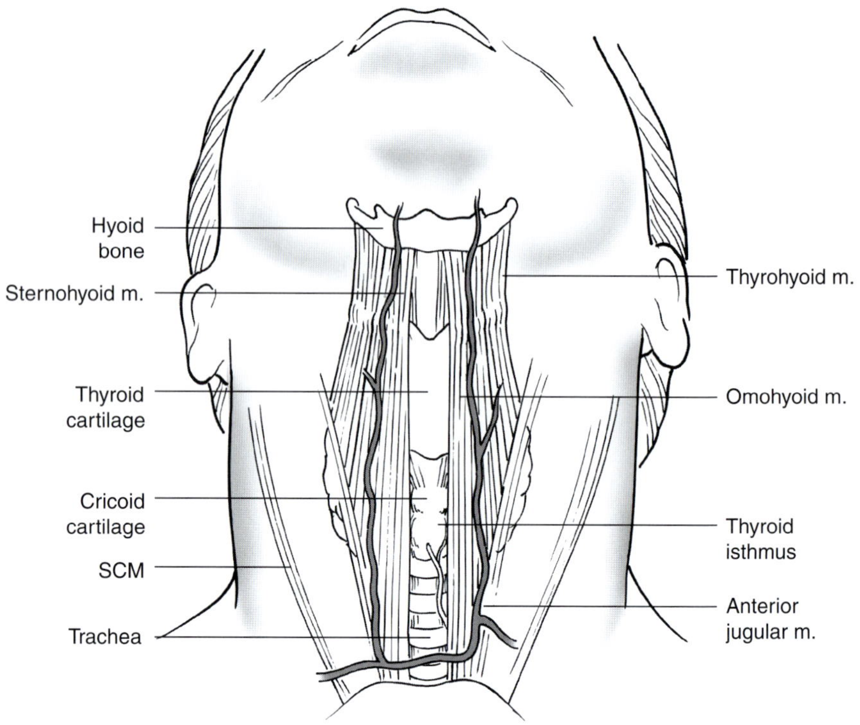

Fig. 28.1 As many as 10% of patients have combined aerodigestive injuries due to the close proximity of structures

For all patients requiring airway control, endotracheal intubation is the preferred route. In stable patients without significant swelling, this can likely be accomplished with direct laryngoscopy. Patients with oropharyngeal swelling, complex facial fractures, or other facial trauma may not be candidates for this technique. In the absence of basilar skull fractures, awake fiber-optic nasotracheal intubation is a safe and effective alternative for airway control. Neuromuscular blockade should be avoided in cases of significant airway compromise, in order to maintain the patient's spontaneous respiratory effort [5]. You should not convert a meta-stable airway (in which the patient is breathing and oxygenating to some degree) to an unstable airway with paralysis. In any case of significant head and neck trauma, intubation should be attempted by the most experienced person available. Sometimes only one attempt at intubation will be possible. It is important to remember that even at teaching institutions, not every case is appropriate to be a teaching case. You should have at least one backup plan if the initial intubation attempt fails. These may include intubation over a gum elastic bougie, supraglottic airway (i.e., Laryngeal Mask Airway [LMA]), or using a videolaryngoscope (i.e., GlideScope).

Should translaryngeal techniques fail, cricothyroidotomy remains the surgical airway of choice. In experienced hands, this can be accomplished quickly and with minimal morbidity to surrounding structures. We prefer to use a vertical incision in this situation although both horizontal and vertical incisions have been described (Fig. 28.2a). Emergency cricothyroidotomy is usually performed in chaotic situations where accurate identification of landmarks may be difficult, if not impossible. A vertical incision allows the flexibility to identify the proper level of the airway, and minimizes bleeding from anterior jugular veins. While a tracheostomy tube is the preferred airway in this situation, an endotracheal tube placed through the cricothyroid membrane is an acceptable alternative when a tracheostomy tube is not available (Fig. 28.2b, c). If you must use a normal endotracheal tube, be sure not to advance it too far, as this is a common error leading to mainstem intubation. Emergent tracheotomy should be reserved for cases of suspected laryngotracheal separation or other cases in which the injury is located below the cricothyroid membrane.

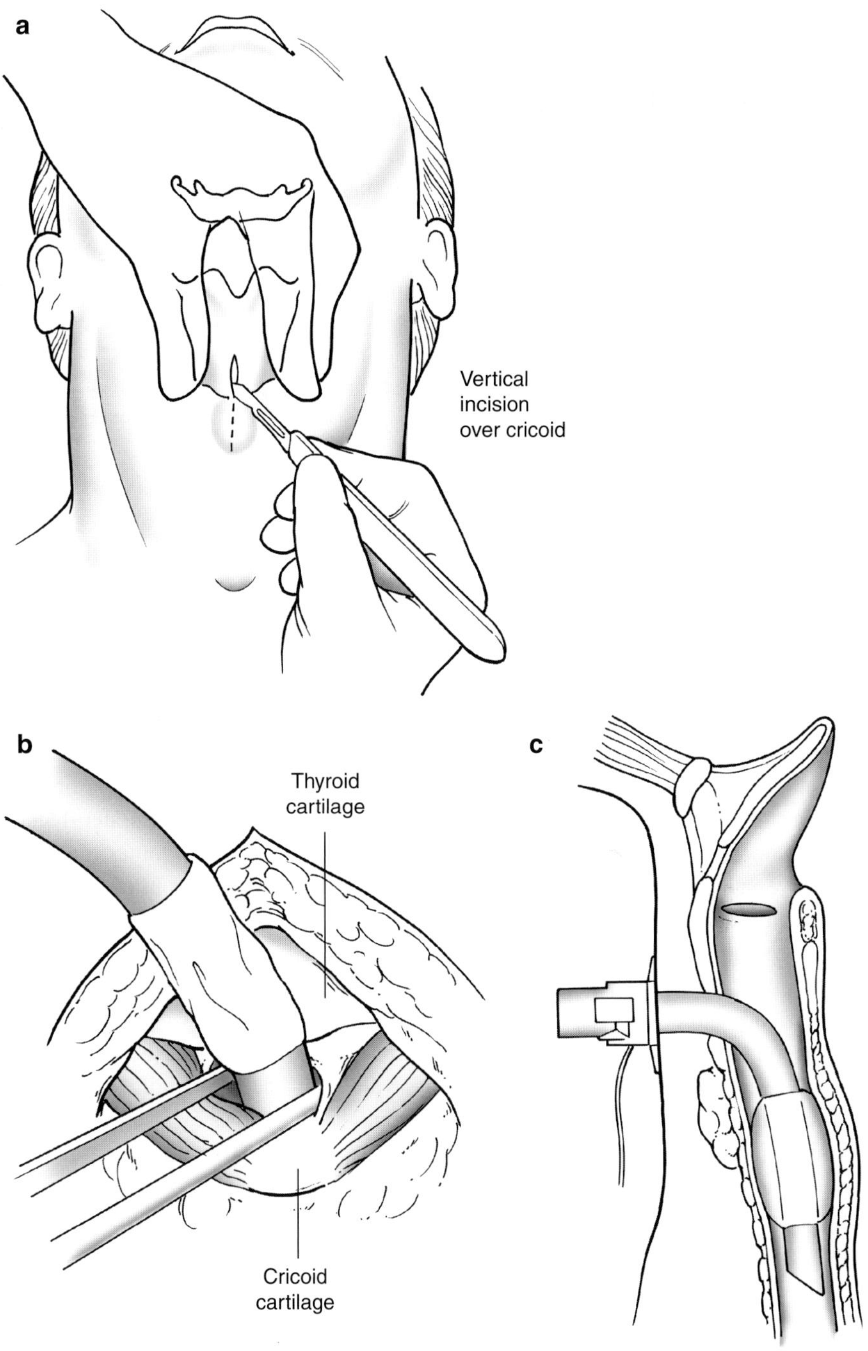

Fig. 28.2 (**a**) Emergency cricothyroidotomy is usually performed in chaotic situations where accurate identification of landmarks may be difficult, if not impossible. A vertical incision allows the flexibility to identify the proper level of the airway, and minimizes bleeding from anterior jugular veins. (**b**, **c**) While a tracheostomy tube is the preferred airway in this situation, an endotracheal tube placed through the cricothyroid membrane is an acceptable alternative when a tracheostomy tube is not available

28.2 Injury Classification

Airway injuries can best be classified based on their location in relation to the vocal cords. Supraglottic injuries, occurring above the cords, are typically associated with vertical fractures of the thyroid cartilage, with or without fractures of the cricoid cartilage. Glottic injuries may also involve the thyroid cartilage, but can also involve the true vocal cords, thyroarytenoid muscles, and aryepiglottic bands. Subglottic injuries involve the lower thyroid and cricoid cartilages. These injuries are particularly dangerous because acute subglottic stenosis related to cricotracheal separation can result in rapid and complete loss of the patient's airway. Such patients require emergent tracheostomy to secure their airway, but will often not even survive long enough to make it to the trauma center. Glottic and supraglottic injures are more complex to repair than subglottic injuries, especially with respect to maintenance or restoration of voice quality. Once the airway is secured, we would recommend further evaluation and treatment by an experienced head and neck surgeon for these types of injuries.

28.3 Decision-Making Process

As stated in the introduction, many penetrating neck injuries can be managed nonoperatively. In a review of 203 patients with penetrating neck trauma, Thoma and colleagues found that 78% of patients could be safely managed nonoperatively [6]. Initial examination will identify so-called hard findings that require urgent operative intervention. Findings requiring urgent intervention include obvious airway compromise, hemorrhagic shock, expanding or pulsatile hematomas, or extensive subcutaneous air. Patients with these findings require urgent airway control and transportation to the operating room for further management. In a review of 223 patients with penetrating neck injuries, Demetriades and colleagues found that no patient that was asymptomatic on initial evaluation required surgical intervention, for a negative predictive value of 100%. Only 4.5% of this population of patients ever required surgery.

In patients without these "hard signs," there are several more subtle findings that suggest more serious injuries, and require additional workup at a minimum. Dysphagia may be a sign of a significant pharyngeal or laryngeal injury. If possible, these patients should undergo direct and/or indirect laryngoscopy to evaluate supraglottic structures. Voice changes can be a sign of significant laryngeal injury, and the vocal cords should be carefully examined. Patients with multiple and/or displaced laryngeal cartilage fractures, or large mucosal lacerations, will likely require operative repair.

Smaller pharyngeal, glottic, and supraglottic lacerations can be managed nonoperatively. These patients should be maintained NPO and be maintained on antibiotic prophylaxis such as clindamycin to allow healing of the mucosa [7]. Minimal edema and small laryngeal hematomas with intact mucosa are also likely to resolve nonoperatively, and require no further intervention. These patients can eventually undergo a fluoroscopic contrast swallow evaluation to identify any persistent pharyngeal leak. Additionally, after repeat evaluation of the larynx to assess for healing, patients should be evaluated by speech and language pathology to ensure adequate swallowing.

28.4 Operative Approach

28.4.1 Incisions

Ideally, you should position the patient supine on the operating table, with a shoulder roll to facilitate neck extension. Depending on the location of the external wound, and possible associated injuries, the neck may be explored from either an anterior or lateral approach. Lateral explorations are useful because they facilitate exposure of vascular structures on the injured side, as well as evaluation of the esophagus when approached from the left. Lateral incisions are placed anterior to the sternocleidomastoid (SCM) muscle, such as you would use for a routine carotid endarterectomy (Figs. 26.1 and 27.2). The SCM as well as the internal jugular vein are retracted laterally. From this approach, the carotid sheath and associated structures may be evaluated (Fig. 26.4). On the left side, posterior to the airway and anterior to the vertebral bodies, the cervical esophagus can be identified and evaluated. Finally, this incision also allows exposure of the cricoid and cervical trachea.

The other main surgical approach to the neck is an exploration via a cervical collar incision, as is often used for thyroid surgery. Typically this is placed approximately two finger breadths above the sternal notch, although a higher incision may be helpful if the suspected injury is more cephalad. You would then raise subplatysmal flaps superiorly and inferiorly, allowing you access to divide the strap muscles along the midline vertically. This exposure allows excellent visualization of the cervical airway, as well as other central neck structures such as the thyroid. If lateral injury is suspected, the midline incision may be extended laterally to either or both sides as described in the previous paragraph, and adequate evaluation of all neck structures can be accomplished (Fig. 27.5).

In addition, if further exposure is needed, you can make a vertical extension from this collar incision to the sternal notch, allowing excellent access to the trachea.

28.5 Laryngeal Repair

The larynx is approached via a high cervical incision and entered through the cricoid membrane. The most important aspect about repair of laryngeal lacerations is to obtain mucosal coverage of exposed cartilage in order to avoid the late complication of granulation tissue. Cartilage fractures can be repaired with absorbable suture such as 4-0 PDS. The mucosa is also repaired with absorbable suture. If the mucosa will not close primarily, a skin graft may be used. You should use flexible endoscopy liberally to fully detect the extent of laryngeal injury. Evaluation of the posterior wall and vocal cords is essential. These types of injuries are relatively uncommon, and repair may be complex. Consultation with an experienced head and neck surgeon can be beneficial to obtain the best functional results.

28.6 Tracheal Repair

As previously described, the trachea may be approached via a lateral or anterior incision. Simple lacerations to the trachea are best repaired primarily with absorbable interrupted suture, such a 4-0 PDS. No tracheostomy is required for postoperative management in the majority of these patients. For patients with larger wounds, where the need for a tracheostomy is anticipated, the tracheostomy may be placed directly through the anterior tracheal wound. Otherwise, you should aim to place the tracheostomy distal to the tracheal injury [5]. Ideally, primary repair with absorbable suture is the goal. You will need to debride all devitalized tissue in order to assure healthy tissue for wound healing. The trachea should be examined endoscopically to evaluate for any posterior wall defects that need repair. If the tracheal defect is large, the distal trachea can be mobilized cephalad simply via the use of the tracheal hook. If necessary, more extensive soft tissue dissection is undertaken to mobilize the trachea. You should do this bluntly in the anterior/posterior planes, rather than lateral, in order to avoid recurrent laryngeal nerve (RLN) injury [8]. The larynx can additionally be brought caudad by mobilizing its suprahyoid connections. Up to 5 cm of trachea can be resected with primary anastamosis. Flexion of the neck will help in closing this gap, which you can facilitate and ensure will be maintained by suturing the chin to the chest with a large suture or steel wire (also see Chap. 33).

28.7 Associated Injuries

In every patient with any aerodigestive injury, you must consider the possibility of associated vascular injury. Although the specific approach to repair of these vascular injuries is outside the scope of this chapter, you must remember to examine all vascular structures (i.e., carotid arteries, jugular veins) intraoperatively and treat any injuries identified with repair, ligation, or reconstruction as indicated. Cervical esophageal injuries are also common in patients with injury to the proximal airway. It is imperative to identify and repair these injuries (also covered in another chapter) since delayed repair is associated with significant mortality. If identified, you must consider the implications of associated injuries when repairing the airway. If the airway injury is associated with either an arterial or esophageal injury repair, you should attempt to separate the suture lines with vascularized tissue in order to avoid fistula formation. You can simply rotate a vascularized flap of SCM or omohyoid muscle placed between the suture lines. Many of these cervical airway injuries may be associated with RLN injury. If RLN injury is suspected at the time of surgery, attempts at direct repair are not recommended at initial exploration [8]. The urgent nature of the surgery, combined with altered anatomy and possible tissue destruction, may lead to inadvertent worsening of nerve damage. Often function may improve with time and observation and if not, patients will likely have better long-term outcomes with delayed repair in a planned setting.

28.8 Complications

In a review of 57 patients with penetrating laryngotracheal injuries, Grewal and colleagues found the overall mortality to be 3.5%. Seventeen percent of patients in this study had voice changes, and 5% suffered from stenosis [2]. Similarly, Demetriades found a mortality rate of 6 out of 223 patients (2.7%), five of which were due to non-neck injuries [9]. Overall, the mortality from penetrating airway injuries is relatively low. However, significant morbidities can occur, particularly in patients who require operative intervention. Cervical abscesses occurred in 3% of patients reviewed by Vassiliu [1]. Another significant contributor to postoperative morbidity is reflux that can injure the repair. Patients should be maintained with the head of bed elevated at all times, and some recommend the use of proton pump inhibitors to decrease acid production [10]. Additionally, they should be NPO until a complete evaluation of their swallowing function can be completed.

Important Points

- Remember ABCs (Airway, Breathing, Circulation) when managing any patient with penetrating neck trauma.
- Consider possible cervical spine injury in all blunt trauma patients.
- Translaryngeal intubation is preferred, when possible.
- Cricothyroidotomy is the primary surgical airway of choice.
- Not all patients will require surgical repair of airway injuries.
- Be aware of the possibility of coexisting digestive tract and/or vascular injury.
- Repair the airway with interrupted, absorbable suture (i.e. 4-0 PDS).
- Use flexible endoscopy liberally to examine the airway and specifically exclude posterior injuries in patients with anterior tracheal penetration.
- Evaluate vocal cord function in all patients with upper airway injuries.
- Use a flap of SCM or omohyoid muscle between the suture lines if repairing multiple adjacent structures.

References

1. Vassiliu P, Baker J, Henderson S et al (2001) Aerodigestive injuries of the neck. Am Surg 67:75–79
2. Grewal H, Rao P, Mukerhi S et al (1995) Management of penetrating laryngotracheal injuries. Head Neck 17:494–502
3. Haut ER, Kalish BT, Efron DT, Haider AH, Stevens KA, Kieninger AN, Cornwell EE 3rd, Chang DC (2010) Spine Immobilization in Penetrating Trauma: More Harm Than Good? Trauma 68(1):115–121
4. Barkana Y, Stein M, Scope A, Maor R, Abramovich Y, Friedman Z et al (2000) Pre-hospital stabilization of the cervical spine for penetrating injuries to the neck – is it necessary? Injury 31:305–309
5. Corneille M, Stewart RM, Cohn SM (2008) Upper airway injury and its management. Semin Thorac Cardiovasc Surg 20:8–12
6. Thoma M, Navsaria PH, Edu S et al (2008) Analysis of 203 patients with penetrating neck injuries. World J Surg 32: 2716–2723
7. Goudy SL, Miller FB, Bumpous JM (2002) Neck crepitance: evaluation and management of suspected upper aerodigestive tract injury. Laryngoscope 112:791–795
8. Dedo HH, Rowe LD (1983) Laryngeal reconstruction in acute and chronic injures. Otolaryngol Clin North Am 16: 373–389
9. Demetriades D, Velmahos GG, Asensio JA (2001) Cervical pharyngoesophageal and laryngotracheal injuries. World J Surg 25:1044–1048
10. Lee WT, Eliashar R, Eliachar I (2006) Acute external laryngotracheal trauma: diagnosis and management. ENT 85: 179–184

Further Reading

National Association of Emergency Medical Technicians (2007) Prehospital trauma life support (PHTLS), 6th edn. Mosby JEMS, St. Louis, p 235

American College of Surgeons Committee on Trauma (2008) Advanced trauma life support (ATLS) student course manual, 8th edn. American College of Surgeons, Chicago. World J Surg. 32(12):2716–2723

Britt LD, Weireter LJ and Cole FJ (2008) Management of acute neck injuries. Trauma. Am Surg. 67(1):75–79

Jordan JD, Stringer SP (2006) Laryngeal trauma. head and neck surgery. Otolaryngology.

Penetrating Injury to the Pharynx and Cervical Esophagus

29

Angela L. Neville and Timothy L. VanNatta

29.1 Anatomic Basics

The region containing the pharynx and cervical esophagus is not an area heavily traveled by the average general or trauma surgeon. Even more, pharyngoesophageal injury occurs in a mere 0.9–6% of penetrating neck injuries [1–3]. Thus, when encountering an injury to this area, knowing a few critical anatomic landmarks can help.

The pharynx originates at the base of the skull and extends to the level of the cricoid cartilage. Its constrictor muscles propel food into the esophagus. The lowermost constrictor comprises the upper esophageal sphincter and sits anatomically at the level of the cricoid and C6 vertebra. (Fig. 29.1) The cervical esophagus descends from there to the thoracic inlet. Thus, the pharynx is the portion of the digestive tube injured in a Zone 2 or 3 injury, and the cervical esophagus is injured in a Zone 1 injury.

The pharynx and cervical esophagus lie deep in the neck and are protected posteriorly by the cervical vertebrae. They are abutted anteriorly by the larynx and trachea. Consequently, the only way to get to the pharyngoesophageal region is via a lateral approach which requires retracting the carotid sheath out of the way. Concomitant (and more deadly) injury to the trachea or vascular structures should be addressed before embarking on a pharyngoesophageal repair.

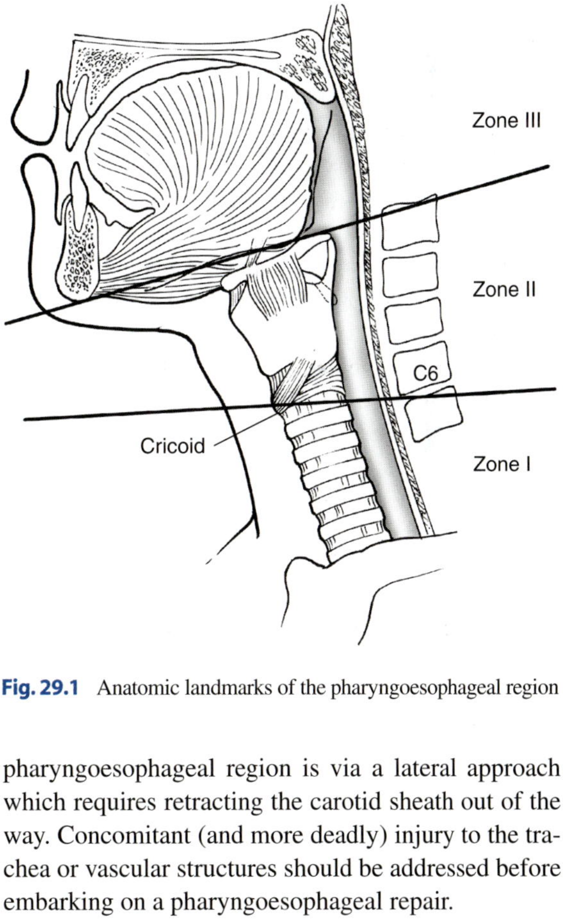

Fig. 29.1 Anatomic landmarks of the pharyngoesophageal region

A.L. Neville (✉)
David Geffen School of Medicine at UCLA,
Division of Trauma, Acute Care Surgery, and Surgical Critical Care, Harbor-UCLA Medical Center,
1000 W. Carson Street, Box 42, Torrance, CA 90509, USA
e-mail: angelane13@gmail.com

T.L. VanNatta
David Geffen School of Medicine at UCLA,
Division of Cardiothoracic Surgery, Division of Trauma, Acute Care Surgery, and Surgical Critical Care,
Harbor-UCLA Medical Center, 1000 W. Carson Street,
Box 42, Torrance, CA 90509, USA
e-mail: timothy.vannatta@gmail.com

29.2 Know When to Go in

There are essentially two scenarios in penetrating neck trauma. The first is a patient with an obvious vascular or tracheal injury who needs to be in the operating

G.C. Velmahos et al. (eds.), *Penetrating Trauma*,
DOI 10.1007/978-3-642-20453-1_29, © Springer-Verlag Berlin Heidelberg 2012

room immediately. Once these injuries are identified and repaired, try to evaluate the esophagus. Trace the trajectory of the bullet. Perform maneuvers to see if there is a hole in the esophagus (on table endoscopy, air in the nasogastric tube, etc.) and repair it. If the patient is too unstable for further exploration, then leave a drain and get out.

The second, more common scenario is a patient who is hemodynamically stable and requires a thorough workup to exclude any injury that should be fixed in the operating room expeditiously. Several retrospective studies have found worse esophageal-specific outcomes in patients who had a preoperative evaluation prior to esophageal repair compared to those who did not [4, 5]. The implication is that delay in repair (while studies are being performed) leads to a worse outcome. The retrospective nature of these studies makes interpretation difficult and no specific time frame has been established, but the take-home lesson is to identify and treat esophageal injury as soon as possible [6].

How to diagnose (and even treat) pharyngoesophageal injury remains a topic of ongoing study and debate. There are no hard signs of pharyngoesophageal injury, but a thorough history and physical examination may give clues that further workup is needed. Symptoms of odynophagia or dysphagia, and signs of subcutaneous emphysema or hematemesis, are indications of pharyngoesophageal injury and warrant further evaluation. In a study of 223 patients with penetrating neck injury, none of the evaluable, asymptomatic patients had an esophageal injury; workup was recommended for symptomatic or unevaluable patients [1]. Still, the potential morbidity associated with a missed injury has led to the recommendation that surgeons have a low threshold for obtaining imaging studies in evaluating penetrating injuries to the neck [6].

If available, helical computed tomography angiography (CTA) has emerged as the single imaging modality with the greatest potential to rule out esophageal, as well as tracheal and vascular, injury [6]. A missile trajectory away from the esophagus (or other vital structures) obviates the need for exploration or additional invasive studies [7]. Beyond this, CTA has not yet proven itself as stand-alone study for diagnosing or excluding pharyngoesophageal injury. In 2003, Gonzales evaluated 42 patients with CTA followed by mandatory esophagogram and operative exploration. Two very small stab wound injuries (<5 mm) were missed both by CTA and swallow study, suggesting that CTA was no better than esophagogram [8]. Inaba subsequently found that CTA "overdiagnosed" aerodigestive injury in four patients with subcutaneous air as the common, nonspecific sign [9]. Two patients had the injuries ruled out by negative contrast swallows and endoscopy. The other two patients underwent negative exploration.

Current recommended workup of pharyngoesophageal injury is by contrast esophagography or esophagoscopy [6]. There is no consensus that one study is preferable to the other and most study protocols seem driven by surgeon preference or institutional availability. If a contrast swallow study is chosen, a majority of authors favor water-soluble esophagogram initially, with thin Barium to follow. The sensitivity of esophagography to detect pharyngoesophageal injury varies widely and is reported between 60% and 100% [2, 6, 10]. Rigid or flexible endoscopy has proven equally, if not more efficacious. Two early studies utilizing rigid esophagoscopy suggested improved sensitivity compared to esophagogram [11, 12]. Since then, flexible endoscopy has been studied with a reported 100% sensitivity (92% and 95% specificity) [13, 14]. As flexible endoscopy does not require general anesthesia or manipulation of the cervical spine, it is a modality that we prefer.

Of importance, multiple authors report successful conservative (nonoperative) management of patients with penetrating pharyngoesophageal injury [3, 10, 15, 16]. In these studies, patients are kept nothing per oral (NPO), given intravenous antibiotics, and maintained on surgical nutrition (enteral or parenteral). Stanley made a compelling argument that penetrating injuries of the upper hypopharynx (above the arytenoids) be managed nonoperatively [15]. He suggested that the anatomy of this area favored spontaneous healing, yet further demonstrated increased complications to the lower pharynx or cervical esophagus if these areas were not surgically repaired. Nel and Yugeros also reported retrospective success of nonoperative management of the pharynx (but did not specify upper or lower) [10, 16]. Madiba successfully managed patients with penetrating injury to the cervical esophagus nonoperatively if their water-soluble contrast study showed contained extravasation (not trickling widely or into the mediastinum) [3]. To date, there are no prospective, randomized studies comparing the role of surgical and nonoperative management for penetrating pharyngoesophageal injury. Based on retrospective data, a nonoperative approach seems feasible in a patient with a contained pharyngeal injury who has no other indication for neck exploration.

To summarize, we recommend physical examination and helical CTA in stable patients with penetrating injuries to the neck. If the examination is negative and the trajectory of the injury away from the pharyngoesophageal area, no further workup is performed. If there is still potential for pharyngoesophageal injury, we recommend expeditious esophagogram. A small, contained pharyngeal leak can be managed nonoperatively, with plans to repeat the swallow study in 3–5 days. A patient with a larger, non-contained injury should be taken immediately to the operating room for primary repair. Flexible endoscopy is our preferred modality in a patient who is already in the operating room, who is already intubated (making the logistics of a swallow evaluation difficult), or whose swallow evaluation is "negative," but whose physical examination or CTA is highly suggestive of a pharyngoesophageal injury.

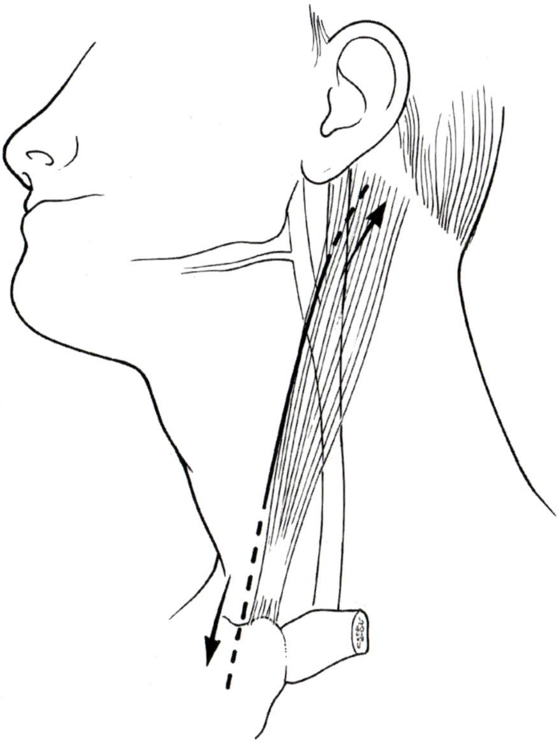

Fig. 29.2 Incision along the anterior border of the sternocleidomastoid muscle

29.3 How to Do the Repair

So you made the decision to operate. Positioning the patient for a complete neck exploration is the first key to success. Place a shoulder roll and tilt the patient's head away from the injury – unless of course, there is concern of a cervical spine injury in which case you will have to keep the head midline. Start your neck exploration on the side that is injured. If the injury is bilateral or you are not sure where the injury originates, start your approach to the esophagus from the patient's left side. The esophagus deviates slightly to left in the neck and there is a lesser chance of injury to the recurrent laryngeal nerve on this side.

Have the anesthesiologist gently place a nasogastric (NG) tube. The NG tube often proves critical in finding your injury when the time comes. Prep and drape both sides of the neck (from the mastoid down) and include the entire chest in the event that mediastinal exploration is warranted. It is also prudent to prepare both groins in case vascular access or saphenous vein harvesting is required.

Start with a generous incision along the anterior border of the sternocleidomastoid muscle (SCM) (Fig. 29.2). If better exposure is required, the incision can be extended all the way up to the mastoid superiorly. Curve posteriorly as you approach the angle of the mandible to avoid injuring the marginal mandibular branch of the facial nerve and the complication of smiling asymmetry. Inferiorly, the incision can be carried down to the sternal notch (and even further if median sternotomy is needed).

Divide the platysma muscle and look for the SCM. The critical next move is dividing the fibrous tissue (superficial cervical fascia) along the anterior border of the SCM (Fig. 29.3). Use a retractor to pull the SCM laterally so you can fully extend the exposure in either direction. This gives you direct access to the carotid sheath.

Put in self-retaining retractors, such as blunt-tip Weitlaners, now. Make sure that the Weitlaner prongs sit below the SCM to retract the entire muscle belly laterally.

You are about to begin your search for the pharyngoesophagus. In order to get to the esophagus, visualize the mantra – "carotid sheath down and thyroid gland up." That is the path you must create to get to your injury. (In actuality, you will retract the carotid sheath posterolaterally and the thyroid/trachea anteromedially,

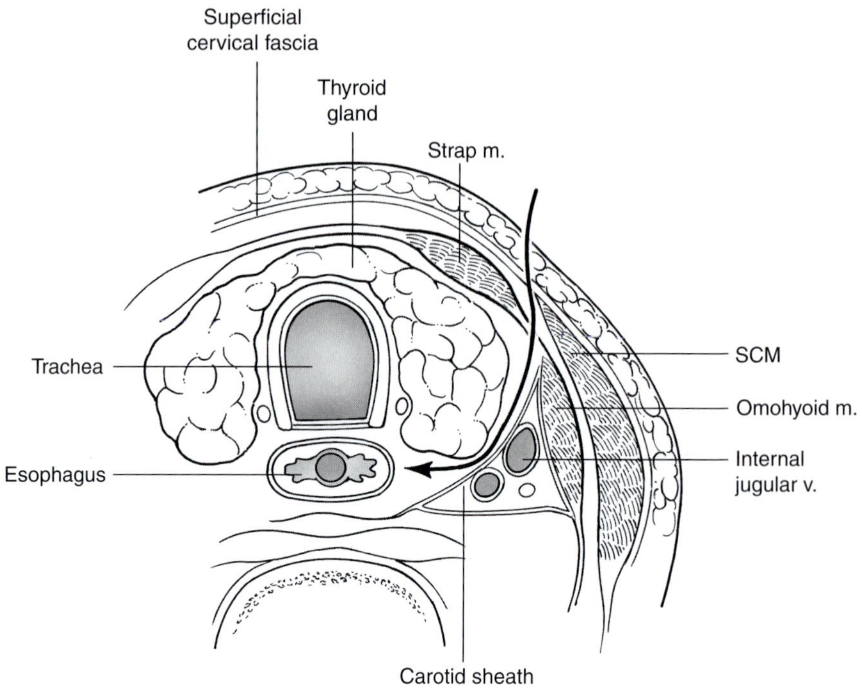

Fig. 29.3 Approach to the cervical esophagus

but that is too hard to say in your head.) To safely and effectively perform this retraction, you will need to open the carotid sheath and ligate some key structures. Tackle any encountered vascular injuries first.

Open the carotid sheath laterally over the big blue internal jugular vein (Fig. 29.4). Stay on the anterior surface of the vein and extend in both directions. As you move superiorly, you are looking for the large facial vein which courses just over the carotid bifurcation. The facial vein is a critical landmark in any neck exploration; once identified, it needs to be ligated and divided. This provides direct access to the carotid bifurcation and also releases the internal jugular for lateral retraction. With the facial vein ligated, you may replace your blunt Weitlaners below the medial aspect of the internal jugular to increase exposure.

Begin to March from superior to inferior along the internal jugular vein to release the thyroid gland and retract it "up" (anteromedially), so you can access the pharyngoesophagus. In your approach, you will sequentially encounter and divide three structures – the middle thyroid vein, the inferior thyroid artery, and the omohyoid muscle (Fig. 29.5). The middle thyroid vein comes directly off the internal jugular and goes into the thyroid gland. Once this is divided, the thyroid gland can be pulled more medially. Next, gently retract

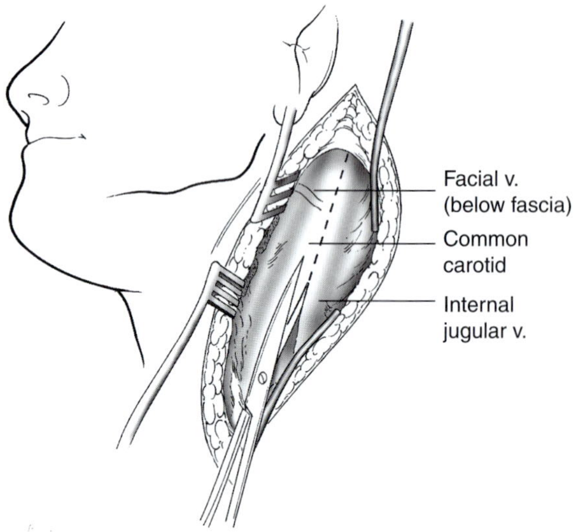

Fig. 29.4 Open the carotid sheath over the internal jugular vein and identify the facial vein

the carotid laterally and you will see the inferior thyroid artery, a branch of the thyrocervical trunk (from the subclavian artery), coursing horizontally posterior to the carotid and entering the posterolateral aspect of the thyroid. Divide this. Note: The inferior thyroid artery is another crucial landmark as it leads you

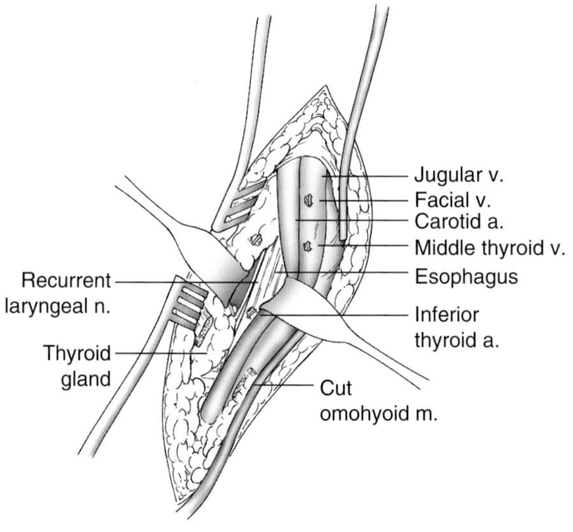

Fig. 29.5 Optimizing exposure of the cervical esophagus

directly to the recurrent laryngeal nerve. Use this opportunity to look for the nerve in the tracheoesophageal groove and avoid it. Finally, carry on inferiorly and divide the superior belly of the omohyoid muscle. You now have maximal exposure to the pharyngoesophagus and are ready to go.

With the thyroid gland retracted "up" and the carotid sheath "down," open the deep cervical fascia. Gentle. The fascia can be thin. You are looking for the longitudinal muscle fibers of the pharyngoesophagus. Technically, the cervical esophagus starts anatomically at the level of the cricoid. Whether your injury is to the pharynx or cervical esophagus is really inconsequential; finding the injury is what matters!!

Start by gross inspection. Identifying an injury in the pharyngoesophagus can be tricky given its lack of a shiny serosal layer, and you may not see a subtle hole in the muscle lying before you (particularly from a stab wound). Here is where the NG tube comes in. The NG tube provides a firm structure to feel for in an area which may have distorted tissue planes. Use your finger to feel for the NG tube. Use careful digital dissection posteriorly in the areolar tissue plane between the esophagus and the spine (Fig. 29.6). Remember the recurrent laryngeal nerve lies anterior to the esophagus in the tracheoesophageal groove, so it is much safer to work posteriorly. Keep your eye on the nerve and avoid it. You can basically hook around the entire esophagus with this blunt maneuver. To avoid injury to the recurrent laryngeal nerves and the membranous trachea, dissect very carefully along the anterior aspect of the esophagus.

Next, utilize air via the NG tube to look for the injury. Have the anesthesiologist pull back the NG tube so that you can feel the tip. Bathe the area with saline and gently push air into the NG tube. The area that bubbles is injured. If you still cannot find the hole, then we recommend intraoperative endoscopy to look for the injury from the inside. While rigid esophagoscopy was traditionally used, we have found flexible endoscopy (a more familiar technique) to be extremely efficacious. Methylene blue insertion in the NG tube is another option, but can color the field and make further

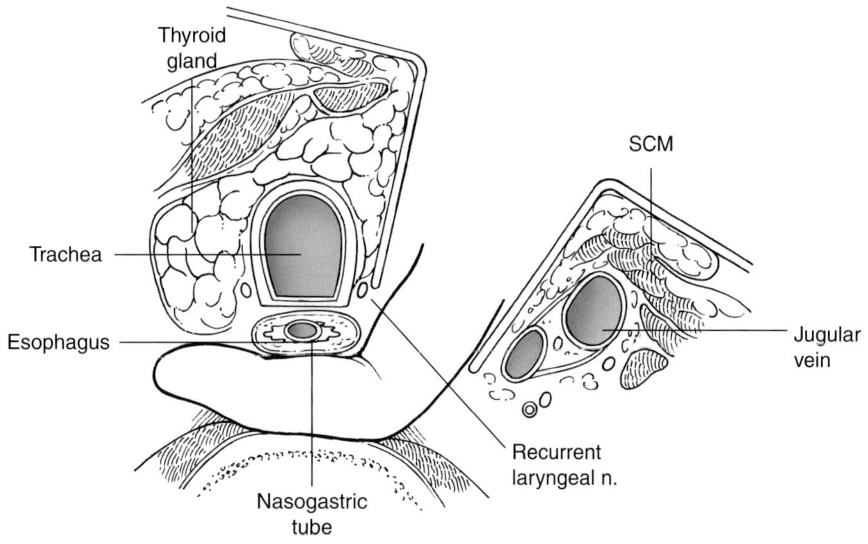

Fig. 29.6 Careful digital dissection posterior to the esophagus to aid in identifying injury

work more difficult; we are less keen on this option. Be diligent in your search for an injury and consider the possibility of a contralateral through and through injury that you might be missing. Make sure you have your trajectory accounted for before you leave the operating room.

With the injury identified, you are ready for repair. Debride esophageal wound edges completely and re-approximate only well-vascularized, healthy tissue. Repair the injury in one or two layers – equally efficacious. In a trauma situation, where time is important and there is often an element of tissue loss, we prefer a solid one-layer closure. Full-thickness, interrupted bites using a 3.0 absorbable monofilament suture is our preference. The submucosa is the strength layer and good mucosal apposition is critical. A second layer can be performed, but take care to avoid narrowing the lumen. We try and perform the repair over a 40-French Bougie to prevent this complication.

For simple injuries, sutures suffice. If the patient has ANY other injury to the surrounding area (laryngotracheal or vascular) or if you are concerned about the repair (tissue viability, tension, etc.), buttress it with a muscle flap! We strongly recommend placing muscle between combined esophageal and airway injuries to avoid a fistula. Use whatever muscle you can easily mobilize – omohyoid, another strap muscle, or sternal portion of the SCM – and make sure that it overlies the esophageal suture line.

Draining your repair is the final crucial step. If you do get a leak, you have it controlled. Leave a closed suction drain (we like the flat-fluted Jackson Pratt) adjacent to your repair. Bring it out away from the carotid sheath. Confirm hemostasis to avoid an urgent trip back to the operating room for a neck hematoma. Irrigate and close.

Note: This operation becomes very disconcerting when you just cannot do the repair. This may be because the patient is too hemodynamically compromised or because the pharyngoesophagus is too mangled. Your bailout option for a smaller pharyngoesophageal injury is to leave a drain. Remarkably, some of these fistulas will heal on their own, or additional procedures may be required once the patient has stabilized. The bailout for a highly destructive pharyngoesophageal injury is to staple across the distal cervical esophagus and construct an esophagostomy (spit fistula). Divide the esophagus as low as possible and bring your distal esophageal stump to a small skin incision. Be sure to also leave a drain. It is not pretty, but your goal is to prevent mediastinitis and save the patient.

29.4 Post-op Care and What to Do If the Repair Falls Apart

There is no gold standard or tried-and-true algorithm for the postoperative care of a pharyngoesophageal repair. Our preference is to leave the NG tube in place and keep the patient NPO for 3–5 days. At this point, we obtain a swallow study to evaluate the integrity of the repair and rule out a subclinical leak. If the repair is solid, we remove the NG tube and start clear liquids with advancement to a soft, dysphagia diet as tolerated.

We favor leaving the NG tube in place early on to provide enteral nutrition usually starting around postoperative day 2. Some authors prefer total parenteral nutrition (TPN) in the perioperative period. We have not found TPN necessary, or had an increase in complications, when feeding via a properly positioned NG tube. The NG tube is removed when the swallow study is negative. Broad-spectrum antibiotics are used empirically until the patient has no clinical signs of infection (afebrile, normal white cell count) and leak has been excluded by swallow study.

We feel the most critical aspect of postoperative care is the drain. The drain should be well secured and maintained until the swallow study confirms no leak and dysphagia diet tolerated for 1–2 days.

But what if there is a problem? Perioperative complications of penetrating pharyngoesophageal injury include neck abscess (and in the worst case, a descending infection leading to mediastinitis), salivary fistula, tracheoesophageal fistula, and swallowing dysfunction.

Neck infection is a complication occurring in both operative and nonoperative management and requires prompt open drainage to prevent descending progression. Madiba reported a single case of local sepsis (6% incidence) in 17 patients with contained cervical esophageal injury who were managed nonoperatively [3]. A multicenter study found the incidence of neck abscess to be 3.3%, esophageal fistula 3.8%, and tracheoesophageal fistula 1.9% in 211 patients with cervical esophageal injuries [2].

Winter and Weigelt reported cervical esophageal fistulas occurring in 9% of 46 penetrating cervical esophageal injuries [17]. In this study, all of the fistulas healed with nonoperative management. This study gave support to the widely practiced dictum that the vast majority of esophageal fistulas will heal on their own. Importantly, this is contingent upon control of local sepsis (which may necessitate opening of the surgical wound) and no distal obstruction. Of note, a much higher incidence of complications has been reported by Stanley who found that 22% of patients with a hypopharyngeal injury and 39% of patients with cervical esophageal injury developed either a neck infection that required drainage or a postsurgical salivary fistula [15]. This group did not discuss their management of these problems, but did report that one of two tracheoesophageal fistulas healed spontaneously at 3 weeks time, and the other required a sternocleidomastoid muscle interposition flap [15].

The consensus is that a majority of esophageal fistulas (to the skin or even to the trachea) will heal spontaneously, but this may require a period of prolonged restricted oral intake. In recent years, endoscopically positioned self-expanding stents have been used to successfully treat iatrogenic, mid-thoracic esophageal perforations. The stent excludes the injury while the body repairs itself; the stent is extracted in approximately one month's time and the patient restudied. Recent literature has now echoed its potential in penetrating esophageal injury [18] and injury to the cervical esophagus [19]. A caveat is that the stent needs to be positioned inferiorly to the upper esophageal sphincter to avoid patient discomfort. We recently managed a large posttraumatic cervical esophageal fistula successfully with a covered plastic stent. Thus, we recommend stenting be considered as an option in a case of persistent fistula.

29.5 At the End of the Day

While it may not be the most familiar or hospitable place for a penetrating injury, expeditious diagnosis and management of a pharyngoesophageal injury is generally very satisfying as the surgeon knows he/she has (hopefully) staved off a future, lethal mediastinitis. Familiarity with the neck exploration as we have described here can aid in success. And with the knowledge that this area can be forgiving as long as postoperative management is vigilant, we hope that you breathe easier the next time this injury rolls through the door.

Important Points

- Initial assessment of penetrating pharyngoesophageal trauma involves history, physical examination, and CTA (if available). A swallow study or endoscopy should confirm or exclude an injury in the stable patient.
- Small, contained pharyngeal injuries can be managed nonoperatively.
- Patient positioning is key – unless there is concern for an unstable cervical spine, place a shoulder roll and turn the head away from the side of injury. If it is unclear which side is more involved, approach the esophagus through the left neck.
- Stay along the anterior border of the sternocleidomastoid muscle and retract it laterally to gain exposure to the neck.
- Open the carotid sheath along the internal jugular vein and ligate the facial vein.
- Retract the carotid sheath down and the thyroid gland up to find the esophagus. You will divide the middle thyroid vein, the inferior thyroid artery, and the omohyoid muscle to maximize this exposure.
- Place an NG tube to facilitate finding the pharyngoesophagus by feel. Find the injury by looking for bubbles. Be vigilant to avoid a missed injury.
- Debride injury to healthy edges and repair it in one or two layers – no tension, over a Bougie if you can.
- Mobilize a muscle flap and interpose this tissue any time you create two suture lines or are concerned about a repair.
- Leave a drain until the swallow study confirms no leak and the patient is tolerating a diet.
- If the repair fails, the vast majority of fistulas will heal spontaneously (or consider use of a temporary stent).

References

1. Demetriades D, Theodorou D et al (1997) Evaluation of penetrating injuries of the neck: prospective study of 223 patients. World J Surg 21:41–48
2. Demetriades D, Velmahos G et al (2001) Cervical pharyngoesophageal and laryngotracheal injuries. World J Surg 25:1044–1048

3. Madiba TE, Muckart DJJ (2003) Penetrating injuries to the cervical oesophagus: is routine exploration mandatory? Ann R Coll Surg Engl 85:162–166
4. Asensio JA, Berne J et al (1997) Penetrating esophageal injuries: time interval of safety for preoperative evaluation – how long is safe? J Trauma 43(2):319–324
5. Asensio JA, Chahwan S et al (2001) Penetrating esophageal injuries: multicenter study of the American Association for the Surgery of Trauma. J Trauma 50(2):289–296
6. Tisherman SA, Bokhari F et al (2008) Clinical practice guideline: penetrating zone II neck trauma. J Trauma 64(5):1392–1405
7. Gracias VH, Reilly PM, Philpott J et al (2001) Computed tomography in the evaluation of penetrating neck trauma: a preliminary study. Arch Surg 136:1231–1235
8. Gonzalez RP, Falimirski M et al (2003) Penetrating zone II neck injury: does dynamic computed tomographic scan contribute to the diagnostic sensitivity of physical examination for surgically significant injury? A prospective blinded study. J Trauma 54:61–65
9. Inaba K, Munera F et al (2006) Prospective evaluation of screening multislice helical computed tomographic angiography in the initial evaluation of penetrating neck injuries. J Trauma 61(1):144–149
10. Nel L, Jones LW, Hardcastle TC (2009) Imaging the oesophagus after penetrating cervical trauma using water-soluble contrast alone: simple, cost-effective and accurate. Emerg Med J 26:106–108
11. Weigelt JA, Tal ER, Snyder WH III et al (1987) Diagnosis of penetrating cervical esophageal injuries. Am J Surg 154: 619–622
12. Armstrong WB, Detar TR, Stanley RB (1994) Diagnosis and management of external penetrating cervical esophageal injuries. Ann Otol Rhinol Laryngol 103:863–871
13. Srinivasan R, Haywood T, Horwitz B et al (2000) Role of flexible endoscopy in the evaluation of possible esophageal trauma after penetrating injuries. Am J Gastroenterol 95: 1725–1729
14. Flowers JL, Graham SM et al (1996) Flexible endoscopy for the diagnosis of esophageal trauma. J Trauma 40(2): 261–265
15. Stanley RB, Armstrong WB et al (1997) Management of external penetrating injuries to the hypopharyngeal-cervical esophageal funnel. J Trauma 42(4):675–679
16. Yugueros P, Sarmiento JM, Garcia AF et al (1996) Conservative management of penetrating hypopharyngeal wounds. J Trauma 40(2):267–269
17. Winter RP, Weigelt JA (1990) Cervical esophageal trauma. Incidence and cause of esophageal fistulas. Arch Surg 123(7):849–851
18. Bazerbashi S, Villaquiran J, Bennett M et al (2008) Stented esophageal transfixion injury. Ann Thorac Surg 86:1367–1369
19. Buscaglia JM, Sherwood JT, Jagannath SB (2007) Endoscopic treatment of a cervical esophageal dissection using a polyflex self-expanding plastic stent. Pract Gastroenterol 31:68–71

Carotid, Jugular and Vertebral Blood Vessel Injuries

30

Dirk Le Roux and Martin Veller

- Trauma to the neck is dangerous and has a high mortality and morbidity.
- Penetrating neck injuries remain challenging, as there are a number of important structures in a small volume. Injury to any of these structures frequently is also not readily apparent.
- The cervical blood vessels are involved in 25% of patients with head or neck trauma, and carotid artery injury constitutes 5–10% of all arterial injuries. The reported mortality for carotid injuries ranges from 10% to 31% with permanent neurological deficit ranging from 16% to 60% and remains high despite advances in diagnosis and treatment.
- The management of penetrating neck trauma has undergone considerable development in recent years. In the 1980s, a policy of routine exploration was slowly replaced by a policy of selective exploration. More recently, treatment strategies have been refined by the introduction of accurate diagnostic modalities in the stable patient (mostly rapid multi-slice CT scanning) and the use of endovascular therapies.

Caveat: Severe vascular injury after neck trauma can be present even in the absence of clinical signs. Liberal Duplex Doppler or angiography after penetrating trauma when cervical vessel injuries cannot be ruled out is indicated. Associated injuries of the cervical spine, airway, and digestive tract must always be considered.

Always stabilise the neck of patients in all types of severe cervical trauma until the entire spectrum of injuries is known.

If the patient is stable, angiography should always be performed in penetrating injuries to zones I and III.

Duplex doppler or angiography should be performed (if available) in order to select between conservative, endovascular and surgical management.

The surgical anatomy of the superior mediastinum and neck is shown in Fig. 30.1, demonstrating the proximity of the vessels and nerves around the aero-digestive tract (Fig. 30.1).

The neck contains many vital structures located in a small volume.

- The important anterior structures of the neck lie deep to the platysma and as a result only injuries that have penetrated through this muscle are clinically significant.
- As a result of the aero-digestive tracts position in the midline and its close relationship to the major blood vessels in the neck injuries, crossing the midline usually causes a greater degree of damage.
- The sternocleidomastoid muscle divides the posterior and anterior triangles of the neck. Within the anterior triangle lie the aero-digestive tract and the major blood vessels supplying the head and face

D. Le Roux (✉) • M. Veller
Division of Vascular Surgery, Charlotte Maxeke Johannesburg Academic Hospital, University of the Witwatersrand Medical School, 7, York Road, Parktown 2193, Johannesburg, South Africa
e-mail: leroux@vascare.co.za; acv@icon.co.za

G.C. Velmahos et al. (eds.), *Penetrating Trauma*,
DOI 10.1007/978-3-642-20453-1_30, © Springer-Verlag Berlin Heidelberg 2012

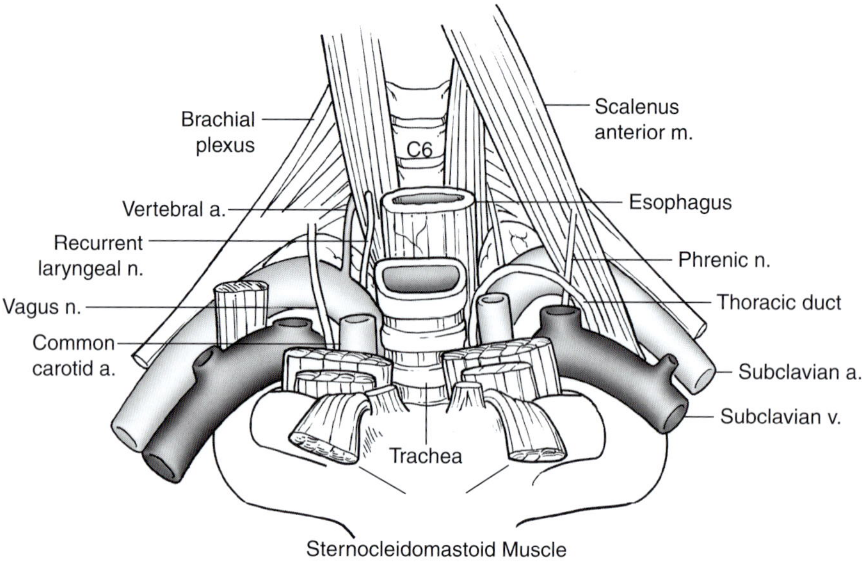

Fig. 30.1 The surgical anatomy of the superior mediastinum and neck with its proximity of the vessels and nerves around the aero-digestive tract

while the posterior triangle contains the nerves and blood vessels to the upper limbs.

- The area of the neck posterior to the cervical vertebral body and the scalene muscles is composed mainly of muscle, bone, and other non-vital structures. The spinal cord is encased in the cervical spine which usually can only be penetrated by gunshots.
- The neck is divided into three zones using anatomic landmarks (Fig. 30.2). The management of injuries in these zones varies due to the vital structures that each zone contains and the manner in which access can be gained.
  - Zone I is the area between the clavicle/suprasternal notch and the cricoid cartilage, encompassing the thoracic outlet structures (Fig. 30.2a). The proximal common carotid arteries, internal jugular veins, vertebral arteries and veins, and subclavian arteries and veins and the trachea, oesophagus, thoracic duct, and thymus are located here (Fig. 30.2b).
  - Zone II is the area between the cricoid cartilage and the angle of the mandible. It contains the internal and external carotid arteries, jugular veins, pharynx, larynx, oesophagus, cranial, sympathetic and recurrent laryngeal nerve, spinal cord, trachea, thyroid, and parathyroid glands.
  - Zone III is the area that lies between the angle of the mandible and the base of the skull. It contains the distal extra-cranial internal carotid and vertebral arteries, the uppermost segments of the jugular veins and a variety of cranial nerves.

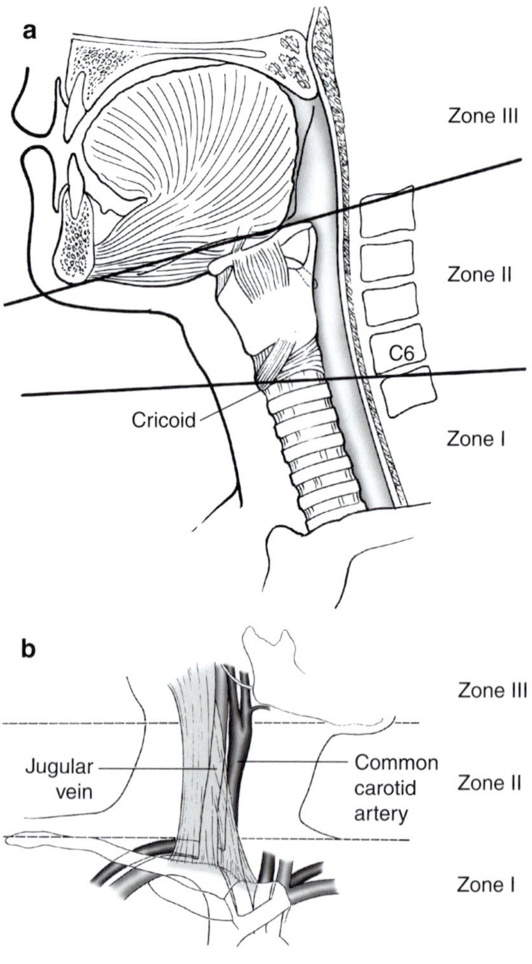

Fig. 30.2 (**a**) Zones of the neck, projected onto the cervical spine. (**b**) Zones of the neck and vascular structures

- Tight fascial compartments of neck structures may limit external haemorrhage from vascular injuries, but it may increase the risk of airway compromise by an expanding haematoma.

30.1 Pathophysiology

Wounding instruments have specific characteristics that affect surgical findings. Two factors in the mechanism of injury or kinematics in penetrating neck trauma determine the extent of damage to the tissue.

- Weapon characteristics
  - Tissue injury results from either a direct impact by the penetrating projectile or tissue displacement from temporary cavitation caused by high-velocity projectiles.
  - Stab wounds typically have a 10% higher rate of negative exploration than injuries from projectiles.
  - Secondary missiles in gunshots frequently add to the injury severity.
- Location of injury and human tissues involved.
  - Wound sites and, if present the wounding agent (retained bullet or stabbing implement), provide an indication of the likely injury complex.
  - Implied wound tract, particularly if it crosses the midline, is of particular value.

Penetrating injuries may cause partial or complete transection with thrombosis of the vessel or pseudoaneurysm. Pseudoaneurysm may have an acute or delayed onset with progressive enlargement causing compression of the surrounding structures. An arterio-venous fistula may develop if there is adjacent perforation of an artery and vein and is often accompanied by a pseudoaneurysm. Intimal injury can be caused by a high-velocity missile shock wave. The vessel is macroscopically intact with minimal bruising, but on opening the vessel, there is an intimal tear with or without a superimposed thrombosis.

The potential neurological consequences of vascular injuries are caused by hypoperfusion (caused by transected or thrombosed vessels) or embolisation from intimal injuries, pseudoaneurysm or AV fistulae.

30.2 Clinical Signs

Rapidly expanding cervical haematoma, absent carotid pulse a bruit or thrill and external bleeding are hard signs indicative of vascular injury. Soft signs which may indicate an vascular injury and warrant further investigation include active or previous bleeding from wounds of the neck or the pharynx, a superficial temporal artery pulse deficit, ipsilateral Horner's sign, IX–XII cranial nerve dysfunction, and a widened mediastinum. Neurological deficit may be present, but obscured due to concomitant head injury, shock or the use of alcohol or drugs. Up to 50% of patients with established blunt injury caused by cavitation to the carotid and vertebral arteries could initially be asymptomatic, but 43–58% of these will eventually develop neurological signs.

30.2.1 Diagnostics in Stable Patient: CT Scan or Equivalent

- Patients with active bleeding and a compromised airway require immediate exploration. Occasionally, such bleeding can be controlled with insertion of a Foley's catheter and thereby converting this extremely dangerous setting to a semi-elective one.
- Haemodynamically stable patients with a patent airway who have the following signs should undergo further appropriate investigations:
  - In gunshot injuries:
    Proximity to vessels
    Evidence of crossing the midline
    Bleeding that has been controlled by Foley's catheter or similar manoeuvre
  - In stab wounds:
    Wound penetrating platysma and with bleeding that has been controlled by Foley's catheter or similar manoeuvre.
- The diagnostic modalities used are:
  - Duplex Doppler examination is useful for investigating zone II vascular injuries. Duplex scanning, however, has its limitations in zones I and II due to anatomical constraints.
  - Multislice contrast CT and CTA has replaced arteriography in recent years as it not only demonstrates vascular anatomy well but also gives substantial additional information about other structures in particular those of the aero-digestive tract. A review by Woo and colleagues reports that the use of CTA is associated with less operative exploration, less negative explorations, and reduced use of invasive studies, such as conventional angiography. Physical examination

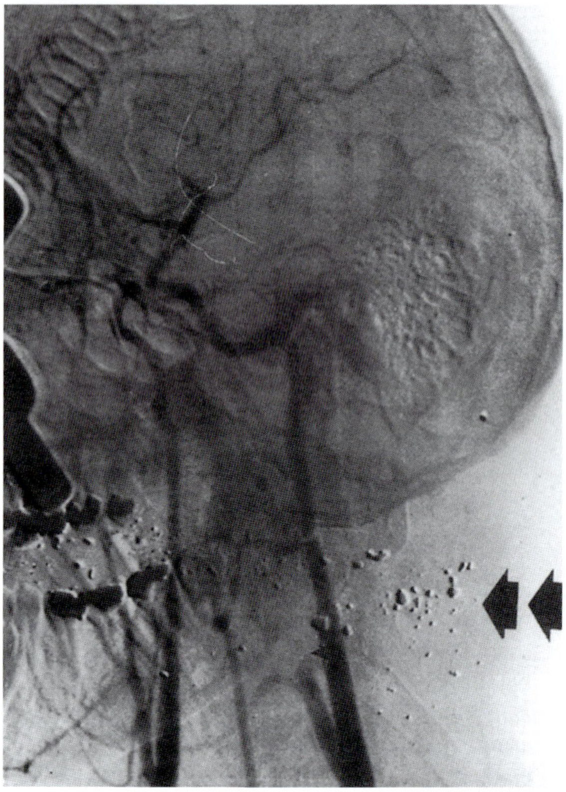

Fig. 30.3 CTA has replaced angiography as the initial study of choice in the vascular evaluation of a neck injury (here in patient with fragmented gunshot neck)

findings supplemented by CTA should have a prominent role in the selective management of penetrating neck injuries. CTA has replaced angiography as the initial study of choice in the vascular evaluation of a neck injury (Fig. 30.3).

- A CT scan of the brain should be obtained to investigate patients with associated head trauma, bone injuries of the spine and skull and those with neurologic deficit. A CT scan of the brain is a good predictor of outcome: Patients who have an infarct on initial CT on admission have a high mortality with poor chance of neurological recovery compared to those patients who have a normal CT on admission.
- Arch angiography remains a good alternative if CTA is not available for the diagnosis of cervico-mediastinal and zone 3 vascular injuries. It gives information regarding suspected injuries to other vessels and evaluation for possible endovascular treatment. Certain centres that have in-house angiographers may perform angiography for injuries in zone I and zone III despite hypotension or haemorrhage. Angiography remains the criterion standard for defining arterial anatomy and injury complexes, with an accuracy close to 100% (Arteriography demonstrates a low yield in asymptomatic patients). Arteriography usually is performed using a digital subtraction angiography (DSA) technique that reduces the amount of contrast required and yields a superior computer-manipulated image for evaluation.
- MR angiography may be valuable in carotid artery and vertebral artery dissection but only in the stable patient.
- Cervical anteroposterior and lateral radiography with bullet markers is used to evaluate for vertebral bony injury; retained foreign bodies; and foreign body deformity, location, size, and number.

30.2.2 Operative Approach in Unstable Patient

Management in the Emergency Department:

ATLS guidelines should be followed for severe cervical vascular injuries. Thus, airway with cervical spine control and respiration have first priority, followed by control of bleeding. Control of bleeding is best achieved by manual compression or application of a Foley's catheter (see later) applied directly to the bleeding site. Blind application of haemostatic clamps should not be attempted because of the risk of injuries to blood vessels as well as to other structures.

The concept of hypotensive resuscitation should be adhered to as hypertension may increase bleeding and also induce progression of a dissection, while severe hypotension will increase the risk for thrombosis and decreased cerebral perfusion.

Intubation should be performed in such a manner as to avoid coughing and increase in blood pressure, which might dislodge thrombus and thus cause haemorrhage or embolisation. Take care not to flex the patient's neck at the intubation because of the risk of associated cervical vertebral fractures or dislocations. The intubation might also be difficult because a haematoma might cause compression of the trachea. Emergency tracheotomy or cricothyroidotomy is then the only alternative, but it may also be complicated by the deranged anatomy and risk of bleeding. The risk of profuse and uncontrolled haemorrhage is greatest if the haematoma is located on the anterior triangle of the neck because the tamponade will be lost when the pretracheal fascia is incised. By using liberal intubation early on and under controlled conditions, loss of airway could be avoided.

30.2.2.1 After Initial Rescuscitation: What Now?

1. Injuries in zone II not penetrating the platysma need no further examination.
2. Immediate operation is indicated for unstable patients with active bleeding not responsive to resuscitation or with a rapidly expanding haematoma or airway obstruction, irrespective of anatomical zone.
3. All others require further diagnostic evaluation to determine whether critical structures have been injured. If angiography or high-quality duplex ultrasound is not available, injuries in zone II need to be surgically explored.

We recommend repair in all patients with penetrating carotid injuries when there is still evidence of prograde flow and the patient has no major neurological symptoms.

For minor injuries to the carotid artery, including those with small but adherent intimal flaps, defects, or pseudoaneurysms <5 mm in size, repair is recommended in symptomatic patients. If the patient is asymptomatic and there is no ongoing active bleeding, a conservative approach has proven to be a safe alternative; however, the patient needs to be followed on an inpatient basis for a couple of days to monitor for the appearance of neurological symptoms. We Employ Duplex Doppler examination repeatedly. Anticoagulation therapy and antiplatelet therapy are routinely initiated.

Management of significant carotid artery injury existing with major neurological deficit and coma is controversial. Some suggest only observation and palliation, especially in patients with CT-verified cerebral infarction, because of the poor prognosis. We advocate repair and are aware of the risk of converting an ischaemic infarct into a haemorrhagic infarct. This strategy however requires extensive experience in carotid surgery and/or endovascular intervention. Most patients with carotid artery injuries are best managed by primary arterial repair, regardless of neurological status. We consider neurological deficit only a contraindication to surgical repair in case of a deeply comatose patient with a dense neurologic deficit, arterial occlusion and a large infarct on cerebral CT scan; these patients have poor outcome regardless of treatment. All other patients with associated neurological deficit would benefit from arterial repair with improved mortality and final neurologic status.

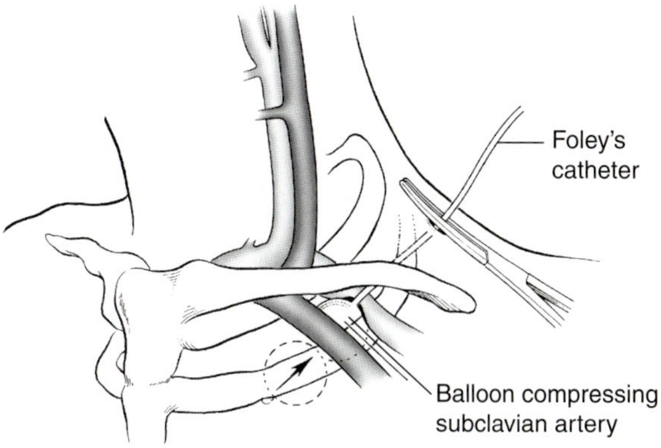

Fig. 30.4 In the unstable patient, a Foley's catheter extraluminally or a Fogarty catheter (intraluminally) can be utilised to tamponade bleeding temporarily while waiting to move the patient to the operating theatre

When the carotid artery is occluded and there are no neurological symptoms, we recommend observation and anticoagulation with heparin and antiplatelet therapy followed by 3–6 months of an oral anticoagulant and antiplatelet irrespective of the type of trauma.

In the unstable patient, a Foley's catheter extraluminally or a Fogarty catheter (intraluminally) can be utilised to tamponade bleeding temporarily while waiting to move the patient to the operating theatre (Fig. 30.4). As a generalised dictum, a liberal sternotomy and clamping of the proximal neck vessels in the upper mediastinum is a safe method to gain proximal vessel control.

South African experience from large series suggests that all penetrations beyond the platysma should at least be evaluated if not explored due to the high morbidity and mortality associated with missed injuries, not only of the vital arteries but also of the aero-digestive tract.

30.3 Operative Technique

Remember that vascular control may be problematic in zone I (proximal control) and zone III (distal control). This consequently leads to the higher mortality rates in patients with vascular injuries in these neck zones.

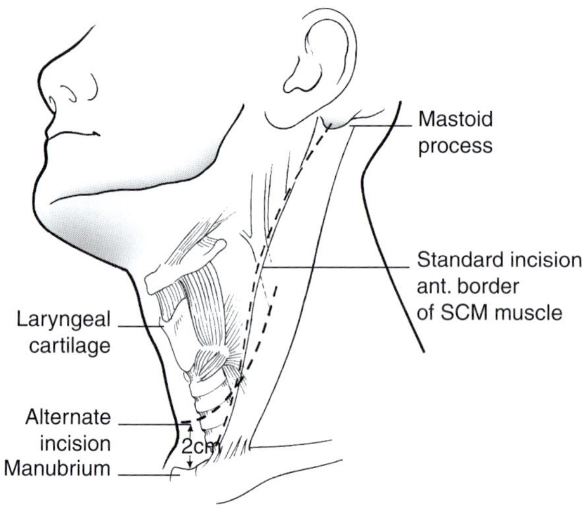

Fig. 30.5 Standard approach to the common carotid bifurcation

General principles of management are:

1. In order to have good exposure, be sure to have the patient in a supine position with a bolster between the scapulae and the neck extended and the head rotated to the contralateral side. The patient must be draped to allow access from the base of the scull to the xiphisternum.
2. Zone II injuries are explored by the standard incision overlying the anterior border of the sternocleidomastoid muscle. Figure 30.5 shows the steps of standard exposure of the common carotid bifurcation.
3. Zone 1 injuries usually require a median sternotomy unless endovascular or similar control of vascular structures can be achieved.
4. Various techniques have been described to improve exposure of the distal internal carotid artery in zone 3 injuries by dislocating the jaw and detaching the Sternocleidomastoid muscle from its insertion on the mastoid process and resecting the styloid process. We use endovascular techniques like over-the-wire Fogarty balloons in conjunction with open surgery.
5. We only make use of intra-luminal shunts during complicated repairs of the internal carotid artery.
6. The external carotid artery can be safely ligated if the internal carotid artery is patent.
7. Internal carotid artery ligation is only allowed when the distal vessel is thrombosed with no back bleeding following extraction of thrombus.
8. Minor venous injuries can be managed by lateral suture repair, but complex venous repair is not indicated as there is a high occlusion rate, and it increases the magnitude of the operative procedure. Ligation of a single jugular vein can be performed without significant sequelae.
9. Protect the vascular repair in the presence of associated injuries to the trachea and oesophagus, by soft tissue interposition (sternocleidomastoid muscle).

An incision anterior and parallel to the anterior border of the sternocleidomastoid muscle is recommended. The incision can be extended dorsal to the ear and down to the sternal notch. As previously stated, preparations need to have been made to allow elongation of the incision into a median sternotomy in order to obtain proximal control of the neck vessels.

A transverse or collar-type incision can be performed for suspected injuries traversing the cervical region, providing exposure to both sides and obviating the need for bilateral neck incisions.

The specific injuries described below must be confirmed and treated during neck exploration. Note that multiple structures frequently are injured from penetrating neck injury because of the numerous vital structures that are contained in a small area.

Carotid artery injuries are the most common, with an incidence of approximately 9%. They also pose one of the most immediate life-threatening situations. The objective of surgery is to arrest haemorrhage yet maintain cerebral blood flow and preserve neurologic function. Arteriorrhaphy, vein patch, or interposition repair with autogenous reversed saphenous vein graft can be performed to repair the injury. Arterial repair is shown to have lower morbidity and mortality rates than ligation. The presence of neurologic deficits, coma, and shock, especially preoperatively, are poor prognostic signs but are not absolute contraindications for carotid artery repair. Carotid ligation is advocated in patients who are comatose with no evidence of antegrade flow in the internal carotid artery. Ligation also can be an option when uncontrollable haemorrhage is present and temporary shunt placement is technically difficult.

Jugular vein injury repair is contingent on the condition of the patient. Repair can be performed by simple lateral closure, resection and reanastomosis, or saphenous vein graft reconstruction, particularly the internal jugular. Repairing at least one side is very important if both internal jugular veins are injured. The external jugular vein can be ligated without any adverse effects.

30.4 Technical Tips

30.4.1 Surgical Exposure of the Carotid Arteries

After the skin has been incised, subcutaneous fat and the platysma is divided. The sternocleidomastoid muscle is retracted laterally, and a dissection plane anterior to the muscle is identified. The next structure overlying the carotid medially is the facial vein and its confluence to the internal jugular vein (Fig. 30.6). This is suture-ligated and divided and is usually a very good landmark because it is located just above the carotid bifurcation (Beware – the hypoglossal nerve may be adherent to the posterior surface of this vein). Dividing this vein allows posterior retraction of the internal jugular vein and exposure of the common carotid and its bifurcation. When preparing the carotid arteries, care must be taken to avoid manipulation of the vessel to avoid the risk of embolisation to the brain. Vessel loops are applied, and the most cranial clamp is applied first to avoid embolisation when the more proximal parts are clamped. Important structures to protect are the hypoglossal and vagus nerves. The former usually crosses over the internal carotid artery 2–3 cm cranial to the bifurcation and is best exposed after cranial retraction of the digastric muscle. The vagus nerve runs parallel, posterior and between to the common carotid artery and jugular vein. The sympathetic trunk runs posterior to the carotid sheath. The ansa cervicalis, often located obliquely over the carotid bifurcation, can be divided to facilitate exposure. We use local heparinised saline solution and not general heparinisation.

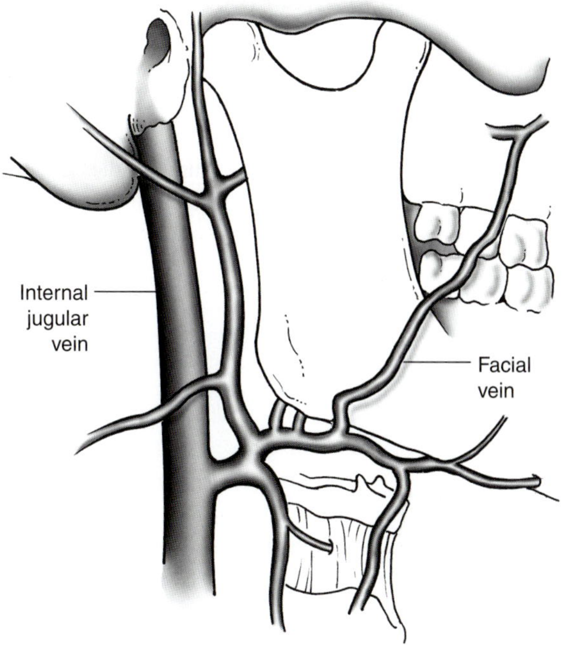

Fig. 30.6 The next structure overlying the carotid medially is the facial vein and its confluence to the internal jugular vein

30.4.1.1 Vertebral Artery Injuries

The incidence of vertebral artery injury is low with the reported incidence in penetrating neck trauma ranging from 1% to 7%. Gunshot wounds are the most common mechanism of injury.

The majority of patients with vertebral artery injuries have associated injuries of the cervical spine, spinal cord, other vascular structures in the neck or the aero-digestive tract. Helical CT angiography has a high sensitivity and specificity for detecting vertebral arterial injury and is being used increasingly in penetrating neck trauma.

Angiographic embolisation is the treatment of choice in the majority of patients with vertebral artery injuries, as access to the vertebral artery may be difficult and time consuming (Fig. 30.7). Operative management is only indicated for severe active bleeding or when embolisation has failed. Haemodynamically stable patients with a thrombosed vertebral artery do not need any intervention.

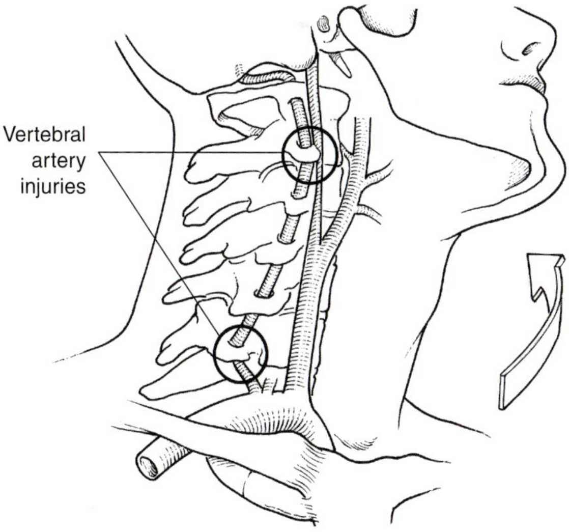

Fig. 30.7 Exposure of the vertebral artery in its canal may be difficult and time consuming

30.4.1.2 Postoperative Procedure

Vascular injuries are managed postoperatively to ensure haemorrhage is stopped and blood supply and drainage to affected organs is adequate. Continually, monitor the neurologic status of the patient. Follow-up angiographic and Doppler ultrasound studies can be performed to evaluate suspected complications with the repaired vessels.

Important Points

1. The neck contains a vast amount of vital structures in a small space.
2. This region illustrates the importance of the stepwise approach used in ATLS resuscitation as it contains the aero-digestive tract and Cervical spine (A), the respiratory system is in close proximity (B), major blood vessels (C) supplying the brain (D). It is important to fully expose the neck anteriorly and posteriorly to asses the extent of the injuries (E).
3. The unstable patient should be explored immediately while the stable patient allows for further investigation.
4. Early airway control is essential as this may be lost at any stage.
5. Proper positioning of the patient allows for adequate exposure of the structures in this region.
6. The use of endovascular techniques to gain proximal and distal control has introduced very useful adjuncts in operating in this field – the so-called hybrid approach.
7. Endovascular techniques are also useful in the definitive treatment of injuries to the vessels – both in accessible and inaccessible regions.

Suggested Reading

Bowley DMG, Degiannis E, Goosen J et al (2002) Penetrating vascular trauma in Johannesburg, South Africa. Surg Clin North Am 82:221–336

Corr P, Abdool-Carim AT, Robbs J (1999) Colour-flow ultrasound in the detection of penetrating vascular injuries of the neck. S Afr Med J 80:644–646

Kumar SR, Weaver FA, Yellin AE (2001) Cervical vascular injuries: carotid and jugular venous injuries. Surg Clin North Am 81:1331–1344

Van Marle J, Le Roux D (2009) Vascular trauma. In: Beard JD, Gaines PA (eds) Vascular and endovascular surgery: a companion to specialist surgical practice, 4th edn. Saunders Elsevier, Chapter 9, pp 147–166

Navsaria P, Thoma M, Nicol A (2006) Foley catheter balloon tamponade for life-threatening hemorrhage in penetrating neck trauma. World J Surg 30(7):1265–1268

Rezende-Neto J, Marques AC, Guedes LJ, Teixeira LC (2008) Damage control principles applied to penetrating neck and mandibular injury. J Trauma 64(4):1142–1143

Robbs JV (1989) Injuries to the vessels of the neck and superior mediastinum. In: Champion HR, Robbs JV, Trunky D (eds) Rob and Smiths operative surgery, 4th edn. Butterworths, London, pp 529–538

Robbs JV (2001) Basic principles in the surgical management of vascular trauma. In: Greenhalgh RM (ed) Vascular and endovascular techniques, 4th edn. WB Saunders Ltd., London, pp 455–465

Robbs J (2003) Penetrating injury to the blood vessels of the neck and mediasternum. In: Branchereai A, Jacobs M (eds) Vascular emergencies. Futura, New York, pp 39–48

Woo K, Magner DP, Wilson MT, Margulies DR (2005) CT angiography in penetrating neck trauma reduces the need for operative neck exploration. Am Surg 71(9):754–758

Part III

Surgical Strategies in Penetrating Trauma to the Chest

Penetrating Trauma to the Subclavian Vessels

31

Daniel Francois Du Toit

The management of penetrating injuries of the subclavian vessels presents a considerable challenge to even the most experienced surgeon [1]. Complex surgical exposures required for conventional open repair contribute to a high morbidity and mortality [2]. The contemporary management of these injuries consists of a combination of open and endovascular surgery. The availability of local expertise, resources, surgeon preference, and clinical presentation will dictate the management of individual cases. A comprehensive knowledge of the anatomy of the subclavian vessels [3] is essential for the selection and execution of individualized patient management.

31.1 Applied Surgical Anatomy (Fig. 31.1)

The subclavian artery: On the right side, the subclavian artery arises from the innominate artery behind the sternoclavicular joint; on the left, it comes directly from the arch of the aorta. Each subclavian artery is divided into three parts for descriptive purposes. The first part extends from its origin to the medial border of the scalenus anterior muscle, the second part lies behind this muscle, and the third part extends from its lateral border to the outer aspect of the first rib where it becomes the axillary artery. The first parts of the right and left subclavian arteries differ with respect to course, length, and relation to neighboring structures and require separate descriptions. The second and third parts of the two arteries are essentially similar and will be described together.

First part of the right subclavian artery: Arising from the innominate artery behind the right sternoclavicular joint, it passes in a supero-lateral direction to the medial border of the scalenus anterior muscle. The extent to which it ascends above the clavicle varies. This can influence the ease with which it can be accessed via a supraclavicular incision. It is covered anteriorly by the skin, superficial fascia, platysma muscle, deep fascia, the clavicular head of the sternocleidomastoid muscle, and the sternohyoid and sternothyroid muscles. It is crossed by the internal jugular and vertebral veins, the vagus nerve, and a loop of the sympathetic trunk. Posterior and inferior lie the pleura and apex of the right lung as well as the sympathetic trunk and first thoracic vertebra. The recurrent nerve winds around its inferior and posterior aspect.

First part of the left subclavian artery: This arises from the aortic arch posterior and lateral to the left common carotid artery and ascends to the root of the neck and then inclines laterally to the medial border of the scalenus anterior muscle. Its anterior relations are similar to the right side and posteriorly lies the esophagus and thoracic duct. Medially lie the esophagus, trachea, thoracic duct, and left recurrent nerve. Laterally, the left pleura and lung are to be found.

Second part of the subclavian artery: This lies behind the scalenus anterior muscle, is short, and is the most superiorly located part of the vessel. The phrenic nerve runs from lateral to medial over the muscle. Posterior to the vessel are the scalenus medius muscle

D.F. Du Toit
Department of Surgical Sciences,
Tygerberg Academic Hospital, University of Stellenbosch,
P.O. Box 19063, Tygerberg 7505, South Africa
e-mail: vascular@netactive.co.za

G.C. Velmahos et al. (eds.), *Penetrating Trauma*,
DOI 10.1007/978-3-642-20453-1_31, © Springer-Verlag Berlin Heidelberg 2012

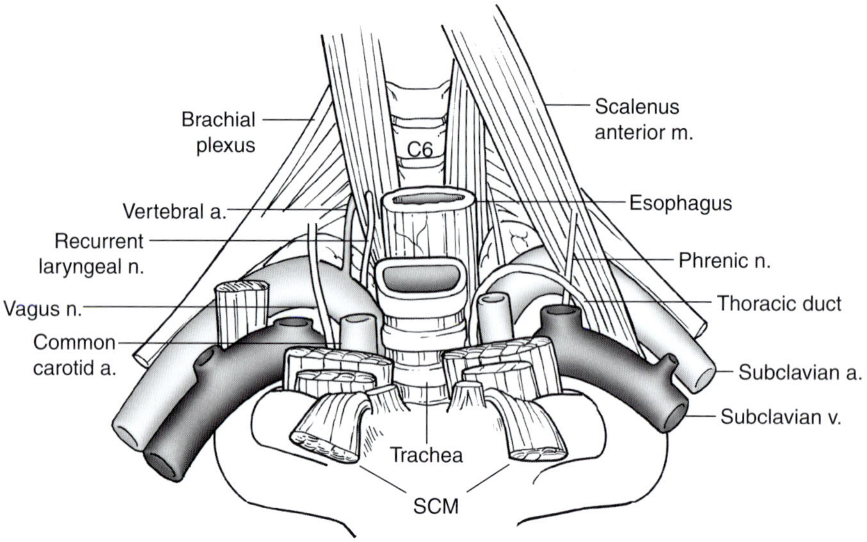

Fig. 31.1 The anatomy of the thoracic outlet showing the relations of the subclavian vessels

and pleura, superior the brachial plexus, and inferior the pleura. The subclavian vein lies below and in front of the artery, separated from it by the scalenus anterior muscle.

Third part of the subclavian artery: This part runs in an infero-lateral direction from the lateral border of the scalenus anterior muscle to the outer aspect of the first rib where it becomes the axillary artery. It is covered by the skin, platysma muscle, supraclavicular nerves, and the deep cervical fascia. The external jugular vein and tributaries crosses anterior and medial to it. The distal part of the artery lies behind the clavicle and the subclavius muscle, with the subclavian vein anterior and at a slightly lower level than the artery. Posteriorly lies the brachial plexus which intervenes between the artery and the scalenus medius muscle. Superiorly and to the lateral side are the upper trunks of the brachial plexus and the omohyoid muscle and inferiorly the first rib.

31.1.1 Branches of the Subclavian Artery

First part: Vertebral artery
  Internal mammary artery
  Thyrocervical trunk
Second part: Costocervical trunk
Third part: Dorsal scapular artery

31.1.2 Anatomical Anomalies

- The right subclavian artery can arise as a separate trunk from the arch of the aorta as a first, second, third, or last branch of the arch.
- If it arises as the last branch, it passes from left to right behind the trachea, esophagus, and right carotid or sometimes between the trachea and esophagus.
- It can pass anterior to the scalenus muscle, perforate it, and can ascend as high as 4 cm above the clavicle.
- The left subclavian artery generally does not reach as high in the neck as the right.

31.1.3 The Subclavian Vein

The subclavian vein is a continuation of the axillary vein, extending from the outer aspect of the first rib to the manubrial head of the clavicle. Here it unites with the internal jugular vein to form the innominate vein behind the manubrio-clavicular joint. Its relations are as follows: anterior: the clavicle; postero-superior: the subclavian artery separated by the phrenic nerve and the scalenus anterior muscle; Inferior: the first rib and the pleura.

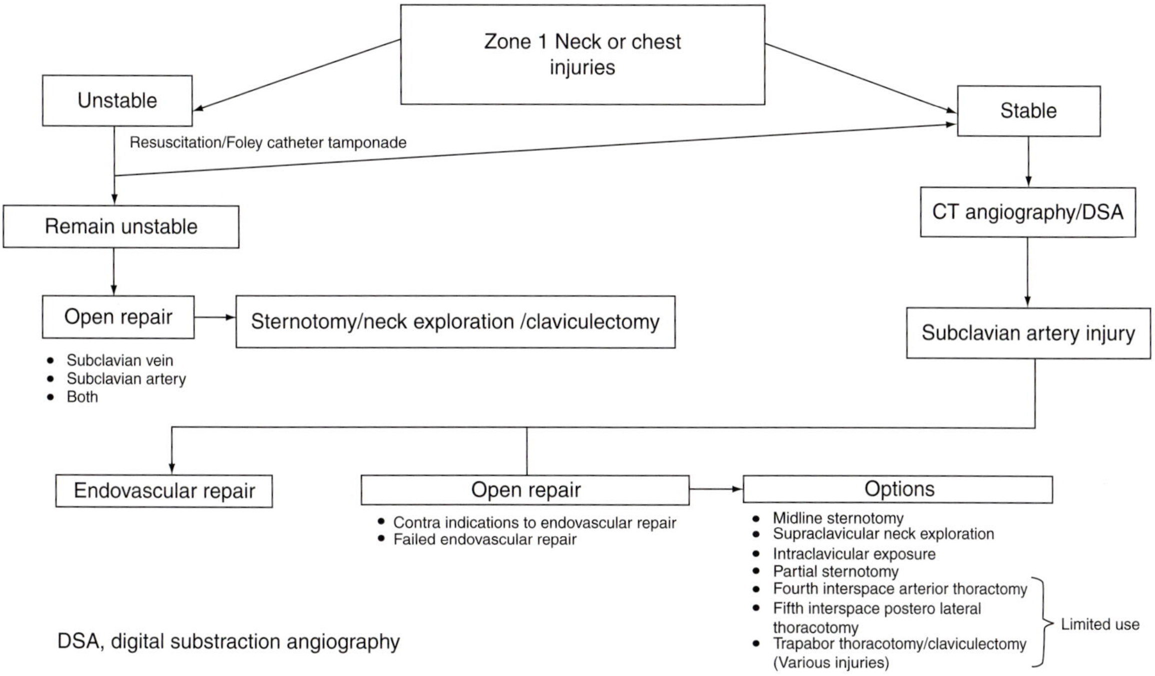

Fig. 31.2 Algorithm for the treatment of patients with potential subclavian vessel injuries

31.2 Clinical Presentation, Preoperative Care, Diagnosis, and Management Principles (Fig. 31.2)

Patients with subclavian vessel injuries can present in hypovolemic shock with active bleeding or in a stable condition with a Zone I or II neck [4] or infraclavicular anterior chest wounds. Zone I is defined as the area between the clavicle and the cricoid cartilage and Zone II the area between the cricoid and the inferior border of the mandible. Resuscitation should be managed according to ATLS guidelines and adjunctive measures to control active bleeding include Foley catheter tamponade (Fig. 31.3) and manual compression. If local control cannot be achieved or if the patient bleeds into the pleural cavity as evidenced by continuous blood loss from a chest drain, the patient should be transferred to the operating room immediately. In this case, we prefer a midline sternotomy, with appropriate extension, if needed, to provide access to most mediastinal and thoracic-outlet structures. Stable patients or patients that remain stable after resuscitation should be evaluated for arterial injury. In the stable or stabilized patient, you should proceed to diagnostic imaging. Controversy exists with regards to routine investigation of these surface wounds if no significant other signs of arterial injury are present [5]. We currently favor routine CT angiography to exclude arterial injuries. When hard signs of arterial injury are present, it allows assessment of the extent of the injury and planning of intervention. When soft signs only are present, it acts as a low morbidity screening investigation to exclude arterial injuries. If an arterial injury is diagnosed in this case, you should note the exact position and extent of arterial injury and evaluate the patient for endovascular or open surgery.

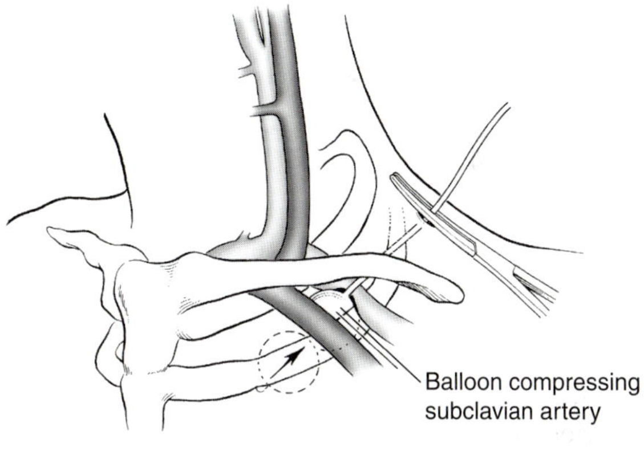

Fig. 31.3 Balloon tamponade controlling bleeding from an injured subclavian artery

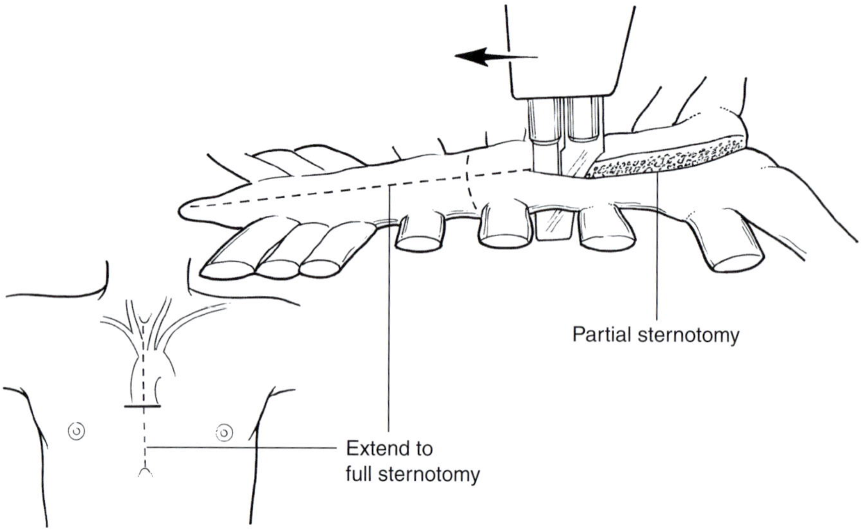

Fig. 31.4 Upper mediastinal access via a partial or full midline sternotomy

In our practice, we prefer endovascular treatment by stentgrafts whenever possible as we believe that it greatly benefits the patient by limiting surgical morbidity and mortality. The relative contraindications that can preclude endovascular management include clinical and angiographic factors [6]. Clinical factors are active uncontrollable hemorrhage, critical limb ischemia, airway or brachial plexus compression, concomitant aero-digestive injuries, and infected wounds. Angiographic factors include excessive luminal discrepancy proximal and distal to the injury, an inability to traverse the lesion by guidewire and a dominant vertebral artery on the injured side. Transfemoral endovascular management is our first choice if no contraindications are present.

If any of the above mentioned are present, consider open surgical repair. The basic approaches available for the exposure and proximal and distal control of subclavian vessel injuries include a full or limited upper median sternotomy, a supraclavicular incision, an infraclavicular incision, a limited anterolateral third-interspace thoracotomy, a full fifth-interspace posterolateral thoracotomy, a medial partial resection of the clavicle, and a trapdoor thoracotomy. The extent of the injury, pathology, the presence of a venous injury, the part of the vessel, and surgeon preference will dictate which approach, or more usually, combination of approaches to be used. In our practice, clavicle resection and trapdoor thoracotomy are very rarely used, only for subclavian vein injuries that cannot be controlled via any of the other approaches. This will usually be an extension of an existing sternotomy and supra-or-infraclavicular incision.

31.3 Surgical Exposures

31.3.1 Midline Sternotomy in the Unstable Patient with No Diagnostic Imaging (Fig. 31.4)

Here the source of bleeding could be from a number of large vessels in the mediastinum and thoracic outlet, or even from the heart. In this scenario, it is best to position the patient for a midline sternotomy with a small sandbag between the scapula, with the ipsilateral arm in 30° lateral abduction, allowing for manipulation of the thoracic outlet and better access to the distal subclavian/proximal axillary arteries. If time permits, it is prudent to clean a proximal thigh for harvesting saphenous vein, should this be required.

This preparation should be effected within minutes. It is also good practice to ascertain that a working pneumatic saw and a vascular instrument tray are available in the operation room. While pressure on or in the wound is maintained you can, with good suction and two Langenbeck retractors, coordinate the release of pressure and a "quick peep" into the wound can sometimes be of value. A visible vessel (subclavian or a large branch) can sometimes be glimpsed and clamped with one or two straight atraumatic vascular clamps. This should happen in seconds and you should not attempt more than two "peeps," otherwise the patient is in danger of exsanguinating. With luck, control, or partial control, can be achieved in this fashion. You can complete the procedure by formal supraclavicular neck exploration.

If control cannot be achieved in this way, the best option is to proceed to a midline sternotomy. A vertical midline incision is made from the suprasternal notch to 2 cm distal to the xiphoid process. You can extend the incision superiorly along the anterior border of the sternocleidomastoid muscle or, in the case of a true subclavian artery injury being identified, continue obliquely over the two heads of this muscle laterally about 2 cm above the clavicle for supraclavicular exposure. The sternal incision is deepened to the periosteum with electrocautery. In the sternal notch, deepen the midline space between the two sternal heads of the sternocleidomastoid muscles with a combination of sharp and blunt dissection. One or two large but unimportant veins may be encountered. Entry to the retrosternal space is effected with blunt finger dissection between the strap muscles, which implant on the posterior aspect of the sternum. Inferiorly the xiphoid is mobilized and a plane should be developed retrosternally, in an upward direction. The anesthesiologist should arrest ventilation in expiration (to prevent lung injury) and the sternum is divided in the midline using a pneumatic saw or Lebsche knife. Bleeding from the sternal edges is controlled by electrocautery and bone wax. The latter is used to prevent infection and impaired wound healing. Insert a sternal retractor and open it carefully, a few turns at a time to prevent sternal and rib fractures.

In the fully retracted position, a divided sternum reveals the structures of the anterior, superior, and middle mediastinum (Fig. 31.5). The thymus gland is encountered first. Divide it vertically to expose the left innominate vein that runs obliquely from the left to its confluence with its right-sided counterpart to form the superior vena cava. This vein can be mobilized by dividing its numerous tributaries, and exposure of the arch can thus be achieved without dividing it. In the emergency situation with active bleeding, you can be divide it and ligate it without any morbidity. The aortic arch with the origins of the innominate artery and the left common carotid is now visible.

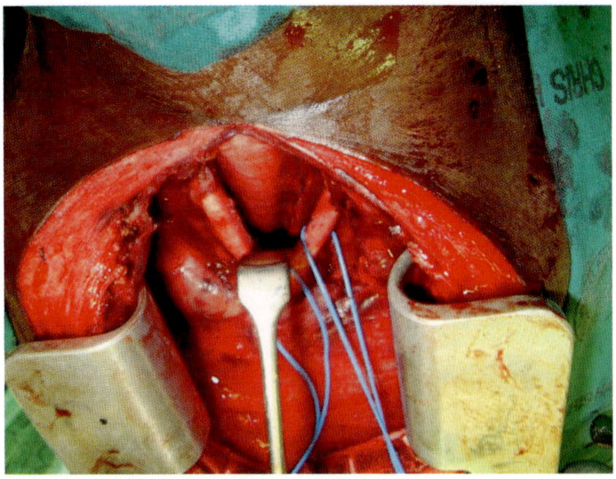

Fig. 31.5 The mediastinal structures exposed at sternotomy. Note blue vascular loops around both common carotid arteries. The trachea can be seen at the back between both vessels

On the right, the origin of the innominate artery at the aortic arch is identified and then carefully followed cranially for about 3–5 cm, where it will divide into subclavian and common carotid arteries. At this bifurcation, the right vagus nerve crosses anterior to the first part of the subclavian artery and then descends into the mediastinum posterior to the right innominate vein. The recurrent laryngeal branch of the right vagus nerve loops around the inferior border of the subclavian artery and ascends medially in the neck between the trachea and the esophagus. When exposing and controlling the short first part of the right subclavian artery, take care to avoid injury to these nerves. In the event of overwhelming bleeding from the right subclavian artery, the origin of the innominate artery can be temporarily clamped to facilitate dissection with immediate transfer of the clamp upon exposure of the proximal subclavian artery. Take care in the case of the "bovine arch" where both the carotid arteries and the right subclavian artery originate from the innominate artery. This congenital anomaly is present in about 10% of cases and can result in major brain damage if the innominate artery is clamped for any extended duration [7].

Depending on the rotation of the aortic arch, the origin of the left subclavian artery can vary from anterior to far posterior in the left half of the sternotomy wound (Fig. 31.6). In the latter situation, it can be difficult to get good exposure of this vessel and you should take

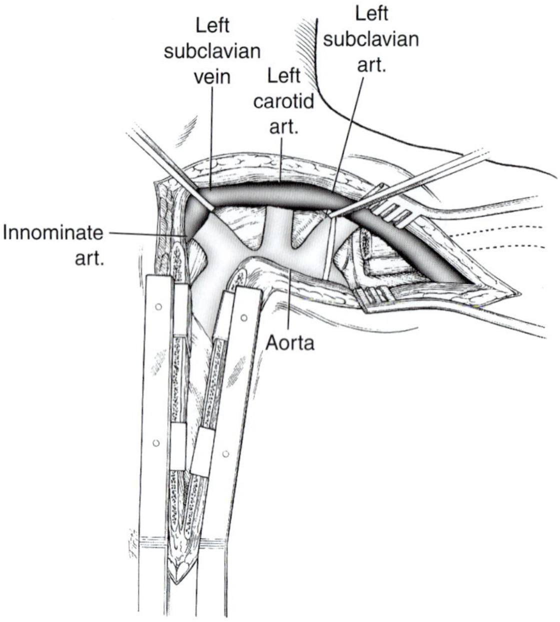

Fig. 31.6 Sternotomy combined with supraclavicular extension and medial resection of the clavicle demonstrating exposure of the proximal left subclavian artery, left subclavian, and innominate vein

care to avoid inadvertent clamping the left common carotid artery, thereby impeding cerebral blood flow. In the acute bleeding situation, the left pleural space can be entered before mediastinal dissection to facilitate compression of a subclavian artery that is bleeding into the pleural space. To locate the origin of the left subclavian artery, you should follow the aortic arch posterolaterally to the left past the origin of the left common carotid artery, taking care to prevent injury to the left vagus nerve as it descends between the carotid and left subclavian arteries to cross anteriorly over the left side of the aortic arch. The left recurrent laryngeal branch passes under the aortic arch and then courses medially to the tracheoesophgeal groove.

In an unstable patient, the relevant subclavian artery should be clamped at its origin and then dissected further to achieve distal control. On the right side, this usually entails a supraclavicular extension of the incision for exposure of the second and third parts of the right subclavian artery. Divide the right-sided strap muscles and the sternal and clavicular heads of the right sternocleidomastoid muscle should be divided to facilitate full exposure of the first part of the right subclavian artery and its branches up to the medial border of the scalenus anterior muscle. The internal jugular vein passes anterior to the subclavian artery, and it can be mobilized or divided if needed. The left subclavian artery has a much longer intrathoracic course which sometimes allows distal control in the chest without supraclavicular extension. Complete control and a bloodless field can be difficult to achieve because branches of the first part of the subclavian artery can cause problematic backbleeding. The vertebral and internal mammary arteries should be preserved if possible. Actual repair of a subclavian artery is described later.

31.3.2 The Midline Sternotomy in the Stable Patient with Imaging

This approach is exactly the same as described for the unstable patient and can be combined with the supraclavicular approach as described above.

31.3.2.1 The Limited Upper or Partial Sternotomy (Fig. 31.4)

This incision should be reserved for stable patients with preoperative imaging diagnosing a subclavian artery injury. The patient is prepped and draped as for a full sternotomy. The upper part of the dissection in the sternal notch is similar as for a full sternotomy, and the vertical midline incision is extended to the level of the third or fourth intercostal space. At this level, dissect the soft tissue overlying the sternum on both sides toward the intercostal spaces with electrocautery. A potential extrapleural space is carefully developed bilaterally dissecting the internal mammary artery away from the transaction plane of the sternum. Then divide the sternum in the midline to the level of this intercostal space using a pneumatic saw. Then divide horizontally the lower end of the sternum forming an inverted T by inserting the saw in the juxtasternal spaces that were created. The remainder of the dissection is exactly as described for the full sternotomy, and access to the aortic arch and its branches can be easily achieved. This approach should not be used for unstable patients as it takes more time and it limits access to the rest of the mediastinal structures.

31.3.2.2 The Supraclavicular Exposure of the Subclavian Artery (Figs. 31.7 and 31.8)

This incision should be used for proximal control in part 2 and 3 injuries or for distal control and repair in

Fig. 31.7 The supraclavicular exposure of the right subclavian artery with division of the scalenus anterior and the clavicular head of the sternocleidomastoid muscles

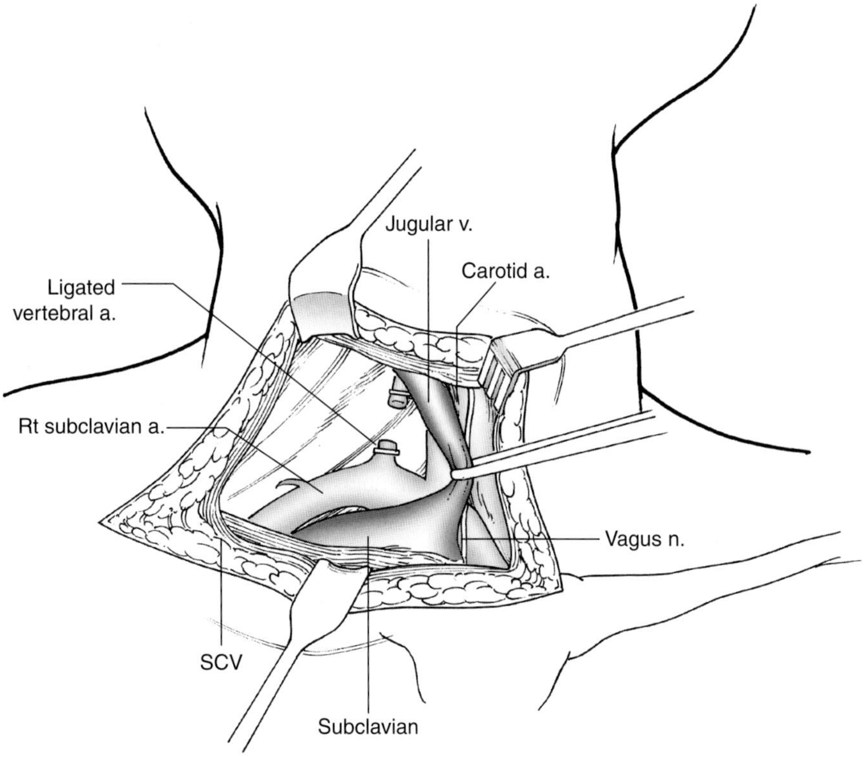

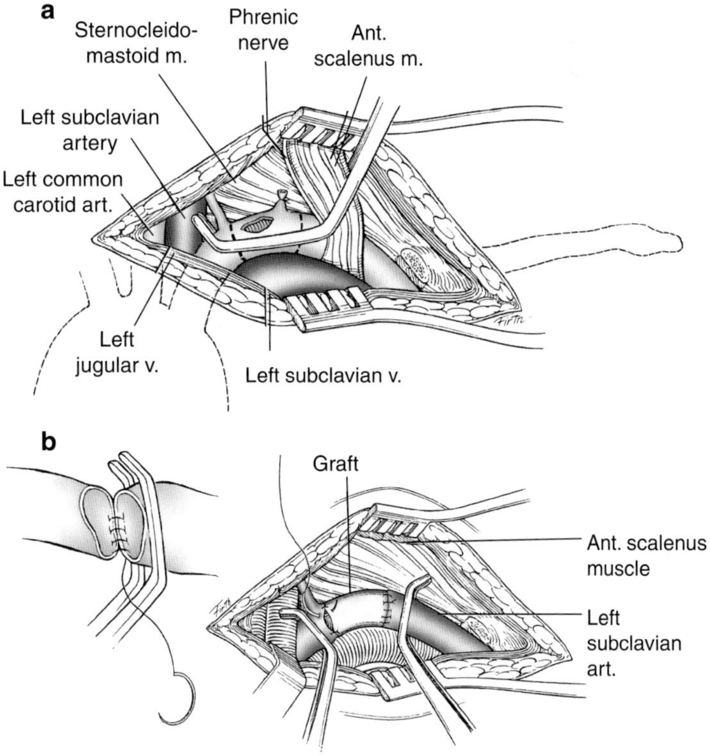

Fig. 31.8 Interposition graft repair of an injury to the second part of the left subclavian artery via a supraclavicular exposure

part 1 injuries. Position the patient as for sternotomy with a small sandbag between the scapulae, the head rotated to the opposite side and if infraclavicular exposure is expected, prep and drape the ipsilateral arm free on a narrow lateral armboard to facilitate this exposure. The neck, anterior chest, and ipsilateral arm should be included in the surgical field. Make a transverse incision 1–2 cm above and parallel to the clavicle, beginning at the sternal notch and extending laterally for about 7 cm. Deepen the incision through the platysma muscle to the scalene fat pad and the external jugular vein divided. The scalene fat pad is divided transversely and it usually contains branches of the thyrocervical trunk and the omohyoid muscle. Take care to divide and control the lymphatic ducts in this area, as on the left; this includes the thoracic duct. In the same horizontal plane, divide the clavicular and sternal heads of the sternocleidomastoid muscle, exposing the carotid sheath with the internal jugular vein enclosed in its lateral edge.

The scalenus anterior muscle will now come into view and care should be taken to preserve the phrenic nerve that courses from lateral to medial over the anterior aspect of this muscle. It should be carefully mobilized and retracted with a thin elastic sling. The scalenus muscle should be mobilized down to its origin from the first rib and carefully divided taking care not to damage the subclavian vein (anterior) or the subclavian artery (posterior). The subclavian artery will now be visible from the lateral border of the internal jugular vein to where it disappears beneath the clavicle. The internal mammary, vertebral, and thyrocervical branches of the first part are usually now visible. You can extend the medial access by retracting the internal jugular vein (or even dividing it) and dividing the lateral part of the strap muscles. The first part of the subclavian artery can be followed into the mediastinum on the left and to its origin from the innominate artery on the right. Care should be taken to prevent injury to the carotid arteries and the vagus and phrenic nerves. Control and/or repair should be achieved and then the wound must be closed in layers over a suction drain if needed. There is no need to repair the scalenus muscle, but the sternocleidomastoid can be repaired using a 2/0 absorbable suture and turning the head to the neutral position. You can use this incision in continuity with the midline sternotomy from its medial end. An infraclavicular incision should always be separate; do not connect these two incisions when used in the same patient. Division of the clavicle for arterial injuries is not advised.

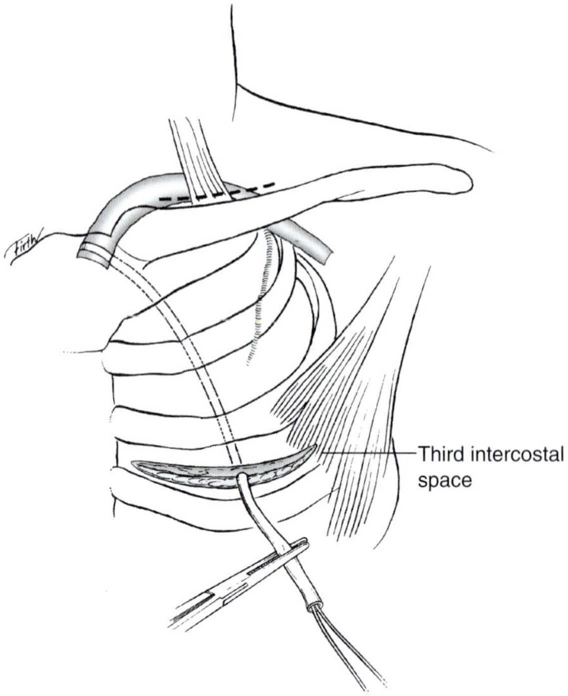

Fig. 31.9 Control of the left proximal subclavian artery via a third-interspace anterolateral thoracotomy. Repair is usually completed via a supraclavicular incision (*dotted line*)

31.3.2.3 The Left Third-Interspace Anterolateral Thoracotomy (Fig. 31.9)

The rationale for this exposure is the fact that the left subclavian artery originates from the posterolateral aspect of the aortic arch and is therefore difficult to access via a midline sternotomy. In a mediastinal bleeding of unknown origin, it is better to do a midline sternotomy because it does not limit your options as this incision does. It is not an easy approach and only allows for limited dissection and clamping of the left subclavian artery. Repair of the injury still needs supraclavicular or more extensive mediastinal dissection. The only scenario where this incision can be used with potential benefit is in a stable patient with a diagnosed left subclavian artery injury.

The patient is placed supine. A sandbag is placed behind the left shoulder. We prefer the third-interspace incision above the nipple line, but some prefer a fourth interspace incision below the nipple. Place the incision

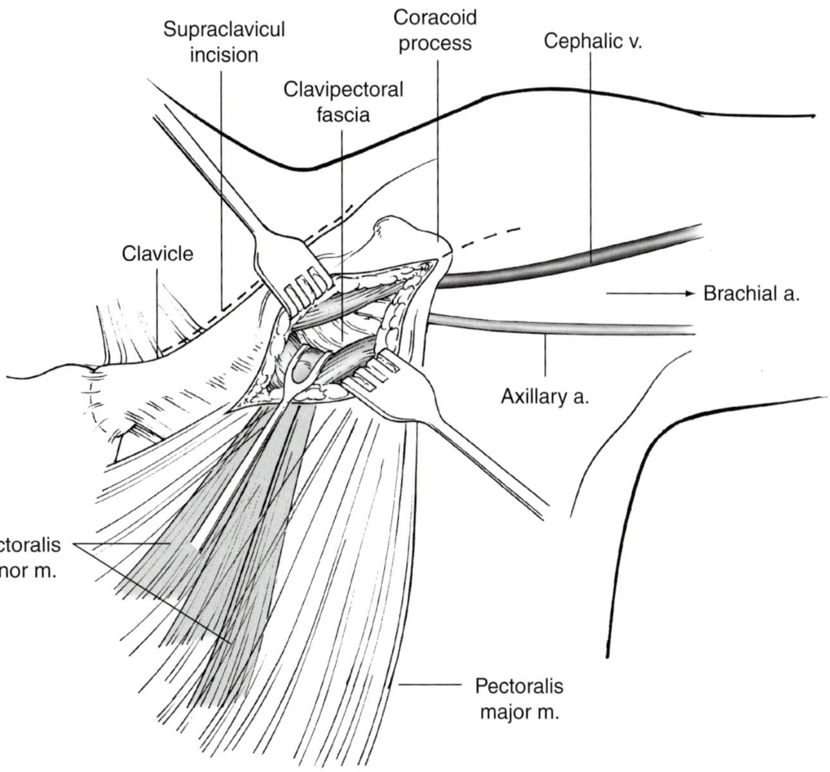

Fig. 31.10 Infraclavicular incision with control of the distal subclavian/proximal axillary artery by splitting the pectoralis major and dividing or retracting the pectoralis minor muscles

horizontally over the superior margin of the fourth rib from the lateral sternal border to the anterior axillary line. Divide the intercostal muscles, staying clear of the neurovascular bundle by entering the parietal pleura along the top of the fourth rib. The lung will collapse away from the chest wall, and the wound is fully opened. Lung collapse can be aided by double lumen tracheal intubation. Care should be taken to prevent injury to the internal mammary artery and vein in the medial aspect of the wound when slowly opening the wound with a rib spreader. Retract the upper lobe of the left lung downward, and then, the aortic arch with the origin and intrathoracic part of the left subclavian artery will be visible and still covered by the parietal pleura. This should be carefully opened, avoiding injury to the left vagus nerve which courses down the medial aspect of the subclavian artery and crosses the anterolateral aspect of the aortic arch. You can now mobilize and encircle with a vessel loop the left subclavian artery ready for clamping. Repair of the injury can then be completed via the supraclavicular incision. Close the wound in layers after insertion of an intercostal drain.

This approach is becoming redundant in the era of endovascular repair and the preference for a midline sternotomy in unstable patients.

31.3.2.4 The Left Fifth-Interspace Posterolateral Thoracotomy

This approach has limited application in the management of left subclavian artery injuries. It is time consuming and it limits options because the patient must be placed in the true lateral position that does not allow access to the neck for supraclavicular exposure. The only possible place for this exposure might be in a stable patient with injury to the first part of the left subclavian artery where proximal and distal control as well as repair can be completed in the chest.

31.3.2.5 The Infraclavicular Exposure of the Distal Subclavian and Proximal Axillary Artery (Fig. 31.10)

This incision is usually used for distal control of a second or more commonly a third part of subclavian artery injury. The classic injury is the one posterior to the clavicle at the junction between the distal subclavian and proximal

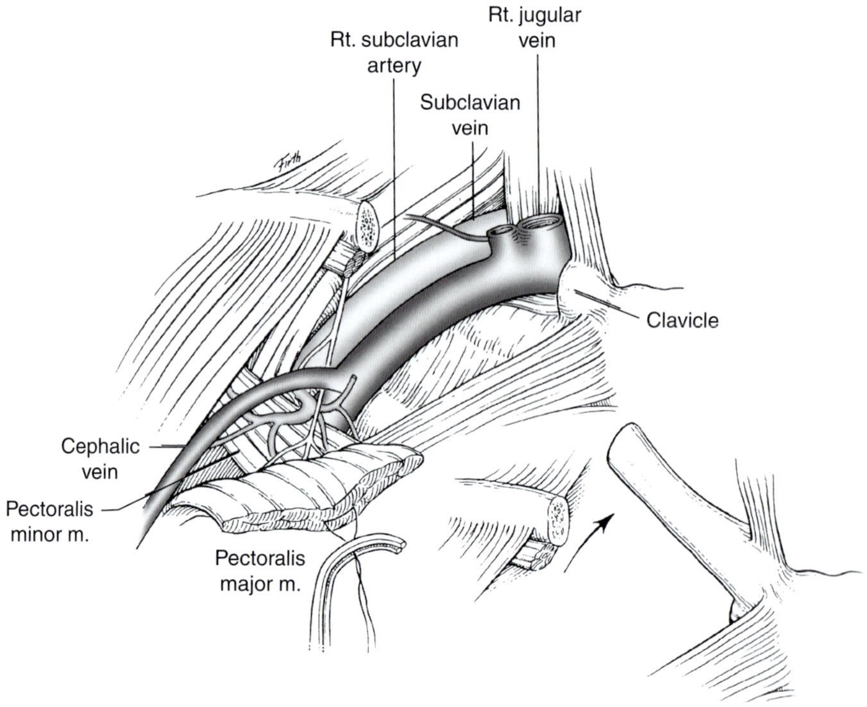

Fig. 31.11 Medial resection of the right clavicle exposing the right subclavian vein and its confluence with the internal jugular vein

axillary arteries. Proximal control can be achieved by the supraclavicular incision as described, but distal control and repair require control of the first part of the axillary artery via an infraclavicular exposure.

Position the patient as for the supraclavicular incision with the arm, chest, neck, and supraclavicular area prepped and draped. The ipsilateral arm should be free, draped 90° abducted on a narrow armboard allowing surgeon and the assistant to stand comfortably close to the operative field. The degree of abduction of the arm can be manipulated during the procedure, thereby facilitating peri-clavicular movement and control of the vessel.

Make a horizontal subclavicular skin incision parallel and 2 cm below the clavicle with its outer third slightly curved in the delto-pectoral groove and the medial part originating at midclavicular level. Deepen the incision through the subcutaneous tissue to the level of the pectoralis major muscle. Pull this muscle downward or split its fibers by blunt dissection, allowing exposure of the clavipectoral fascia. This fascia should be entered by sharp dissection and the axillary sheath will become visible below the clavicle. Exposure can be enlarged by encircling the pectoralis minor muscle in the lateral aspect of the wound and either retracting or dividing it. The first part of the axillary artery usually lies superior and deep to the vein and anterior to the cords of the brachial plexus. It should be carefully explored by division of venous branches and encircled with a vessel loop. Attain control by careful placement of a vascular clamp, avoiding inadvertent clamping of the brachial plexus.

A "behind the clavicle" injury is usually not amenable to primary repair, and the vessel should be controlled and transected above and below the clavicle. Repair of the defect will then need an interposition graft with the proximal anastomoses being performed end-to-end above the clavicle. The graft must then be tunneled posterior to the clavicle, and the distal anastomosis is performed below the clavicle in an end-to-end fashion to the axillary artery. The arm should be in 90° abduction when deciding on the length of the graft.

The clavicle should not be divided as all injuries can be managed by working around the clavicle as described. Division of the clavicle takes time and can result in major venous bleeding from the subclavian vein lying posterior to it.

This wound should be closed in layers with or without a suction drain in place.

31.3.2.6 The Trapdoor Thoracotomy and Partial Resection of the Clavicle (Figs. 31.6 and 31.11)

This incision combines the supraclavicular exposure, the partial midline sternotomy, and a fourth intercostal space anterolateral thoracotomy. This approach is rarely used as it has limited advantages, if any, over the standard full midline sternotomy combined with a supraclavicular approach. It is a complex exposure, takes a lot of time, the pleural space is entered, and it has a propensity for excess bleeding. It is not a routine option in the unstable patient with an undiagnosed injury, but might be of limited benefit in subclavian vein injuries where more lateral exposure needs to be achieved to access the vein behind the clavicle. Resection of the medial half of the clavicle in combination with a midline sternotomy is preferred for better exposure and control of venous injuries. A partial medial claviculectomy is time consuming but increases exposure of this area significantly.

31.3.2.7 The Surgical Repair of the Subclavian Vessels

The subclavian artery is a friable elastic artery, and the principles of repair for all arterial injuries should be adhered to. This includes proximal and distal control via the surgical approaches as described, control of branches, and debridement of the injured area. You should do a proximal and distal embolectomy with a number 3 Fogarty catheter and, in case of an isolated injury with no coagulopathy, you should administer systemic heparin (70 U/kg). Prophylactic antibiotic, such as 1 g of cefazolin, should be given intravenously. Attain control as close as possible to the injured area as major branches especially of the first part can cause substantial backbleeding if not isolated. These branches can be temporarily controlled or it can be ligated if necessary. The vertebral artery is an exception and you should preserve, if at all possible. If it was demonstrated to be a dominant vessel on preoperative imaging, it should be revascularized during the repair. In the rare case of the internal mammary artery being a bypass conduit of a previous coronary bypass, it should also be protected or repaired at all cost.

The local pathology can also influence the type of repair needed. Large false aneurysms and arteriovenous fistulae mandate more extensive dissection for wider proximal and distal control, as well as arterial and venous control in the latter. The extent of the arterial defect will dictate the type of repair needed. The basic principles are debridement of all damaged arterial wall and to then establish a tension-free repair. This can include mobilization of the artery with primary repair by lateral suture using 60 polypropylene suture materials in continuous or interrupted fashion. If the defect is too extensive, an interposition graft is required. The options are autologous saphenous vein or synthetic material such as PTFE or Dacron. Vein grafts tend to be favored, but, in this location, no clear long-term benefit has been demonstrated. Disadvantages include the availability and time delay especially in the unstable patient, the risk of kinking, impingement between the clavicle and the first rib, and potential size discrepancy. It is, therefore, reasonable to use externally reinforced PTFE or Dacron grafts of appropriate size. No clear inferior long-term patency or significantly higher sepsis rate has been reported in the literature, when compared to vein grafts.

In case of proximal subclavian artery injuries close to the origin, interposition grafting from subclavian to subclavian artery might not be possible. Proximal takeoff of the graft might then be from the ascending aorta, innominate artery, or the adjacent carotid arteries. Transpositions of the debrided subclavian artery to the ipsilateral carotid arteries are also a possibility. In extreme cases where the procedure is seen as a damage control situation, the subclavian artery should simply be ligated proximal and distal to the injury. This is usually well tolerated and repair can be deferred to when the patient is stable or if he/she develops upper limb claudication.

31.3.2.8 Endovascular Management (Fig. 31.12)

This is our treatment option of choice for all stable patients with subclavian artery injuries. This treatment modality is now well established as a safe alternative to open surgery with less morbidity, shorter hospitalization, less blood loss, and acceptable short- and long-term follow-up results [6]. Absence of local expertise and angiography facilities as well as surgeon preference might influence the choice of management options. Patient selection is based on clinical presentation and diagnostic angiography. Clinical and radiological factors precluding stentgraft treatment were already mentioned.

The procedure is performed in an arteriography suite or a hybrid operating room equipped for general anesthesia and conventional surgery. Intravenous heparin (50 units/kg) and prophylactic cefazolin were routinely administered before stentgraft deployment and empirically continued for 24 h, at a dosage of 5,000 units subcutaneously and 1 g intravenously respectively, every 8 h. Transfemoral arterial access is attained under

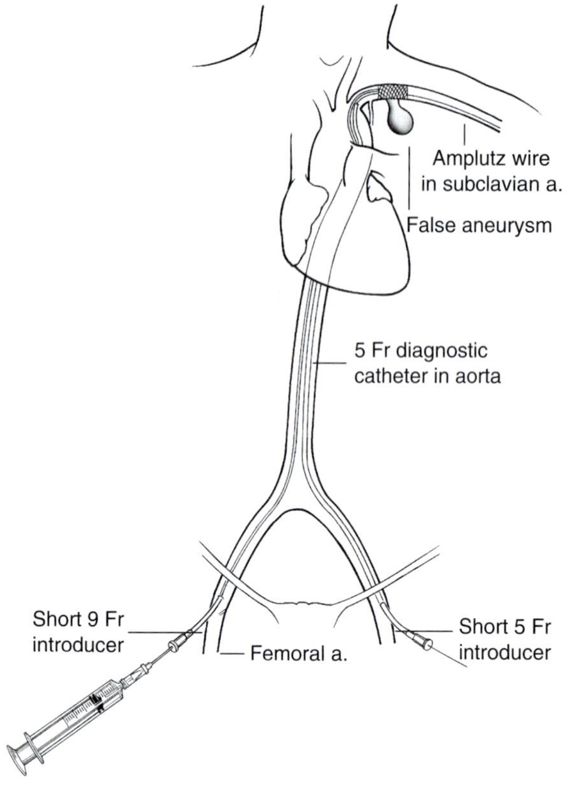

Fig. 31.12 Stentgraft repair of a false aneurysm of the left subclavian artery by using a double femoral puncture technique

local anesthesia. Anatomical location of lesions and proximal and distal vessel diameters are determined with routine angiography and a final decision regarding stentgraft treatment then taken. If a preoperative CT-angiogram was done, a more directed approach is possible.

The stentgraft is placed via a percutaneous transfemoral approach. Bilateral transfemoral access (5-F and 9-F Cordis® [Johnson & Johnson, Waterloo, Belgium] introducer sheaths) is obtained. Engage the subclavian artery to be stented with a diagnostic catheter (5F Headhunter). Do a diagnostic run and measure the diameter of the subclavian artery. Choose a stent graft 1–2 mm larger than the subclavian artery and covering at least 1 cm proximal and distal to the lesion. If the vertebral artery has to be covered, the presence of a good quality contralateral vertebral artery has to be confirmed. It is usually unnecessary to coil-embolize subclavian artery branches in the area to be stented unless they clearly contribute to an AV fistula. Using a roadmap, pass the subclavian artery lesion with a steerable hydrophilic guidewire and steer the wire to the mid-brachial artery. Advance the diagnostic catheter over the guidewire into the brachial artery and exchange for a stiff wire (Amplatz®).The appropriate stentgraft is introduced via the 9-F sheath (11 cm in length) over a stiff guidewire, crossing the lesion, and angiographic control for precise deployment was provided by a diagnostic catheter (via the 11 cm 5-F sheath) positioned in the proximal subclavian artery or aortic arch. Alternatively, a single long introducer sheath (9-F, 100 cm in length) can be used. It has the advantage of only one femoral puncture providing stentgraft access and angiographic control of deployment, but in very proximal injuries, achieving a stable position may be difficult. Furthermore, contrast injection may be problematic necessitating an even larger sheath and a cutdown might be needed. The stentgrafts that are commercially available include the Hemobahn® endovascular prosthesis (W.L. Gore), the Wallgraft® (Boston Scientific, Target Therapeutics, Fremont, CA 94538 USA), the Fluency® (Bard, Murray Hill, NJ, USA). Sheaths are removed 60–90 min after intravenous heparin and hemostasis is obtained with digital compression. The patient is observed overnight and can be discharged the next day, barring other injuries requiring continued hospitalization. No long-term anticoagulation or antiplatelet drugs are prescribed. Figure 31.13 depicts the successful endovascular management of a left subclavian artery false aneurysm.

31.4 Venous Injuries

Clinically significant subclavian vein injuries are an uncommon occurrence. Many penetrating neck and chest wounds might involve the subclavian veins, but few will need treatment. The venous system has a low pressure and these injuries are usually self-limiting, as hypotension and soft tissue tamponade cause local thrombosis with healing over time.

Clinically, significant subclavian vein injuries are the result of a large open laceration of the skin and soft tissue surrounding the vein with an equally large injury to the vein. Under these circumstances, local tamponade is compromised and massive external bleeding can occur. You can control this by manual compression and/or Foley catheter tamponade. Diagnostic imaging

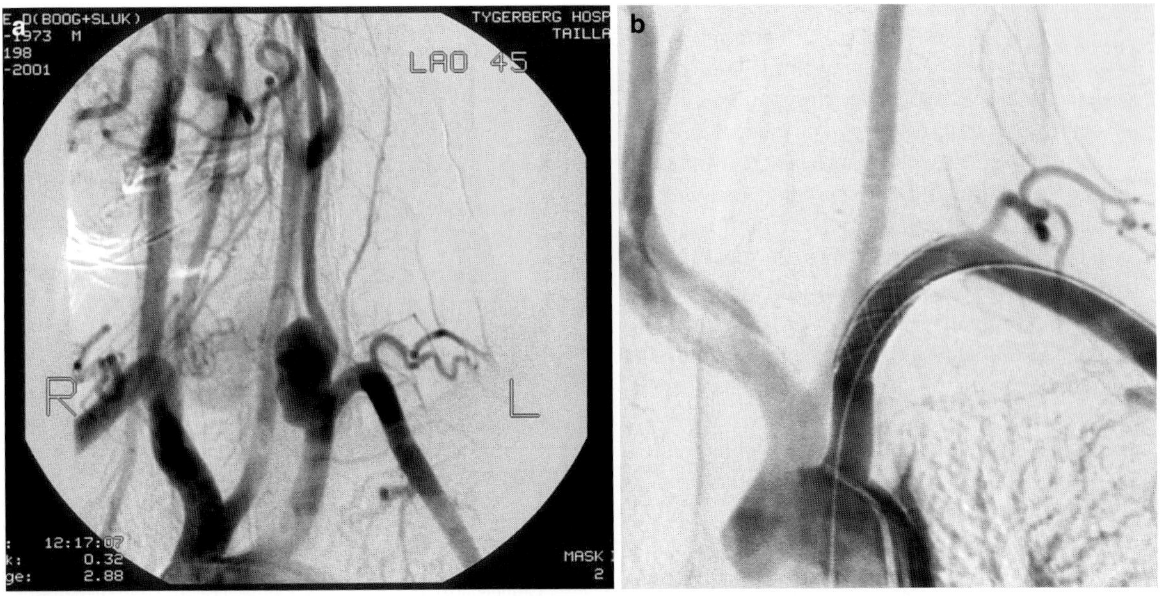

Fig. 31.13 Endovascular treatment of a left subclavian artery false aneurysm. (**a**) Initial angiogram demonstrating the false aneurysm. (**b**) Completion angiogram showing exclusion of the false aneurysm after preoperative coil embolization of the participating vertebral artery to prevent an endoleak

can then exclude arterial injuries and the catheter should be left in place for 24–48 h before careful removal. If no bleeding recurs, you can suture the wound and observe the patient for another 48 h in hospital before discharge. If bleeding recurs, the catheter should be re-inflated and exploration should be done. Fortunately, this happens very seldom.

The other scenario is the patient bleeding actively from a supraclavicular wound with an unknown vessel injury that cannot be stabilized by Foley catheter tamponade. You should take this unstable patient to the operating room with manual compression of the wound and careful local exploration with a low threshold to do a midline sternotomy. The color of the blood is usually not a good indication of the source of the bleeding as in these patients, venous oxygen saturation is high on 100% oxygen ventilation. If a venous injury is diagnosed, careful handling of this injury is the key to success. Proper exposure can at times be a nightmare especially if the subclavian vein is damaged posterior to the clavicle and if its confluence with the internal jugular vein to form the innominate vein is involved. A midline sternotomy with supraclavicular extension is usually the exposure to start with, but although time consuming, resection of the medial part of the clavicle with or without the corresponding half of the manubrium can provide excellent exposure of the subclavian vein. When handling the vein, manual compression with proximal and distal control is essential. The vein should always be handled with great care as it tears easily and a small injury can quickly become a massive problem if grabbed with traumatic clamps. Soft straight vascular clamps should be used to gently clamp the injured area. This will achieve partial control and the vessel can be gently pulled up by these clamps. A curved vascular clamp should now be passed behind these clamps and the vessel is secured in a horizontal fashion controlling the injury. The vein can now be mobilized and repaired as needed. Extensive efforts to properly repair the vein are not encouraged as ligation is a safe alternative.

The subclavian vein injury can also present as a stable arteriovenous fistula where it communicates with an adjacent arterial injury. This can pose a great challenge as arterial and venous bleeding and collaterals complicate surgery. This is the ideal lesion to treat by endovascular techniques. A stentgraft should be used to treat the arterial injury while venous patency is maintained [8].

Important Points

- In unstable, actively bleeding patients, try to control bleeding by Foley catheter tamponade and stabilize patients for preoperative imaging and evaluations for endovascular treatment or planning of open surgery.
- Clinically significant venous injuries usually present with active bleeding and can be managed conservatively with Foley catheter tamponade followed by angiography and balloon deflation after 48 h if no arterial injury is detected.
- Unstable patients with uncontrollable hemorrhage should always undergo open surgery. A controlled "peep" in the neck wound might reveal a superficial bleeder or allow vascular clamping of the injured vessel. A low threshold for a midline sternotomy with extensions as needed should be maintained
- If at sternotomy, the subclavian vein is revealed to be the source of bleeding and control is not possible via this exposure, adding a medial claviculectomy might be of great assistance.
- Stable subclavian artery injuries should all be considered for endovascular management if no contraindications are present.
- We do not advise division of the clavicle or the trapdoor thoracotomy for arterial injuries.
- The friable elastic subclavian artery should be carefully repaired with fine 60 polypropylene sutures. Primary repair is preferable, but interposition vein grafting is often needed. You should not hesitate to use reinforced PTFE if the vein is too small or if the patient's condition dictates expedient conclusion of the procedure.
- Connecting the supraclavicular exposure and the median sternotomy entails the division of the both heads of the sternocleidomastoid muscle and the strap muscles, taking care not to damage the contents of the carotid sheath and the phrenic nerve.

References

1. Robbs JV, Baker LW (1984) Cardiovascular trauma. Curr Probl Surg 21(4):1–84
2. Demetriades D, Chahwan S, Gomez H et al (1999) Penetrating injuries to the subclavian and axillary vessels. J Am Coll Surg 188:290–295
3. Moore KL, Dalley AF (2005) Neck. In: Clinically oriented anatomy. Lippincott Williams & Wilkins, Philadelphia 211-265
4. Demetriades D, Theodorou D, Cornwell E et al (1997) Evaluation of penetrating injuries of the neck: prospective study of 223 patients. World J Surg 21:41–48
5. Eddy VA (2000) Is routine arteriography mandatory for penetrating injuries to zone 1of the neck? J Trauma 48: 208–214
6. du Toit DF, Lambrechts AV, Stark H et al (2008) Long-term results of stent graft treatment of subclavian artery injuries: management of choice for stable patients? J Vasc Surg 47: 739–743
7. Layton KF, Kallmes DF, Cloft HJ et al (2006) Bovine aortic arch variant in humans: clarification of a common misnomer. Am J Neuroradiol 27:1541–1542
8. du Toit DF, Leith JG, Strauss DC et al (2003) Endovascular management of traumatic cervicothoracic arteriovenous fistula. Br J Surg 90:1516–1521

Penetrating Trauma to the Thoracic Oesophagus

32

Elias Degiannis, Tugba H. Yilmaz, and Lisa A. Burnell

Penetrating trauma to the thoracic oesophagus is a rare injury. There are several reasons for that. The thoracic oesophagus is too deep for most stab wounds and penetrating trauma that inflicts injury to the mid-thoracic oesophagus is also likely to involve the heart and the mediastinal vessels and therefore be fatal.

Start with a plain x-ray. Remember that the patient's survival with this type of injury is directly related to the time interval between injury and repair, therefore have a high index of suspicion so that you come to an early diagnosis. Pleural effusions are present in a significant number of patients with oesophageal injury, and in their presence you should insert intercostal drains. Apart from pleural effusions, a plain chest radiograph will quite frequently demonstrate subcutaneous emphysema, pneumomediastinum, pneumothorax and mediastinal air fluid levels. Investigate trans-mediastinal gunshot wounds with a CT scan if the patient is physiologically stable. See the bullet tract and proceed to further investigations if it is in close proximity to the oesophagus. Contrast studies are very helpful. Start with a barium swallow since barium is relatively inert and is better than gastrografin in showing hollow viscus leaks. Remember that water-soluble contrast agents like gastrografin can cause severe pneumonitis if aspirated and can miss small leaks. If the level of consciousness of patient is low but has still got a good gag reflex, administer the contrast carefully through a Foleys catheter that you insert high in the oesophagus and inflate its balloon to prevent aspiration of the material. If your patient is intubated, you can administer the contrast via a nasogastric tube positioned near the suspected area. You can also confirm oesophageal leak by asking the patient to swallow methylene blue and see it leaking from a previously inserted intercostal drain (for pleural effusion on chest x-ray). Although pathognomonic of the presence of oesophageal defect, it cannot localise its exact site.

It is worth mentioning that CT scan can also demonstrate mediastinal complications secondary to oesophageal perforation as paraoesophageal air and mediastinal collections.

If you still suspect oesophageal injury in the presence of a normal swallow, proceed to flexible oesophagoscopy. Remember that oesophageal injuries are likely to be missed if you do not properly inflate the oesophagus so that you can have a good look at the lumen of the oesophagus with completely flattened mucosal folds. Impressive bubbling in an intercostal drain bottle every time you inflate the oesophagus during the oesophagoscopy is pathognomonic of an oesophageal leak but again does not localise accurately its site.

As mentioned the prognosis of penetrating oesophageal injuries has been shown to be directly related to the

E. Degiannis (✉)
University of the Witwatersrand Medical School, Chris Hani Baragwanath Academic Hospital, Trauma Directorate, 7 York Road, Parktown, 2193 Johannesburg, South Africa (RSA)
e-mail: degiannis@yebo.co.za

T.H. Yilmaz
Department of Surgery, Baskent University, 6371 Sokak No: 34, Bostanli, Izmir 35540, Turkey
e-mail: tugba.yilmaz@deu.edu.tr

L.A. Burnell
Trauma Directorate, Department of Surgery, Chris Hani Baragwanath Academic Hospital, University of the Witwatersrand Medical School, 7 York Road, Parktown, Johannesburg 2193, Republic of South Africa
e-mail: mburnell@iafrica.com

G.C. Velmahos et al. (eds.), *Penetrating Trauma*,
DOI 10.1007/978-3-642-20453-1_32, © Springer-Verlag Berlin Heidelberg 2012

time interval between injury and repair as the morbidity and mortality dramatically increase if it is more than 24 h. It is advised in many trauma books to approach the upper two thirds of the oesophagus by a right and the distal third by left thoracotomy. We always proceed with a right thoracotomy choosing the level of the incision according to the site of the injury. Approaching the oesophagus from the right gives you the ability to mobilise the oesophagus for as far as it is necessary without having the descending aorta in the way. If during the operation we have to access the abdominal oesophagus, we proceed to laparotomy with an upper midline incision. Try to convince the anaesthetist to use a double lumen tube. It is worth tuckling his resistance as a deflated lung is of paramount importance to make the surgeon's life easier and the repair more sound. In any case, operating to the oesophagus is not the same as operating for bleeding, so he can take as long as he needs to intubate the patient with a double lumen tube. Use a small sand bag to elevate the patient's right side to 30° with right arm abducted and suspended by the anaesthetic screen cephalad to the surgical field. Prepare the neck, chest and abdomen in case you find yourself in a situation that you must extend your surgery to these anatomical areas. If you find yourself to extend your operation in the neck or the abdomen, you simply have to rotate the operating table until the abdomen or the neck is parallel with the floor. Make an incision along the intercostal space that is appropriate for the expected level of the site of the injury, from the sternum to the posterior axillary line in men. Needless to say that in women, your incision should be at the infra-mammary fold and you should choose the space after elevation of the breast. Incise the pectoral and the anterior serratus muscle at the selected level. Use high coagulation current and go very slowly, 'charcoaling' the muscles. It is worth being patient and going slowly than having bleeding later on. Divide the intercostal muscles along the upper border of the lower rib of the selected space (remember that for counting the ribs, you should put your hand under the elevated scapula. The highest palpable rib is usually the second rib). Look for the internal mammary artery and ligate it (although you can keep your incision laterally to it). Enter the pleura carefully, making sure that you do not damage the underlying lung (or if you damage it, you do not overdo it!) and divide the cartilage of the rib at the cephalad of the incision after ligating its neuromuscular bundle. This cartilage severance will make the wound incision bigger and the operating field more accessible. If this is not done, you should be very patient while screwing open the rib spreader in steps so that you avoid fracture of the ribs. Remember that intraoperative access to an oesophageal leak does not have the same urgency as that of operating for thoracic bleeding, so breaking ribs is not acceptable as it can negatively influence the patient's postoperative course. Look for the area of injury; if this is not obvious, you will see a yellow discoloration under the posterior mediastinal pleura. If neither of the above two is present, divide transversely the mediastinal pleura where the oesophagus is expected to be and expose it. Then divide the pleura longitudinally, proximally and distally to expose at the surface of the oesophagus. Completely mobilise the oesophagus for about 3 cm proximally and distally to the area of the injury. If you have not mobilised the oesophagus before in your life, use a pledgelet to create a groove at the lateral and medial aspects of the oesophagus. Then take a large Babcock and gently grab transversely as much of the muscular tube as possible and again gently elevate it from its bed. You will see that there is tissue posteriorly that holds the oesophagus in its bed. Take a large right-angled Lahey and penetrate this tissue and encircle the oesophagus with a ribbon. Do the above 3 cm proximally as well as 3 cm distally to the site of the injury. Mobilise the oesophagus in between (the part that includes the defect) by meticulously dividing the tissue that holds it in its bed – remember that in this tissue, runs the small arterial branches that supply blood to the oesophagus. It is usually easier to divide these branches between haemoclips.

If the azygous vein is in your way, divide the pleura superficially to the vein and then divide and transfix it. Then lift the proximal stump of the vein from the underlying oesophagus by dividing the pleura transversely on both sides of the vein. This will make your life easier if you need to mobilise these areas. We always split longitudinally the pleural peritoneum along the whole length of the anterior aspect of the oesophagus irrespective of mobilisation or not. As with every septic wound, proceed with drainage of any collection, washout of the area and debridement of the wound. Remember that the majority of the gunshot wounds are due to low-energy bullets. Therefore, your debridement should be limited. It is common in the oesophagus the wound in the muscle layers to be smaller than that of the mucosa that also tends to retract. It is of paramount importance to increase the size of the muscle wound so that you identify fully the margin of the mucosa. Remember that the oesophageal mucosa looks white and it is most important to include it in your repair in as it is the toughest layer of the oesophageal wall.

Have a good look around the circumference of the oesophagus at the site of the injury to make sure that there is no second one. The management of injuries that present themselves within 24 h is different than the ones that present later, as the chances of wound dehiscence following primary repair are unlikely in the first case and significant in the second. If the injury has been present for less than 24 h, washout, debridement, primary repair and drainage suffice. There are many methods of repairing the oesophagus, meaning that none of them have any advantage to the rest and is free of 'mishaps'. We repair the oesophagus in one layer of intermitted horizontal mattress sutures (Fig. 32.1a). We choose a stitch with high-tensile strength, not because we expect our sutures to break, but because usually they are quite thick and therefore less likely to cut through the oesophageal tissue while approximating the tissue edges and making the knots and later on when some tissue swelling develops. We are 'old fashioned' and use Nr 1 silk or vicryl that the scrub sister makes sure is wet so that it slips through the tissue. Include 4 mm of the oesophageal mucosa in each bite. This method of suturing results in everted oesophageal repair edges. This does not make any difference – remember that when using staplers, all margins are everted without that resulting in more complications than in inverted suture lines. We tie the mattress sutures at the end after all of them have been inserted in place and we do not cut the edges. Then we reinforce our suture line by putting a 2.0 interrupted silk or vicryl stitch in the space between two consecutive horizontal mattress sutures and then cut all the stitch ends (Fig. 32.1b).

Do a barium swallow at the seventh day after the repair and if there is a small leak that presents itself as a small sinus, we can ignore it and start the patient on liquid diet after 7 days.

If the gap is too large to approximate the edges of the damaged oesophagus, and/or the patient is physiologically unstable, proceed to a bail-out solution by proximal drainage of the oesophagus via a NG tube and insertion of an intercostal drain to convert the free perforation into a controlled fistula. This can also apply in situations when the injury is older than 24 h and the repair precarious or the surgeon not experienced with

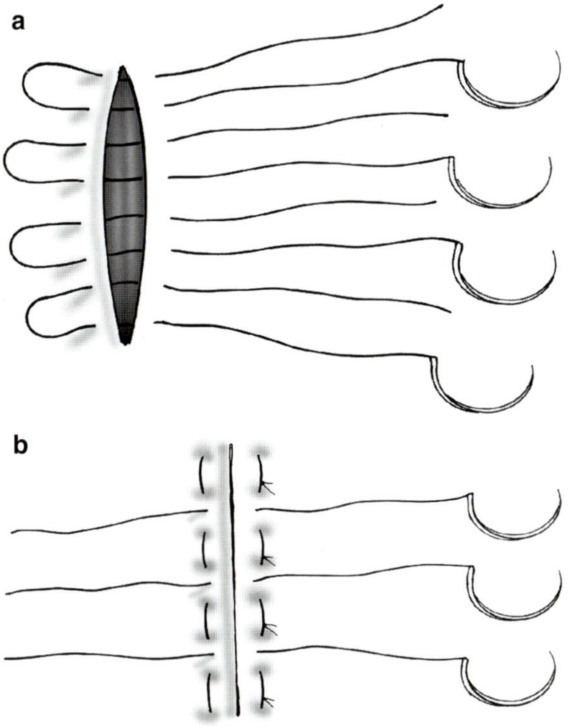

Fig. 32.1 (**a**) We repair the oesophagus in one layer of intermitted horizontal mattress sutures. (**b**) Then we reinforce our suture line by putting a 2.0 interrupted silk or vicryl stitch in the space between two consecutive horizontal mattress sutures and then cut all the stitch ends

tackling an injury in this anatomical area. After the bailout, a different procedure can be considered if appropriate. If there is significant defect or contamination, you can do T-tube drainage (22–24 French). Very large defects may require use of tracheal T-tube with a chest tube intussuscepted over the end of the T-tube. If possible, approximate the edges of the hole around the drain. Drain the pleural cavities with separate tubes. Obtain an oesophagogram after 10 days if there is no clinical leakage; if not start the patient on liquid diet and then full diet and remove the T-tube after 5–6 weeks by oesophagoscopy to avoid widening of the tract.

When the injury is present for more than 24 h, there is significant infection present that together with the swelling of the oesophageal tissue makes primary repair precarious. There is a variety of methods described for tackling this difficult problem, none of them are complication-free. If it is possible to repair the defect, attempt doing it. As far as we are concerned, this should be the one case where your repair should always be done with interrupted sutures and not continuous, as

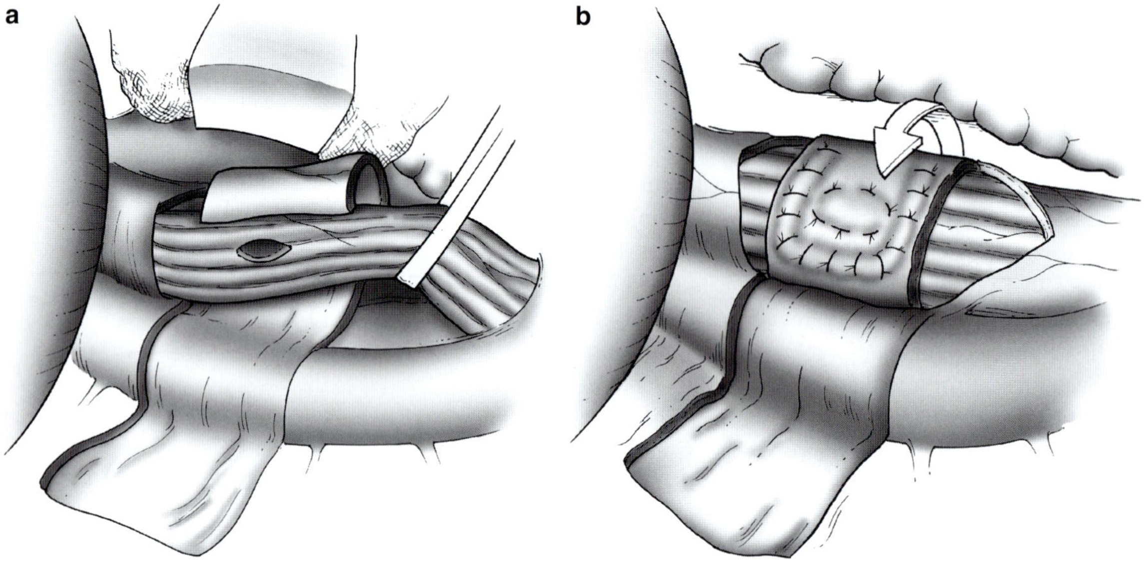

Fig. 32.2 (**a**, **b**) We prefer to mobilise the pleura, which due to inflammation is thickened, and wrap it 'tightly' around the repair in immediate contact with the oesophagus but not very 'tight' so that it becomes obstructed

failure of the suture line is a real threat with stitches cutting through the tissues. The chances of complete opening of the repair in the presence of continuous stitch is higher than if you use interrupted, as hopefully some of them will stay intact and therefore keep the defect smaller than the original one. It is wise to buttress the repair. We prefer to mobilise the pleura, which due to inflammation is thickened, and wrap it 'tightly' around the repair in immediate contact with the oesophagus but not very 'tight' so that it becomes obstructed (Fig. 32.2a, b). This should be about 5-cm long. Books describe wrapping (buttressing) with pericardium but in our experience, it does contribute to acceptable outcomes. We avoid it as in case of failure of the oesophageal repair, the infection can spread into the pericardial sac. If the oesophageal injury is just above the hiatus, create a diaphragmatic flap and oversew it on the oesophagus, covering the suture line. The base of this flap should start of 2 cm from the periphery of the hiatus and extend radially to about 6 cm or even longer if more length is needed to reach the defect site. Rotate the flap upwards from its base, towards the oesophagus, cover the repair or gap and close the diaphragmatic defect by interrupted sutures (Fig. 32.3a, b). There are cases that buttressing of the oesophagus will probably not be enough to support the integrity of the suture line. In these cases, it is worth considering isolating the injured area. Distal exclusion of the oesophagus has been practised on the basis that it controls the gastric secretions from not being refluxed to the area of the injury. We avoid stapling the distal oesophagus in the chest. We prefer to staple the oesophagus intra-abdominally close to the gastro-oesophageal junction. Mobilise the abdominal oesophagus via an upper abdominal incision exactly the same way as you mobilise for truncal vagotomy. Apply and fire the TA stapler at the gastro-oesophageal junction making sure that you do not include the vagi. Fashion a gastrostomy or probably a jejunostomy. In most cases, this staple line will open by itself as is the case with pyloric exclusion. If this is not the case and the oesophagus has healed, the staple line can be resected, and the oesophageal injury can be re-implanted at the anterior aspect of the fundus of the stomach.

The issue of proximal isolation is more complex. It has been suggested by certain authors that proximal exclusion should be done by stapling intra-thoracically above the site of the injury. We discard it as obsolete as the proximal part of the oesophagus will act as a dead-end oesophageal pouch, an undrained 'sack' that will be the source of ongoing sepsis and aspiration and can kill the patient. The alternative of fashioning of a loop cervical oesophagostomy has been disappointing in our hands. We find it difficult to mobilise the cervical oesophagus to obtain enough length to construct a tension-free loop oesophagostomy. Usually in the next

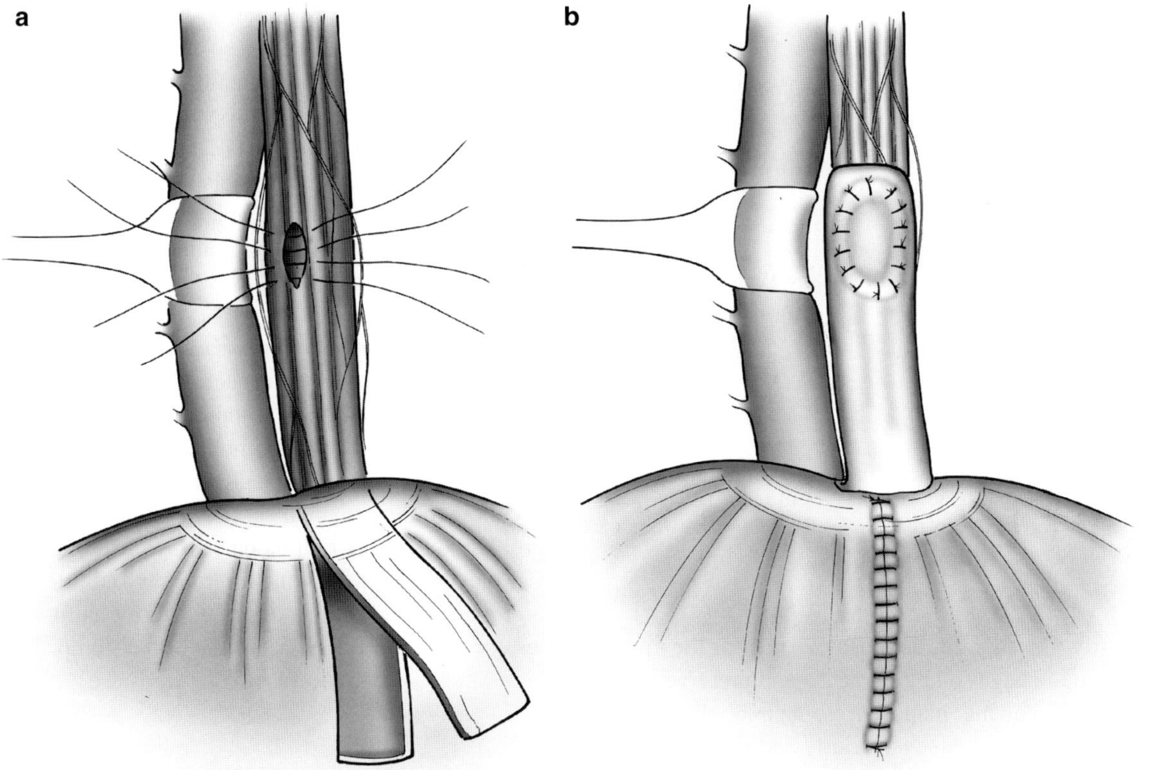

Fig. 32.3 (**a**, **b**) Rotate the flap upwards from its base, towards the oesophagus, cover the repair or gap and close the diaphragmatic defect by interrupted sutures

few days, the stoma retracts to the extent that it almost closes. It is also very difficult to apply a drainage bag around the retracted stoma. If it is combined with a blind oesophageal loop after intrathoracic stapling of the oesophagus above the injury, it does not really overt the blind oesophageal loop complications. Overall its presence does not make the presence of a blind oesophageal loop inside the oesophagus less deleterious.

If you consider a proximal diversion, the best solution is to proceed to fashioning of an end-oesophagostomy. This should also be done if at the initial operation, the damage of the oesophagus is beyond repair, or if you get yourself into the vicious circle of doing re-look thoracotomies for sepsis. In that case (if the patient is physiologically stable), proceed to removal of the thoracic oesophagus at an early stage and bringing out the proximal part as a stoma (if not physiologically stable, perform the damage control – bail-out procedure that was mentioned previously). To perform an end-cervical oesophagostomy, do a left cervical incision at the anterior margin of the sternocleidomastoid muscle. Incise the investing fascia along the sternomastoid muscle while retracting it laterally. Identify and divide the omohyoid muscle as it passes laterally deep to the sternomastoid muscle. Divide the rest of the strap muscles, close to the clavicle and identify the carotid sheath. And retract it laterally while simultaneously retracting the larynx medially. Create a plane between the two with your fingers and you will feel as you dissect posteriorly the bodies of the vertebrae. The musculotubular structure anterior to this is the cervical oesophagus. You create a plane between the oesophagus and the body of the vertebra with a right-angled Lahey – distally to the level of the cricoid cartilage. Then insert your hooked right index finger in this plane and push downward as you are standing on the patient's left side. In this way, you strip off the posterior aspect of the oesophagus from the cervical vertebral column. Now you must mobilise the anterior aspect of the oesophagus from the posterior aspect of the trachea. Remember that the oesophagus at that level deviates slightly to the left. It will be useful if you first divide the inferior thyroid artery and middle thyroid vein.

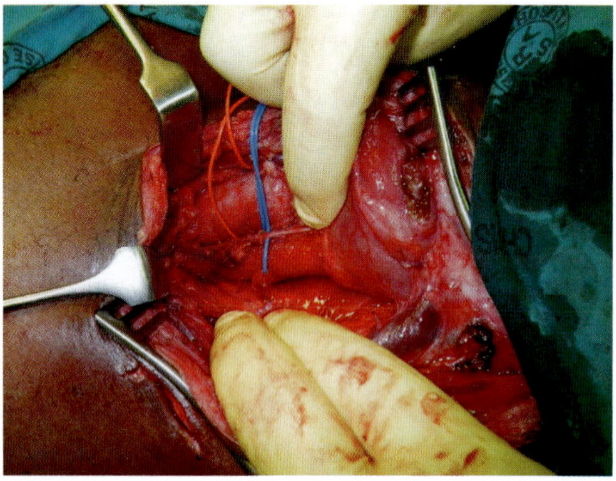

Fig. 32.4 The cervical trachea has been encircled with red and the cervical oesophagus with blue vessel loop. The recurrent laryngeal nerve is seen running in the groove between the viscera

Identify the recurrent laryngeal nerve near the groove of the oesophagus and the trachea and preserve it during the following manoeuvres. Retract the trachea slightly to the right and superiorly and the oesophagus slightly inferiorly. Then keeping the tension to the two structures; use your scissors and by cutting with its tip, open a plain between the oesophagus and the posterior wall of the trachea. After this plane has been 'deepened', you can use a right-angled Lahey to complete the separation of the two viscera. Further distal separation can now take place, by blunt dissection with your hooked right index finger swiped distally between the two, always taking care of the recurrent laryngeal nerve (Fig. 32.4). Pull then the remnant of the thoracic oesophagus through the thoracic inlet. Usually, if adequate dissection has been done from the chest, the proximal oesophageal stump can be easily brought into the field with minimal, if any, dissection. Tend to save as much thoracic oesophagus as possible as you will see that a lot of its length is consumed in your effort to externalise it and many times you find its length rather short to do that. Having a decent length of cervical oesophagus for the construction of a cervical oesophagostomy will also later on make reconstruction of the continuity of the GI tract easier by being able to anastomose a decent length of oesophagus to the stomach or to the large bowel. If the oesophageal stump is short, although a later stage anastomosis is still feasible, it will be problematic from the function point of view. If the cervical oesophageal stump is very short, you can even find yourself anastomosing to the pharynx with the patient possibly becoming physiologically crippled. It is preferable to make the stoma over the anterior chest wall by creating a subcutaneous tunnel rather than through or near the cervical incision in the neck as application of stomal appliances is much easier over the relatively flat surface area of the chest than the uneven surface of the neck. However, if proximal oesophageal length is compromised through the necessity of the resection, do no hesitate to bring out the stoma through the cervical incision. Usually the blood flow to the proximal cervical oesophagus is not a problem due to the rich blood supply of the submucosal plexus supplied by the inferior thyroid arteries, therefore creating a stoma over the anterior chest wall does not usually result in ischaemia of the stump.

Important Points

1. Have a high index of suspicion in oesophageal injury.
2. Liberal use of CT scan of the chest and proceed to swallow, oesophageoscopy if the CT scan shows track proximity to the oesophagus.
3. Buttress repair in late presentation.
4. Liberal drainage in all explorations and repairs.

Recommended Reading

Degiannis E, Benn CA, Leandros E, Goosen J, Boffard K, Saadia R (2000) Transmediastinal gunshot injuries. Surgery 128(1): 54–58

Karmy-Jone RC, Wagner JW, Lewis JW Jr (1998) Oesophageal injury. In: Trunkey DD, Lews FR (eds) Current therapy of trauma, 4th edn. Mosby, St. Louis

Smakman N, Nicol AJ, Walther G, Brooks A, Navsaria PH, Zellweger R (2004) Factors affecting outcome in penetrating esophageal trauma. Br J Surg 91:1513–1519

Pulmonary and Bronchotracheal Trauma

33

Elias Zigiriadis, Peter Loogna, and Tugba H. Yilmaz

The majority of penetrating thoracic trauma can be managed non-operatively. Only 15% of the penetrating chest trauma requires thoracotomy.

The thoracic cavity can hold up to 3 L of blood. A haemothorax results from lacerations or rupture of any thoracic structure following blunt or penetrating trauma. Remember that intra-abdominal injuries can sometimes result in a haemothorax, when blood traverses a diaphragmatic injury. The same is true with penetrating injuries to the base of the neck that may also bleed into the pleural space. A haemothorax is called massive when there is more than 1,500-mL blood in the pleural space. Usually massive haemothorax is caused by laceration of the intercostal arteries, internal mammary vessels, central lung injuries, heart or great vessel injuries. Bleeding from the lung parenchyma is rarely massive due to the low systolic pulmonary artery pressure and the high thromboplastin levels in the lungs. A large haemothorax may restrict ventilation and impair the venous return.

E. Zigiriadis (✉)
Division of Cardiothoracic Surgery,
Charlotte Maxeke Johannesburg Academic Hospital, University of the Witwatersrand Medical School,
7, York Road, Parktown 2193, Johannesburg, South Africa
e-mail: zigigabriel@hotmail.com

P. Loogna
Surgical Department, Sophiahemmet, Vallhallavägen 91,
S-114 86 Stockholm, Sweden
e-mail: ploogna@hotmail.com

T.H. Yilmaz
Department of Surgery, Baskent University,
6371 Sokak No: 34, Bostanli, Izmir 35540, Turkey
e-mail: tugba.yilmaz@deu.edu.tr

Drain any haemothorax that is bigger than the amount required to obscure the costophrenic angle or is associated with a pneumothorax.

If there is still a haemothorax despite a functioning intercostal chest drain (preferably a curved one), insert an additional drain. Always do a post-insertion chest x-ray. Be alert of malfunctioning drains (i.e., drain occluded or drain holes outside chest cavity in subcutaneous tissue) when an initially high volume loss suddenly ceases. In cases of inadequate drainage of the haemothorax by chest tubes, a thoracotomy or thoracoscopy is performed within 4 days. A minimal haemothorax such as blunting of the costophrenic angle can be managed conservatively.

33.1 Thoracotomy

Most haemothoraces are managed with insertion of intercostal drains. However, if the initial drainage after placement of a chest drain is >1,500 mL blood or the blood loss continues at a rate of 300 mL/h for 3–4 h post insertion, this is an indication for thoracotomy. Furthermore, a patient that is unstable despite aggressive volume resuscitation may also need a thoracotomy. Always repeat the CXR to make sure that there is no retained clot in the pleural cavity giving you the false impression that bleeding has stopped. There is no data supporting decreased haemorrhage or mortality by clamping the chest tube while preparing the patient for surgery. Consider autotransfusion of blood from the chest cavity to reduce the need for donor blood.

G.C. Velmahos et al. (eds.), *Penetrating Trauma*,
DOI 10.1007/978-3-642-20453-1_33, © Springer-Verlag Berlin Heidelberg 2012

33.2 Access to the Thoracic Cavity

33.2.1 Choice of Incision

Without doubt, access to the pleural cavity is best achieved first by a posterolateral and then an anterolateral thoracotomy, usually via the fifth or sixth intercostal space. A right posterolateral incision permits access to the trachea, right bronchus, carina, proximal 3 cm of left bronchus right lung, right chest wall and the whole of the oesophagus. The left posterolateral incision provides access to the aorta, proximal left subclavian artery (only for initial control in exceptional circumstances), the distal left bronchus, the left lung and the distal oesophagus. However in case of haemodynamic instability, need to access heart or the other side of thoracic cavity an anterolateral incision is more appropriate.

33.3 Posterolateral Thoracotomy

The patient should be in a full lateral position. The lower leg is flexed and the upper leg is straight. A pillow separates the legs. For better stability and spreading of the ribs, place a pillow beneath the chest perpendicular to the patient, this splays the thoracic cavity open. The upper part of chest is then strapped at the shoulders with either an elastoplast or strapping belts. The same is done at the hips to hold the lower body in position. The upper limbs are flexed and elevated in such a way that the endotracheal tube sits in between the arms and the lateral chest wall is fully exposed and there is ample space for your assistant to stand. Stand behind the patient and make a curvilinear incision extending from anterior to the tip of scapula – one fingers breadth below it – and curving posteriorly towards the vertebral column but stopping short of it approximately 5 cm. Start dividing the muscles individually.

Elevate the scapula with a scapular retractor away. The plane between the scapula and the chest wall is avascular. Now slide your hand under the scapula to the apex of the chest and begin to count the ribs. The first rib could be difficult to feel and usually the highest palpable rib is the second one. (On identifying the first or the second rib, keep in mind that usually there is a step between these two ribs that is not present between the second and the third). Count the ribs this way and find the fifth or sixth rib that is normally the level that you should to enter the chest. Then continue division of the muscles onto the rib surface followed by division of the intercostal muscle onto the superior border of the rib. At this point, if the patient has been intubated with double lumen endotracheal tube, you notify your anaesthetist to isolate the respective lung. Divide the intercostals muscles by diathermy at the upper border of the corresponding rib, gently followed by penetrating the pleura into the thoracic cavity.

Watch out for: A lung that is not isolated or a lung that is adherent to the pleura due to a previous pleuritis or inflammatory process. Being alert of these two circumstances will prevent any unnecessary injury to the lung.

Spread the ribs by a Finochietto retractor. Do that gradually so that you avoid iatrogenic rib fractures. In the case that the patient is bleeding torrentially, fracturing of the ribs is unavoidable. Make sure that you or your assistants avoid injury from the spikes.

Insert two intercostal drains at the end of the operation. One in anterior position at the apex and the other, a curved one, in posterior position at the base of the thorax. Insert the drains through low stab incisions and connect them to underwater seal bottles or autotransfusion drainage systems. Place them on Gomko suction once in the intensive care or high care unit.

Close the thoracotomy by using a few figure-of-eight sutures, passing above the superior border of the upper rib followed by the superior border of the lower rib. Use no. 1 vicryl suture on a round body needle. The muscles are approximated by continuous suturing in layers.

33.4 Anterolateral Thoracotomy

Place the patient in an oblique lateral position with a sandbag supporting behind the posterior chest. The upper arm is supported to the anaesthetic screen with the elbow flexed in 90° angle. You stand behind the patient.

The skin incision starts below the breast approximately over the fifth rib along the inframammary skin crease to end 2 cm below the inferior angle of the scapula.

The incision is deepened and the anterior portion of the latissimus dorsi is divided. Incision is deepened by division of the muscles. Entering the pleural cavity, inserting the intercostal drains and closing are the same as for posterolateral thoracotomy.

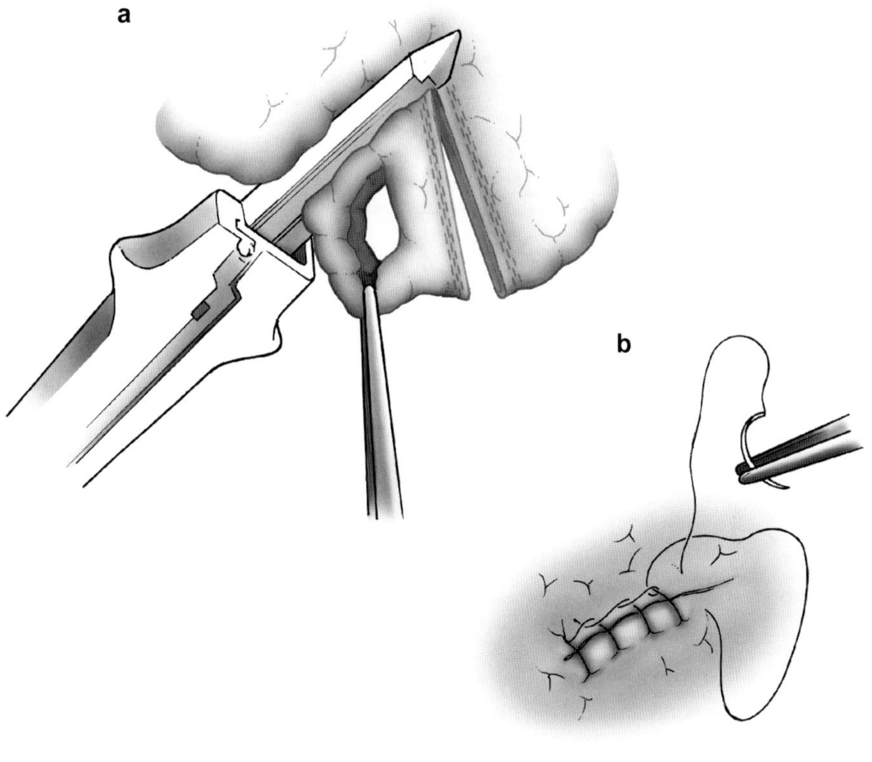

Fig. 33.1 (**a**, **b**) Repair of pulmonary laceration. Main sketch: wedge excision with stapler

If you decide to also access the opposite thoracic cavity, you can proceed by transecting the sternum. Remember always to ligate the internal mammary arteries. Sometimes due to severe hypovolemia, they are not actively bleeding during the operation just to start to bleed in the postoperative care unit.

33.5 Injuries to the Lung Parenchyma

When performing surgery on the chest, it is advisable to isolate the respective lung by inserting a double lumen endotracheal tube.

When treating bleeding from the lung parenchyma, always try to use the technique with the least possible physiologic insult. The inflated lung can easily be injured if you handle it forcefully. Always use big gauze and your palms when handling the lungs. If needed divide the inferior pulmonary ligament by concurrently palpating and freeing the ligament between your thumb and index finger by a gentle rolling action. Avoid excessive pulling and jerking.

Superficial parenchymal lacerations are preferably managed with the lung isolated i.e., deflated. This avoids any unnecessary tears of the friable parenchyma during suturing. The laceration depending on the extent can be repaired with either pledgetted 4/0/prolene SH (larger needle) or a running suture in two layers, firstly a horizontal mattress followed by an 'over-and-over' suture. Open superficial missile tracts with electrocautery and ligate individual vessels individually with ties or liga clips depending on their size. Open bronchioles are ligated for control. Do not close and liberally irrigate. You can also manage peripheral injuries with a stapled wedge resection either with GIA (newer products available are also reinforced with pericardium – this adds to the integrity of the stapled surface and reduces the incidence of air leaks postoperatively especially if your patients will be ventilated receiving the additional insult of positive pressure ventilation) or TA stapler (Fig. 33.1). Avoid the use of staplers with a fully inflated lung. Ask the anaesthetist to stop ventilating the lung; apply pressure to partially deflate it, and then staple. Then check the staple line for bleeding and air leaks, and if necessary reinforce it with a figure-of-eight suture of prolene (less friction in the easily lacerated lung parenchyma). An alternative to this technique is to use two soft bowel clump wedged

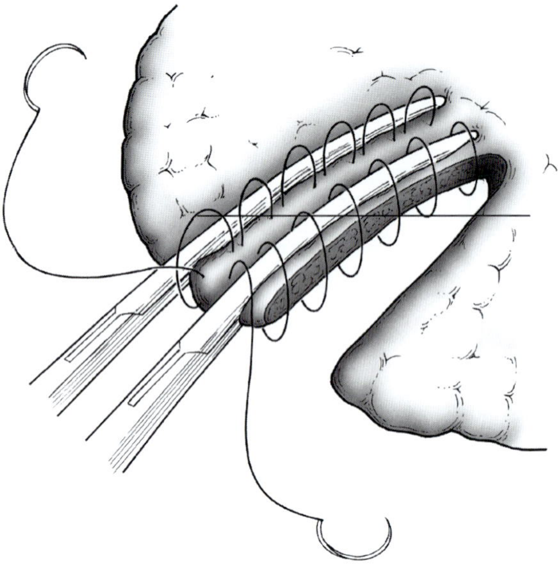

Fig. 33.2 Wedge excision using soft bowel clamps

on either side of the part of the lung to be resected. A mattress suture is used under the clamp and the repair is then completed by a continuous locking stitch at the resected end (Fig. 33.2).

33.6 Tractotomy

Deep parenchymal laceration can be controlled by a non-anatomic exposure of the laceration tract by tractotomy. Insert clamps or the limb of a linear stapling device along the tract and divide it (Fig. 33.3). Before using the staplers, ask the anaesthetist to stop ventilating the lung and apply pressure to partially deflate it. If vessels or small bronchi are not effectively included in the suture line, oversew them by figure-of-eight monofilament sutures such as polypropylene. Always be aware that when the lung re-inflates, the staples may give way. In those cases, overrun the suture line with a continuous locking suture. Beware of placing superficial sutures in deep lacerations that are bleeding, as this can lead to an intrapulmonary haematoma, infection and air-embolism.

33.7 Pulmonary Resections

Central injuries may need anatomical lobectomy. Very rarely a pneumonectomy might be needed. The mortality rate in the latter is high.

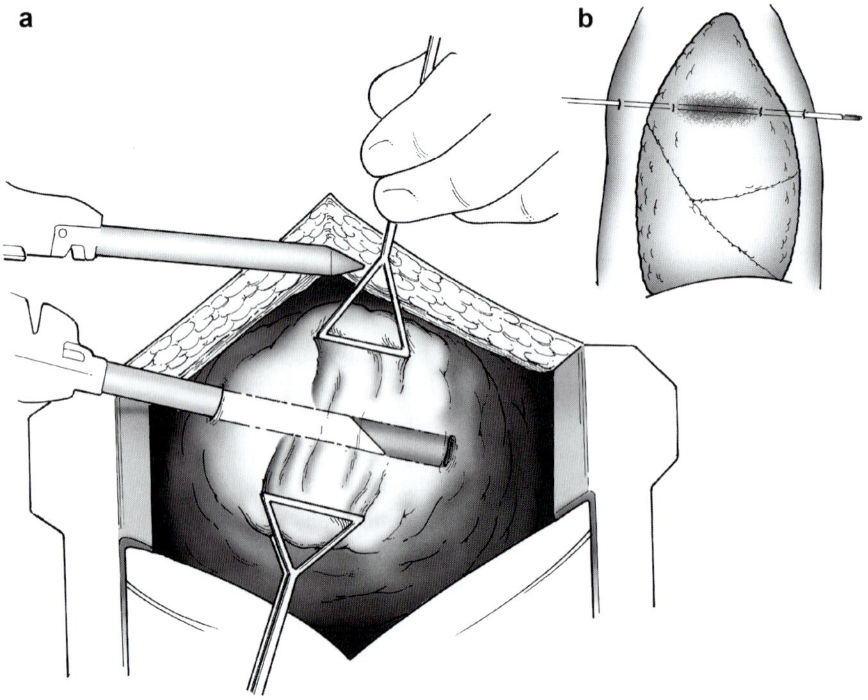

Fig. 33.3 (**a**, **b**) Insert: Bullet track in pulmonary tissue. Main sketch: tractotomy using staplers

33.8 Lobectomy

33.8.1 Intubate with Double Lumen Endotracheal Tube if Time Permits

It is imperative to gain access of the pulmonary vasculature. Remember that both the arteries and veins are fragile and tear easily. Use large gauze on palms when manipulating the lungs, to facilitate traction. Open the adventitial plane anterosuperiorly to isolate either the right or left pulmonary artery. This is achieved with blunt dissection using an angled Lahey and is encircled with no. 1 tie. This is a life-saving manoeuvre should there be any further injury to the vasculature while mobilising. Isolating the left pulmonary artery is different as one has to dissect inferior to the aortic arch. Look for the left recurrent laryngeal nerve that is in close proximity. Identify the segmental braches and ligate depending on which lobe is to be resected with a vascular clamp and oversewn with 3-0 monofilament as a running over-and-over stitch together with two proximal suture ligatures that overlap. The assistant must relax the traction of the lung when these ligatures are being tied. You can alternatively use vascular staples.

Division of the bronchus must be close to the trachea or adjacent lobar bronchus to avoid future formation of bronchopleural fistula. This can be closed either with staples or sutures. If with sutures, use simple interrupted sutures of your choice. Try and cover the bronchial stump with a pleural flap or other tissue if possible.

33.9 Pneumonectomy

In desperate cases, pneumonectomy may be required for massive hilar injuries. The same principles as for a lobectomy are applied.

33.10 Control of Hilum of the Lung

Massive bleeding from pulmonary injuries can temporarily be controlled by clamping of the hilum with a large vascular clamp (Fig. 33.4). For applying the vascular clamp i.e., the Satinsky, hold the hilum between the index and third finger and apply the Satinsky proximally to your fingers. Adhesions may be present in and around the hilum secondary coexisting inflammatory disease, such as tuberculosis. Dissect the vessels initially using blunt dissection with the aid of Lahey swab (gauze on a Roberts forceps). Identifying the pulmonary veins may be difficult, and in this case, you can access them by opening the pericardium (intrapericardial mobilisation).

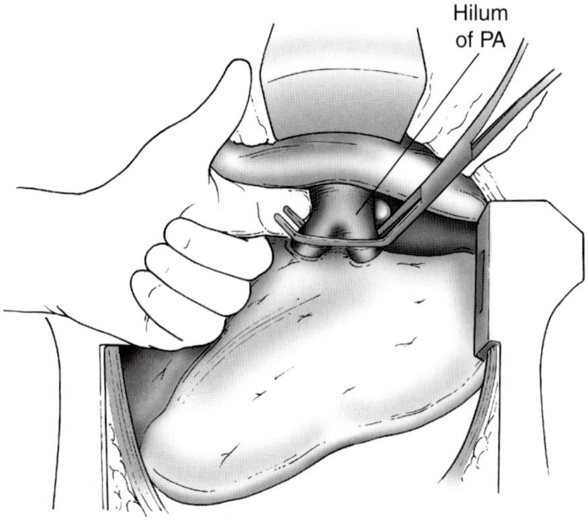

Fig. 33.4 Clamping of the hilum

33.11 Tips

- Before opening the chest, ensure you have all your various vascular and bronchial clamps ready and inspected.
- Try to have a cell saver available for rapid reinfusion of patient's own blood.
- Be aware of the three major life-threatening surgical complications: (1) injury to major vessel with massive haemorrhage, (2) cardiac arrhythmias and (3) contralateral pneumothorax.
- Pulmonary arteries are thin and careful initial dissection from their fibrous sheaths with a pair of blunt tipped scissors in the long axis is best done before attempting mobilisation.
- Remember that a right upper lobectomy is more complex than any other lobe and arterial anomalies are more common. (In approximately 80% of individuals, right upper lobe is partially or completely fused to the middle lobe.)
- On the right side, at the azygocaval junction, a lymph node is present and can be used as a landmark to identify the upper border of the pulmonary artery.

- Be careful when dissecting medially the right inferior pulmonary ligament, a lymph node will be noted anteriorly and will alert you to the inferior pulmonary vein.

33.12 Tracheobronchial Injuries

These injuries are rare and may involve the trachea or bronchi from the level of the cricoid cartilage to the division of lobar bronchi. They are associated with a 30% mortality rate and are often associated with injuries to other vital structures as well. Oesophageal and vascular injuries are common with penetrating tracheal injuries. In up to 80%, the penetrating injuries involve the cervical trachea. In contrast, blunt trauma causes in more than 80% of cases a tracheobronchial rupture within 3 cm from carina.

The clinical presentation is variable and spreads from asymptomatic to those patients with stridor, dyspnoea, haemoptysis, hypoxia and subcutaneous emphysema. Often the patient has a massive air leak via the chest tube and a second chest tube could be required to overcome it. Always suspect a tracheobronchial injury when the lung does not expand with the chest tube drainage with concomitant subcutaneous emphysema and pneumomediastinum.

Chest x-ray may show pneumomediastinum, pneumothoraces and pleural effusions. Occasionally air surrounding a bronchus and the 'fallen lung sign' can be seen. This latter sign is pathognomonic of a complete disruption of a mainstem bronchus. The bronchus is transected and the affected lung may drop down onto the diaphragm with the apex of the lung sitting at the level of the pulmonary hilum. CT scanning may assist with the diagnosis of tracheal and bronchial injuries. Still most recommend a bronchoscopy for definitive diagnosis. A flexible bronchoscope may miss the injury if passed through an endotracheal tube that itself traverses the injury. A rigid bronchoscopy has the benefits in that it allows ventilation through the instrument and it is easier to evacuate blood and debris through it.

Approaches to the trachea include:

- Suprasternal Collar incision
- Sternotomy – mobilising aorta to left and superior vena cava to right gives you access to lower trachea (with or without cardiopulmonary bypass).
- Left or right thoracotomy for the carina or bronchi

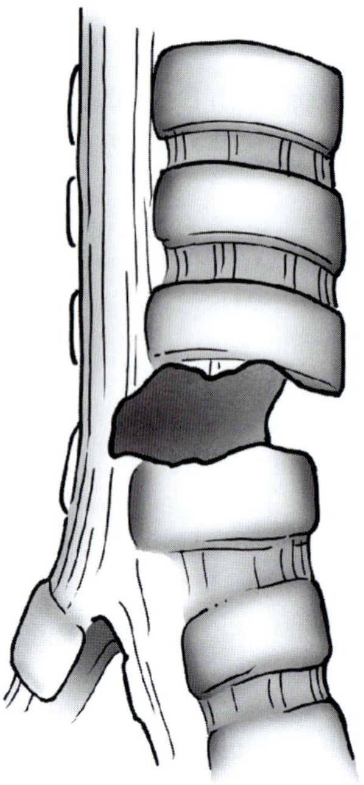

Fig. 33.5 Injury of trachea to be resected

33.13 Tracheal Resection and Reconstruction

The tracheal resection and reconstruction procedure is as follows:

For reconstructing the upper trachea: Position patient in supine position with a soft pillow behind the chest and the neck extended if there are no cervical spine injuries, patient is intubated via the oropharyngeal route with the tip of tube distal to the tracheal injury.

Incision: Transverse collar incision 1–2 fingers breadth above sternal notch and separation of the underlying fascial and muscular planes – stay in the midline by noting a whitish fascial plane running longitudinally while separating the muscles.

Remember the trachea is about 10–12 cm and almost 50% can be resected with the various releases that can be done.

Avoid extensive dissection of trachea up or down as blood supply is segmental, and in addition preserve the recurrent laryngeal nerve.

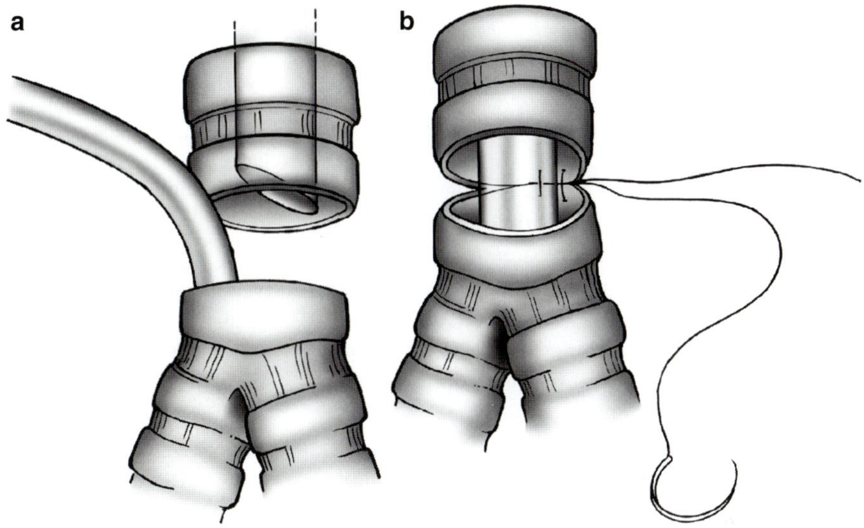

Fig. 33.6 (**a**) Pulling of oropharyngeal endotracheal tube proximally and reintubating of the proximal trachea. (**b**) Interrupted sutures placed at posterior wall of trachea, removal of distal endotracheal tube and advancement of the oropharyngeal endotracheal tube

Encircle the tracheal segment involved, warn the anaesthetist to ensure the endotracheal tube bulb is not penetrated accidently.

Resect the involved segment having placed stay sutures at the 3 o'clock and 9 o'clock positions distal to the resection margin (Fig. 33.5).

Now, the oropharyngeal endotracheal tube is pulled back gently after deflating the cuff and reintubating the lower distal trachea with a sterile cuffed tube of a slightly smaller size if possible, this makes it easier to work with when placing sutures posteriorly (Fig. 33.6a, b). At this point one can also suction the trachea and bronchi with a suction tube to remove any blood or secretions after temporarily removing the tube.

Sutures are placed starting at the 6 o'clock position using 4/0 PDS interrupted sutures posteriorly and ensuring the knot is outside. Take 2–3-mm bites at the membranous portion of the trachea. The anterior half of the trachea 3/0 PDS sutures are used in the same fashion (single interrupted around the tracheal rings and not through) (Fig. 33.7). All sutures are then gently pulled together with constant tension after flexing the neck and removing the tube. At this point, the anaesthetist has prepared another cuffed endotracheal tube and advances it beyond your suture line. Start by tying the posterior sutures in alternate fashion from each end.

At the completion, place a silk suture from the chin to manubrium for 7–10 days.

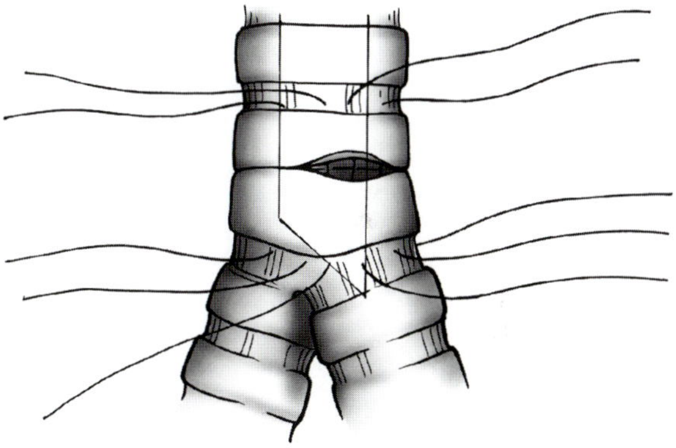

Fig. 33.7 Placement of anterior wall of trachea sutures

If possible it is always better to extubate the patient on the table and avoid any excessive coughing.

Reconstruct the lower trachea is via a right thoracotomy, and in a similar fashion, the distal trachea is transacted and traction sutures placed and the left main bronchus reintubated with a sterile tube.

Certain manoeuvres help to avoid excessive tension on the trachea include flexing the neck, releasing the inferior pulmonary ligament and hilar release.

Avoid any tension on the trachea, any failure is devastating.

For repair of main bronchi, follow the same principles.

Important Points

- Most haemothoraces/haemopneumothoraces can be managed by chest drains with Gomko or gentle wall suction.
- Never remove chest drains if lung is incompletely expanded or drain bottle still bubbling.
- The decision for operative treatment of a haemothorax is determined by the physiologic status of the patient.
- Manage pulmonary lung lacerations with the technique that cause the least physiologic insult of the patient.
- Do not just oversew the lung surface in case of a seep bleeding laceration as the result can be a large parenchymal haematoma.
- Always try to deflate the lung before you use the stapler device.
- Do a bronchoscopy in patients with suspected airway injuries.
- A bronchial injury can be repaired by end-to-end anastomosis with mucosa-to-mucosa apposition.
- Use absorbable sutures when repairing bronchial defects to reduce the risk of stitch granuloma inside the airway.

Recommended Reading

Huh J, Milliken JC, Chen JC (1997) Management of tracheobronchial injuries following blunt and penetrating trauma. Am Surg 63:896–899

Jameel A, Med M, Wan Q (1995) Effectiveness of chest tube clamping in massive hemothorax. J Trauma 38(1):59–63

Loogna P, Bonanno F, Bowley DM et al (2007) Emergency thoracic surgery for penetrating, non-mediastinal trauma. ANZ J Surg 77(3):142–145

Powell RJ, Redan JA, Swan KG (1990) The hilar snare, an improved technique for securing rapid vascular control of the pulmonary hilum. J Trauma 30:208–210

Velmahos GC, Baker C, Demetriades D et al (1999) Lung-sparing surgery after penetrating trauma using tractotomy, partial lobectomy, and pneumonorrhaphy. Arch Surg 134:186–189

Wall MJ, Hirschberg A, Mattox KL (1994) Pulmonary tractomy with selective vascular ligation for penetrating injuries to the lung. Am J Surg 168:665–669T.H. Yilmaz
Department of Surgery, Baskert University,
6371 Sokak No: 34, Bostanli, Izmir 35540, Turkey
e-mail: tugba.yilmaz@deu.edu.tr

Mediastinal Vessels

34

Philip R. Calderbank, Nigel R. M. Tai,
and Douglas M. Bowley

The resting cardiac output of the average adult is approximately 5 L/min. Coupled with venous return and the pulmonary circulation, large amounts of blood pass through the mediastinal vessels each minute. Following a penetrating injury to any of these vessels, exsanguination may occur within moments; but those patients that do survive the initial bleed and transport to hospital are salvageable if treated swiftly and decisively. Whilst deterioration may often be rapid and access difficult, the right operation performed at the right time can set the conditions for patient survival. The difficulty is in gaining control whilst the patient still has sufficient physiological reserve. The aim of this chapter is not to list every possible technique of repair for penetrating injuries to the mediastinal vessels, nor give exhaustive details of the steps entailed. Instead, it aims to describe a system that will allow the surgeon to make the right choice, at the right time, from admission to definitive care, in order to give the best chance of success.

34.1 Patterns of Injury

Penetrating trauma to the mediastinal vessels is rare, with injuries of the thoracic great vessels occurring in about 5% of all gunshot wounds and 2% of all stab wounds to the chest. Table 34.1 documents the expected incidence of injury types after penetrating injury to the chest, and it is always worth remembering that a high proportion of patients with penetrating chest injury will have diaphragmatic penetration and intra-abdominal injuries (Table 34.2).

34.2 Iatrogenic Injury

Percutaneous central venous catheter placement may damage mediastinal vessels as well as the surrounding pleura. Unguarded placement of chest tubes, with or without a trocar, may also damage the mediastinal vessels, along with any other organ within reach. Metal stents placed in nearby structures such as the oesophagus may erode causing mediastinal vessel damage, sometimes with catastrophic results. The use of intra-aortic balloon pumps and other cardiac instrumentation has the potential to damage the mediastinal vessels. These patients are usually older and have more co-morbidity than those injured due to stabbing or ballistic injury. Underlying management principles remain similar: the first step is to suspect the presence of mediastinal vascular injury, as late detection is usually associated with a poor outcome. Consider the possibility of mediastinal vascular injury in any patient who becomes unstable following the above type of interventions and act accordingly.

34.3 Management Strategy

34.3.1 Principles

Patients who survive to reach hospital after penetrating mediastinal vascular injury represent a self-selected, potentially salvageable cohort. Existing data suggests

P.R. Calderbank • N.R.M. Tai • D.M. Bowley (✉)
Academic Department of Military Surgery and Trauma,
Royal Centre for Defence Medicine, Birmingham Research Park,
Vincent Drive B15 2SQ Birmingham, UK
e-mail: info@militarysurgery.org.uk

G.C. Velmahos et al. (eds.), *Penetrating Trauma*,
DOI 10.1007/978-3-642-20453-1_34, © Springer-Verlag Berlin Heidelberg 2012

Table 34.1 Most frequent major injuries from penetrating chest trauma

Injury	Incidence (%)
Pneumothorax	19
Haemothorax	23
Haemopneumothorax	34
None	11
Cardiac wound	14

Table 34.2 Other major injuries associated with penetrating chest trauma

Injury	Incidence (%)
Diaphragm	26
Liver	20
Major vascular	11
Stomach	10
Colon	5
Small intestine	4
Kidney	3
Spinal cord	3
Extremity	3
Pancreas	2

that up to 60% of the patients will be in an unstable condition on arrival and the overall mortality is in the order of 50%. Urgent assessment and simultaneous management is a necessity. Initial assessment is aimed at gauging the probabilities of injury and at determining the degree of physiological compromise. The only question to ask is: is the patient stable? Definitive diagnosis is unnecessary as this will waste time to definitive haemorrhage control; all that is required is a management strategy. Please also remember that 'stability' cannot be decided upon from single time-point measures.

34.3.2 Assessment and Resuscitation

Simultaneous assessment and treatment (along ATLS® guidelines) should begin immediately, and the triage process begun (see below). Information should be sought from the transferring team, patient (where possible) or accompanying witnesses about the timing and circumstances of the incident. Of particular consideration is mechanism of injury; the path of any projectile or penetrating object should never be assumed, nor should the anatomy of the patient. Careful examination of the external surfaces of the body much be done in every case. Small stab wounds and even small calibre GSW are surprisingly easy to overlook, particularly in the axillary folds or on the back. Unpaired injuries after GSW should be assumed to represent a retained projectile which may be in a body cavity remote from the site of injury (very rarely due to the phenomenon of bullet embolus [see below]). Attending staff must discipline themselves not to make assumptions about whether any particular GSW is an entrance or an exit wound. It is easy to make mistakes and such assumptions can cause clinical and then later medico-legal difficulty.

Any injury that passes in proximity to the mediastinum (including upper abdominal) should be assumed to have injured the great vessels (and/or heart). Likewise any injury below the level of the nipples anteriorly or inferior borders of the scapulae posteriorly should be assumed to have entered the abdomen.

34.3.3 Categorisation of Patients After Primary Survey

For patients with penetrating chest injury that are *in extremis*, the primary survey must rule out tension pneumothorax (as the life-threatening condition that can be most easily treated). The next aim of the primary survey is to triage patients into the three simple management categories; remember that definitive diagnosis is not required.

Categorisation of patients with suspected penetrating mediastinal vessel injury

1. Patients that require immediate surgical intervention
2. Patients that require or potentially require urgent intervention (surgical or endovascular)
3. Patients that do not currently require surgical or endovascular procedures

The triage process consists of four sequential steps which will assist in categorisation:

1. Initial assessment and resuscitation
   - (a) Stable patients proceed to further assessment
   - (b) Unstable patients proceed to thoracotomy
     - (i) In-extremis: Emergency resuscitative thoracotomy
     - (ii) Other patients: proceed to OR
2. Further assessment; History, Examination, CXR, +/– tube thoracostomy
   - (a) Mediastinal injury suspected, patient stable, proceed to CTA

(b) Mediastinal injury not suspected, patient stable, proceed to investigate and treat other injuries
(c) Unstable patients proceed to thoracotomy

3. Contrast-Enhanced Helical Computed Tomography Angiography (CTA)
   (a) Negative CTA: Admit for observation/discharge according to injury burden
   (b) Positive CTA: Proceed to intervention, with or without other investigations
   (c) Equivocal CTA: proceed to Intra-Arterial Digital Subtraction Angiography (IADSA)
4. IADSA
   (a) Where positive CTA but more information required (for consideration of endovascular repair)
   (b) Where equivocal CTA and more information required

If at any point, the patient becomes unstable, then investigation should be curtailed and the patient submitted to surgery. Where no injury is detected by CTA, or the injury is deemed trivial enough not to require operation, stable patients should be observed closely in a high dependency setting. Other injuries, where present, should be managed accordingly. Invasive monitoring is advisable, and its use will depend on resource availability. Where early intervention has occurred, care should be taken to ensure a tertiary survey (head-to-toe examination of the patient and review of imaging) is completed to avoid missed injury.

34.3.4 Clinical Examination

A thorough initial examination can elicit signs of possible mediastinal great vessel injury. Possible indications of a great vessel injury include:

- 'Proximity' wounds: stab wounds, fragment or GSW to the chest with signs of shock
- Expanding thoracic outlet haematoma
- Massive haemothorax
- Suspicion or evidence of pericardial penetration
  - Proximity wound in presence of shock
  - Muffled heart sounds
  - Congested neck veins
  - Pulsus paradoxus
- Precordial 'machinery shunt' murmur
- Discrepancy in pulse/BP – right vs. left arm, upper vs. lower limbs
- Lateralising neurological signs; signs of brachial plexus or spinal cord injury.

34.3.5 Recognition of the Shocked or 'Unstable' Patient

Recognition of the 'shocked' patient is surprisingly difficult. We find it helpful to use the shock index (SI); this is a very simple clinical tool with a reliable base of evidence to support its use. Divide the patient's heart rate by the systolic blood pressure; if the resultant SI is >0.9, then the patient can be said to be 'shocked'.

Apart from simple failure to recognise the shocked patient, the other big error is to be lulled into a sense of security by initial response to resuscitation; patients with penetrating trauma to the major vascular structures of the chest almost always continue to bleed with fatal results if no action is taken. The difference between a stable and an unstable patient can be a matter of minutes, and constant awareness of the patient's physiology is essential. Any suspicion of a great vessel injury 'must' be resolved before transferring the patient to a ward.

'Unstable' patients are characterised as follows:

- Shock index (pulse/systolic blood pressure): >0.9
- Other signs of shock (class I–IV shock...revise your ATLS® manual)
- Nil or only transient response to volume resuscitation
- Continued blood loss >200 mL/h (where measured e.g. chest drain)
- Continued external haemorrhage
- Acidosis, elevated base excess

34.4 Chest Radiograph (CXR)

The supine antero-posterior chest radiograph is an important first-line investigation. In a study of penetrating transmediastinal gunshot wounds, physical examination and CXR together were shown to correctly identify mediastinal injury in 90% of patients. This simple investigation is increasingly overlooked in the era of rapidly available CT; however, it may be the only investigation you need to make a correct management decision, so do not forget to order it! Prior to the CXR, we typically will tape an unfolded paperclip over penetrating wounds; these so-called bullet markers can be a helpful guide to make a first judgement about trajectory and the likelihood of thoraco-abdominal injury.

Evidence of mediastinal great vessel injury on chest radiograph includes:

- Widening of the mediastinum
- Loss of the aortic knuckle
- Tracheal deviation away from the site of injury
- Massive haemothorax
- Pneumomediastinum

34.5 Contrast-Enhanced Computed Tomographic Angiography (CTA)

Improvements in CT have increased speed and accuracy whilst reducing the dose of ionising radiation. Its place as a first-line investigation in penetrating injuries of the mediastinum is now well documented. In addition, the same CT sequence can be used to screen for injuries in other anatomical regions. Incorporation of CT as first-line investigation has been shown to reduce cost compared to previous protocols and reduces the need for other investigations. As such CTA is effectively displacing angiography as the initial and definitive investigation of choice in suspected aortic/great vessel injuries. CTA sensitivity for mediastinal vascular injury is reported at >96%, with specificity and accuracy almost 100%.

The disadvantages of CTA may include the need to transfer the patient away from the resuscitation area, and the exposure of the patient to a period of time in the scanner where therapeutic input may be minimal. No matter what the physical layout of the trauma area and the scanner are, doctors have a duty to continue resuscitation and active treatment in the scan room.

CTA relies on the interpretation of its images, and the specialist input of a radiologist competent in trauma radiology interpretation is usually helpful. Where doubt about extent of injuries exists, formal angiography, oesophagoscopy, thoracoscopy and bronchoscopy may be useful. Combining CTA with judicious use of further investigations can reduce the rate of missed injury to negligible levels. Where CT is negative, further investigation is unwarranted, and such patients generally proceed on to active observation.

34.5.1 Formal Angiography

Digital subtraction angiography (DSA) provides detailed information on the nature of arterial injury, but is invasive and requires specialist logistical infrastructure. The frequency with which this investigation is used for the delineation of blunt aortic injury has dropped to <10% in most modern units. Some studies have suggested that conventional angiography following an indeterminate CT is unlikely to show further injury, but where significant doubt exists following an equivocal CTA, we would still order DSA.

34.5.2 Resuscitation

34.5.2.1 Initial Manoeuvres

Resuscitation should follow standard ATLS® guidelines. All patients should receive high-flow oxygen and multiple large bore venous access points; the intraosseous route can be used until venous access is established. Prompt intubation and ventilation are necessary for those *in extremis*. Remember to take blood samples for the normal trauma screen and cross match, arrange six units of packed cells and six of plasma from the blood bank for patients with signs of major injury. Shocked patients should undergo transfusion with O negative or type specific blood rather than be exposed to a delay for cross-matched blood. We try and avoid resuscitation with large volumes of crystalloid. Insertion of 6 French 'shock lines' via the large central veins is counter-productive if mediastinal vascular trauma is suspected. Our priority is haemorrhage control and replacement of lost blood with packed cells and plasma. Broad-spectrum prophylactic antibiotics should be administered as early as possible. Where it is available, we auto-transfuse salvaged blood obtained from chest drainage where massive haemothorax is present.

34.6 Emergency Room Thoracotomy (ERT)

The ideal place to perform definitive care remains the operating room or endovascular suite. ERT should be reserved for *in extremis* patients or those in cardiac arrest following penetrating chest injury. ERT is more likely to be successful when tamponade rather than exsanguination is the reason for circulatory collapse. Contraindications to ERT are debated, but generally relate to the likelihood of positive outcome, the main determinant being cerebral hypoperfusion. Where there is evidence of severe cerebral injury, or prolonged pre-hospital CPR, thoracotomy is likely to be futile. A guideline of pre-hospital CPR of 10 min intubated, 5 min non-intubated has been suggested as a cut-off.

The aim of the ERT is to stabilise the patient until formal repair and definitive haemostasis can be undertaken in more desirable surroundings and with the necessary equipment. As such this is a part of resuscitation, not of definitive management, and excessive time attempting to find the specific injury in a stabilised patient should not be undertaken. The main aims of the procedure are to relieve (or exclude) tamponade by pericardiotomy, arrest massive exsanguination via clamping, lung twist or manual pressure on the appropriate vessel e.g. descending aorta, pulmonary vein/artery and to perform effective internal cardiac massage if required. Assuming the circulation can be re-established, the patient should be transferred immediately to the operating theatre for further surgical evaluation and treatment as required.

34.6.1 Operative Action

The key logistic requirements should be anticipated and requested during the resuscitative phase. This may include mobilisation of a cell-savers, setting out of thoracic instruments, call-in of perfusionists, radiologists or cardiothoracic surgeons, and making arrangements for post-operative critical care. Our standard operative approach depends on the stability (or otherwise) of the patient. We usually choose a median sternotomy to approach injuries of the mediastinal vessels; however, clam-shell thoracotomy provides great access and can be combined with sternotomy to provide spectacular anatomical exposure. Do not be afraid to use composite (or multiple) incisions to access the injuries.

34.7 Cardiopulmonary Bypass (CPB)

Injuries to the arch branches of the aorta, or of the aorta itself, require surgical isolation in order to effect haemorrhage control and repair. This may entail clamping of the proximal thoracic aorta and significant systemic ischaemia. In such circumstances, cardiopulmonary bypass mitigates against complications such as spinal cord and visceral ischaemia. However, CPB is infrequently used in critical patients due to the necessity to use heparinised circuits (in the case of full bypass) and logistic constraints in summoning timely cardiothoracic assistance.

34.8 Damage Control

The use of sterile plastic tubing to restore distal perfusion across an injured vessel is an established technique, and is particularly useful in dealing with injuries to the proximal carotid and brachiocephalic vessels in order to maintain cerebral perfusion. Placement of a shunt is a demanding procedure to effect without damaging the delicate vessel intimal surface, and can only be undertaken after appropriate exposure and proximal-distal control has been gained. Once inserted and secured (we tie in shunts with 2-0 silk rather than use sloops), shunts can be left in situ for hours if the principle condition for definitive repair (physiological stability) has not yet been met. Other damage control measures include ligation of vascular structures rather than attempting repair. The consequences of this depend upon the vessel to be ligated and the degree of collateral circulation – subclavian arterial ligation rarely results in critical arm ischaemia and venous ligation is generally better tolerated than arterial; however, if needs must consider ligation.

34.9 Endovascular Repair

Endovascular repair obviates the requirement for morbid incisions and allows direct intervention following angiographic diagnosis. Guided catheters can be introduced remotely and used to position intraluminal balloons to lessen haemorrhage or achieve proximal control at the thoracic inlet, or to allow placement of covered stents across a breach in the vessel wall. Data with penetrating injuries is limited to short case series with relatively short follow-up; although for proximal subclavian arterial injuries, we definitely favour the endovascular approach in stable patients.

Suitability of a lesion for intraluminal repair depends on a variety of factors, not least of which is the experience and capability of the individual practitioner. Further factors include length of vessel defect to be crossed – with longer lesions being more difficult to bridge with a guidewire, and whether stent placement risks compromising the ostia of branch vessels. Complications include damage to the target vessel or end-organ (stroke), infection, embolisation, thrombosis and structural failure; patients in whom stent-grafts have been used require life-long follow-up.

34.10 Specific Injuries

34.10.1 Ascending Aorta and Aortic Arch

These injuries are best approached via midline sternotomy. Major injuries such as partial or complete transection are invariably incompatible with life; those presenting to the surgeon are often amenable to treatment, with survival rates of 50–80%. For injuries to the arch, superior extension to the neck may be necessary to expose the damaged segment, which may be obscured by a large pulsatile haematoma. Open the pericardium so that you get access to the ascending aorta and ligate the innominate vein to allow access to the arch. As true proximal control is not really feasible, before going near the haematoma, make sure you have a large side-biting vascular clamp available; as when the haematoma is explored, rapid and frightening bleeding usually occurs; control with digital pressure and then swift application of the clamp, this allows maintenance of distal blood flow. We always try to wear a mask with a visor if we anticipate cardiac or major vascular injury! Pledgeted sutures of 3-0 prolene should be used to repair the defect and a piece of pericardium may be used for the pledgets, if suitable prosthetic material is not immediately to hand. Posterior lacerations or complicated composite injuries may require cardiopulmonary bypass although the likelihood of such injuries presenting in salvageable patients is low. If the mechanism of injury involved a small projectile, just consider the possibility of distal embolisation of a projectile or fragment.

34.10.2 Descending Aorta

If patient stability permits, a left posterolateral thoracotomy at the fourth intercostal space provides optimal access. Achieve proximal and distal control in the immediately adjacent aorta 'upstream' and 'downstream' of the injury to maximise intercostal and spinal perfusion, with 'windowing' of the overlying pleura to allow application of a vascular clamp and careful dissection of the injured aorta away from adjacent viscera. Avoid damage to the posteriorly sited intercostals vessels as these are very difficult to control once injured. Upon initial clamping, pharmacological vasodilatation may be necessary to counteract the profound afterload and resultant strain this will place on the heart, although the requirement for this depends upon the initial volume status of the patient. Use simple aortorraphy for small lacerations, which may be controllable by application of a side-biting clamp, but larger and more complex injuries will require partial resection and graft interposition. Paraplegia may result if clamp times are prolonged.

34.10.3 Innominate Artery

Access is via midline sternotomy, with right supraclavicular extension if necessary. Once again, exposure is only effective after division of the innominate vein. Obtain proximal control at the base of the vessel before breaching the haematoma. Simple partial lacerations may be repaired with running lateral arteriorrhaphy with 4-0 or 5-0 prolene. Complete disruption or other complex injuries can be temporised with a shunt prior to reversed vein bypass grafting

34.10.4 Pulmonary Arteries

Planned access to proximal injuries should be via midline sternotomy. The right pulmonary artery requires dissection of the superior vena cava away from the ascending aorta to achieve adequate exposure. These injuries are associated with massive blood loss, with significant mortality (reported in excess of 70% in the literature). Because of the flow involved, anything other than simple injuries may require cardiopulmonary bypass.

Distal pulmonary artery injuries require approach via ipsilateral posterolateral thoracotomy. If the injury extends to involve the hilum, and injury is extensive, rapid progression on to pneumonectomy may be necessary. To obtain haemostasis, we find it easiest to rotate the lung around the hilum by 180° (divide the inferior pulmonary ligament first to improve mobility), or else cross-clamping of the whole hilum before continuing on to pneumonectomy using a 90 mm gastrointestinal stapler; we always oversew the suture-line with 3-0 prolene running stitch.

34.10.5 Innominate Vein

The innominate vein can be readily sacrificed, and if damaged should be ligated.

34.11 Vena Cava

Access is via median sternotomy when possible. Isolation of the IVC injury requires interruption of the venous return to the heart with critical effect on cardiac output. In these circumstances, use of a side-biting clamp is desirable if possible. Alternately repair can be better effected via imposition of cardiopulmonary bypass. Large defects, where present, may require synthetic patch or graft interposition.

34.12 Pulmonary Veins

Access is difficult in these injuries, and depends on the exact location involved. Proximal injuries may be addressed from within the pericardium. Distal injuries often require occlusion of the entire hilum in the first instance for haemostasis. Unless a simple lesion that is easily repairable is present, ligation of the pulmonary vein may be necessary and subsequent resection of the appropriate lobe of the lung.

34.13 Internal Mammary Arteries

Internal mammary artery (IMA) injuries may produce massive haemothorax and patients often appear as if they have cardiac tamponade. Treatment of the transected IMA is by ligation (of both ends!).

34.14 Azygous Vein

The azygous vein bleeds copiously and injuries are associated with high mortality. Often not considered until other sources have been ruled out following thoracotomy or sternotomy, persistent venous type bleeding from the right posterior mediastinum should alert the surgeon to the possibility of azygous injury. Management is to consider the possibility of azygous vein injury and then ligate it.

34.15 Foreign Body Embolisation

Foreign body embolisation is a problem peculiar to penetrating trauma. There are two different injury patterns:

- Systemic to central embolus (foreign bodies entering the circulation and embolising to pulmonary veins)
- Central to systemic embolus (foreign bodies entering a mediastinal vessel or within the heart and embolising systemically)

Approximately one third of central emboli are symptomatic. In the first instances, patients may present with symptoms of pulmonary embolus. The classically described CXR finding is of a blurred, out-of-focus object overlying the cardiac shadow when all other structures are in focus.

In the stable patient, and depending on location, these can be removed via endovascular snare. If open removal is required, this should be performed under bypass and the injured side should remain dependant using tilting of the operating table, to prevent it dislodging and passing contralaterally. Intra-operative radiological screening is invaluable in locating errant projectiles.

The second type of injury is often even more difficult to locate. In penetrating injuries due to projectiles without an obvious exit wound, the location of the missile should be sought, usually with plain x-radiographs or CT. However, the propensity of bullets particularly to break apart within the body means that this can happen even in the presence of an exit wound. Action depends on the individual location of the foreign body, and may be suitable for endovascular removal, or even left in situ.

34.16 Air Embolus

Air embolus is a potentially life-threatening problem. Its cause can be iatrogenic from the insertion of central venous catheters or intra-operatively, or in the presence of combined major vascular and bronchial injury. Where massive air embolus is suspected, the patient should proceed to immediate thoracotomy. The source of the air should be removed (e.g. cross-clamping of the hilum, clamping of any catheters). The patient should be placed in the Trendelenburg position and air aspirated from the left ventricle and aorta, with or without open cardiac massage. Without prompt action, these patients undergo cardiac arrest and/or stroke, but correct management can significantly affect outcome. In a dying patient, in the presence of vascular and major lung injury, the surgeon must consider this diagnosis and take appropriate action.

34.17 Thoracic Duct

Injuries to the thoracic duct may be visualised during surgery, but most often present post-operatively with persistent chyle leak in the chest drain. This phenomenon may well be iatrogenic, caused particularly when mobilising the descending aorta. Initially commencement of a fat-free diet and a 3-week conservative trial may be all that is required. Where this is not successful, a thoracic surgeon should undertake Video-Assisted Thoracoscopic Surgery (VATS) in order to locate the specific injury and ligate the duct.

34.18 Other Injuries

Arterio-venous fistulas, or other great vessel fistulas, can frequently occur with penetrating trauma, and may present late. If the patient remains stable, adequate imaging can be undertaken to allow planning of the correct procedure. Access is via the usual incision to approach the vessels, although endovascular stenting is an option. Mediastinal injuries seldom occur in isolation, and the surgeon must be alert to other injuries involving the myocardium or lung. Incisions may need to be extended or refined in order to secure haemorrhage or air-leak from the lungs, or to address injuries in the neck or abdomen.

34.19 Outcomes

Overall mortality associated with penetrating injury to mediastinal great vessels is significant (up to 55%). Important predictors for mortality include injury to the aorta, thoraco-abdominal injury, associated major neurological injury, gunshot wounds, unrecordable blood pressure on admission and the need for ERT. Complications are also possible after these injuries and are summarised in Table 34.3.

Table 34.3 Complications of penetrating mediastinal injuries

Common complications of penetrating mediastinal vessel injuries
Pulmonary • Atelactasis • Pneumonia • ARDS • Empyema • Bronchial stenosis
Vascular • Great vessel or other AV fistula • Ischaemia/infarction • Thromboembolism
Mediastinum • Mediastinitis • Pericarditis
Neurological • Brain injury • Paraplegia • Brachial plexus injury • Phrenic nerve injury • Recurrent laryngeal nerve injury
Other • Thoracic duct injury • Graft failure/infection/migration

Important Points

- Consider mediastinal vascular injury in your initial assessment of a patient with penetrating chest injury; they are rare, but will need an operative (or endovascular) procedure to fix them.
- Perform a rapid, focused clinical assessment.
- Commence resuscitation.
- Think about tension pneumothorax and decide whether the patient needs ERT (to relieve or exclude cardiac tamponade).
- Do not give too much crystalloid; if you think the patient has bled massively, or there is ongoing major bleeding, give blood and plasma early.
- Decide which category the patient falls into: shocked or not-shocked.
- Next decide if they can wait for more imaging … or if they need surgery straight away.
- CT angio is the best form of imaging (but further investigations may be required).

- Do not hesitate to shunt or ligate vessels in a critical patient … think 'damage control'.
- If you are struggling to access the injury through your first incision, make another one.
- Endovascular stenting is a possibility for certain carefully selected patients … if the expertise exists in your hospital.
- Do not forget the possibility of injury to other mediastinal structures (major airway/oesophagus) and always consider the possibility of injury in an adjacent body cavity.

Further Reading

Burack JH, Kandil E, Sawas A et al (2007) Triage and outcome of patients with mediastinal penetrating trauma. Ann Thorac Surg 83(2):377–382; discussion 382

Degiannis E, Benn CA, Leandros E et al (2000) Transmediastinal gunshot injuries. Surgery 128(1):54–58

Demetriades D (1997) Penetrating injuries to the thoracic great vessels. J Card Surg 12(2 Suppl):173–179; discussion 179–180

Demetriades D, Theodorou D, Murray J et al (1996) Mortality and prognostic factors in penetrating injuries of the aorta. J Trauma 40(5):761–763

Deneuville M (2000) Injury of the pulmonary artery and its branches due to penetrating chest trauma. Ann Vasc Surg 14(5):463–467

du Toit DF, Odendaal W, Lambrechts A et al (2008) Surgical and endovascular management of penetrating innominate artery injuries. Eur J Vasc Endovasc Surg 36(1):56–62

Fulton JO, de Groot KM, Buckels NJ et al (1997) Penetrating injuries involving the intrathoracic great vessels. S Afr J Surg 35(2):82–86

Hanpeter DE, Demetriades D, Asensio JA et al (2000) Helical computed tomographic scan in the evaluation of mediastinal gunshot wounds. J Trauma 49(4):689–694; discussion 694–685

Ibirogba S, Nicol AJ, Navsaria PH (2007) Screening helical computed tomographic scanning in haemodynamic stable patients with transmediastinal gunshot wounds. Injury 38(1):48–52

Marin ML, Veith FJ, Panetta TF et al (1994) Transluminally placed endovascular stented graft repair for arterial trauma. J Vasc Surg 20(3):466–472; discussion 472–463

McGrath EE, Blades Z, Anderson PB (2010) Chylothorax: aetiology, diagnosis and therapeutic options. Respir Med 104(1):1–8

Michelassi F, Pietrabissa A, Ferrari M et al (1990) Bullet emboli to the systemic and venous circulation. Surgery 107(3):239–245

Pate JW, Cole FH Jr, Walker WA et al (1993) Penetrating injuries of the aortic arch and its branches. Ann Thorac Surg 55(3):586–592

Renz BM, Cava RA, Feliciano DV et al (2000) Transmediastinal gunshot wounds: a prospective study. J Trauma 48(3):416–421; discussion 421–412

Roye GD, Zorn GL, McGiffin DC et al (1995) Acute repair of aorta-innominate vein fistulas. J Trauma 39(4):753–756

Schonholz CJ, Uflacker R, De Gregorio MA et al (2007) Stent-graft treatment of trauma to the supra-aortic arteries. A review. J Cardiovasc Surg(Torino) 48(5):537–549

Stassen NA, Lukan JK, Spain DA et al (2002) Reevaluation of diagnostic procedures for transmediastinal gunshot wounds. J Trauma 53(4):635–638; discussion 638

Subramanian A, Vercruysse G, Dente C et al (2008) A decade's experience with temporary intravascular shunts at a civilian level I trauma center. J Trauma 65(2):316–324; discussion 324–316

Wall MJ Jr, Mattox KL, Debakey ME (2006) Injuries to the azygous venous system. J Trauma 60(2):357–362

Yee ES, Verrier ED, Thomas AN (1983) Management of air embolism in blunt and penetrating thoracic trauma. J Thorac Cardiovasc Surg 85(5):661–668

Penetrating Cardiac Trauma

35

Elias Degiannis, Tugba H. Yilmaz, and Dietrich Doll

In the last three decades, there have been numerous publications on the subject of penetrating cardiac injuries including a number of large series. Controversial issues remain; they relate to the diagnostic procedures that may be indicated and the therapeutic strategy best suited to each patient. These controversies are partly a reflection of differences in personal surgical preferences and logistical organization of trauma care. To a large extent, however, they stem from a lack of consistent stratification of patients. An elaborate scoring system for the purpose of predicting outcome has been devised, but attempts as classifying patients to involve rational management decisions have been rare and incomplete. In our clinical practice, we classify our patients in five categories:

35.1 Category 1: Lifeless

In this category, we include patients presenting with a thoracic wound who are becoming unconscious with no sign of life (no respiratory effort, palpable pulse, or recordable blood pressure) and who have not intubated and started on CPR after a witnessed cardiac arrest 5 min before arrival to our emergency department.

35.2 Category 2: Critically Unstable

We include patients who have a penetrating thoracic injury and present with profound hypotension and in pending cardiac arrest. The clinical picture is accounted for by either massive hemorrhage from the heart or severe tamponade.

35.3 Category 3: Cardiac Tamponade

These patients present with a thoracic wound and a clinical picture typical of cardiac tamponade (slight-to-severe hypotension and raised central venous pressure in the absence of tension pneumothorax).

35.4 Category 4: Thoracoabdominal Injury

Patients have a high epigastric wound or multiple lacerations of the trunk, often from gunshot or shotgun injury. The diagnosis of cardiac tamponade is clouded by the presence of an obvious abdominal injury.

E. Degiannis (✉)
University of the Witwatersrand Medical School,
Chris Hani Baragwanath Academic Hospital,
Trauma Directorate, 7 York Road, Parktown,
2193 Johannesburg, South Africa (RSA)
e-mail: degiannis@yebo.co.za

T.H. Yilmaz
Department of Surgery, Baskent University,
6371 Sokak No. 34, Bostanli, Izmir 35540, Turkey
e-mail: tugba.yilmaz@deu.edu.tr

D. Doll
University of the Witwatersrand Medical School,
Chris Hani Baragwanath Academic Hospital,
Trauma Directorate, 7 York Road, Parktown,
2193 Johannesburg, South Africa (RSA)

Department of Visceral, Vascular and Thoracic Surgery,
Phillips-University of Marburg,
Baldingerstraße, D-35043 Marburg, Germany
e-mail: ddoll@gmx.de

G.C. Velmahos et al. (eds.), *Penetrating Trauma*,
DOI 10.1007/978-3-642-20453-1_35, © Springer-Verlag Berlin Heidelberg 2012

35.5 Category 5: Benign Presentation

Patients present with penetrating thoracic wound but are hemodynamically stable and without symptoms or signs of either hemorrhage or cardiac tamponade.

35.6 Management

35.6.1 The Lifeless Patient

Treatment consists of immediate intubation followed by thoracotomy and cardiorraphy in the resuscitation area. No procedure short of this heroic intervention would be adequate. However, reserve the emergency department thoracotomy for the lifeless patient whose vital signs have been preserved, at least for some time in the prehospital period.

35.6.2 The Critically Unstable Patient

This patient presents with signs of life, but the clinical picture is dominated by profound hypotension and impending cardiac arrest. As in the previous category, diagnostic procedures a part from FAST performed immediately in the resuscitation area would be detrimental. Immediate endotracheal intubation and fluid replenishment are required. Some of these patients may regain sufficient hemodynamic stability and allow urgent thoracotomy in the operating room while others may remain unresponsive to resuscitation and require thoracotomy in the resuscitation area. It is clear from the literature that emergency room thoracotomy is more successful in this category of patients than in those who are "lifeless." It is less clear however even better results might not be achieved by expeditious transfer to the operating room. There is some evidence that thoracotomy in critically unstable patients is attended by a significantly greater mortality rate in the emergency room than in the operating room, but this conclusion is based on small numbers of non-randomized patients. A decision on this matter must take into account the logistics of trauma care in the particular institution involved.

35.6.3 The Patient with Cardiac Tamponade

A high degree of suspicion based on the location of the thoracic wound in relation with this syndrome is usually sufficient to suggest the diagnosis of penetrating cardiac injury. The presence of both tracheal deviation and hyper-resonance of the chest will rule out tension pneumothorax. A number of diagnostic methods have been recommended to increase clinical accuracy. The globular heart on the chest x-ray is present in less than 40% of cases. There is no place for needle pericardiocentesis as a therapeutic measure. We believe like many others that except for the rapid requisition of a chest radiograph in the resuscitation room, any other diagnostic maneuvers are time consuming and therefore dangerous except if FAST is immediately available in the resuscitation room. Even a young patient with mild cardiac tamponade may deteriorate rapidly and have a cardiac arrest. In experienced hands, clinical judgment combined with a low threshold for intervention results in an extremely low rate of negative thoracotomy in patients with a clinical picture of cardiac tamponade.

35.6.4 The Patient with Thoracoabdominal Injury

The diagnosis of cardiac tamponade may be masked by the presence of obvious abdominal signs due to peritonitis or more often by hemorrhage. An accurate preoperative diagnosis is often difficult, but is sometimes made, particularly if FAST is available in the emergency department. The clinician must then exercise clinical judgment in deciding which lesion is addressed first or whether a two team approach is indicated. In our experience, intra-abdominal hemorrhage usually takes precedence over cardiac tamponade. In some cases, the cardiac tamponade is suspected only on completion of the laparotomy, either because the surgeon is worried about the presence of a precordial wound or because control of the intra-abdominal bleeding does not result in the expected improvement of the patient's condition. In this situation, a diagnostic pericardial window before closure of the abdomen has been shown to be safe and reliable.

35.6.5 The Patient with the Benign Presentation

A number of patients with a penetrating precordial injury present with no symptoms or clinical signs of either cardiac tamponade or intra-thoracic hemorrhage:

Nevertheless, the alert clinician should be concerned about the presence of a thoracic wound especially in the precordium. The chest x-ray may be normal. All these patients should be investigated by cardiac echo or even a CT angio of the mediastinum. Two arguments may be adduced in favor of aggressive management for all patients with penetrating cardiac injury, however minor. The first is the uncertainty about the long-term outcome of patients with an undrained hemopericardium. The entity of posttraumatic chronic constrictive pericarditis has been described in both the experimental and clinical settings. The second is the danger of sudden and irremediable deterioration (even under hospital observation) which may occur several days after the initial injury. We do not share the view that clinical observation alone is sufficient for this patient; therefore, we proceed to the abovementioned investigations. In cases of doubt, we support assessment via a sub-xiphoid pericardial window.

Always be very alert with the patient who has sustained penetrating trauma to the cardiac box and he lies very quietly looking unwell or becomes aggressive trying to lift himself off the bed. This is a clinical picture that in our experience could well be related to cardiac injury.

35.7 Operative Management

There are several incisions that can be applied in patients with penetrating cardiac trauma and which one you are going to choose depends on the urgency of the situation. In the patient who has catastrophic physiological deterioration in the emergency department, proceed immediately to an emergency room thoracotomy. In that case, remember that it is of paramount importance to ensure adequate precautions to safeguard yourself and the rest of the staff from bloodborne infections. The stress of the situation and the tendency to show heroism from your side is not an excuse to risk lives of the health personnel. Neglecting the use of protective gear particularly of the eyes when the patient has "bled out" and has "no blood pressure" is foolish. It is common on opening the chest for rapid decompression to have blood sprayed from traumatized lung tissue (due to the insult itself or due to iatrogenic injury on opening the chest), particularly if the patient is ventilated.

On performing an emergency department thoracotomy(the anterior-lateral incision), incise the skin at the 5th intercostal space, always keeping in mind the female anatomy. Going through the female breast is not only aesthetically unacceptable but also makes access to the thoracic cavity more time consuming and bloody. Ask your assistant to pull the breast upward and proceed to a sub-mammary incision. Get another assistant or any member of your team to raise the arm to 90°. That will enable you to extend the incision laterally toward the axillary line. When you insert the rib retractor, make sure that you do not limit your access through your incision. Place the joint of the retractor away the sternal side of the incision, so that you do not limit your ability to extend your incision laterally if you decide to. The emergency department thoracotomy, always performed in patients who are in extremis, is always coupled with abrupt opening of the retractor and therefore always leads to rib fractures. As it is always related to the procedure, cannot be considered as a pitfall. Instead of that, the pitfall lies if you omit to cover the edge of your incision with large abdominal swabs and you do not warn your assistant of the possibility of injury himself from rib spikes. With this thoracotomy, you have a satisfactory access (although not ideal to the heart). Most times it is enough to repair the heart in an absolute emergency, taking into consideration that most of the heart lies left of the chest. On the other hand, there will be situations that it is difficult to access the further right aspect of the heart and that necessitates for you to split the sternum transversely. In the books, it is recommended that the transverse division of the sternum should be performed with a Gigley saw or bone cutter. We find both of them time consuming as it is easy to do it with the use of a pneumatic, or in its absence a Libscher knife and hammer. When you decide to divide the sternum with this method, you should pay attention to two things. First accidental injury to the heart as the intact pericardium holds its contents in close proximity with the posterior aspect of the sternum. To avoid that, apply upward traction of the pneumatic saw or the Libscher knife, coupled with a forward and upward rotation of the distal saw/blade tip. Do not forget that with this incision, you cannot avoid severing the mammary arteries. In the patient who is in his extremis – always related to non-palpable pulse and a blood pressure in his boots – there is a good chance that these arteries will not bleed to the extent that they draw your attention. There are even cases that they will contract and clot and you will only remember that you forgot to look for them when you have to take the patient back to theater for bleeding after you have performed a successful thoracotomy and repair of the heart. It is important to find and ligate the four edges of the severed internal mammary arteries in the loose tissue lateral to the sternum even if they appear not to be actively bleeding.

In situations that the patient is not in extremis (and you have time to transfer him from the resuscitation area to theater), it is preferable to get access to the heart by performing a median sternotomy. This is the ideal incision not only for repairing the heart, but also the arch of the aorta and its proximal branches. The most common pitfall of this incision is to miss the midline on splitting the sternum. Make the skin incision first and use the diathermy to extend the incision deep to the anterior aspect of the sternum from sternal notch to xiphoid, marking the midline of the sternum with the diathermy. Then divide the intraclavicular ligament so that you create a small retrosternal space at the retrosternal notch either using a diathermy or a right-angled Lehay. When you do this procedure or the lower down description of splitting the sternum, you should place yourself at the left of the patient if you are right handed and on the right if you are left handed. You will find that the intraclavicular ligament is very tough, and for most of us, it is quite difficult to perforate with the tip of a closed right-angled Lehay when we are using one hand. Grab the Right-Angled Lehay with your two hands: the right hand (if you are right handed) on the vertical part quite close to the tip and the left hand grabbing the handle. Position the tip of the right-angled Lehay just posteriorly to the sternal notch and push the tip at the retromanubrial space with a rotational movement, the force of the movement applied by your right hand. There is a characteristic giving way and noise as the tip of your clamp goes through the tough ligament. As it is difficult to perforate the ligament, it is also difficult then to open the limbs of your right-angled Lehay so that you create the space for the introduction of the pneumatic saw or the tip of the Libscher knife. Hold the two arms of your clamp separately (one arm in each hand) and then open the clamp. This maneuver can sometimes lead to alarming bleeding from the area that it is difficult to control due to its limited access. Do not panic! There is always a worry that you have injured a large vessel, remember that the only large vessel in this area is the innominate vein which in any case lies too deep to be injured with this maneuver.

If rapid opening of the sternum is of paramount importance and the bleeding from this area is too much, pack the area, apply some pressure, and perform a medial sternotomy by starting from the xiphisternum upward. If this option is chosen be very careful as the caudal part of the sternum is thinner and therefore as you put force on splitting it, it is quite easy to miss the midline and start dividing the intercostals cartilages. In any case, irrespective of from which direction you open the sternum, make sure that you do not miss the midline.

Open the sternum along the diathermy line using a pneumatic saw or a Libscher knife and hammer following religiously the diathermy line, making sure that you apply only the necessary force to split the sternum. If you apply more force than necessary, you may feel a sudden giving way of the resistance of the sternum resulting in loss of the midline. If you use the Libscher knife and hammer on opening the sternum from a manubrium to xiphoid direction that is the recommended route, make sure that you have placed a sand bag between the shoulder blades of the patient and have his neck extended and his face turned away from you. The hammer should initially hit the Libscher knife at an angle of 30° with the horizontal plane so as to avoid hitting the patient's jaw (we have seen it happen). After splitting the manubrium, there is enough distance from the jaw so that the sternum is split by hitting the hammer on the knife horizontally. This problem of course does not arise if you use a pneumatic saw, but it is always advisable to have a Libscher knife on standby as it happens sometimes to be let down by "technology" when you most need urgent access to the mediastinum. Your sternal retractor should be placed into the sternotomy including the distal portion of the manubrium, therefore minimizing the risk of fracturing the sternum on rapidly opening the retractor.

On opening with a preoperative diagnosis of penetrating trauma to the heart (which many times is a clinical diagnosis), inspect the pericardium to confirm tamponade, unless there is an obvious source of active bleeding not related to the heart and you misdiagnosed it as cardiac injury. If this is the case, of course you divert your attention to the site of torrential bleeding and you control it. Haemopericardium may be recognized by the presence of a bulging, tense pericardium, or sometimes only by the white bluish color of the underlying clot. A classic mistake is to leave the pericardium unopened due to its normal appearance from the outside. It is amazing how often you can have a pericardial sack containing a significant amount of blood from injury to the heart or intrapericardial mediastinal vessel, which is not visible through the intact pericardium. Take a scalpel and make a small nick in the pericardium if there is a clot underneath or use two Mosquitoes to lift the pericardium and then make a nick with the scalpel if you cannot see any blood between the pericardium and the heart. Insert the tip of your scissors inside the hole and open the pericardium in a vertical direction avoiding injury of the phrenic nerve, which should run parallel and to the left of your pericardial incision. The phrenic nerve is significant in size and it is most unlikely to damage it. On the other hand, if you transect it in the heat of the moment, proceed with your life-saving procedure without too much grief about the nerve. Patients (particularly the young ones as it is in most cases of penetrating cardiac trauma) can have perfectly normal lives with one paralyzed diaphragm. If further access to the heart is required, add a transverse pericardial incision at the caudal end of your vertical incision (an inverted "T"). Start internal cardiac massage if you find the heart in asystole or ventricular fibrillation while inserting some "fast" stitches to close the defect. The pericardial incision should be extensive enough for you to be able to insert not one but both of your hands. Never do intrapericardial massage by using the palm of one hand and compressing the heart against the spine. This traumatizes the heart and it becomes apparent from the extensive bruising from the heart seen thereafter. The correct way of massaging the heart is to put one palm posterior to it, palm facing upward, fingertips toward the base of the heart and the other hand palm facing downward on the anterior aspect of the heart. Then start doing cardiac massage, by compressing the heart between your two palms maintaining good firm contact between the heart and the palms at all times, minimizing the chance of potential injury from the application of the cardiac massage. In the presence of non-perfusing ventricular arrhythmia, shock the heart with 20 J with one internal paddle behind the heart and the other in the front. If required, repeat the defibrillation by shocking the heart with a maximum of 50 J. Never defibrillate the heart that is at a complete standstill as this will only further damage the myocardium.

When a penetrating injury to the anterior aspect of the heart occurs, the operation is not complete if you do not check for a posterior wall injury – the patient my leave theater only to return because of re-accumulation of a haemopericardium. For checking the posterior aspect of the heart, you must lift the heart out of the pericardial sack. Do that by putting the tips of your fingers as proximally as you can, right at the base of the heart, so that you do not "kink" the heart but you lift it "en block" (Fig. 35.1). The heart is always unhappy with this maneuver, so you should repair the posterior injury as quickly as possible as the heart rapidly develops bradycardia that can lead to asystole. As soon as you see bradycardia developing, drop the heart back into the pericardial sack even if you have not succeeded to completely repair the posterior injury yet. Lift up the heart again to proceed with the repair when the rhythm returns to normal. During this piecemeal repair of the posterior wound, the heart is very irritable and may develop a nonresponsive bradycardia even though you replace it to its bed. In this case, it is very useful to pour very warm saline on the heart which results in the heart starting to beat normally again, sometimes even developing tachycardia.

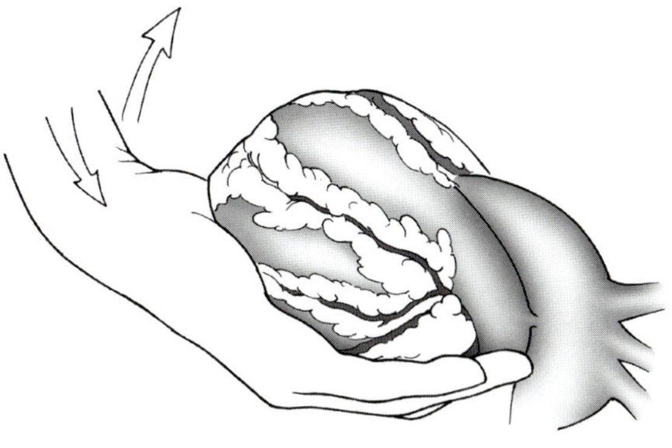

Fig. 35.1 Lift the heart en bloc to minimize arrhythmias

Use a 2.0 silk (when available) and the biggest atraumatic needle you can find when it comes to stitching up the heart. We prefer silk because it is easier for the first knot to hold, and the last thing you want when you repair hearts is to have loose knots – if silk is not available, use a similar size PDS. While your assistant is controlling the bleeding by applying pressure with a swab on the side of the injury, you position your needle at the needle holder in such a way that the needle holder is very close to the posterior end of the needle. The reason is that in your first through-and-through bite of the heart, you want to insert as much length of needle as possible inside the heart cavity so that you can grab the tip of the needle through the opening of

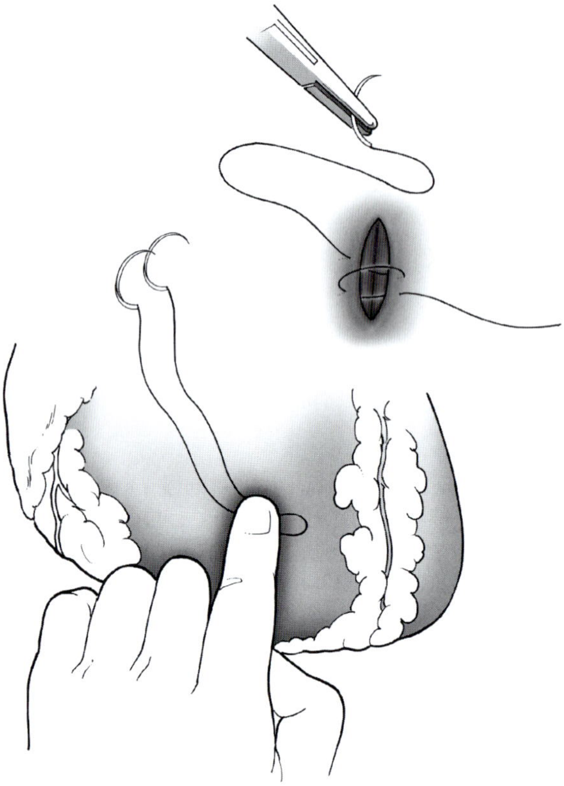

Fig. 35.2 Stitch closure technique of myocardial defect

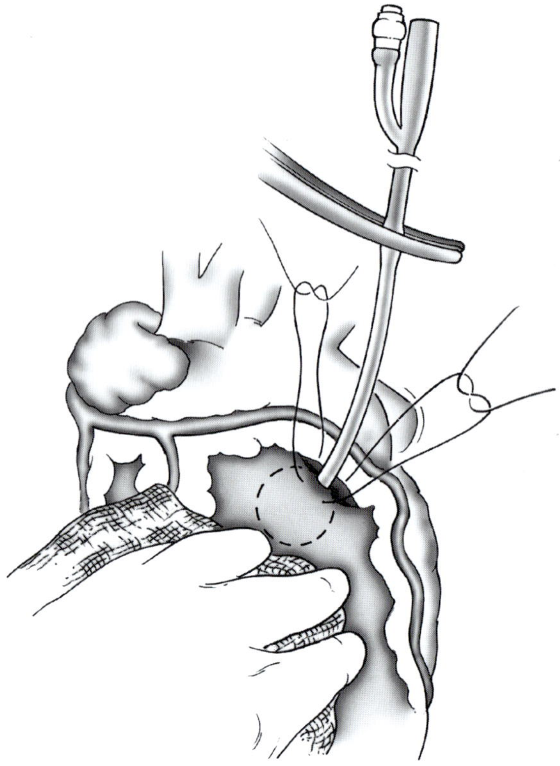

Fig. 35.3 Just gently lift up the Foley catheter with inflated balloon; otherwise, the small tear will convert into a large tear

the heart with your needle holder as easily as possible. While inserting your first bite on one side of the defect, there will be a lot of blood spurting out from the heart; keep your cool and insert the tip of your needle holder at the base of the column of the spurting blood and pull your needle out of the defect making sure that your move coincides with the curve of the needle so that you do not slash the myocardium. Reapply your needle on your needle holder while you assistant again controls the bleeding by pressure and insert your needle at the opposite side of the defect. After this bite, things become easier. Hold with your left hand both ends of the stitch and lift them upward. You will see that the two edges of the defect are in this way approximated and you have a spectacular reduction in the amount of blood that is leaking through it. So by holding the initial stitch up, you reapply another stitch so you complete a figure-of-eight stitch (Fig. 35.2). Continue closing the defect by putting more figure-of-eight sutures. It is quite common if your patient is "young at heart" to have a very powerful myocardium that sometimes contracts so forcefully that it kicks away the tip of your needle as you go to insert it inside the myocardium. In this case, hold the handle of your needle holder with both hands and make a fast curved move as you insert the needle inside the myocardium, trying to take advantage of the diastolic period of the heart. It is described in the books that if the defect is not too large, you can insert a Foley's catheter and inflate the balloon, therefore controlling the hemorrhage. It does work! Grab the distal 1 cm of the Foley's catheter with a clamp and insert it inside the cavity. It is much easier to do that than holding the tip of the catheter with your fingers as you will find that the column of blood escaping from the defect is under a lot of pressure and it is difficult to insert the tip of the catheter inside the cavity and inflate the balloon. As soon as you inflate the balloon, apply slight upward traction so that you occlude the defect, make sure that you do not overdo it; otherwise, you can make it even bigger (Fig. 35.3). This is the part that the balloon catheter helps in stitching up a cardiac wound. What you will

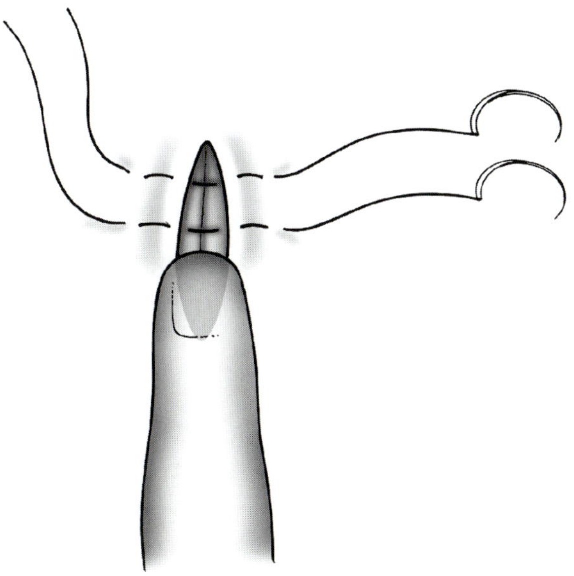

Fig. 35.4 It is easier to insert the suture than to tie the knot in cardiac injuries. Digital pressure exposes just the edge of the wound that you work on

see in the books – stating that you can push the balloon inside, put your sutures, and then apply traction at the balloon and occlude your defect again and then repeat the process and complete the repair of the defect – is not feasible. The initial obstruction of the defect by the balloon only gives you time to concentrate, probably stabilize the patient and get ready for the insertion of the first bite. Be prepared: As soon as you insert your first bite, you will hear a popping sound and the balloon will break and you will find again yourself in the situation of having a spurt of blood coming out of the defect. Continue inserting your sutures in a figure of eight as already discussed.

There are times that the length of the injury is such and the hemorrhage so brisk that it is difficult to control the bleeding promptly by inserting sutures with the above methods. As it is in such instances, you can gain digital control of the hemorrhage by occluding the long defect by applying pressure on it with the length of your assistant's index finger. You can then put multiple sutures beneath the occluding finger. Then you can tie your knots as he slowly withdraws his finger (Fig. 35.4). This is a method that is full of risks for the surgeon to hurt his assistant with the needle, and we also apply it in injuries with inaccessible occasions as the posterior aspect of the left ventricle. If you have a similar situation of a very long and widely open defect in the anterior aspect of the heart, use a 2.0 stitch on a colt needle and rapidly apply figure-of-eight sutures closing en masse from one side to the other. The size of the needle is a great advantage for stitching rapidly. On the other hand, you must keep in mind that the half centimeter of the tip of the needle is "cutting." Therefore, when you insert the needle inside the myocardium, make sure that it is in phase with the diastole, otherwise if the tip is caught inside the myocardium at the time of contraction, the myocardium will be slashed. If you are caught with the tip of the needle at the time of contraction, take your hands rapidly away from the needle so that its tip does not pivot at your fingers and concentrate to push the needle through at one of the consecutive cycles of diastole.

If the injury is near the coronary arteries, make sure that you repair the defect by inserting horizontal mattress sutures that pass beneath the coronaries and around the injury, thereby controlling the hemorrhage but not occluding the artery. It is convenient if you use a double-arm suture (Fig. 35.5). There are cases in practice that the bleeding is so extensive that there is no time for these "fancy" sutures. In this case, insert the standard figure-of-eight sutures (that will of course occlude the coronary arteries) and control the bleeding. Next to that, you insert the recommended mattress sutures under the coronaries, remove the figure-of-eight sutures with a size 11 blade and tie up the mattress sutures. We have done this maneuver many times without having any problems with the coronaries. We are wondering if this happens because most of our penetrating cardiac trauma patients are young and the coronaries are quiet "soft" and can take a short interval of compression without being damaged.

Do not use skin staples for definite repair of the myocardium. First of all, it is impossible to use them even in small lacerations if the gap created by the escaping blood is significant so that the skin staples cannot get the wound edges and approximate them. Use skin staplers as a temporary measure to control the bleeding from tiny defects and then insert appropriate sutures at your leisure.

Repair small needle puncture wounds of the coronary arteries with a 6.0 or 7.0 with a polypropylene suture. Ligate distal injuries. Proximal injuries to the coronary arteries may devascularize significantly large areas of myocardium and you should contact the cardiothoracic surgeons for emergency aorto-coronary bypass as soon as you control the hemorrhage.

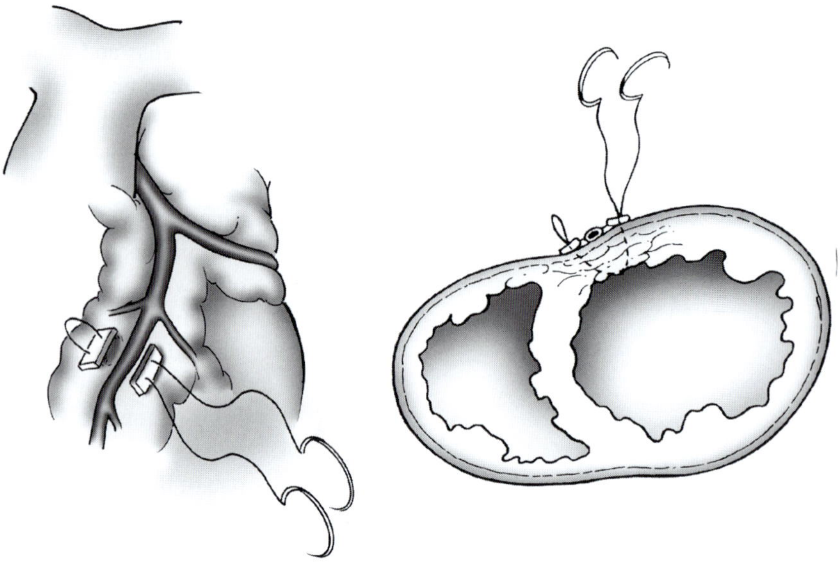

Fig. 35.5 Horizontal mattress sutures are inserted to avoid inclusion of the coronaries

This bypass should ideally be performed not longer than 2–3 h after time of injury.

If you encounter injury to the atria, apply a small Satinsky and close it proximally to the defect so that you can control the bleeding and repair the defect with a continuous 5.0 prolene suture (Fig. 35.6). If needed, buttress your sutures with small pieces of pericardium. During the repair, your assistant should religiously control a Satinsky. You should make sure that he does not apply any traction on the wall of the atrium in his effort to facilitate your suturing and also make sure that at no time, he lets the clamp fall free. Both of the above can rip off the atrium and convert a repairable injury a non-repairable one.

It is important to close the pericardium as non-closure or partial closure can lead to herniation of the heart. Close the pericardium with a running stitch making sure that you leave a 2-cm gap at the distal part of your closure and insert a tube drain right at the front of the gap. This will hopefully act as a safety valve and will prevent the formation of a tension hemopericardium in case of postoperative bleeding from the heart. Insert a tube drain via a midline incision just distally to the distal end of the sternotomy incision and connect it with under-water drain. The tip of the tube should be in front the pericardial gap. Be particularly meticulous when you close the proximal part of the pericardium as small gaps left behind by inserting your stitches in big steps can lead to herniation of the auricles through them. Sometimes it is not possible to close the pericardium because of overdistension of the heart. This is usually related to overtransfusion of fluids by an anesthetist not experienced to deal with cardiac trauma. Ask your anesthetist to administer furosemide to your patient and attempt to close the pericardium after 20 min. In very rare cases, the pericardium cannot be closed because of primary swelling of the cardiac muscle, a situation that cannot really be dealt with acutely and in this case you have to leave it open. Remember that patients who were operated for penetrating trauma to the heart can return to theater in the future for a new injury of the mediastinum or they can undergo cardiac surgery not related to trauma. If you as a trauma surgeon find yourself in such a situation, be extremely careful on opening the sternum as the anterior aspect of the heart can be "stuck" on the posterior aspect of the sternum and can be inadvertently damaged, resulting even in the death of the patient. Probably in a situation like that, an anterior-lateral thoracotomy will give you safer access to the heart.

On closing the sternotomy, if you are not experienced with the procedure, you will see that getting the needle and the wire through the sternum may be quite taxing. Insertion of the needle can be facilitated by applying the needle holder not in the recommended junction of the middle and distal third of the needle, but rather at the junction of the proximal and middle third of the needle, and advancing in a vertical direction rather than the usual rotational movement. As pressure is applied with the needle on the sternum, it is not uncommon for

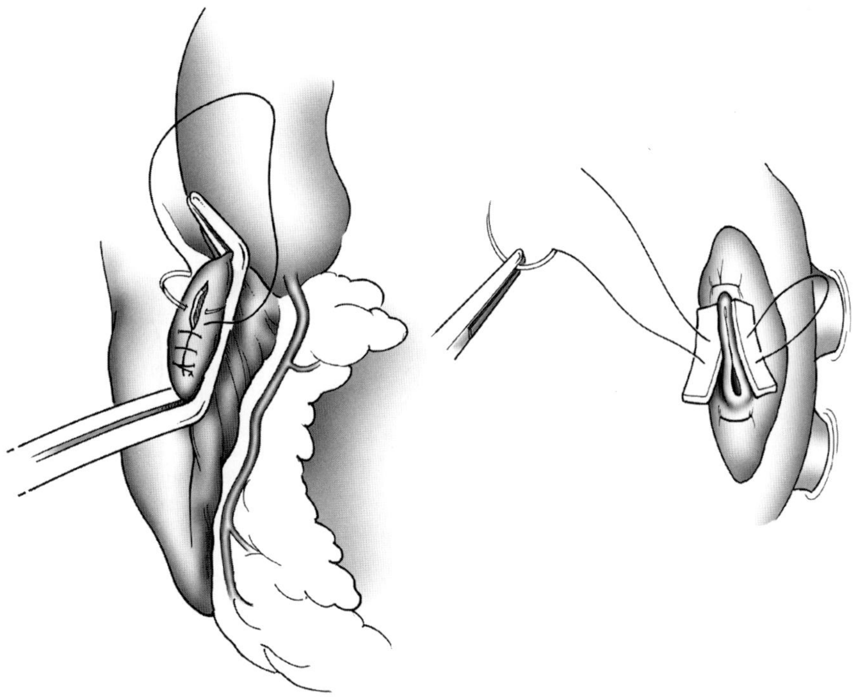

Fig. 35.6 Suture of the cardiac atrium with Lahey in place

the sternum to give way and the needle to go through suddenly, damaging underlying structures. Use a soup spoon with the concavity facing upward, applied under the sternum at the expected point of penetration. This will safeguard against inadvertent injury of mediastinal structures. Control the bleeding from the edges of the divided sternum by applying bone wax or electrocautery. Make sure that you apply only as much wax as necessary, as excess application is related to increased risk of infection of the sternum. Approximate the edges of the divided sternum well, as good approximation is also of paramount importance to avoid sternal infection. This is sometimes difficult to achieve particularly when inserting the wires through areas of the sternum that are technically difficult or when the two halves of the sternum do not approximate easily on tying the wires. In this case, after you insert an initial wire through the manubrium, apply wires to the body, not through the sternum, but around it. If you still find difficulty in approximating the two halves of the sternum, ask an assistant or even the anesthetist to place both his/her hands on the scapulae facing upward. By flexing his/her fingers, the scapulae are lifted forward, transmitting force upward and medially, approximating the two sternal edges and giving you the opportunity to twist the wires under less tension. Remember to make sure that you have not damaged the internal mammary arteries as your needle goes around the body of the sternum.

Use a sub-xiphoid pericardial window in cases that you cannot exclude pericardial blood collection clinically or via investigations. On performing your pericardial window, start with a 5-cm incision from the xiphisternum distally and open the linea alba. You should restrain yourself from opening the peritoneum. The plane to work is that of the pre-peritoneal fat. Insert your scissors proximally, tip facing, in the pre-peritoneal fat space under the xiphisternum in a horizontal plane and open the limbs of your scissors. You will then see the pericardium right in front of you. Raise the pericardium with two Burkett's and divide it in between. If there is any blood, aspirate it and if the pericardial window was performed after a recent injury proceed to sternotomy. If there is delayed presentation and there is no further bleeding after aspiration insert a Pencil drain and close the pericardial incision around it. You can remove the Pencil, drain within 48 h if no recurrence of bleeding occurs. If on opening the pericardium and aspirating, there is still blood collecting in the pericardial sack, convert to a median sternotomy, and deal with the problem. We do not recommend a trans-diaphragmatic pericardial window. It is surprising how easy it is to fail to locate the pericardium on opening the diaphragm through the abdomen. Therefore, the whole process becomes frustrating and time consuming.

Before discharging your patient home, you must make sure that there is no injury of the cardiac septae or the valves. Auscultate daily your patient's pericardium for murmurs, and even if they are absent, do a routine cardiac echo as soon as convenient before discharge.

Important Points

- Avoid volumes of fluid preoperatively into the patient presenting with cardiac and tamponade.
- In the grossly physiologically unstable patient, proceed with left anterior thoracotomy.
- Always consider the possibility of a second posterior wound.
- On inspecting the posterior aspect, replace the heart in pericardial sac as soon as it develops bradycardia.
- Check if the coronaries are included in your stitches.

Recommended Reading

Degiannis E, Smith MD (2008) Pot pouri of heuristics in penetrating trauma to the chest. ANZ J Surg 78(12):1103–1105

Degiannis E, Zinn RJ (2008) Pitfalls in penetrating thoracic trauma (lessons we learned the hard way…). Ulus Travma Acil Cerrahi Derg 14(4):261–267

Degiannis E, Bowley DM, Westaby S (2005) Penetrating cardiac injury. Ann R Coll Surg Engl 87(1):61–63

Degiannis E, Loogna P, Doll D, Bonanno F, Bowley DM, Smith MD (2006) Penetrating cardiac injuries: recent experience in South Africa. World J Surg 30(7):1258–1264

Navsaria PH, Nicol AJ (2005) Haemopericardium in stable patients after penetrating injury: is subxiphoid pericardial window and drainage enough? A prospective study. Injury 36:745–750

Saadia R, Levy RD, Degiannis E, Velmahos GC (1994) Penetrating cardiac injuries: clinical classification and management strategy. Br J Surg 81(11):1572–1575

Velmahos GC, Degiannis E, Souter I, Saadia R (1994) Penetrating trauma to the heart: a relatively innocent injury. Surgery 115(6):694–697

Velmahos GC, Degiannis E, Souter I, Allwood AC, Saadia R (1995) Outcome of a strict policy on emergency department thoracotomies. Arch Surg 130(7):774–777

Penetrating Injuries to the Diaphragm

36

Elmin Steyn

Penetrating injuries of the diaphragm are often not immediately apparent, as the inevitably present concomitant injuries usually receive diagnostic priority. In the acutely injured patient, identification and treatment of the occult injury eliminates the risk of late complications, and in the patient who presents late, prompt diagnosis may reduce mortality from further complications.

36.1 Pathophysiology

Diaphragmatic injuries are commonly associated with penetrating injuries of the trunk, especially left thoracoabdominal injuries, but may be notoriously difficult to diagnose in patients who have no immediate indication for laparotomy. Missed injuries, however small, have a risk of intestinal herniation, often presenting after many years with bowel loops incarcerated in the chest, potentially leading to life-threatening sepsis. This is due to the constant movement of the diaphragm and the negative pressure gradient between the chest and abdominal cavities. The overall incidence of diaphragmatic injuries associated with penetrating thoracoabdominal injuries (as reported by Murray et al. 1997) is 42% (59% for gunshot wounds, 32% for stab wounds). Associated intra-abdominal injuries are common, determine the initial outcome and are often the reason for surgical exploration and intra-operative diagnosis of the diaphragmatic wound.

After recovery from the acute injury, the patient may be asymptomatic for many years while gradual herniation of abdominal contents into the chest cavity takes place. Late presentation is usually with obstruction of the incarcerated intestine, complicated by strangulation, gangrene and possibly perforation of stomach, small bowel, or colon. Herniation may be massive, causing lung compression, cardiac tamponade or diaphragmatic splinting. The smaller hernias are also capable of significant complications, as they present with minimal abdominal signs, leading to late diagnosis. The reported morbidity and mortality rates of late presenting diaphragmatic hernias are 30% and 10% respectively.

36.2 Clinical Assessment

All penetrating torso injuries, generally caused by stabs or gunshots, potentially may involve the diaphragm together with adjacent structures in the chest or abdominal cavities. Few signs and symptoms are specific to diaphragmatic injury and few noninvasive investigations can reliably exclude a small penetrating diaphragmatic injury.

Clinical assessment should firstly be directed at abnormalities of airway, breathing, and circulation. Attention should be paid to possible signs of injury on the contralateral side of the diaphragm. The incidence of associated injuries is high, typically presenting with peritonism or a hemopneumothorax. However, in a review of patients with proven penetrating diaphragmatic injuries, 31% had no abdominal tenderness, 40%

E. Steyn
Department of Surgery,
Christiaan Barnard Memorial Hospital,
Cape Town, Republic of South Africa
e-mail: esteyn@mweb.co.za

G.C. Velmahos et al. (eds.), *Penetrating Trauma*,
DOI 10.1007/978-3-642-20453-1_36, © Springer-Verlag Berlin Heidelberg 2012

had a normal chest roentgenogram, and only 49% had an associated hemopneumothorax (Murray et al. 1997).

Diaphragmatic injury may be suspected based on the location of the external wound(s), on the basis of a predicted trajectory of the injury, or on abnormal findings involving both cavities. All stab wounds below the tip of the scapula at the back or below the nipple line in front should be considered as possibly involving the diaphragm and could be associated with intra-abdominal injuries. Stab wounds of the chest accompanied by local subcostal tenderness (not necessarily including peritonism or generalized tenderness) warrant laparotomy, or at least laparoscopy. In patients with lower chest injuries in the absence of subcostal tenderness or peritonism, even repeated clinical assessment may not be sufficient to identify all cases of diaphragmatic penetration. It is estimated that 30% of such injuries are missed on routine evaluation, and therefore, laparoscopic, thoracoscopic, or MRI assessment of these cases is recommended.

Right-sided penetrating injuries of the diaphragm are inevitably associated with liver injury and the clinical findings may vary from massive hemorrhage into the chest or abdomen, to benign injury amenable to conservative management. As most small penetrating right-sided diaphragmatic injuries are effectively sealed off by the liver, the risk of late bowel herniation is small.

36.3 Radiological Assessment

Chest radiographs are notoriously unreliable for diagnosis of the small penetrating diaphragmatic injury, and normal chest radiographs were found in 40% of diaphragmatic injuries, according to Murray et al. (1997). In the presence of any gunshot wounds of the trunk or pelvis, a diaphragmatic injury should be considered, based on the estimated trajectory of the bullet. This requires radiological assessment of the chest, abdomen, and pelvis as indicated, with metal markers (such as paper clips) identifying the entrance and exit (if present) wounds. Gunshot injuries should always be assessed to find wounds in pairs (or to pair an entrance wound and a retained bullet), although it should be kept in mind that bullets do not always travel in straight lines. Lodox is useful for rapidly identifying the position of retained bullets and foreign bodies in all types of penetrating injuries, facilitating the identification of missile trajectories.

36.4 Contrast Studies

Contrast studies outlining the stomach or colon may be useful to diagnose diaphragmatic rupture due to blunt trauma in the acute setting, or penetrating injuries with gut herniation at a later stage, but are of no value in demonstrating the typical acute penetrating injury.

36.5 Ultrasound

Ultrasonography is commonly utilized in trauma cases and may visualize large diaphragmatic disruptions or herniation; however, small penetrating injuries may be missed. FAST may be useful to demonstrate pleural fluid associated with a penetrating abdominal injury or intraperitoneal fluid in the presence of a penetrating chest injury.

36.6 Diagnostic Peritoneal Lavage (DPL)

A positive DPL in a patient with isolated penetrating chest injury is conclusive evidence that the diaphragm has been traversed. Contrary to the applications of DPL in blunt abdominal trauma, very small amounts of blood in the peritoneal cavity (in the presence of a supra-diaphragmatic wound) should be considered significant. Therefore, a more sensitive criterion such as 10,000 RBC/mm^3 should be used. DPL may be false-negative if the penetrating chest wound extends directly into the lesser sack. Drainage of lavage fluid from the chest tube indicates a positive result.

36.7 Computed Tomograpy (CT)

CT is a poor diagnostic tool to demonstrate the diaphragmatic injury as such, but can provide indirect evidence of injuries above and below the diaphragm. MDCT (Multi Detector CT with 64 slice technology or more) has a sensitivity of 87.2% to demonstrate diaphragmatic injury and accurately rules out diaphragmatic injury with a specificity of 72.4%. The overall accuracy is reported as 77% (Stein et al.). When MDCT is equivocal, further investigation is required to evaluate the diaphragm.

36.8 Magnetic Resonance Imaging (MRI)

MRI is able to demonstrate the diaphragm and may be used in a stable patient with equivocal findings and no indication for laparotomy, or for late diagnosis.

36.9 Laparoscopy

Diagnostic laparoscopy provides a vital tool for detecting occult diaphragmatic injury among patients who have no other indications for formal laparotomy. Patients with left lower chest penetrating wounds and no clinical or radiological evidence of diaphragmatic perforation should have a laparoscopic assessment of the left diaphragm. Diagnostic laparoscopy and video-assisted thoracoscopy have improved the diagnosis of occult injuries. Laparoscopic examination of the diaphragm in high-risk cases reduces the risk of negative or non-therapeutic laparotomies. Friese et al. report the specificity, sensitivity, and negative predictive value of laparoscopy as 100%, 87.5%, and 96.8%, respectively and conclude that in asymptomatic hemodynamically normal patients with penetrating thoracoabdominal injury, laparoscopy alone is sufficient to exclude diaphragmatic injury. Diaphragmatic penetrating injury, once diagnosed laparoscopically, may be amenable to laparoscopic repair; however, laparoscopic assessment for other intra-abdominal injuries is not universally reliable. In all but expert hands, laparoscopic identification of a diaphragmatic injury should be followed by laparotomy, to safely rule out occult bowel injury.

36.10 Thoracoscopy and Video-Assisted Thoracoscopic Surgery (VATS)

VATS has been used for patients with penetrating chest trauma to visualize the diaphragm when an injury is suspected and laparotomy is not clinically indicated. Out of 171 patients undergoing VATS assessment of a hemidiaphragm, 60 patients (35%) were found to have a diaphragmatic injury (Freeman et al.). The true benefit of thoracoscopy and laparoscopy for assessment of left-sided diaphragmatic injury is the reliable negative predictive value.

Fiber-optic thoracoscopy has been demonstrated to be useful for the diagnosis of diaphragmatic injury in children.

36.11 Treatment

36.11.1 Surgery

All diaphragmatic injuries benefit from early detection and repair. The route of access will be determined by the cavity requiring exploration, which invasive diagnostic procedure has been performed, and whether the diagnosis is made late or early.

Penetrating thoracoabdominal injuries, especially gunshot injuries, often require laparotomy for bleeding or peritonism. Those with no overt abdominal findings may require thoracoscopic or laparoscopic assessment of the diaphragm. When clinical findings such as peritonism or ongoing bleeding mandate laparotomy, the diaphragmatic wound should be sought and repaired.

It must be emphasized that any penetrating diaphragmatic injury diagnosed thoracoscopically or laparoscopically usually mandates laparotomy to exclude sub-diaphragmatic visceral injuries.

The left diaphragm is assessed by pressing down the stomach and transverse colon, while the assistant robustly retracts the left upper abdominal wall and/or sternum. Once the diaphragmatic perforation has been identified, it is brought into vision using Babcock or Allis forceps and repaired in a single full-thickness layer with a nonabsorbable suture.

If there is contamination or bleeding in the chest, the pleural cavity should be washed out or suctioned via the opening in the diaphragm, which may be enlarged if required. A chest drain should be placed, if not already present. If the lung is collapsed or significantly atelectatic, it may be manually expanded by the anesthesiologist as the final diaphragmatic suture is closed.

Late presentation of a diaphragmatic hernia with incarcerated abdominal structures can be approached from the chest or abdomen. An abdominal approach may facilitate the process of resection and re-anastomosis of bowel if required. A thoracic approach may facilitate the release of pleural and lung adhesions to the herniated viscera. Again pleural washout and adequate drainage should be provided, together with broad-spectrum antimicrobial therapy if visceral ischemia is present.

Important Points

- Penetrating diaphragmatic injuries are diagnostically challenging, and need to be actively sought and excluded.
- Invasive diagnostic procedures such as laparoscopy or thoracoscopy are the most sensitive modalities to definitively exclude small penetrating injuries.
- Multislice CT scanning, FAST, and DPL are strongly contributory in identifying high-risk cases.
- Early diagnosis and surgical repair of all left-sided diaphragmatic hernias is essential to reduce the morbidity and mortality of late complications.

Recommended Reading

Degiannis E, Levy RD, Sofianos C, Potokar T, Florizoone MG, Saadia R (1996) Diaphragmatic herniation after penetrating trauma. Br J Surg 83(1):88–91

Freeman RK, Al-Dossari G, Hutcheson KA, Huber L, Jessen ME, Meyer DM, Wait MA, DiMaio M (2001) Indications for using video-assisted thoracoscopic surgery to diagnose diaphragmatic injuries after penetrating chest trauma. Ann Thorac Surg 72:342–347

Friese RS, Coln CE, Gentilello LM (2005) Laparoscopy is sufficient to exclude occult diaphragm injury after penetrating abdominal trauma. J Trauma 58:789–792

Murray JA, Demetriades D, Cornwell EE III, Asensio JA, Velmahos G, Belzberg H, Berne TV (1997) Penetrating left thoracoabdominal trauma: the incidence and clinical presentation of diaphragm injuries. J Trauma 43(4):624–626

Murray JA, Demetriades D, Asensio JA, Cornwell EE III, Velmahos GC, Belzberg H, Berne TV (1998) Occult injuries to the diaphragm: prospective evaluation of laparoscopy in penetrating injuries to the left lower chest. J Am Coll Surg 187(6):626–630

Nel JH, Warren BL (1994) Thoracoscopic evaluation of the diaphragm in patients with knife wounds of the left lower chest. Br J Surg 81:713–714

Petrone P, Leppaniemi A, Inaba K, Soreide K, Asensio JA (2007) Diaphragmatic injuries: challenges in the diagnosis and management. Trauma 9(4):227–236

Pitcher G (2001) Fiber-endoscopic thoracoscopy for diaphragmatic injury in children. Semin Pediatr Surg 10(1):17–19

Powell BS, Magnotti LJ, Schroeppel TJ, Finnell CW, Savage SA, Fischer PE, Fabian TC, Croce MA (2008) Diagnostic laparoscopy for the evaluation of occult diaphragmatic injury following penetrating thoracoabdominal trauma. Injury 39(5):530–534

Shaw JM, Navsaria PH, Nicol AJ (2003) Laparoscopy-assisted repair of diaphragm injuries. World J Surg 27:671–674

Stein DM, York GB, Boswell S, Shanmuganathan K, Haan JM, Scalea TM (2007) Accuracy of computed tomography (CT) scan in the detection of penetrating diaphragm injury. J Trauma 63(3):538–543

Thoracoabdominal Injury 37

Elias Degiannis, Tugba H. Yilmaz, and Dietrich Doll

Thoracoabdominal injuries in penetrating trauma are very important for two reasons. Firstly, they are characterized by a high morbidity and mortality due to the significant physiological impact on the patient. Secondly, it is often difficult to come to a conclusive decision on which cavity needs to be operated on, or, if both cavities have to be opened, which one takes priority. Therefore, it is difficult to give clear-cut guidelines, but certain aspects can render the decision-making process more error proof. Having said that, the surgeon should still have the flexibility to move from one cavity to the other if his initial decision was wrong, or if life-threatening developments present intraoperatively from the other cavity.

The following course of action maybe followed for patients presenting with thoracoabdominal injury:

- Once the patient has arrived at the resuscitation room, place bullet wound markers in the correct location and proceed with X rays of the chest and abdomen. This will give an idea of the trajectory and apart from confirming the thoracoabdominal nature of the injury, this information will also help you to see if the bullet crossed the midline (if there is no obvious entry and exit wound).
- Insert an intercostal drain (ICD) at the side of the injured chest cavity, if you have not already done so on admission to resuscitation area.
- Do a FAST to make sure that the ICD is serving its purpose and pleural cavity has been properly evacuated.

With the use of FAST, assess the pericardial cavity for cardiac tamponade and/or the peritoneal cavity for free fluid. Laparoscopy in the physiologically stable patient can help with the diagnosis of diaphragmatic injury. Patients with clinical signs of peritonitis will have to be operated without any further investigations of the abdomen.

Several lines of thought can help decision making. For example: Should only one cavity, or both, be opened and which one should be operated first. It is important to know that in 85% of patients with penetrating chest trauma, insertion of an ICD is all that is needed.

Also remember that the two cavities – the thoracic and the peritoneal – communicate through a diaphragmatic defect sometimes smaller sometimes large but in all cases large enough to have blood moving from one cavity to the other.

Assuming that we have a functioning ICD, the chance of blood migrating from the thoracic cavity via the diaphragmatic defect to the abdomen and resulting in a large hemoperitoneum is small. On the other hand,

E. Degiannis (✉)
University of the Witwatersrand Medical School,
Chris Hani Baragwanath Academic Hospital,
Trauma Directorate, 7 York Road, Parktown,
2193 Johannesburg, South Africa (RSA)
e-mail: degiannis@yebo.co.za

T.H. Yilmaz
Department of Surgery, Baskent University,
6371 Sokak No: 34, Bostanli, Izmir 35540, Turkey
e-mail: tugba.yilmaz@deu.edu.tr

D. Doll
University of the Witwatersrand Medical School,
Chris Hani Baragwanath Academic Hospital,
Trauma Directorate, 7 York Road, Parktown,
2193 Johannesburg, South Africa (RSA)

Department of Visceral, Vascular and Thoracic Surgery,
Phillips-University of Marburg,
Baldingerstraße, D-35043 Marburg, Germany
e-mail: ddoll@gmx.de

G.C. Velmahos et al. (eds.), *Penetrating Trauma*,
DOI 10.1007/978-3-642-20453-1_37,

it is quite feasible for intraperitoneal fluid to be sucked into the chest through the diaphragmatic defect and present itself as ICD output.

Having these two latter points to consider, it is clear how useful it would have been to be able to close the communication between these two cavities and assess them separately. Unfortunately, this is not possible. Therefore, we have to rely on our "good Clinical Judgment" and be flexible and convert from one cavity to the other if the intraoperative findings do not fit the physiological status of the patient or if developments at the other cavity become clinically evident in case of operation. It is important to close the diaphragmatic defect as soon as possible. You should consistently monitor the output of the ICD during the laparotomy. Remember that there will be times when we will have to perform a pericardial window to a patient who is undergoing a laparotomy. Importantly, the anesthesiologist is the (at least in this case) "surgeons' best friend." He does not only contribute in keeping the patient alive but he can also draw your attention to any significant increase in ICD output, difficulties with ventilating the patient, and unexplained physiological instability.

From experience, it is evident that in the majority of cases, the best bet is to start by opening the abdominal cavity. Even though there is no "silver bullet," we recommend the following in an attempt to standardize the operative approach.

- Small amounts of ICD output combined with large amount of intraperitoneal fluid on FAST. (Operate on the abdomen.)
- Large amount of ICD output combined with large amount of intraperitoneal fluid on FAST. (Operate on the abdomen with open mind to shift to chest.)
- Small amount of ICD output combined with small amount of intraperitoneal fluid on FAST. (Operate on the abdomen.)
- Large amount of ICD output combined with small amount of intraperitoneal fluid on FAST. (Operate on the chest.)

Quite often you may find that you were wrong and, unfortunately, even with extensive experience in trauma and gut feeling, you could be let down. On the other hand, intraoperative alertness and flexibility can save the day and your patients' life.

Loss of the Chest Wall

38

John C. Mayberry

38.1 Field Management of Chest Wall Loss and Open Pneumothorax

Significant loss of the chest wall occurs in a variety of trauma scenarios including high-velocity rifle bullet penetrations, close-range shotgun blasts, explosions with secondary projectiles, industrial mishaps, and impalements during a fall or vehicular crash. Many patients with chest wall loss do not survive more than a few minutes because of exsanguination from within the thorax and/or associated injuries. This chapter outlines recommended field, emergency department, and operating room procedures that will be effective in those patients who are discovered alive. A damage control operative strategy with the goal of ultimate closure of the defect with minimal risk of infection and with preservation of as much of the chest wall's mechanical integrity as possible will be described. These injuries in their severest form are rare, and therefore, no single surgeon has a vast experience. Surgeons are thus encouraged to tailor these recommendations to fit the particular scenario.

Most patients with traumatic chest wall loss will be in acute respiratory distress from the incompetent pulmonary mechanics associated with the open pneumothorax. As the patient attempts to breathe, air preferentially flows through the defect into the pleural space and the patient's ability to inspire air into their airway and expand their lungs is greatly compromised.

J.C. Mayberry
Department of Surgery,
Oregon Health and Science University,
Trauma/Critical Care/EGS/L611, Portland, OR 97239, USA
e-mail: mayberrj@ohsu.edu

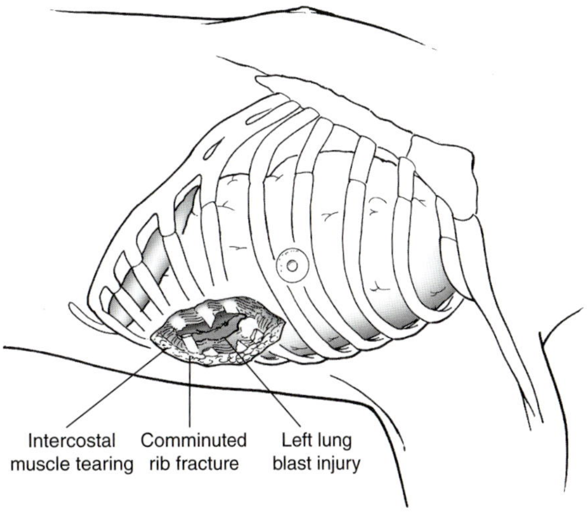

Fig. 38.1 Chest wall defect 5–10 cm in diameter with open pneumothorax, comminuted rib fractures, intercostal muscle tearing, and underlying pulmonary injury

Lesser degrees of chest wall loss, e.g., an open pneumothorax with a chest wall defect 5–10 cm in diameter (Fig. 38.1), may be tolerated for a short transport by an otherwise healthy patient, but for most patients, qualified providers in the field should provide an airway and respiratory support. Chin lift, jaw thrust, oropharyngeal or nasopharyngeal airways, and bag-valve-mask ventilation are effective temporizing measures until you can place an endotracheal tube. If the defect is on the left chest wall and there appears to be a pulmonary laceration with air loss, attempt a blind right mainstem bronchus intubation (deep intubation) in order to exclude the severely injured lung from ventilation. This maneuver will not only prevent unnecessary air loss from the injured parenchyma and tracheobronchial

G.C. Velmahos et al. (eds.), *Penetrating Trauma*,
DOI 10.1007/978-3-642-20453-1_38, © Springer-Verlag Berlin Heidelberg 2012

tree but may also prevent venous air embolism. If endotracheal intubation is not successful, a multilumen esophageal airway or laryngeal mask airway are less desirable alternatives.

After airway management, examine the edges of the chest wall defect for significant bleeding. Many experienced first responders are capable of clamping an arterial or venous bleeder in the chest wall, assuming they have an appropriately sized clamp. It does not make sense to embark on a significant transport to a higher level of care while an easily accessible vessel continues to hemorrhage. The chest wall contains numerous named arteries and veins, e.g., the intercostal arteries and veins as well as the muscular branches of the subclavian and axillary vessels, any of which can exsanguinate the patient. Any continuous bleeding during transport can lead to a coagulopathy that will be difficult to reverse even once the patient arrives at a hospital. Only the most obvious sites of hemorrhage should be clamped and not more than 3 min should be spent under austere conditions. First responders would not be expected, however, to try to clamp a pulmonary laceration within the thorax or attempt to control a source of mediastinal hemorrhage. In the case of severe pulmonary or mediastinal bleeding, however, following airway control, the hemithorax should be tightly packed with gauze in the hope of at least slowing the hemorrhage.

You should cover the defect itself with a sterile or clean dressing, e.g., dry gauze, petrolatum gauze or plastic wrap, and secure on three sides only so that accumulating pleural air, e.g., from a pulmonary or tracheobronchial laceration, can escape from the pleural space. This measure will prevent the development of a tension pneumothorax and will also prevent further contamination of the wound from the outside.

Because these patients have a high risk of deterioration and will likely require immediate surgery, transport to a designated trauma center should not be further delayed. During transport, a hypotensive strategy of resuscitation should be employed to minimize blood loss, dilutional coagulopathy, and pulmonary edema [1].

38.2 Emergency Department Management

For a patient with a larger and more destructive chest wall injury, the emergency department (ED) should be bypassed for direct transport to the operating room (OR). If an OR is not ready, ED management should be limited to life-saving procedures that cannot wait until an OR is available. For example, you can address exsanguinating hemorrhage from the edges of the defect, within the pulmonary parenchyma, or in the mediastinum. Hilar clamping or the pulmonary hilar twist are effective means of temporarily controlling pulmonary hemorrhage. Time spent in the ED can also be used to obtain a blood specimen for type and cross, to ensure adequate venous access, and to begin blood product transfusion. Chest radiographs or CT scans will not change surgical therapy and are therefore unnecessary and time wasting.

If the chest wall defect is smaller and hemorrhage is controlled, you can start a search for associated injuries in the ED prior to operative repair. In cases where the chest wall defect resulted from an explosion or a severe blunt mechanism, extra-thoracic injuries may take precedence in the treatment plan.

38.3 Operative Management

You can safely and effectively manage the smaller defect of 5–10 cm in diameter (Fig. 38.1) with minimal contamination of dirt and debris in 1–3 serial operations. Administer to the patient prophylactic intravenous antibiotic coverage for gram-positive organisms. The first operation consists of wound cleansing and debridement of devascularized skin, subcutaneous fat, muscle, and bone. If the defect involves only the intercostal muscle between two ribs and wound contamination is nil or very minimal, debride the defect and close it in a single operation. The intercostal muscle defect is closed by approximating the two ribs together with absorbable suture taking care not to entrap the intercostal nerve. The best way to approximate the ribs without nerve entrapment is to drill four holes in each rib and cerclage the two ribs together with figure-of-eight ties. Then close the skin over a bulb suction drain.

If the defect involves comminuted rib fractures, tissue loss, and contamination, then at least two operations are necessary. Excise the portions of rib that are partially devoid of muscular attachments because devascularized bone will not survive and will later become a nidus for osteomyelitis. If contamination is nil or minimal, a biologic tissue patch derived from human or porcine dermis can be sutured

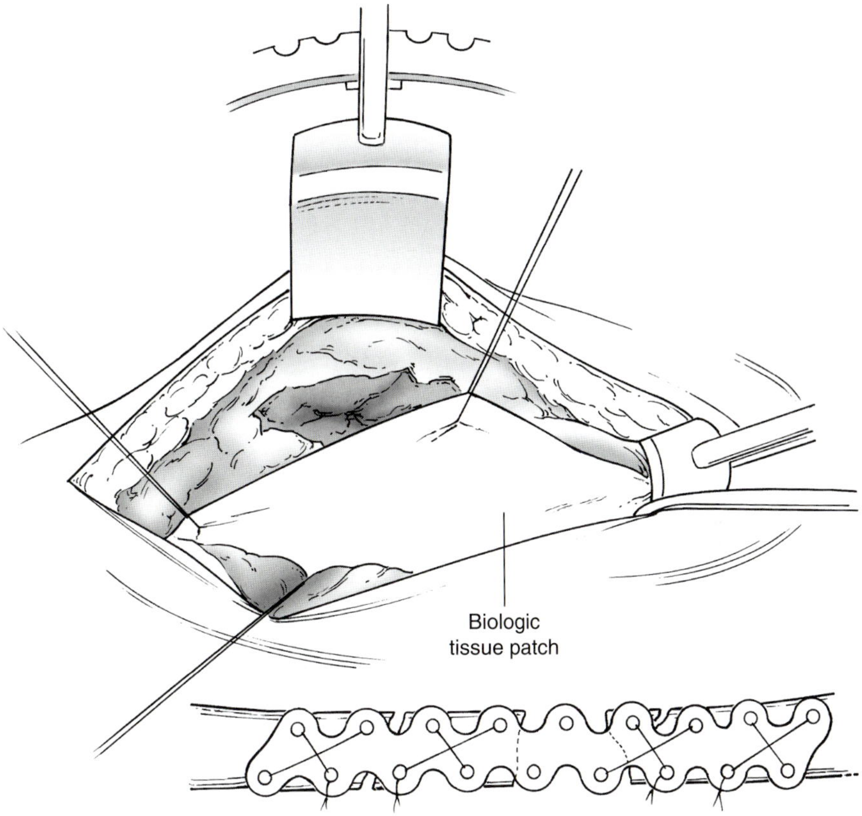

Fig. 38.2 A biologic tissue patch derived from human or porcine dermis is sutured circumferentially to the defect. If a comminuted rib fracture is present, an absorbable plate is affixed to the rib to provide a stronger edge to which to anchor the patch (insert). Partially devascularized bone should be excised

circumferentially to the defect in the first operation (Fig. 38.2). Such tissue patches provide protection to underlying lung, effectively bridge the defect with a firm yet flexible platform, and are less prone to infection than nonbiologic prostheses. If along one of the edges of the defect, a rib fracture or even a comminuted rib fracture with a small tissue gap is present, affix an absorbable, polylactide fracture repair plate to the rib to provide a stronger edge to which to anchor the patch (Fig. 38.2 insert) [2].

Place an anterior 32 or 36 French chest tube, either straight or right-angled, to underwater seal/wall suction to drain air and fluid that will accumulate. Dress the wound with a vacuum suction dressing over the biologic patch (Fig. 38.3) for at least 2 and as long as 3 days. The patient can be extubated postoperatively depending on the extent of the pulmonary injury and any associated injuries. The vacuum dressing can be expected to provide an adequate degree of chest wall stability for this smaller sized defect.

At the second operation, examine the wound for persistent contamination or dead tissue that must be

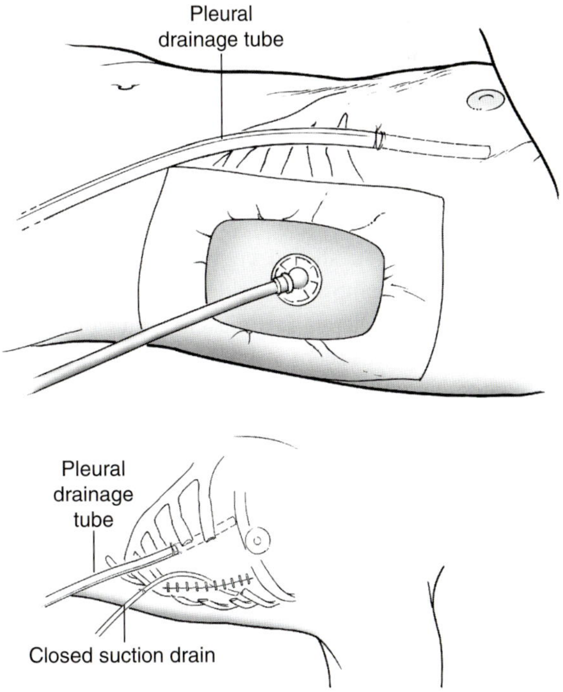

Fig. 38.3 A vacuum suction dressing is placed over the biologic patch

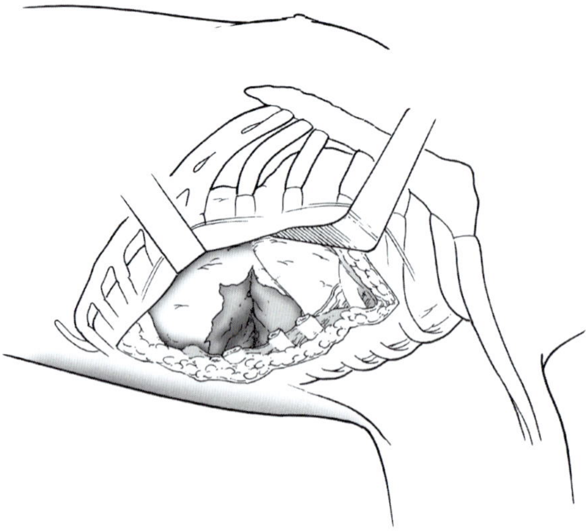

Fig. 38.4 Large chest wall defect, >10–15 cm in diameter, with underlying pulmonary laceration

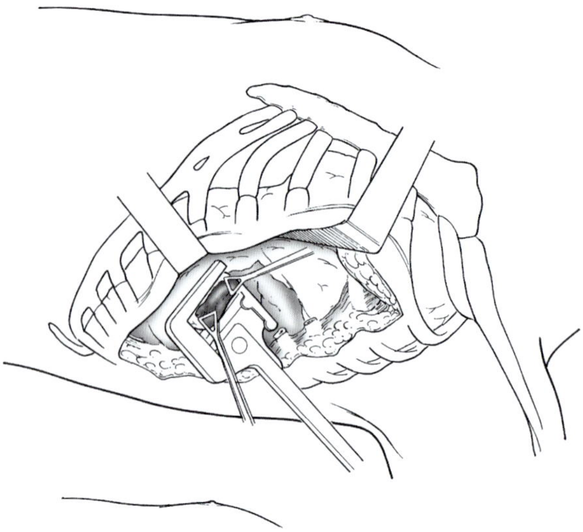

Fig. 38.5 Nonanatomic pulmonary resection with stapling device

debrided. The surgeon decides whether an additional 2–3 days of vacuum dressing are necessary or whether the wound can be closed by undermining skin and subcutaneous tissues and closing over a bulb suction drain.

The larger chest wall defect, >10–15 cm in diameter, is considerably more challenging to repair (Fig. 38.4). Depending on the mechanism of injury, it is much more likely that a significant pulmonary injury will be present, such as a large laceration, contusion, or intraparenchymal hematoma. You will have to manage this pulmonary injury simultaneously. Nonanatomic surgical resection may be necessary to control bleeding and air leak (Fig. 38.5). As in the smaller defect, you should commence immediately with wound cleansing and debridement of devascularized skin, subcutaneous fat, muscle, and bone. The defect resulting will seem formidable, but you can set up a good outcome by following the basic principles of debridement and damage control. At the conclusion of the first operation, place a 32–36 French chest tube through an anterior stab incision into the pleural space and tuck a plastic sheet under the chest wall defect in the same fashion as described for an open abdominal defect (Fig. 38.6) [3]. Pack the wound with moist gauze (Fig. 38.6 insert) and apply a vacuum suction dressing. In this case, do not extubate the patient postoperatively since the extent of chest wall loss will preclude effective, non-assisted pulmonary mechanics.

Depending on associated injuries, you should take back the patient to the OR at 2–3 day intervals for debridements and surgical management of the underlying pulmonary injury as necessary. When the wound is clean and the pulmonary injury stable, a large biologic tissue patch is sutured to the chest wall with absorbable suture in a similar fashion to the smaller defect shown in Fig. 38.2. The wound is again dressed with a vacuum dressing and attempts are made to wean the patient from the ventilator. A tracheostomy may be indicated for ventilator weaning if after 5–7 days, weaning progress has stalled. When the patient's pulmonary status is substantially improved and the wound is stable (7–14 days), a latissimus dorsi vascularized muscle flap is used to fill the defect and cover the biologic patch (Fig. 38.7). A bulb suction drain should be placed between the biologic patch and the muscle flap to prevent seroma formation and allow the muscle to adhere to the patch. A split-thickness skin graft will be necessary to cover the external surface of the muscle flap since the patient's own chest wall skin will have been debrided very significantly (Fig. 38.7 insert).

Removal of drains should follow standard surgical principles of ≤200 cc fluid per day and no air leak for tube thoracostomies and ≤30 cc fluid per day for bulb suction drains. You should tailor the antibiotic management to the amount and type of contamination, but in general, 48 h of gram-positive coverage should be sufficient.

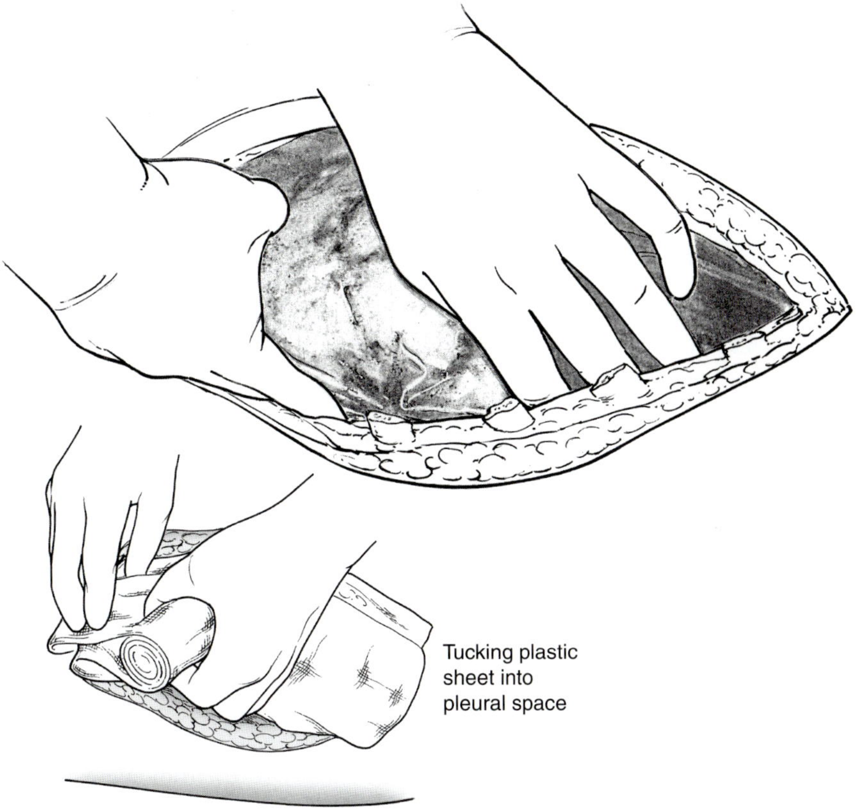

Fig. 38.6 A plastic sheet is tucked under the chest wall defect. The wound is then packed with moist gauze (insert) and a vacuum suction dressing is applied

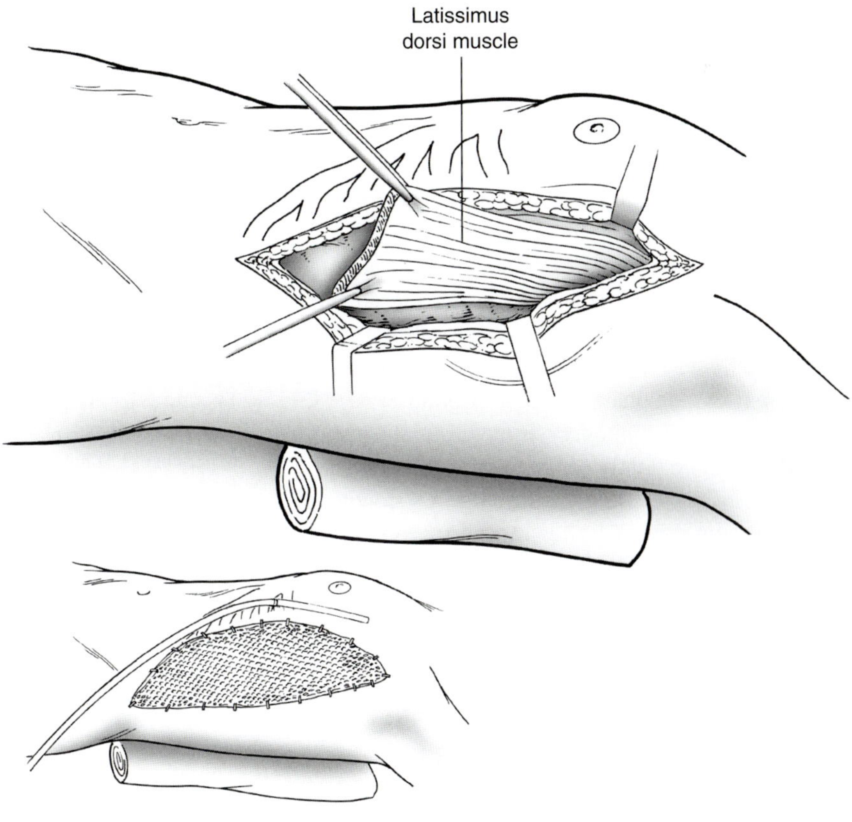

Fig. 38.7 A latissimus dorsi vascularized muscle flap is used to fill the defect and cover the biologic patch. A split-thickness skin graft is used to cover the external surface of the muscle flap (insert)

38.4 Recovery and Rehabilitation

Patients with smaller defects repaired may have little functional loss of their pulmonary mechanics and should recover completely. They will always, however, be at risk for pulmonary hernia development over months to years that may need elective repair. Larger defects will require longer intensive care unit and hospital stays and more days on the ventilator. These patients will be at higher risk for pulmonary hernia development. Chest wall replacement with more rigid prostheses should wait, however, for several months until the risk of prosthetic infection returns to that expected for a clean, noncontaminated, nontraumatic operation. If a tracheostomy was required, it can be downsized and eventually removed when the patient can tolerate tracheostomy plugging for 1–2 days without respiratory decompensation.

Important Points

1. Most chest wall loss patients will need immediate airway and ventilatory control. If the defect is on the left chest wall and there is a pulmonary laceration, blind right mainstem bronchus (deep) endotracheal intubation should be attempted.
2. Patients with lesser sized chest wall defects, e.g., <5 or 10 cm diameter, who are otherwise stable and cooperative, can be supported with intermittent bag-valve-mask ventilation during transport.
3. If able, the first responder is advised to briefly try to clamp intercostal arterial or venous bleeding or other chest wall muscular vessel bleeding from which the patient may exsanguinate during transport.
4. Significant pulmonary or mediastinal bleeding can be tightly packed with gauze and an occlusive dressing in the hope of slowing the hemorrhage during transport.
5. In the field, the defect is covered with a dressing and secured on three sides only so that accumulating pleural air can escape. This will prevent the development of a tension pneumothorax and will also prevent further contamination of the wound from the outside.
6. Chest radiographs or CT scans will not change surgical therapy and are therefore unnecessary and time wasting.
7. For a patient with a large, destructive chest wall injury, the emergency department (ED) should be bypassed for direct transport to the operating room (OR).
8. A destructive chest wall defect will seem formidable, but the surgeon can set up a good outcome by following the basic principles of debridement, damage control, and staged operations.
9. Portions of rib that are partially devoid of muscular attachments should be excised because devascularized bone will not survive and will later become a nidus for osteomyelitis.
10. Biologic mesh should be used to bridge the defect because of the lesser risk of prosthetic infection compared to standard prosthetic mesh. For a larger defect, a vascularized muscle flap will be necessary to fill the defect.

References

1. Bickell WH, Wall MJ Jr, Pepe PE et al (1994) Immediate versus delayed fluid resuscitation for hypotensive patients with penetrating torso injuries. N Engl J Med 331(17): 1105–1109
2. Mayberry JC, Terhes JT, Ellis TJ, Wanek S, Mullins RJ (2003) Absorbable plates for rib fracture repair: preliminary experience. J Trauma 55(5):835–839
3. Barker DE, Green JM, Maxwell RA et al (2007) Experience with vacuum-pack temporary abdominal wound closure in 258 trauma and general and vascular surgical patients. J Am Coll Surg 204(5):784–792

Part IV

Surgical Strategies in Penetrating Trauma to the Abdomen and Pelvis

39 Access to the Abdomen: Emergency Laparotomy

George C. Velmahos

The emergency laparotomy includes tasks and strategies that are drastically different than the elective laparotomy. The surgeon is constantly fighting an unforgiving foe: time. A moderately longer operation has little effect in outcome on a patient who is physiologically stable and not losing blood. On the other hand, every intraoperative minute counts on patients in metabolic disarray and hemodynamic collapse. Therefore, the entire philosophy of emergency abdominal access is dominated by the focus on minimizing time, while not compromising adequate exposure and technique. A standardization of tasks will prevent missed injuries, wrong procedures, or retained sponges, all of which are associated with emergency operations.

39.1 Position and Preparation

Always place the patient supine on the operating table. There is really no other choice. Left and right lateral positions may offer better access to specific retroperitoneal structures under elective circumstances, but do not allow adequate exploration of the entire abdomen and are time consuming for opening and closing. If there is a suspicion that a thoracotomy may be used (as it may happen with a thoracoabdominal penetrating injury), then a pillow under the patient's relevant hemithorax will offer enough area for an adequate anterolateral thoracotomy. Under emergency conditions, a postero-lateral thoracotomy is not advisable.

Prep the patient from neck to mid-thighs. One never knows what cavity should eventually require access. A variety of injuries, for example, require access on multiple areas: a thoracoabdominal injury producing significant injuries across the diaphragm; a retrohepatic inferior vena cava injury, requiring total liver isolation and clamping of the intrapericardial cava through a sternotomy; a thoracic or abdominal vascular injury, requiring a saphenous vein graft for the groin, etc.

Similarly, the drapes should be placed in such a way that will allow access to multiple areas. A narrow surgical field is the wrong principle for an emergency operation.

39.2 Incision

It is commonly suggested that the only proper way to explore the abdomen is a long midline incision from the xiphoid to the pubic symphysis. This certainly stands true for many cases. Nothing can be more frustrating for the surgeon and unsafe for the patient than trying to find and repair injuries through an inadequate exposure. On the other hand, the length of incision correlates with postoperative pain and complications. Therefore, not every incision needs to stretch from top to bottom. I see little reason to extend an upper midline incision far beyond the umbilicus in a thoracoabdominal wound with a clear high upper abdominal trajectory. Similarly, there is little justification for doubling the length of a lower midline incision made for a bladder rupture by extending it over the umbilicus. Having said that, you should have a very low threshold of

G.C. Velmahos
Harvard University Medical School,
Massachusetts General Hospital ,
Division of Trauma, Emergency Surgery
and Surgical Critical Care,
165 Cambridge Street, Suite 810, Boston, MA 02114, USA
e-mail: gvelmahos@partners.org

G.C. Velmahos et al. (eds.), *Penetrating Trauma*,
DOI 10.1007/978-3-642-20453-1_39,

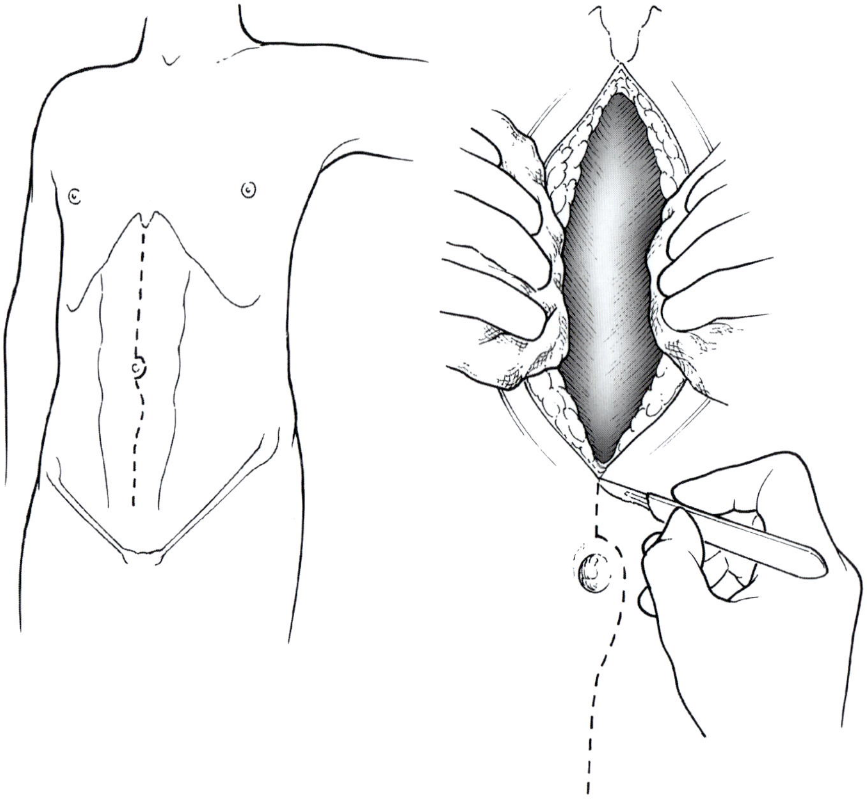

Fig. 39.1 Skin and subcutaneous tissue incision with the scalpel, while countertraction is applied on the two edges of the wound

extending an incision, if the exposure is inadequate, a satisfactory exploration cannot be achieved, or the repair is compromised.

There is hardly any other incision for entering the abdomen than a midline laparotomy for a traumatic emergency. Infrequently, there are reports of using subcostal incisions to access the liver or spleen for a subacute traumatic condition, as it would be with a splenic necrosis and abscess following embolization for trauma. This is acceptable although the benefits of the midline laparotomy are hard to match. In true emergency situations, enter the abdominal cavity in the following steps:

1. Incise the skin and subcutaneous tissue with the scalpel. Ignore the bleeding. Typically, if you place a gauze at the edges of the incision to retract the skin laterally, most of the bleeding will have stopped by the end of the incision. There is no reason to create a large thermal wound by electrocoagulating every possible small vessel (Fig. 39.1).
2. Incise the linea alba with the scalpel. Remember that the linea alba is narrow close to the xiphoid and wide close to the umbilicus. Incise it first in the immediate supraumbilical area. With incremental cuts of your knife, extend the linea alba incision upward. Do not yet cut through the preperitoneal fat and peritoneum that lies under the linea alba (Fig. 39.2).
3. Grasp the left side of the fascia with a Kocher clamp mid-way between the xiphoid process and the umbilicus and with a gauze bluntly dissect the preperitoneal fat away from the overlying fascia moving laterally. You will realize that the thick fatty tissue lying under the midline transitions to a thin and almost transparent peritoneal layer lying under the fascia laterally to the midline. You can usually enter into the peritoneal cavity bluntly by pushing your digit through this thin peritoneal layer (Fig. 39.3).
4. Under direct vision, incise the peritoneum up and down.
5. Insert your hand to protect the bowel, and with electrocoagulation extend the incision below the umbilicus. As opposed to the supraumbilical midline, on

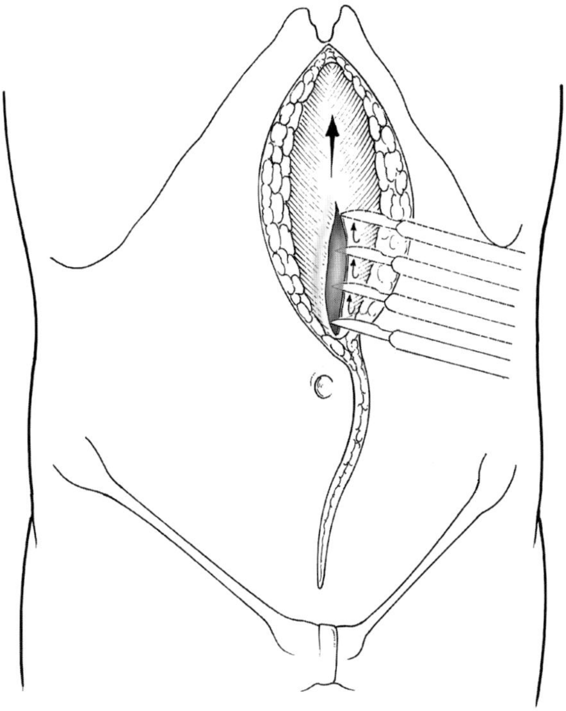

Fig. 39.2 Incising the linea alba with incremental cuts upward

which the fascia fuses in the relatively avascular linea alba, below the midline, there is no linea alba and electrocoagulation will help in minimizing bleeding from the muscle (Fig. 39.4).

6. It is now time to check for any major bleeding from the walls of the incision. Usually, there is none, but if any, use electrocoagulation to control it.

If the operation is not a true emergency, more time can be spent to open the abdomen along elective operation principles. In general, I dislike the attempts to control every small and temporarily bleeding subcutaneous vessel with electrocoagulation, as this causes an extensive thermal burn. If you place a gauze while retracting the edges of the wound laterally, the bleeding stops. At the end of the incision, you can electrocoagulate only the few remaining sites which continue to bleed.

39.3 Bleeding and Contamination Control

The standard teaching is to pack the four quadrants as soon as you enter in the peritoneal cavity. I believe that blind packing is ineffective and unnecessary. Suction the blood that is in the abdomen and localize its source. Then, pack this area meaningfully to achieve temporary control. It makes little sense to pack the entire abdomen, if the bleeding comes from the spleen!

Once you have packed, and with the bleeding controlled, make sure there is no other bleeding site. Often, there are more than one. You do not want to pack only the spleen, when an insidious mesenteric tear continues to shed blood in the pelvis, and fail to discover it before a substantial amount of blood is lost.

Your focus now should shift to the control of contamination. Have a *quick* look to check for perforations of any hollow viscus. If there is any, control it by placing a Babcock clamp or a quick occluding suture.

With the bleeding and contamination temporarily controlled, it is time to return to the bleeding site. Unpack carefully and check the extent of the injury. If there is something that can easily be repaired or ligated, then do so. Otherwise, repack, as your next step is to explore the entire abdomen.

39.4 Systematic Exploration

The exploration of the abdominal cavity should be performed systematically, following a routine that avoids missing injuries. I always start from the left upper quadrant and visualize the stomach, spleen, left diaphragm, and left lobe of the liver. Then, I move to the right upper quadrant, retracting the liver and visualizing its superior and inferior surfaces, the right diaphragm, the duodenum, and the hepatic hilum.

At this point, the assistant holds up the transverse mesocolon and the surgeon pulls all the small bowel toward the right side. This exposes the ligament of Treitz and the exploration of the small bowel begins by "running" it segment by segment, while flipping it over every time to inspect the anterior and posterior surfaces of it up to the ileocolic area. Then, the colon is inspected in detail all the way to the rectum and the peritoneal reflection. The pelvis is checked for retroperitoneal hematomas.

I do not routinely open the mesocolic ligament to inspect the pancreas and posterior surface of the stomach, unless if there is a specific indication.

Missed injuries occur if the above routine changes or if the described maneuvers are not performed diligently. I list below areas which I have frequently seen to be inadequately explored, resulting in missed injuries:

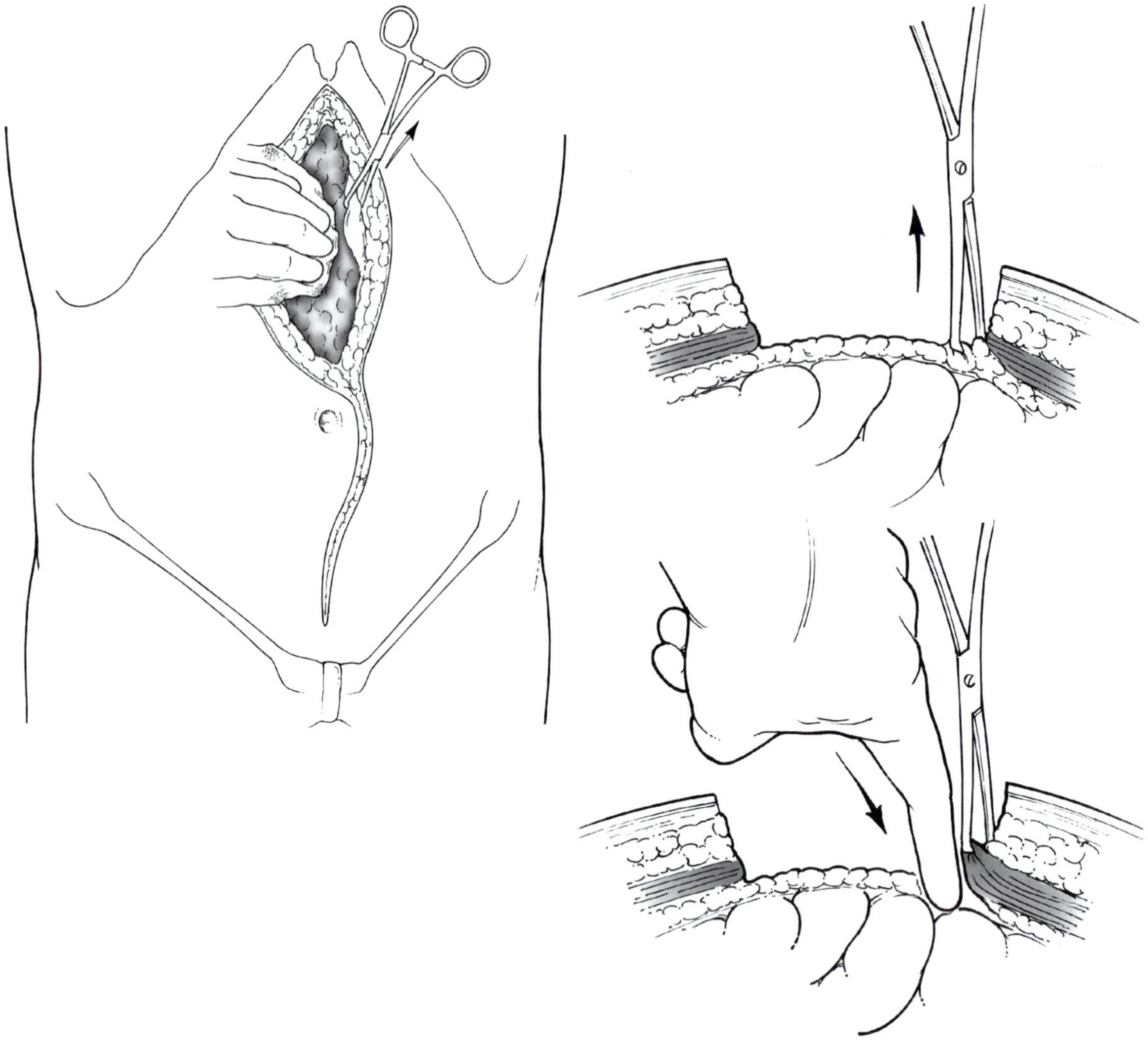

Fig. 39.3 Peritoneum laterally to the midline becomes thin and can easily be violated by pushing a digit through it

(a) The diaphragms: The stomach, colon, and spleen on the left side and the liver on the right side must be manually pushed downward in order to reveal the diaphragms. Injuries can easily be missed, particularly in the posterior portions of the diaphragms, if this is not done.

(b) The colon (particularly, the transverse colon): A small perforation can be missed in an obese person with large amount of fat tissue around the colon. In particular, omental attachments or the gastrocolic ligament may conceal a hole. Small hematomas close to the colon wall should be carefully explored. The gastrocolic ligament should be divided, if necessary to look in the posterior site of the transverse colon. Upon appropriate indications, the peritoneal attachments should be incised to check the retroperitoneal colon. In penetrating injuries, the rule is that there should be an even number of holes in the lumen of a hollow viscus. If the number is odd, search hard for the missing through-and-through perforation.

(c) The posterior side of the stomach: The rule of even holes applies here too. If there is a perforation of the anterior wall of the stomach, open the gastrocolic ligament to inspect the posterior wall.

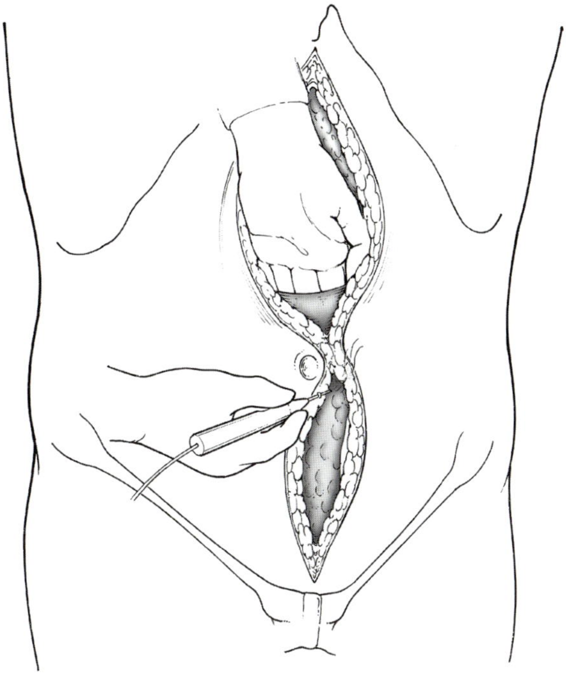

Fig. 39.4 With one hand in the abdomen, protecting the viscera, incise the muscle under the umbilicus with electrocoagulation

(d) The retroperitoneum: Although the retroperitoneal structures do not routinely require direct inspection, you should inspect the retroperitoneal areas and explore, as needed. As a general rule, retroperitoneal hematomas after blunt trauma should be explored if they lie centrally and left alone if in the pelvis or the lateral aspects. Retroperitoneal hematomas after penetrating trauma should be explored, unless there is a very high degree of confidence that no significant injury is present. There are exceptions on both rules. A blunt pelvic retroperitoneal hematoma could be explored for a known transaction of a major vessel. On the other hand, a blunt retrohepatic hematoma that is stable may be best left undisturbed. Similarly, a penetrating injury to the lateral edge of the kidney that causes a lateral hematoma may be safely observed without exploration.

39.5 Closure

Close the midline laparotomy in a single layer. I routinely use a single, long, running monofilament suture, starting from the lower end and finishing at the upper end. Having the left lobe of the liver under the incision when I am placing my last few sutures with limited visualization is much safer than having loops of bowel. For this, I always end my fascial suturing at the upper side. I never use subcutaneous sutures and close the skin routinely with staples.

Damage Control Surgery

40

Frank Plani and Riaan Pretorius

Damage Control is one of the key concepts to have emerged in the management of severe trauma in the past 25 years.

Other concepts which we have embraced in managing trauma are the following:

- The development of trauma systems
- The presence of senior surgical staff in the emergency room
- Hypotensive resuscitation
- The development of advanced haemostatic agents

Some forms of Damage Control surgery have been used in the last 90 years, beginning with Pringle in 1908 and Halstead in 1913 by means of liver packing; however, their popularity had waned, and was only resurrected in the 1970 for complex liver injuries.

In 1983, Stone and colleagues showed improved outcomes when an abbreviated laparotomy was used in many other unstable patients. The actual term 'Damage Control', however, was first used in 1993 by Rotondo and colleagues, borrowing it from naval terminology.

F. Plani (✉) • R. Pretorius
Trauma and Burns Unit, Chris Hani Baragwanath Hospital, University of the Witwatersrand Medical School, 7 York Road, Parktown, 2193 Johannesburg, Republic of South Africa
e-mail: frankplani@bigpond.com

40.1 Definition and Pathophysiology

What do we mean by Damage Control Surgery in 2010?

Most trauma surgeons would agree that it refers to an abbreviated staged surgical procedure anywhere in the body (laparotomy, shunting of vessels, external fixation, etc.) done on a patient in physiological extremes in order to minimize the insult of the surgery.

Your aim in damage control is to prevent the so-called lethal triad (acidosis, hypothermia, and coagulopathy) and to minimize the inflammatory response and multiple organ failure.

40.1.1 Acidosis

We often encounter metabolic acidosis in trauma as the consequence of hypovolemic shock (Ivatury, Chap 12, Damage Control) from blood loss and third space losses. Our patients end up with inadequate perfusion, anaerobic metabolism, and lactic acidosis.

Severe acidosis ($pH < 7.20$) reduces myocardial response to catecholamines and is partly responsible for initiating coagulopathy, thus worsening bleeding and worsening shock.

40.1.2 Hypothermia

We must take meticulous care in ensuring that our patients do not become hypothermic. We define hypothermia as a core temperature below 36°C and 32°C as the crucial temperature where below the enzymes stop being functional.

G.C. Velmahos et al. (eds.), *Penetrating Trauma*,
DOI 10.1007/978-3-642-20453-1_40, © Springer-Verlag Berlin Heidelberg 2012

Therefore, it is our practice to implement damage control measures "ab initio" at the critical temperature of 34°C.

The way hypothermia causes tissue hypoxia and acidosis is via the following mechanisms:

- Shivering – increased oxygen consumption
- Hypoventilation
- Peripheral vasoconstriction
- Oxygen dissociation curve shift to left

Hypothermia causes coagulopathy through enzyme failure that compromises platelet function: platelet-fibrin clots are not sustained and fibrinolytic activity is increased. This will cause a prolongation of both prothrombin and partial thromboplastin time.

Thus hypothermia plays a vital role in the worsening of the acidosis and coagulopathy and the fatal cycle of the lethal triad.

40.1.3 Coagulopathy

We encounter coagulopathy as the result of both intrinsic and extrinsic factors.

Intrinsic factors:

- Extensive tissue injury, release tissue factors resulting in consumption coagulopathy
- Activation of the inflammatory cascade due to hypoperfusion
- Hemodilution due to mobilization of extracellular fluid
- Effects of acidosis and hypothermia
- Decrease in calcium

Extrinsic factors:

- Large amount of clear fluids
- Effects of massive transfusion

We recommend considering thromboelastometry and recombinant factor VIIa as components of damage control as suggested by Bartal and Yitzhak.

They go hand in hand, as thromboelastometry may guide you to whom and when rFVIIa could be administered. Evidence shows that rFVIIa may delay or even decrease our need for surgery, although it does not seem to influence mortality. We need further studies to determine exact roles and endpoints for it.

40.2 Indications for Damage Control Surgery

As pointed out above, we must always be on the lookout for the development of the deadly triad of coagulopathy, acidosis, and hypothermia both pre- and intra-operatively in order to be ready to implement damage control surgery as soon as needed.

Just concentrating on surgical operative tasks is never enough when you perform trauma surgery: On the contrary, during any operation you should pay attention to your patients' physiological parameters to detect downwards spirals in the patients' conditions and plan early damage control before descending into the deadly spiral.

40.3 Stages of Damage Control

Through continual involvement in patients' physiological requirements Rotondo was able to describe three stages of damage control:

1. Surgical control of hemorrhage and contamination
2. Correction of acidosis, hypothermia, and coagulopathy in ICU
3. Reoperation with definitive surgical management of pathology

More recently, we have expanded this concept to a five-stage classification, and we feel that awareness of each stage is essential to establish optimal outcome for the patient:

Stage 1: Patient selection
Stage 2: Operative control of hemorrhage and contamination
Stage 3: Resuscitation in ICU
Stage 4: Definitive surgery
Stage 5: Abdominal wall reconstruction (and other reconstructive interventions)

40.3.1 Stage1: Patient Selection

For a good outcome we need to select the correct patient at the right time. We should make our decision to use damage control before we enter the lethal triad but also guard against overusing damage control, as this would also be detrimental.

Indications for Damage Control:

The questions that we should ask ourselves are:

- What is the injury pattern?
- What is the severity of the trauma burden?
- What are the physiological parameters?
- What are the trauma systems in place?

We must look out for the factors that predict that our patient is becoming coagulopathic and acidotic and require an abbreviated laparotomy:

Injury severity score >25

Systolic blood pressure <70 mmHg

Temperature <34°C

pH < 7.10

Other factors that should make you consider employing Damage Control as the procedure of choice include the following situations:

- Inability to achieve hemostasis
- Combined vascular, solid and hollow organ injury
- Inaccessible major venous injury (retro hepatic IVC)
- Anticipated need for time-consuming procedure in severely injured
- Injuries treated non-operatively (pelvic fractures, angio-embolization)
- Desire to reassess organs (relook)
- Evidence of decline of physiological reserve as exemplified by these findings:
  - Temperature <34°C
  - pH < 7.2
  - Serum lactate increasing
  - Prothrombin time >16 s
  - Partial thromboplastin time >60 s
  - >10 units blood
  - S-BP < 90 mmHg for more than 60 min
  - Operating time >60 min
  - Need for emergency room thoracotomy

Make sure you maintain good communication with the anesthetist, since continued re-evaluation and good judgment are needed to give a patient the best benefit from damage control. Surgeons need to know when to step back and treat the patient and not just the local pathology.

40.3.2 Stage 2: Operative Control of Hemorrhage and Contamination

40.3.2.1 General Principles

- Warm operating theatre to prevent hypothermia
- Patients with torso injuries need to be prepared from chin to knees
- Good access lines, ideally above and below the umbilicus (femoral and subclavian)
- Prepare autologous blood recovery system (cell saver)

In the past, penetrating abdominal injury with bowel contamination was a contraindication to blood salvage from the peritoneal cavity. Many trials have proved that blood salvage even with bowel contents can be used safely. Bowley, Barker and colleagues used 44 patients with penetrating torso trauma, hypotension that needed a laparotomy and divided them in 23 control group and 21 in cell save. All patients received prophylactic antibiotics. Intraoperative blood salvage led to significant reduction in allogenic blood usage although there was no effects on postoperative infections or mortality.

Institute Massive Transfusion Protocol

Hemorrhage Control: repair or ligation of accessible vessels

- Occlusion of inflow into bleeding organ
- Tamponade using wraps or packs
- Intra-operative or post-operative embolization
- Intravascular shunting

Control Contamination:

- Ligation or stapling of bowel

Temporary Closure of the Abdomen:

Close the abdomen to prevent hypothermia and to protect the viscera. Various techniques are available:

- Towel clips
- Bogota bag
- Vacuum dressings
- Skin closure only
- Mesh closure

You must continue to resuscitate actively intra-operatively and post-operatively until all parameters have been corrected. Sometimes it is very difficult to determine if bleeding is due to ongoing bleeding or due to coagulopathy: when in doubt, rather re-open and re-pack.

You will often find significant unsuspected bleeders from muscle bellies and venous branches, amenable to suture-ligation.

It is important not to transfer patients to ICU if there is ongoing bleeding to avoid worsening coagulopathy, deteriorating physiological parameters and then having to transfer patients back to theatre, but sicker.

40.3.2.2 Chest

Most thoracic damage control surgery allows definitive procedures, and, more often than not, definitive closure.

The injuries should be assessed as soon as you get into the chest cavity.

Start with packing, particularly for bleeding from the chest wall, then clamping the hilum of the affected lung.

In terms of emergency incisions, you should apply the most suitable incision for the injures and the location you suspect.

Median Sternotomy

We recommend sternotomy for anterior penetrating injuries between the nipple lines, for the heart or the anterior mediastinum, and for access the arch of the aorta and the roots of carotids and subclavian vessels. In an emergency situation you may not have an oscillating sternal saw available, hence familiarity with the Lebsche knife and mallet is recommended; it is best used starting from the xyphoid at the bottom of the incision.

Antero-Lateral Thoracotomy

This is the default incision in most emergency thoracotomies, be they performed in the emergency room or the operating theatre: it allows for better access to peripheral and posterior injuries and can be easily extended across the sternum into a clamshell.

Postero-Lateral Thoracotomy

This is the only incision that allows you to place a graft for a ruptured thoracic aorta, and offers better access to structures in the posterior mediastinum.

Lung Injuries

The key maneuver is to divide the inferior pulmonary ligament avoiding the inferior pulmonary vein.

You must try to control bleeding with manual pressure, hemostatic suture, or rapid resection of injured segment but if all fail the hilum could be clamped or lung can be twisted around his hilum.

Peripheral lung injuries can usually be managed with stapled nonanatomical resection or a stapler can be used to open the tract and individual bleeders can be ligated with prolene or PDS sutures.

Central injuries are very difficult life-threatening injuries to manage.

Expose the hilum and control bleeding by compression between your thumb and index finger.

Proximal control can then be obtained by passing a sling, normally a urinary catheter or strong rubber tubing around the hilum and if that fails you must open the pericardium and apply a clamp to the pulmonary vessels.

In the very unlikely event that repair is not possible use a 90 mm linear vascular stapler and do a stapled pneumonectomy. Control the bleeding with running sutures. We tend to use the new haemostatic products, such as "TachoSil" and others, as a way of minimizing bleeding and leaks.

Sometimes we need to pack the chest cavity and just close the skin at the first operation.

Cardiac Injuries

Release of tamponade and temporary occlusion can sometimes be achieved with a Foleys catheter, skin staples or, for atrial injuries, with a Satinsky clamp.

Then you must affect the repair with 3-0 Prolene or PDS with pledgets or with a figure of eight sutures.

Tracheobronchial Injuries

You should repair these as soon as they become clinically obvious, as demonstrated by non-expanding lung parenchyma despite significant bubbling from the intercostals drains, often within the first couple of hours since presentation.

There are no shortcuts in tracheobronchial injuries, and they require early thoracotomy, adequate exposure, debridement and primary repair, ideally followed by early extubation.

Stents have been used in tracheobronchial conditions, but have not been tested adequately to recommend them as temporizing measures in damage control situations.

Esophageal Injuries

If you have to apply damage control to esophageal injuries, you may have to just drain the mediastinum and create a controlled fistula, with or without esophageal exclusion and gastrostomy.

In less desperate situations, an esophageal stent may be used to bridge a gap temporarily.

Vascular Injuries in the Chest and Neck

You should start by assessing which external compression maneuver achieves the best results and ensure it is maintained until the patient is scrubbed on the operating table.

Sometimes you can manage to tamponade the bleeding with inflated Foleys catheters, but you have no control on what you are compressing, and how effectively.

When faced with a deteriorating patient you should ligate veins and shunt arteries as in other regions. Thanks to rich collateral circulation, however, you can often ligate carotid and subclavian arteries as long as there is good back-flow.

For the same reason, small defects can be repaired by lateral arteriography even if this leads to some narrowing of the lumen.

You can ligate a badly damaged common carotid in most circumstances, thanks to the good back flow and collateral circulation.

40.3.2.3 Abdomen

Carry out a generous midline laparotomy from xiphisternum to pubis, pack all four quadrants immediately, evacuate and try to cell-save all excess blood, and let the anesthetist catch up with fluid resuscitation.

Control hemorrhage and contamination and then decide on damage control or definitive procedures.

Our practice is to take injury patterns into account, and we would encourage you to carry out damage control in the following situations, even if a patient is deemed to be "stable":

- Combined major vascular and hollow visceral injuries
- Very large central injury with hematoma
- High-grade liver injuries
- Pelvic fracture with expanding hematoma
- Injuries in multiple cavities

Consider damage control as an option also in stable patients with correctable injuries, but when your resources are overwhelmed by the number of patients' still awaiting theatre, such as in multiple patient or mass casualties' incidents, when the need for speed relates to the number of operations that need to be carried out in the shortest time possible.

Hollow Organ Injuries

Our aim is quick and effective control of contamination.

Traditionally, the options have centered on bowel interruption, either with resection or not, and using ties or staples to close the cut ends of bowel.

There are concerns that intestinal ligation in a shocked patient as part of damage control leads to increased bacterial translocation and inflammatory response. It may be beneficial to staple or tie the site of perforation and try to preserve some lumen if possible.

Accepted practice for colonic injuries post damage control and open abdomen has been to always bring out colostomies as part of definitive surgery. Miller, Chang and colleagues recently demonstrated that delayed anastomosis in colonic surgery is a safe option. The choice of patients that qualify for delayed anastomosis still needs to be clarified.

Biliary Tract Injuries

In situations demanding damage control, there are usually many associated injuries and only drainage of the biliary tree by a T-tube is indicated.

As with the case with massive injuries to other hollow structures, you can ligate the common bile duct at the time of damage control followed by re-implantation into a Roux-en-Y at a subsequent relook laparotomy.

Spleen

Splenectomy is the only safe option for significant splenic injuries in a damage control setting.

On the other hand, if faced with minor but persistent bleeding at the initial operation, you could pack around the spleen in the same fashion as packing a liver and leave the definitive treatment for the next relook laparotomy.

Liver Injuries

Liver injuries are initially packed and manually compressed to allow the anesthesiologist time to catch up with resuscitation. A Pringle maneuver must be used to isolate the liver if bleeding cannot be controlled with compression.

After stabilization you should divide the falciform ligament to avoid tearing the liver while packing and retracting the abdominal wall with a Doyen retractor. This step is crucial in order to give good exposure of the upper abdomen.

With the Pringle maneuver in place, look for and suture-ligate obvious vessels within the liver parenchyma.

Most but not all bleeding would stop with approximation of the edges with liver sutures or a Vicryl mesh wrap, but obvious large vessel will bleed through.

Apply balloon tamponade early for bleeding from a GSW tract, using a Sengstaken Blackmoor tube, which you should make available before any suspected liver case.

Liver Packing

You can pack the liver in a number of ways: we usually recommend packing the liver back to its natural position against the diaphragm, and therefore avoid packing above the liver: however, you should use your discretion according to type of injuries.

One of the key points to remember is to minimize compression of the inferior vena cava, in order to maintain venous return to the heart.

You should always consider wrapping the liver rather than trying to push it too hard against the IVC: We often achieve this with a couple of vascular swabs tied around the liver after sufficient mobilization, but you can also use self-locking name tags, thick tape, or soft rubber tubing: this technique often requires fewer packs around the liver.

In a similar fashion, try and wrap the liver with a Vicryl mesh: even if you cannot do it fully in an incompletely mobilize liver, just doing a partial wrap may be sufficient.

We tend to carry out angiography and possible embolization after the first damage control operation. If the patient is too unstable, though, we prefer to re-pack the patient after 48–72 h, in the ICU if necessary, and leave the embolization to when the patient is stable enough.

In patients with complex liver injuries, a delayed liver resection may need a subsequent relook, just removing obviously necrotic and easily accessible damaged liver.

With retrohepatic IVC the liver should not be mobilized as much, and packing and cobbling tissue together is often enough to control the hemorrhage.

You would need to carry out a more extensive mobilization if you plan to use an atrio-caval shunt, which may be a life-saving intervention, but then you should have learned this maneuver well in simulation before trying it on a living patient.

Pancreaticoduodenal Injuries

Treat the central abdomen with respect, since there are often multiple large vessels involved, such as the mesenteric vessels and the portal vein as well as often complex duodenal and pancreatic injuries.

For major lacerations to the left of the superior mesenteric vessels you should carry out a distal pancreatectomy while you should usually drain lacerations to the right of the vessels.

Initially you can control bleeding from the pancreas by local pressure, haemostatic sutures or packing. When packing you must also leave a drain, since packing without drainage has been associated with an increased mortality.

You should try and manage duodenal injuries with primary repair. In extreme cases the edges should be approximated over external drain. Primary repair is the best option in most cases since it does not require a number of different anastomosis.

We tend to manage severe duodenal injuries with primary repair or pyloric exclusion with gastrojejunostomy. It is debatable whether not excluding the pylorus makes the procedure safer or not.

Pancreatico-duodenectomies are very seldom indicated or used in severe trauma cases.

Renal and Ureteral Injuries

You can safely drain or tube-stent ureteric injuries at the initial damage control procedure; definitive repair can be delayed for days, as long as the area does not become septic.

If you are faced with a Zone II retroperitoneal hematoma that is expanding, bleeding or pulsatile, it needs to be explored and if the kidney or renal vessels are involved you should do a nephrectomy.

Ascertain the function of the contralateral kidney by palpation and by monitoring the urine output. Oozing but no active bleeding can be controlled by packing of the kidney.

If the zone II retroperitoneal hematoma does not warrant exploration a post-op CT scan-IVP can be done to assess the kidneys.

Abdominal Vascular Injuries

You will not be able to perform any true damage control procedure for the suprarenal aorta, and rapid definitive repair is needed, by suturing even if it leads to reduction in diameter.

Primary repair of the infrarenal aorta is the best option but if not possible you must consider other choices, such as shunting or ligation with extra-anatomical bypass.

Celiac artery and inferior mesenteric artery can be ligated, but the superior mesenteric artery needs to be repaired or shunted.

You can ligate the portal vein, but if the hepatic artery is also involved one of the two needs to be reconstructed.

External iliac arteries can be shunted, repaired, or ligated with an extra-anatomical bypass to prevent limb ischemia. You can safely ligate a unilateral internal iliac artery and it appears that even ligating both may be tolerated.

You can ligate the infrarenal inferior vena cava in damage control, but you must be prepared for significant swelling in both lower limbs and the lower abdomen.

You must try and avoid ligating the suprarenal inferior vena cava: ligation of suprarenal IVC is associated with a high morbidity and mortality. For this reason, avoid exploring a non-expanding supra-renal retroperitoneal hematoma and find yourself with an irreparable venous injury.

40.3.2.4 Pelvis

You must stabilize unstable pelvic fractures with a sheet or pelvic binder tied around the pelvis at the level of the greater trochanters.

You can get good results from a C-clamp but only if adequately trained and experienced on how to use it.

If angiography is immediately available you should investigate the possibility of angio-embolization as a first therapeutic as well as diagnostic modality, otherwise the patient who is still unstable after binding the pelvis should be taken to the operating room for packing and to rule out intra-abdominal injuries. You should familiarize yourself with the technique of extra-peritoneal packing, since this has been shown to be more effective than packing the intraperitoneal pelvis.

40.3.2.5 Extremity Injuries

You have two options in the damage control of extremity injuries:

1. Debridement, packing and back slabs
2. Debridement and external fixation

In any case you should stabilize most extremity injuries in order to minimize movement and bleeding but with limited surgical insult.

Multiple studies have proven that intramedullary instrumentation increases intracranial pressure and this could be detrimental for patients with severe head and severe lung injury, since there is also a higher pulmonary embolic load with intramedullary fixation.

However, the effect on the coagulation system and the inflammatory response is the same for both internal and external fixation.

You should be able to shunt most vascular injuries of the extremities down to elbow and knee, accompanied by distal fasciotomies.

Vascular shunts have become mainstream, and you should consider them as a first maneuver whenever there are combined vascular and orthopedic injuries.

They were first described in 1952 but still considered somewhat experimental by 1994.

In Northern Ireland, temporary shunting has been the norm since the early 1980, with dramatic improvement in survival and amputation rates. They have however mainly been used within the same operative procedure, while waiting for orthopedic surgery to be completed.

In 1989, the first report of long distance air travel with a shunt in a severely ischemic leg ended up with an amputation eventually. However, reports from the recent Iraqi conflicts on their use in long distance transfers highlight their beneficial use even in very perilous circumstances.

In a 6-month experience, transfers took up to 9 h to definite vascular surgery with none of the 19 temporary shunts placed at Theatre Hospital becoming dislodged or suffered shunt complications, and succeeded in saving 94% of limbs thus operated.

This is particularly impressive in view of the type of injuries seen at present. In a series of 3,057 soldiers evacuated for medical evaluation, 1,524 (50%) sustained battle injuries. Known or suspected vascular injuries occurred in 107 (7%) patients.

Sixty-eight (64%) patients were wounded by explosive devices, 27 (25%) were wounded by gunshots, and 12 (11%) experienced blunt traumatic injury.

This has led to recommendations for temporary shunts to be used routinely in civilian trauma, be it blunt or penetrating, where a combination of bony and vascular injuries coexist.

Fox et al. took 16 patients with 20 vascular repairs (3 upper 17 lower extremities) with isolated limb injuries. All were acidotic (pH 7.27 ± 0.1), hypotensive (BP 105/60 ± 29/18) and coagulopathic (INR 1.3 ± 0.4). 95% were repaired with vein grafts. Most (75%) received recombinant factor VIIa in the ED and theatre. They found that aggressive damage control resuscitation allow for complex limb salvage revascularization with excellent limb salvage and graft patency.

With this in mind, your approach to the above-mentioned combined injuries should probably be: fasciotomy, vascular exploration, embolization, heparinised saline flushing, temporary shunting for artery and vein, orthopedic intervention, definitive vascular procedure, angiogram.

In situations where revascularization is delayed, and both arteries and veins are involved, you should consider anastomosing the artery first, getting rid of all the blood accumulated in the venous system, and only then perform your venous anastomosis.

40.3.2.6 Spine

You should consider damage control for spinal injuries as well. In most cases of severe bleeding from the spine and surrounding tissues, this will mean packing and relooking after 24–48 h.

You can certainly position freshly injured casualties prone to have access to the spine, which will also improve ventilation.

What happens next is mainly related to availability of expertise and theatre time.

One recent study favorably compared polytrauma patients having immediate total repair (<24 h) or delayed repair after they recovered from other injuries. It is postulated the former method might increase ventilator-free days, decrease length of ICU and hospital stay, complications, neurological status, and functional recovery.

40.3.2.7 Brain

Unilateral craniectomy with a wide trauma flap to evacuate hematomas is a life-saving surgery and should be carried out within 4 h of an injury. Massive subdural hematomas can bleed torrentially, and you would be well advised to have enough blood, fresh frozen plasma and platelets in such cases.

Lately, "Decompressive bi-fronto-temporal craniectomy" (DECRA) is being used as an isolated operation to control intracranial hypertension following trauma not amenable to unilateral; craniectomy or craniotomy.

The final results from a large multicentre study show increased mortality and poor functional outcomes at 6 months with this technique, but further studies are in progress.

40.3.3 Stage 3: Resuscitation in ICU

Your priorities in ICU are:

- Restore body temperature
  - Passive rewarming using warm fluids and blankets
  - Active rewarming with cavity lavage
- Correct the clotting profile:
  - Use INR, PTT, and platelet count to direct resuscitation
  - You can also make use of thromboelastography (TEG)
  - Transfuse packed cells and FFPs at a ratio of 1:1 and platelet as indicated or for every ten units of cells.
  - Give calcium and other blood products
- Correct acidosis to pH > 7.3 by optimization of oxygen delivery:
  - Volume loading
  - Bring the hemoglobin up to >10 g/dL
  - Measure and correct lactic acidosis to <2.5 mmol/L
  - Give inotropic support as needed

Continue resuscitation actively in ICU: Physiological parameters must be corrected as much as possible, certainly within 12 h but ideally within 6 h, in order to avoid multiple organ failure.

Damage control with an open abdomen is not a contraindication to enteral feeding. If there is no hollow viscus immediate enteral nutrition appears to be safe, with no effect on abdominal closure rate and a decrease in pneumonia.

It is vital that you recognize the indications for unplanned re-exploration.

The two major indications are ongoing bleeding and abdominal compartment syndrome.

Suspect ongoing or new bleeding with large amount of blood in drains, worsening lactic acidosis, increasing requirement of inotropic support, decrease in hemoglobin despite transfusion and deteriorating coagulopathy despite measures to correct it. It might be very difficult to differentiate severe coagulopathy from active bleeding but the earlier recognized and corrected the better the outcome.

Any suction drain with an open abdomen encourages bleeding, and one of your first interventions should be to stop the suction. Bleeding will have often started from abdominal wall or more infrequently, omental bleeding: One of the first useful interventions, long before blaming it on coagulopathy, is to open the dressings and stitch-tie any obvious bleeders or entire areas.

Abdominal compartment syndrome is usually but not necessarily avoided by not closing the fascia or skin during damage control. It presents with decreased BP and urinary output, high intravesical pressures and depending on mode of ventilation either decreased volume (pressure ventilation) or increased pressures (volume ventilation). As in bleeding, the best initial treatment is to have a look, at the bedside, undo tight vacuum assisted dressings, and loosely reapply dressings to the open abdomen.

Be aware, however, that a tighter abdomen might mean intraabdominal bleeding, which you must be prepared for with a large number of abdominal swabs being ready before you go in.

40.3.4 Stage 4: Definitive Surgery

You must take patients back to the operating theatre at the correct time, not too soon, and certainly not too late, within 24–48 h.

Timing is determined by:
- The indication for damage control
- The injury pattern
- The physiological response on resuscitation

Ideally you should be taking patients back to the operating theatre when the end points of resuscitation are achieved such as normalization of lactate, base excess, temperature, and clotting profiles. Unnecessary delay will cause ARDS, SIRS, and sepsis.

A relook should be a thorough laparotomy or other operative intervention, looking for previously undiagnosed injuries. The definitive stages involve removal of packing, more precise evaluation of injuries, and establishing bowel, biliary tract, genitourinary tract, and vascular continuity.

If physiological parameters deteriorate, bleeding is still present or concerns over viability of tissues, further damage control should take place.

40.3.5 Stage 5: Abdominal Wall Reconstruction

After definitive surgery the abdominal wall can be closed. Methods include:
- Primary closure
- Closure of the sheath, leaving skin open
- Bogota bag with delayed closure
- Mesh closure

The method of closure will be determined by the underlying injuries and the timing from initial laparotomy to definitive surgery. Patients with multiple relook laparotomies are usually closed with mesh, but if in any doubt about ongoing sepsis, rather allow the wound to granulate without introducing any foreign bodies.

40.4 Outcome

Sutton et al. did a prospective study to look at the long-term impact of damage control surgery. They collected 56 patients with mean age 31 ± 11 years, mean ISS of 33 ± 13 with equal blunt and penetrating injuries. The overall mortality was 27%. The time spent in the ICU and hospital was 17 ± 13 and 30 ± 19 days, respectively. The most common causes for readmissions were infection, ventral hernia repair and fistula management. Find comparisons with non-damage control.

There is significant morbidity and costs involved with damage control surgery but the survival benefit is undisputable. Cumulative studies suggest a mortality of 50% and a morbidity of 40%; but this has to be balanced against an expected mortality approaching 100% had damage control not been carried out.

40.5 Controversies and New Developments

There are still unresolved issues, 13 years after its first description, among which are the following:
- Overzealous selection of patients for damage control
- Prolongation of life in clearly non-salvageable situations
- Delays in the application of damage control in very unstable patients
- Incomplete control of arterial bleeding
- Excessive numbers of open abdomens and reoperations

It is important that you decide early on the intention to carry out a damage control operation, and not only once the triad of coagulopathy, acidosis and hypothermia have already set in: sometimes, as described by Hirschberg and others, just assessing on CT scan what structures bullets may have traversed may give you some indication of the expected damage to be found and might help you with decision making.

40.6 Conclusions

Damage control has become entrenched as an essential tool in the surgery of major trauma, despite the lack of level I evidence, but supported by good level II evidence.

Damage control saves lives, but must be applied early in order to avoid the deadly triad of hypothermia, acidosis, and coagulopathy.

It is based on a staged approach to the trauma patient alternating resuscitation and interventions, and accepting delayed definitive interventions.

From its original application to abdominal surgery, it has come to encompass all aspects of trauma care, from neurosurgery to orthopedic to ophthalmology.

The main future challenges are to fine tune the various restorative procedures that follow the initial surgery and resuscitation.

Important Points

1. Damage Control Surgery is any form of emergency surgery where temporizing measures are used in preference to definitive procedures for speed and simplicity in unstable patients.
2. It is associated with high mortality and morbidity, but less than if definitive procedure is unwisely attempted.
3. The initial procedure is followed by a short period of intensive resuscitation to correct hypothermia, acidosis, and coagulopathy, after which the patient is returned to the operating theatre for completion of the surgical interventions.
4. Damage control surgery is mainly carried out in the abdomen and pelvis but can be applied anywhere else, including chest, neck, extremities, and in neurosurgical and vascular injuries.
5. Specific temporizing ways of maintaining lumen continuity rather than ligation are the mainstay of damage control in bowel, ureteric, and vascular injuries.
6. The main areas where caution is needed are in relation to the following:
   (a) Suction systems in the open abdomen phase
   (b) Timing and choice of anastomosis versus stomas after damage control for colonic injuries
   (c) Timing and tissue cover after temporary stenting for vascular injuries

Recommended Reading

Sutton E, Bochicchio GV (2006) Long term impact of damage control surgery: a preliminary prospective study. J Trauma 61(4):831–834

Winter CD, Adamides A (2005) The role of decompressive craniectomy in the management of traumatic brain injury: a critical review. J Clin Neurosci 12(6):619–623

Pape HC, Grimme K (2003) Impact of intramedullary instrumentation versus damage control for femoral fractures on immunoinflammatory parameters: prospective randomized analysis by the EPOFF Study group. J Trauma 55(1):7–13

Stahel PF, Flieri MA (2009) Advocating "spine damage control" as a safe and effective treatment for unstable thoracolumbar fractures in polytrauma patients: a hypothesis. J Trauma Manag Outcomes 3:6

Fox CJ, Gillespie DL (2008) Damage control resuscitation for vascular surgery in a combat support hospital. J Trauma 65(1):1–9

Bowley DM, Barker P (2006) Intraoperative blood salvage in penetrating trauma: a randomized, controlled trial. World J Surg 30(6):1074–1080

Hirschberg A, Mattox KL (2006) Top knife: the art and craft of trauma surgery. tfm Publishing Ltd, Castle Hills Barns

Cameron JL (2008) Current surgical therapy, 9th edn. Mosby & Elsevier, Philadelphia

Mohr AM, Asensio JA (2005) Guidelines for the institution of damage control in trauma patients. Int Trauma Care 15(4):185–189

Moeng MS, Loveland JA, Boffard KD (2005) Damage control: beyond the limits of the abdominal cavity. Int Trauma Care Fall:189–196

Rotondo MF, Schwab CW et al (1993) "Damage Control": an approach for improved survival in exsanguinating penetrating abdominal injury. J Trauma 35:375–383

Scott BG, Welsh FJ, Wall MJ Jr, Mattox KL, Hirschberg A (2006) Early aggressive closure of the open abdomen. J Trauma 60(1):17–22

Shapiro MB, Jenkins DH, Schwab CW, Schwab CW (2000) Damage control: collective review. J Trauma 49(5):969–978

Wang P, Wei X et al (2008) Influences of intestinal ligation on bacterial translocation and inflammatory responses in rats with hemorrhagic shock: implications for damage control surgery. J Invest Surg 21(5):244

Cothren CC, Moore EE (2006) Emergency department thoracotomy for the critically injured patient: objectives, indications, and outcomes. World J Emerg Surg 24:1–4

Hirschberg A, Wall MJ Jr, Mattox KL (2002) Bullet trajectory predicts the need for damage control: an artificial neural network model. J Trauma 52(5):852–858

Holcomb JB, Helling TS, Hirshberg A (2001) Military, civilian, and rural application of the damage control philosophy. Mil Med 166(6):490–493

Butler FK, Hagmann J, Butler EG (1996) Tactical combat casualty care in special operations. Mil Med 161(Suppl):1

Rodas EB, Ivatury RR (2005) Hyper acute abdominal compartment syndrome: an unrecognized complication of massive intraoperative resuscitation for extra-abdominal injuries. Am Surg 71(11):977–981

Glover JL, Smith R, Yaw PB (1978) Autotransfusion of blood contaminated by intestinal contents. JACEP 7(4):142

Barros D'Sa AA, McIlrath E (2006) The Belfast approach to managing complex lower limb vascular injuries. Eur J Vasc Endovasc Surg 32(3):246–256

Johansen K, Hedges G (1989) Successful limb reperfusion by temporary arterial shunt during a 950 mile air transfer. J Trauma 29(9):1289

Gillespie DL, O'Donnell SD, Rich NM (2005) Contemporary management of wartime vascular trauma. J Vasc Surg 41(4):638–644

Ertel W, Trentz O (2001) Control of severe hemorrhage using C-Clamp and pelvic packing in multiply injured patients with pelvic ring disruption. J Orthop Trauma 15(7):468

Moore EE, Smith WR (2005) Retroperitoneal packing as a resuscitation technique for hemodynamically unstable patients with pelvic fractures. J Trauma 59(6):1510–1514

Bach A, Bendix J et al (2008) Scand J Trauma Resusc Emerg Med 16:4

Kataoka Y, Soma K (2005) Iliac vein injuries in hemodynamically unstable patients with pelvic fracture caused by blunt trauma. J Trauma 58(4):704

Ertel W, Platz A, Trentz O (2000) Incidence and clinical pattern of the ACS after damage control laparotomy in 311 patients with severe abdominal and/or pelvic trauma. Crit Care Med 28(6):1747

Dyer GS, Vrahas MS (2005) Review of the pathophysiology and acute management of haemorrhage in pelvic fracture. Injury 37(7):602–613

Rotondo Mf, Zonies DH (1997) The damage control sequence and underlying logic. Surg Clin N Am 77:761–777

Rosenfeld JV (2004) Damage control neurosurgery. Injury 35:655–666

Abdominal Esophagus and Stomach

41

Clay Cothren Burlew and Ernest E. Moore

41.1 Initial Evaluation in the Trauma Bay

The initial management of seriously injured patients consists of the primary survey, concurrent resuscitation, the secondary survey, diagnostic evaluation, and prioritized definitive care. Although penetrating trauma to the abdominal esophagus and stomach may not be a direct threat to life within the "golden hour," associated thoracic or vascular injuries may result in hemodynamic compromise. Appropriate evaluation of the trauma patient, therefore, begins with the standard "ABCs" (*A*irway with cervical spine protection, *B*reathing, and *C*irculation). Remember that due to its location high in the abdomen, any patient sustaining penetrating trauma to the stomach is at risk for thoracic trauma as well. Therefore, after ensuring a patent and secure airway, you rule should out thoracic injury and ensure adequate oxygenation and ventilation. A combination of physical exam, focused abdominal sonography for trauma (FAST), and chest radiography should determine if the patient has an associated pneumothorax (tension, open, or simple), hemothorax, or cardiac tamponade.

The abdomen is a diagnostic black box. Fortunately, with few exceptions it is not necessary to determine which intra-abdominal organs are injured, only whether an exploratory laparotomy is necessary. As a rule, minimal evaluation is required prior to laparotomy for gunshot or shotgun wounds that penetrate the peritoneal cavity, because over 90% of patients have significant internal injuries. In contrast to GSWs, SWs that penetrate the peritoneal cavity are less likely to injure intra-abdominal organs. You can explore under local anesthesia in the emergency department anterior abdominal SWs (from costal margin to inguinal ligament and bilateral mid-axillary lines) in patients without evidence of shock or peritonitis to determine if the fascia has been violated. Injuries that do not penetrate the peritoneal cavity do not require further evaluation, and the patient is discharged from the ED. You need to further evaluate for intra-abdominal injury in patients with fascial penetration, as there is up to a 50% chance of requiring laparotomy. The optimal diagnostic approach remains debated between serial examination, diagnostic peritoneal lavage (DPL), and CT scanning [1].

Abdominal SWs of three body regions require a different diagnostic approach: thoracoabdominal SWs, right upper quadrant SWs, and back/flank SWs. You should try and rule out occult injury to the diaphragm in patients with SWs to the lower chest, particularly the left side. Remember that patients undergoing DPL evaluation have different laboratory value cut-offs than standard anterior abdominal stab wounds. You should consider a RBC count of more than 10,000/μL as positive, and an indication for laparotomy while patients with a DPL RBC count between 1,000/μL and 10,000/μL should undergo laparoscopy or thoracoscopy. SWs to the RUQ can undergo CT scan to determine trajectory and confinement to the liver for potential non-operative care [2]. SWs to the flank and back should undergo triple-contrast CT to detect occult retroperitoneal injuries of the colon, duodenum, and urinary tract [3].

C.C. Burlew (✉) • E.E. Moore
Department of Surgery, Denver Health Medical Center, University of Colorado School of Medicine, 777 Bannock Street, MC 0206, Denver, CO 80204, USA
e-mail: clay.cothren@dhha.org; ernest.moore@dhha.org

G.C. Velmahos et al. (eds.), *Penetrating Trauma*,
DOI 10.1007/978-3-642-20453-1_41, © Springer-Verlag Berlin Heidelberg 2012

41.2 Abdominal Exploration and Identification of Injuries

Administer antibiotics to all injured patients undergoing an operation. You should determine the type of antibiotic by the anticipated source of contamination in the abdomen or other operative region; additional doses should be administered during the procedure based on blood loss and the half-life of the antibiotic. You may consider extended postoperative antibiotics for patients with significant intraabdominal contamination with delayed recognition. Perform the abdominal exploration in adults using a generous midline incision. For children under the age of 6 years, a transverse incision may be advantageous. The incision is faster with a scalpel compared to an electrosurgical unit; ignore incisional abdominal wall bleeding until you control the intraabdominal sources of hemorrhage. Evacuate liquid and clotted blood promptly with multiple laparotomy pads and suction so that you identify the major source(s) of active bleeding. After localizing the source of hemorrhage, direct digital or vascular clamp occlusion (vascular injury) or laparotomy pad packing (solid organ injury) is used to control bleeding.

Once you control overt hemorrhage, you turn your attention to identifying sources of enteric contamination. The anterior and posterior aspects of the stomach should be inspected, which requires opening the lesser sac and lifting the stomach cephalad for complete visualization. Full decompression of the stomach with a nasogastric tube facilitates mobilization. You should unroof associated hematomas to rule out adjacent bowel injury. If the trajectory of the injury is in the region of the gastroesophageal (GE) junction, one should mobilize the esophagus circumferentially away from the diaphragmatic cruce with care to avoid injury to the vagus nerves. Mobilization of the lateral segment of the left lobe of the liver facilitates exposure of the GE junction. Dividing the short gastric vessels will aid in mobilization of the gastric fundus and prevent iatrogenic injury to the spleen. The serosa of the stomach can be tightly adherent to the splenic capsule of the upper pole; therefore, take care with dissection. The most common missed gastric injury is the posterior wound of a through-and-through penetrating wound. Injuries can also be overlooked if the wound is located within the mesentery of the lesser curvature or high in the posterior fundus. To delineate a questionable injury, you can digitally occlude the stomach at the pylorus while you instill methylene blue–colored saline via the nasogastric tube. Alternatively, you can insufflate the stomach via the nasogastric tube while submerging the stomach in saline; any leakage of air bubbles will identify a missed injury. If the "leaking or bubbling" injury cannot be found, intraoperative endoscopy may be required. Following identification of injuries, the use of damage control techniques versus primary repair of injuries is based upon the patient's intraoperative physiologic status.

41.3 Treatment of Specific Injuries

Gastric injuries can be oversewn with a running single-layer suture line or closed with a TA stapler. Prior to closure, you must be debride devitalized tissue. If you chose a single-layer closure, take full thickness bites with a 2-0 PDS suture to ensure hemostasis from the well-vascularized gastric wall (Fig. 41.1). If the injury is in proximity to the pylorus, be careful not to narrow the channel with your repair. Performing an associated pyloroplasty with transverse repair may be warranted. A tangential injury to the anterior wall of the stomach can be both excised and closed simultaneously with a TA stapler. Using Babcock clamps to approximate the edges of the gastrotomy, place the TA stapler beneath the opening in the gastric wall (Fig. 41.2). You may be able to perform a wedge resection using a GIA stapler for small defects in the body of the stomach (Fig. 41.3). Alternatively, you may need to perform a partial gastrectomy for complex or destructive injuries to the central body or antrum of the stomach (Fig. 41.4a); resections of the body, distal antrum or pylorus may be reconstructed using a Billroth I or II procedure, based upon local anatomy and a tension-free anastomosis technique (Fig. 41.4b). You should add a drainage procedure such as a pyloroplasty in patients with injuries that damage both nerves of Latarjet or vagi.

Gastro-esophageal junction injuries are usually more challenging to repair. For simple anterior stab wound to the abdominal esophagus, you should repair these with a transverse single layer of interrupted PDS sutures. You can then perform either a partial fundoplication to buttress your repair (Fig. 41.5). If the injury is a through and through injury, primary repair may result in a stenotic segment. Consider resecting the injured segment and pulling up the stomach for a

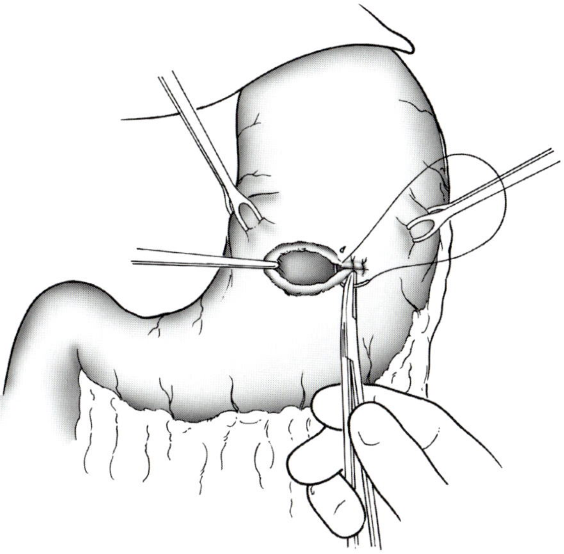

Fig. 41.1 Gastric injuries may be repaired with a running single-layer closure; full thickness bites of the stomach will ensure hemostasis from the well-vascularized gastric wall

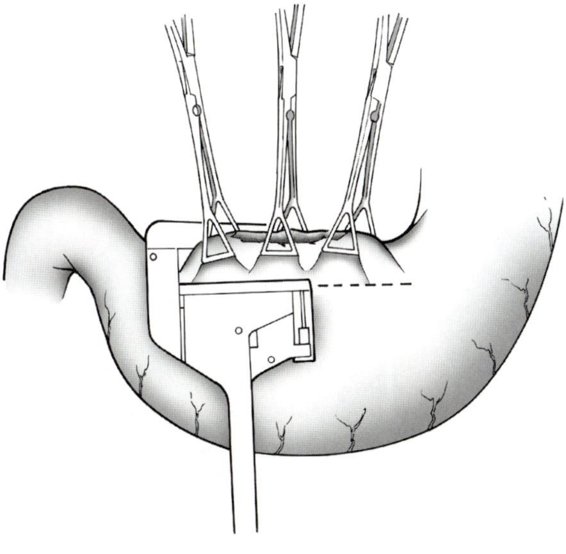

Fig. 41.2 Tangential injuries to the anterior wall of the stomach can be both excised and closed simultaneously with a TA stapler. Babcock clamps are used to approximate the edges of the gastrotomy, placing the TA stapler beneath the opening in the gastric wall

primary end-to-end anastomosis; a wide Kocher maneuver will ensure your anastomosis is tension-free, and performing a pyloroplasty is necessary due to transection of the vagi (Fig. 41.6).

In the multi-system trauma patient, you should consider enteral access via a needle-catheter jejunostomy.

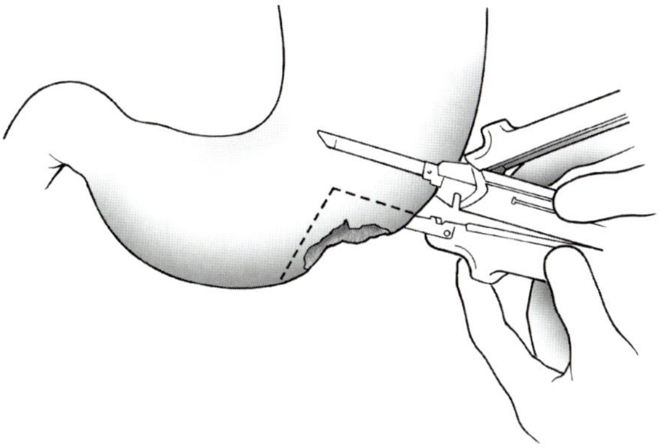

Fig. 41.3 Small defects in the body of the stomach may be repaired by performing a wedge resection using GIA staplers

a

b

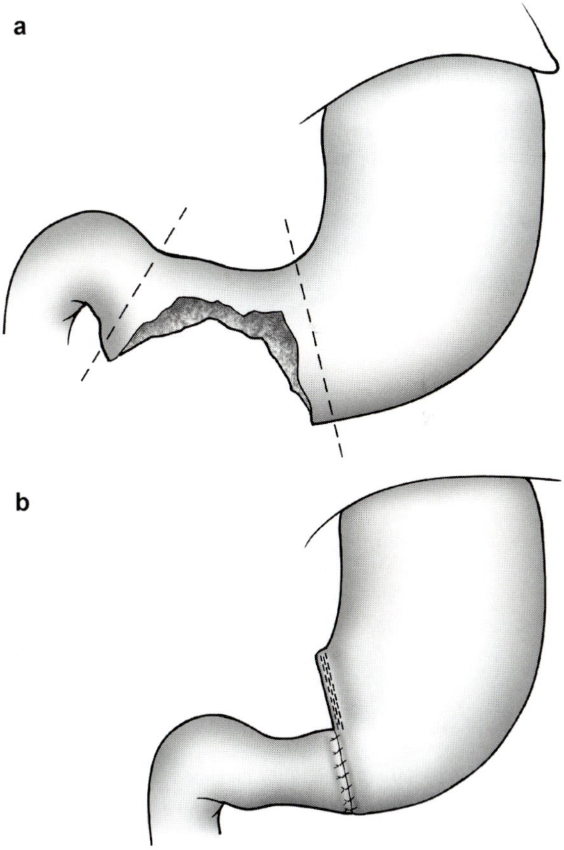

Fig. 41.4 Complex injuries to the central body or antrum of the stomach may require a partial gastrectomy (**a**) with reconstruction using either a Billroth I or II anastomosis (**b**)

Following gastric repair, avoid insertion of a gastrostomy tube as it will likely put tension on the suture/staple line. If abdominal closure is indicated after

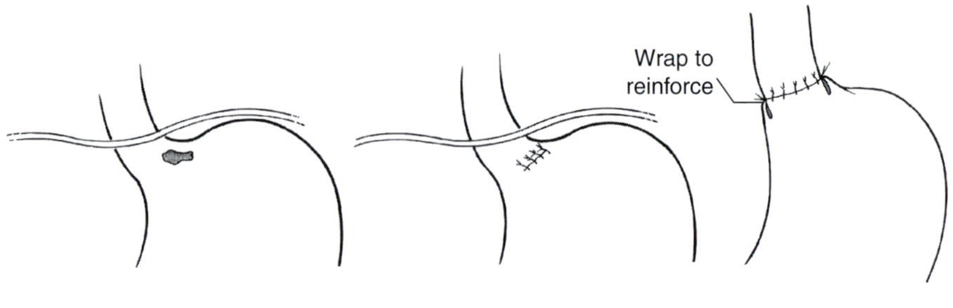

Fig. 41.5 Anterior traumatic gastrotomies may be repaired using a single layer closure followed by a buttressing partial fundoplication

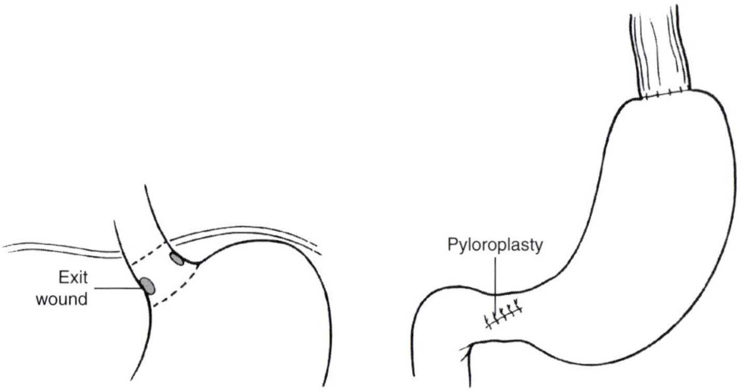

Fig. 41.6 Complex injuries at the gastroesophageal junction often require excision of the injured segment with a primary end-to-end esophagogastrostomy; if the vagus nerves are transected, a pyloroplasty is performed

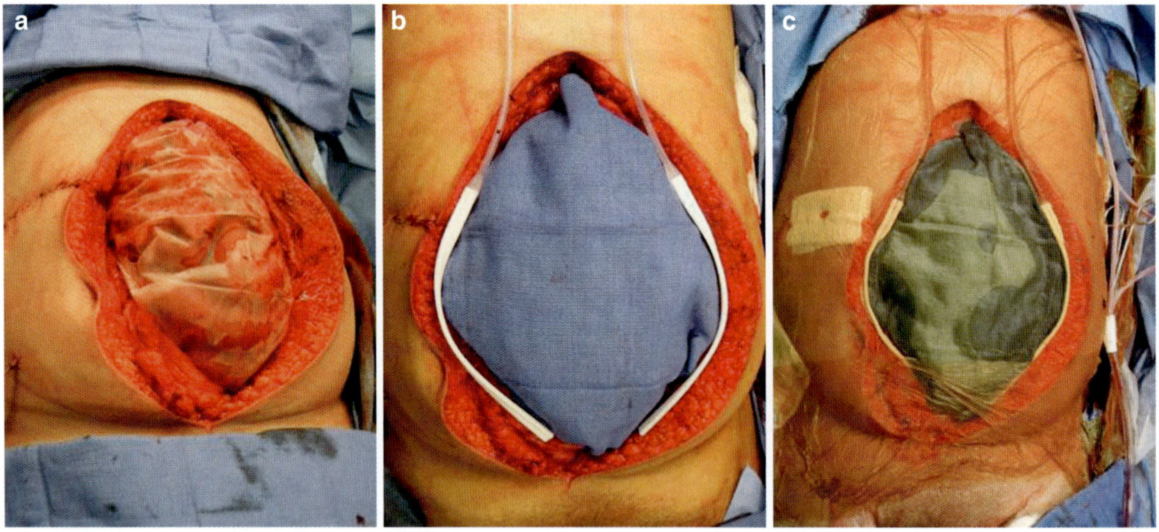

Fig. 41.7 Temporary closure of the abdomen is attained by covering the viscera with a fenestrated, subfascial 1,010 steri-drape (**a**). Two Jackson-Pratt drains are placed along the fascial edges (**b**). The steri-drape and drains are covered using an ioban, allowing closed suction to control reperfusion-related ascitic fluid egress while providing adequate space for bowel expansion (**c**)

addressing the patient's injuries, irrigate the abdomen with warm saline and close the midline fascia with a running heavy suture. Close the skin selectively based upon the amount of intraabdominal contamination.

Damage control surgery techniques should be considered in any patient with a temperature <35°C, arterial pH < 7.2, base deficit < 15 mmol/L (or <6 mmol/L in patients over 55 years of age), and INR or PTT > 50% of normal [4]. The goal of damage control surgery is to control surgical bleeding and limit gastrointestinal spillage. The operative techniques employed are temporary measures, with definitive repair of injuries delayed until the patient is physiologically replete. Gastric lacerations can be controlled with a rapid whipstitch of 2-0 prolene. Segmental damage to the stomach is controlled using a GIA stapler, with resection of the injured segment, leaving the proximal and distal ends of the stomach in discontinuity.

Before returning to the SICU, close the abdomen temporarily. Currently, ioban closure of the abdomen is performed for temporary closure (Fig. 41.7a, b, c). In this technique, the bowel is covered with a fenestrated subfascial 1010 steri-drape (3M Health Care, St. Paul, MN) and 2 Jackson-Pratt drains are placed along the fascial edges; this is then covered using an ioban, allowing closed suction to control reperfusion-related ascitic fluid egress while providing adequate space for bowel expansion to prevent ACS. Return to the OR in 12–24 h for definitive repair of injuries is planned, once the patient's physiology is restored, including normothermia, normalization of coagulation studies, and correction of metabolic acidosis.

41.4 Postoperative Care

Following repair of gastrointestinal injuries, there is an obligatory postoperative ileus. Return of bowel function is noted by a decrease in nasogastric tube output. Although early enteral nutrition is the goal, due to its impact in reducing septic complications [5], you should be wary if the patient has sustained hemorrhagic shock. Evidence of bowel function should be established prior to advancing to goal tube feeds. Overzealous jejunal feeding can lead to small bowel necrosis in the patient recovering from profound shock. While there is some reluctance to initiate TEN in patients with an open abdomen, tube feeding, by any route, may be started within 24 h of abdominal closure, as over 90% of patients will tolerate TEN. Moreover, in patients relegated to an open abdomen, TEN is frequently tolerated at low volumes, i.e. trophic tube feeds (25 cc/h) while actively attempting to close fascia.

In general, wounds sustained from trauma should be examined daily for progression of healing and signs of infection. Complex soft tissue wounds of the abdomen, such as shotgun wounds, may be difficult to manage. Following initial debridement of devitalized tissue, wound care includes wet to dry dressing changes twice daily, or application of the wound VAC. Repeated operative debridement may be necessary, and early involvement of the Reconstructive Surgery service for possible flap coverage is advised. Midline laparotomy wounds are inspected 48-h postoperatively by removing the sterile surgical dressing. If an ileostomy or colostomy was required, one should inspect it daily to ensure it is viable. If your patient develops high-grade fevers, inspect wounds sooner to exclude an early necrotizing infection. If you identify a wound infection – evidenced by erythema, pain along the wound, or purulent drainage – open the wound widely by removing skin staples. After ensuring the midline fascia is intact with digital palpation, the wound is initially managed with wet-to-dry dressing changes. The most common intraabdominal complications are anastomotic failure and abscess. Percutaneous versus operative therapy will be based on the location, timing, and extent of the collection.

Important Points

- Evaluation of the trauma patient begins with the standard "ABCs" (*A*irway with cervical spine protection, *B*reathing, and *C*irculation).
- After localizing the source of hemorrhage, direct digital or vascular clamp occlusion (vascular injury) or laparotomy pad packing (solid organ injury) are used to control bleeding.
- Bowel wall associated hematomas should be unroofed to rule out adjacent enteric injury.
- The most common missed gastric injury is the posterior wound of a through-and-through penetrating wound. To fully evaluate the stomach for injuries, the lesser sac should be opened and the stomach lifted cephalad for complete visualization.
- To delineate a questionable injury, the stomach can be digitally occluded at the pylorus while methylene blue–colored saline is instilled via the nasogastric tube. Alternatively, you can insufflate the stomach via the nasogastric tube while submerging the stomach in saline; any leakage of air bubbles will identify a missed injury.
- If a gastric injury is suspected but cannot be found, intraoperative endoscopy should be employed.
- Prior to repair of a gastric injury, devitalized tissue must be debrided.
- Gastric repair should not narrow the pyloric channel; performing a pyloroplasty with transverse repair may be indicated.

- If a penetrating injury damages both nerves of Latarjet or vagi, a drainage procedure such as a pyloroplasty should be added to your primary procedure.
- Damage control surgery techniques should be considered in any patient with a temperature <35°C, arterial pH < 7.2, base deficit >15mmol/L (or >6 mmol/L in patients over 55 years of age), and INR or PTT > 50% of normal.

References

1. Biffl WL, Kaups KL, Cothren CC et al (2009) Management of patients with anterior abdominal stab wounds; a western trauma association multicenter trial. J Trauma 66:1294
2. Demetriades D, Hadjizacharia P, Constantinou C et al (2006) Selective nonoperative management of penetrating abdominal solid organ injuries. Ann Surg 244:620
3. Boyle EM Jr, Maier RV, Salazar JD et al (1997) Diagnosis of injuries after stab wounds to the back and flank. J Trauma 42:260
4. Moore EE (1996) Staged laparotomy for the hypothermia, acidosis, and coagulopathy syndrome. Am J Surg 172:405
5. Todd SR, Kozar RA, Moore FA (2006) Nutrition support in adult trauma patients. Nutr Clin Pract 21:421

42 Duodenum

George C. Velmahos

The management of duodenal trauma remains challenging not only because of the organ's close anatomic relationship with vascular structures and other organs but also because of its retroperitoneal location which may mask the initial symptoms and cause delays in diagnosis with dire consequences. The grading of the duodenal injuries has been developed by the American Association for the Surgery of Trauma and provides a straightforward way to communicate the severity of injury and plan the operation. A simplified version is shown in Table 42.1.

42.1 General Rules of Operative Strategy

You should always use a midline laparotomy to approach duodenal injuries. Other incisions usually compromise the ability to explore the rest of the abdominal cavity adequately and are more time-consuming to open and close. There are two extremely important issues to which you should pay attention at the beginning of the operation:

(a) *Mobilize the duodenum fully by a Kocher maneuver* (Fig. 42.1). The duodenum must be brought at the surface of the abdominal wound. Avoid working in the depths of the abdominal cavity. For non-trauma operations, the Kocher maneuver is typically limited to the C-loop of the duodenum. I strongly discourage this. Because it is rare that only the duodenum is injured and because adjacent structures are involved and need exploration, you should mobilize the right colon and the duodenum widely toward the midline. Incise the peritoneum at the ileocecal junction and carry the incision with scissors lateral to the cecum and descending colon along the white line of Toldt. Use your fingers to create tissue planes as you incise the soft tissues layer by layer and gently retract the colon medially. Stay away from the mesocolic vessels to avoid inadvertent bleeding and interruption of blood supply to the colon. Navigate laterally around the hepatic flexure and mobilize it similarly toward the midline. At this point you have the entire colon elevated from the duodenum, which is lying attached to the retroperitoneal space. Incise the peritoneum around the lateral surface of the duodenal C-loop and gently mobilize the duodenum (with the attached pancreatic head) toward the midline too. Your Kocher maneuver should be wide and include the entire duodenum from its first to its fourth portion. The duodenum and pancreatic head should be easily inspected anteriorly (Fig. 42.2a) and posteriorly (Fig. 42.2b). The inferior vena cava lying posteriorly and slightly laterally to the second portion of the duodenum should also be inspected for hematomas. There is no need to sceletonize it, if no hematoma exists.

G.C. Velmahos
Harvard University Medical School,
Massachusetts General Hospital,
Division of Trauma, Emergency Surgery
and Surgical Critical Care,
165 Cambridge Street, Suite 810, Boston, MA 02114, USA
e-mail: gvelmahos@partners.org

G.C. Velmahos et al. (eds.), *Penetrating Trauma*,
DOI 10.1007/978-3-642-20453-1_42, © Springer-Verlag Berlin Heidelberg 2012

Table 42.1 Duodenal injury grading (modified from the original version and simplified)

Grade	Description
I	Hematoma of one portion or partial thickness laceration
II	Hematoma of more than one portions or laceration <50% of circumference
III	Laceration 50–75% of circumference
IV	Laceration >75% of circumference or involving ampulla
V	Massive destruction of pancreatoduodenal complex

Similarly, the portal triad can be inspected for hematomas – although again not necessarily requiring full dissection in the absence of suspicion for injury. Only if the duodenum is mobilized in this extensive fashion you will be sure to never miss an injury and have the ability to fix it comfortably if one is present.

(b) *Control temporarily the DI but explore the entire abdominal cavity before performing a permanent repair*. Although an atraumatic clamp or quick suture can be temporarily placed to control contamination from the duodenal perforation, the definitive operation should not be planned before the abdomen is fully explored. It is in this way that the decision is made to proceed to a long operation versus abbreviating the procedure along damage control principles. The extent of the duodenal injuries, presence and severity of other injuries, and the physiologic condition of the patient will dictate the ultimate intraoperative plan.

42.2 Grade-Specific Operative Management

42.2.1 Grade I

The majority of these injuries are managed non-operatively with success. Duodenal hematomas have been reported with a higher frequency among pediatric

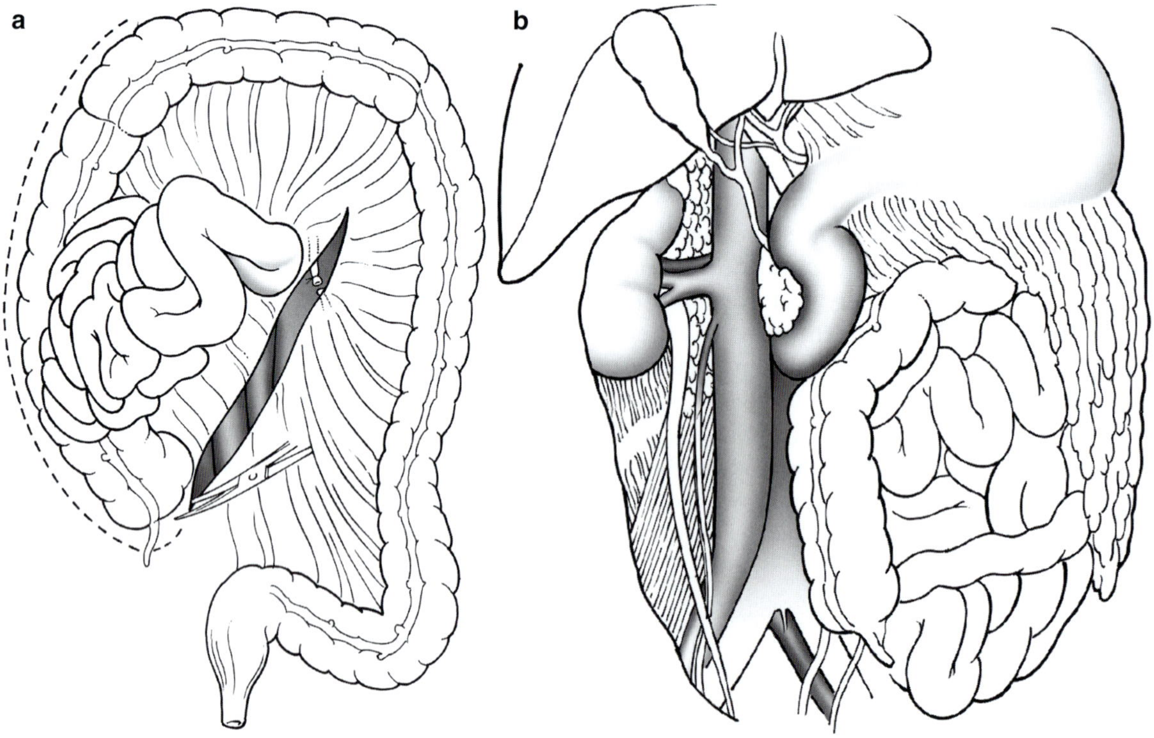

Fig. 42.1 (**a**) Extended Kocher maneuver. Note that the peritoneal incision starts at the distal ileum and the entire right colon is reflected medially. (**b**) The duodenum is fully mobilized, making it possible to inspect the pancreas, IVC, and retroperitoneal space

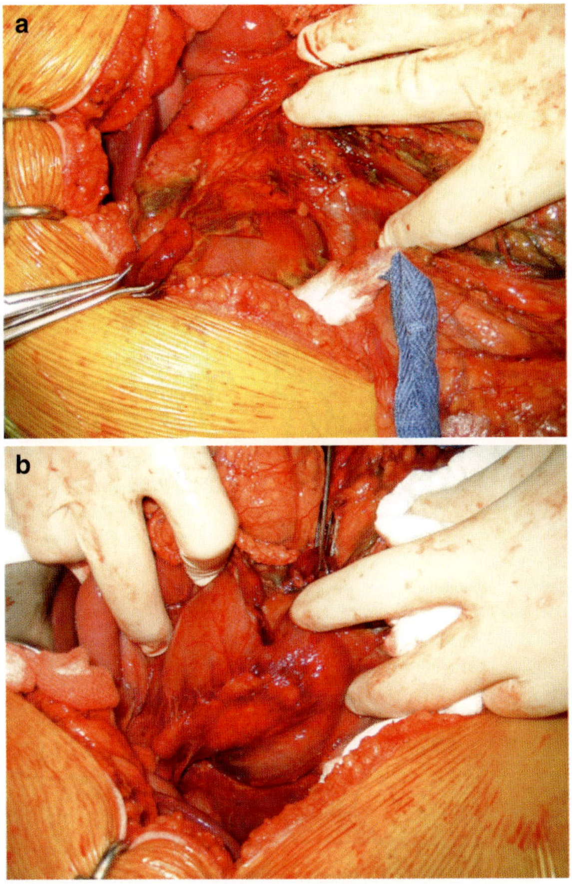

Fig. 42.2 (**a**) Full mobilization of the duodenum revealing the anterior surface of the head of the pancreas. Note the clamp that closes the laceration temporarily to control contamination. (**b**) The posterior surface of the duodenum and head of the pancreas are also easily inspected after the Kocher mobilization

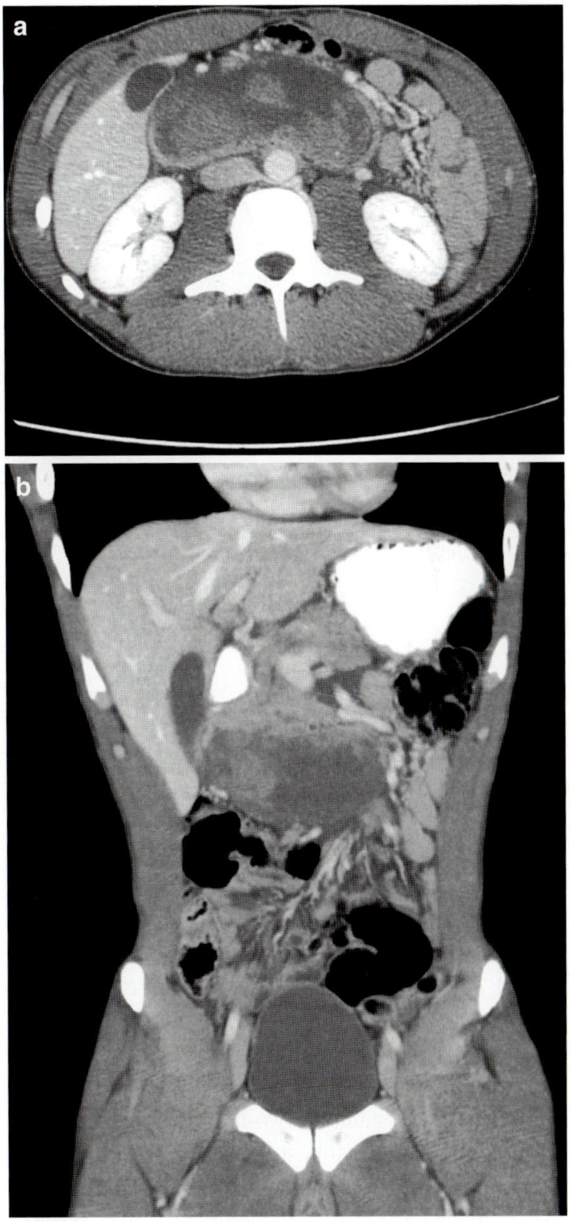

Fig. 42.3 (**a**, **b**) Axial and coronal cut of a massive duodenal hematoma. Despite its size the patient had no complaints except mild epigastric pain and gastric outlet obstruction. He was managed non-operatively with nasogastric tube drainage and the obstruction eventually resolved on post-trauma day 23

than adult patients. They are usually discovered on CT scan and on occasions are totally obstructing the lumen. The majority of them are absorbed with time and the lumen reopens. Two issues need to be clarified when a grade I injury is detected: (a) Is it indeed only a hematoma or is the hematoma covering a full-thickness laceration? A careful inspection of the CT scan for extraluminal air or oral contrast resolves the dilemma in most patients evaluated by new-generation scanners (16- or 64- slice). If not, a formal contrast swallow will show whether the contrast remains within the duodenal contour or leaks extraluminally. (b) How long should one wait before decompressing a totally occluding hematoma? There is no clear answer to this question. Most hematomas will be absorbed -at least partially- within 7–10 days and the patency of the bowel lumen will be restored. I certainly consider it acceptable to wait up to 15 days with a nasogastric tube in place before surgical decompression is considered and have personally waited for 23 days before a massive hematoma was reabsorbed and the lumen became patent again (Fig. 42.3).

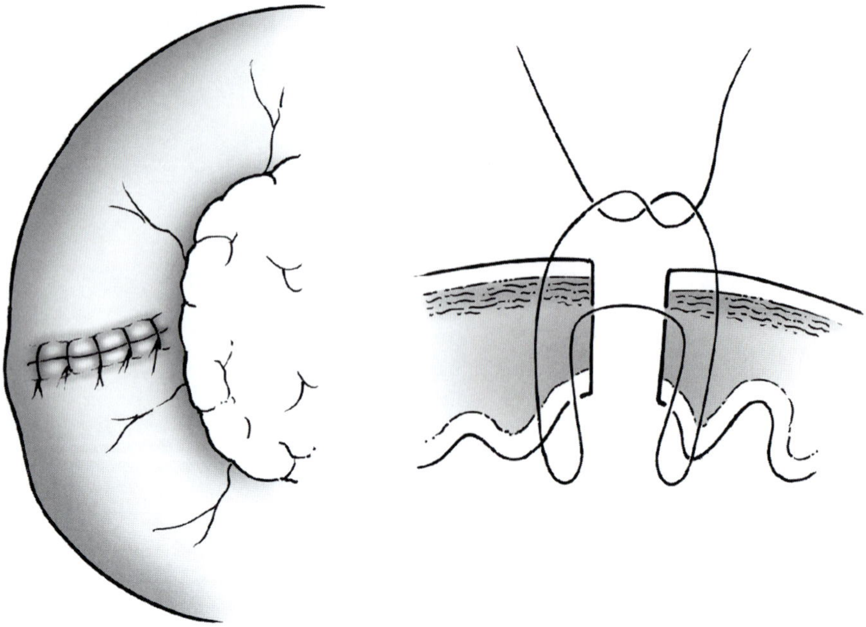

Fig. 42.4 Closure of simple duodenal laceration (after debridement of the edges) with a Gambee suture

42.2.2 Grade II

Such injuries are produced either by very large hematomas or – more frequently – by simple lacerations of the duodenum that occupy less than 50% of the circumference. The management of hematomas is not different than what was described previously. Duodenal lacerations are sutured primarily. Debridement of the rugged edges is important to make sure that well-vascularized tissue is present. Then, close the perforation in one layer with interrupted invaginating Gambee stitches (Fig. 42.4) using a 3-0 non-absorbable or slowly absorbable suture. A two-layer closure – typically with a running absorbably suture and a second layer of interrupted non-absorbable sutures – is also acceptable, although I typically use only one layer only in repairing any part of the intestine. It is important that the line of closure is perpendicular to the axis of the lumen in order to avoid stenosis. Drain the area per routine. No other procedures are necessary.

42.2.3 Grades III and IV

There is a debate about the correct management of grade III injuries which lie in between grades I and II, managed either nonoperatively or with simple repair, and grades IV and V, managed usually with more complex techniques. These techniques include pyloric exclusion, serosal patch, duodeno-jejunal anastomosis, and resection with anastomosis.

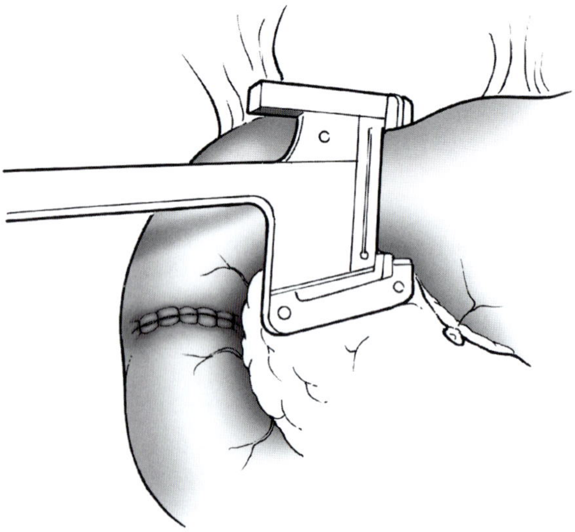

Fig. 42.5 Exclusion of the pylorus by firing a TA stapler at the pyloric ring

Pyloric exclusion aims to divert all supra-duodenal secretions from the repair, not only to prevent distention by the volume of fluids, but also to avoid activation of pancreatic enzymes by gastric contents. Before pyloric exclusion, the duodenal laceration must be sutured, per the techniques described above. Then, exclude the pylorus by either firing a TA stapler at this level (Fig. 42.5) or opening the stomach at the antrum

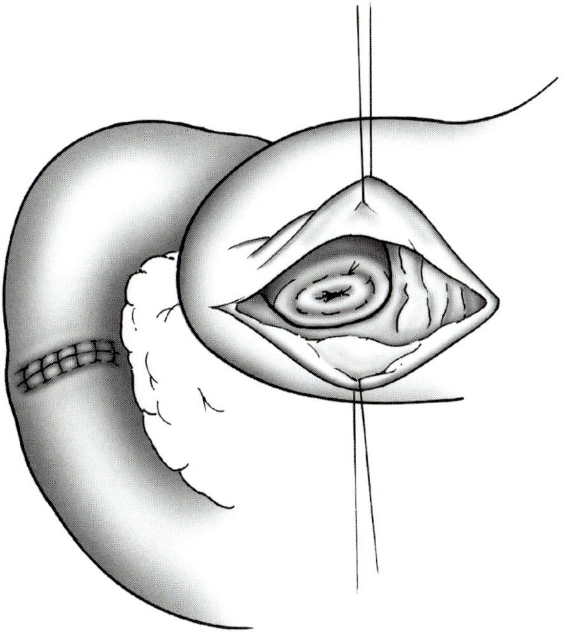

Fig. 42.6 Exclusion of the pylorus by making a gastrotomy in the near vicinity and placing a suture at the pyloric ring level

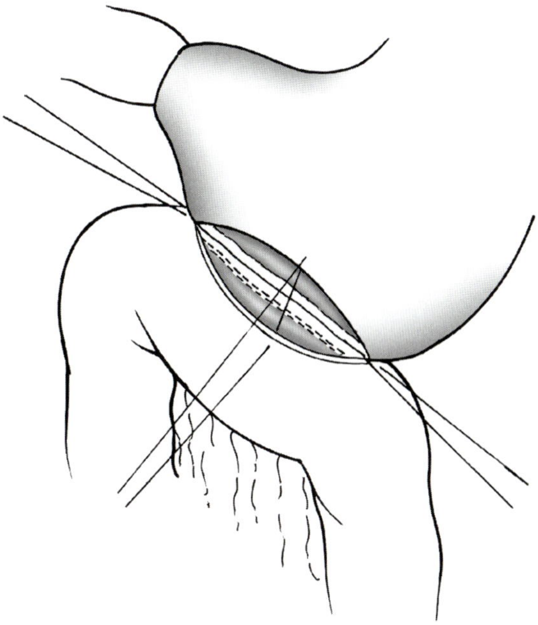

Fig. 42.7 Standard gastro-jejunal anastomosis (preferably retrocolic) by using the gastrotomy site of the pyloric exclusion

and suturing the pylorus from the inside (Fig. 42.6). The gastrotomy should be placed at the most dependent position of the stomach in order to serve as the site of the gastrojejunostomy. Through the gastrotomy, grasp the pylorus with an atraumatic clamp to bring it close to the gastrotomy. Then, place either a pursestring or an interlocking running suture using non-absorbable or slowly absorbable material. It has been suggested that non-absorbable sutures are allowed because the pyloric exclusion almost always opens with time under the continuous peristaltic force of the stomach. In any case, leave a long tail on your suture, so that it can be identified, grasped, and cut via gastroscopy, if this is deemed appropriate in the future. Following the pyloric exclusion, a jejunal loop is brought at the gastrotomy site to function as the new gastric outlet (Fig. 42.7). A retrocolic gastrojejunostomy is performed per routine (Fig. 42.8).

In large injuries of the duodenum, primary closure of the defect may be undesirable because it produces stenosis or places the suture line under great tension. In this situation, the defect can be sealed by bringing a loop of jejunum and suturing its serosal surface on the debrided duodenal wound (Fig. 42.9). This is commonly referred to as a Thal patch. A second circumferential line of interrupted seromuscular sutures

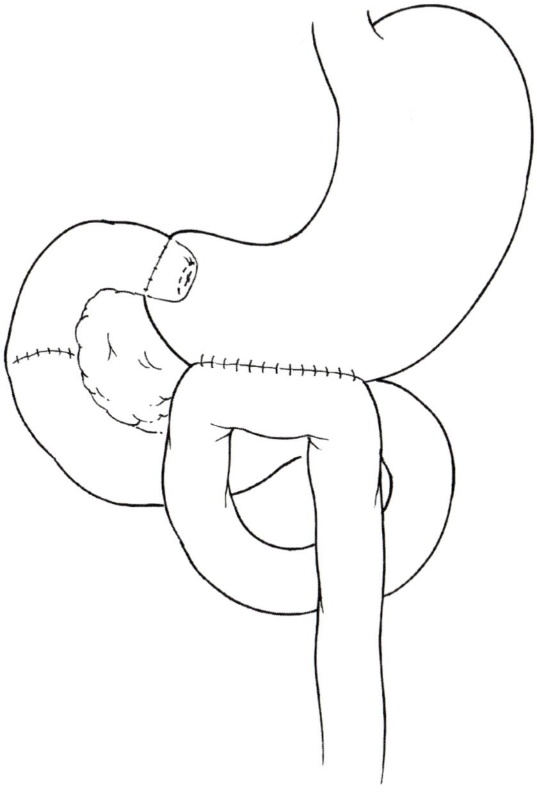

Fig. 42.8 Completed pyloric exclusion with gastro-jejunal anastomosis

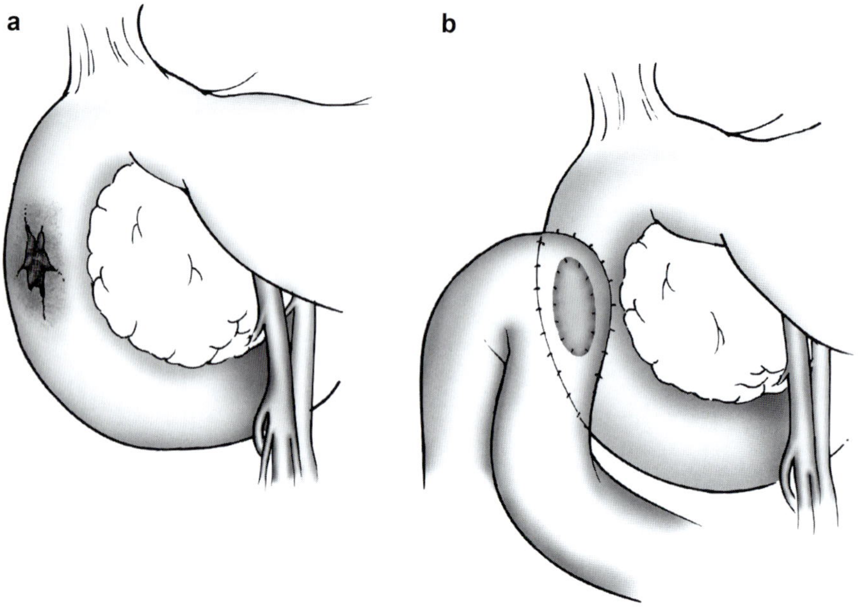

Fig. 42.9 Serosal patch on large duodenal perforation by suturing a loop of uninvolved bowel to the edges of the laceration

is placed between the jejunum and duodenum all around the first line of repair in order to diminish the tension at the first suture line and prevent leaks.

On occasions, even a Thal patch may produce stenosis at the injury level. Under these circumstances a loop of jejunum may be brought and opened to create a side-to-side Roux-en-Y duodeno-jejunal anastomosis (Fig. 42.10). Finally, for extensive injuries of the fourth or even the third portion of the duodenum, resection and primary end-to-end anastomosis is possible (Fig. 42.11). This is easier done at the fourth portion which is more mobile after dissection of the ligament of Treitz. It becomes more challenging in the third portion, as adequate mobilization of the medial portion of the duodenum to provide a tissue margin for anastomosis can be hard. The duodenum is attached to the pancreas and dissection of its medial side requires ligation of small vessels, which may compromise the blood supply to the anastomotic line. The feasibility of resection and a safe anastomosis clearly relies on careful intra-operative assessment of the anatomical conditions and the proximal extent of the injury.

When a complex repair is necessary, strongly consider adding a pyloric exclusion to offer extra protection at the injury repair suture line. Also, consider a feeding jejunostomy, as the complication rate is

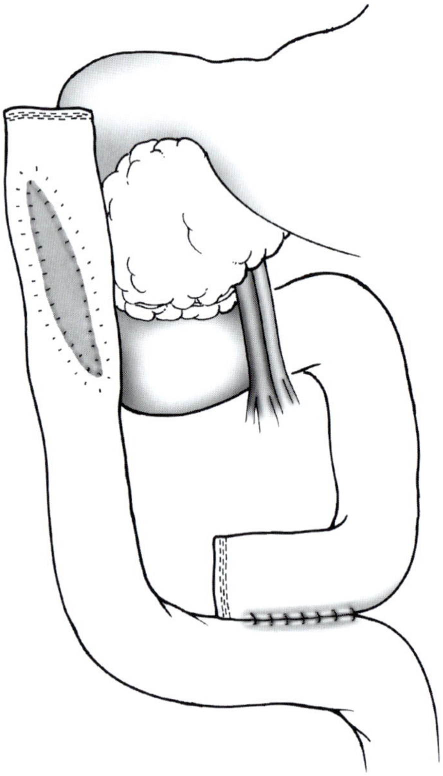

Fig. 42.10 Duodeno-jejunal anastomosis to treat a large perforation of the duodenum, which would produce stenosis of the lumen if closed primarily

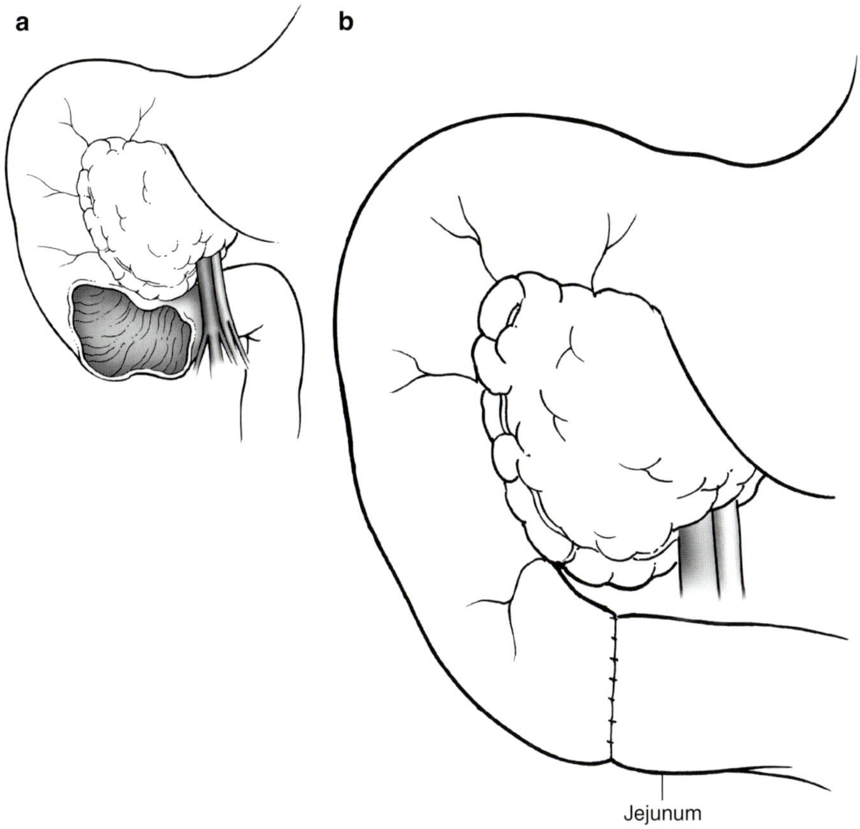

Fig. 42.11 Resection and primary anastomosis of the third/fourth part of the duodenum. This technique is not performed for proximal duodenal injuries

substantial and enteral feeding may not be possible if not directed distally to the repair.

In desperate situations the duodenal injury is so large that it simply cannot be repaired. Then, a pacreatoduodenectomy (Whipple procedure) may be appropriate and will be discussed below. If the patient is not stable for such an extensive procedure, the insertion of a large-bore mushroom-tipped tube in the duodenal lumen and closure around the tube with a pursestring may be the only remaining choice, even if far from optimal (Fig. 42.12). The tube is brought out through the skin to create a directed lateral duodenal fistula. Drains should be placed around the area, as the leak rate after this procedure is high.

As mentioned, there are no clear guidelines about using simple repair or complex techniques. It has been shown that as the grade of injury increases, complex techniques should be used more liberally to prevent complications. I tend to manage the majority of grade III injuries with a simple repair, whereas grade IV injuries usually require complex techniques.

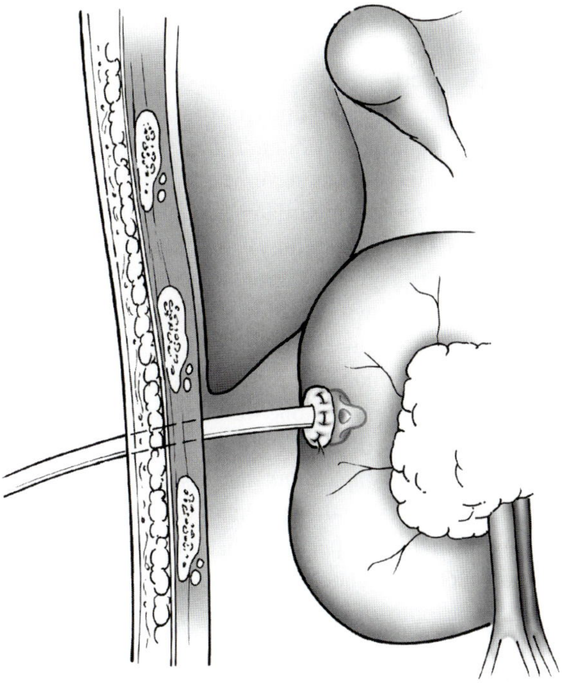

Fig. 42.12 Directed duodeno-cutaneous fistula by insertion of large tube into duodenal perforation

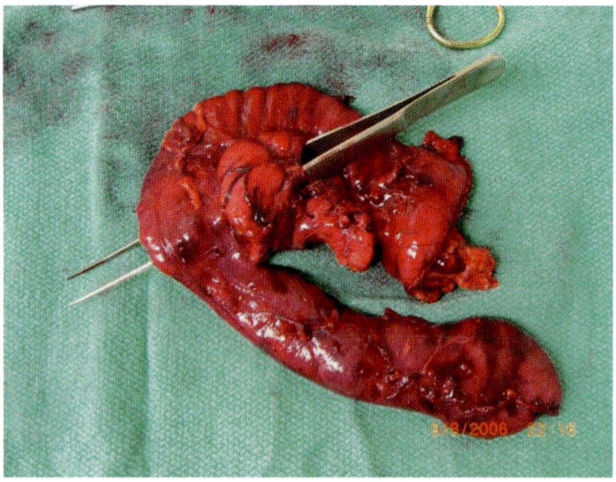

Fig. 42.13 Gunshot wound injury through the head of the pancreas and pancreatoduodenectomy specimen

42.2.4 Grade V

These are the worst possible injuries as they involve the pancreas and quite frequently other peripancreatic vessels and structures. The surgical strategy for this type of injuries obeys in the rule of "all or nothing". If the patient's intra-operative hemodynamic condition allows and in the presence of violation of the ampulla or the major pancreatic duct, a formal pancreatoduodenectomy may be necessary. This is the "all" approach. Start, as always, with the wide Kocher maneuver. Identify the injury of the major pancreatic duct and/or ampulla of Vater. This is not always easy. A variety of techniques have been described, including cannulating the ampulla or cannulating the cystic duct (after cholecystectomy) and injecting contast. The sensitivity and specificity of these techniques are completely unknown. I believe that they are not much better than a careful dissection and inspection of the structures. If in doubt, err toward doing less. If not in doubt about injury to one of the abovementioned structures, proceed! Divide the antrum and proximal jejunum with a stapler and the distal common bile duct sharply. Elevate the specimen off the retroperitoneum and divide the pancreas distal to the injury, saving as much pancreatic mass as possible (Fig. 42.13). Three anastomoses follow, including the pancreato-jejunal, biliary-jejunal, and gastro-jejunal suture lines (Fig. 42.14). Numerous techniques have been described for each one of these anastomoses, and the detailed description of these techniques goes beyond the scope of the chapter. I prefer a telescoping two-layered pancreato-jejunal anastomosis, a one-layered biliary-jejunal anastomosis after "fish-mouthing" the usually narrow common bile duct (no stents are placed in the anastomosis), and a standard gastro-jejunal anastomosis.

On the other hand, a hemodynamically unstable patient should never have a Whipple procedure. Instead, one should have an abbreviated damage-control operation. This I call the "nothing" approach only to contrast it with the time-consuming pancreatoduodenectomy but with no intent to minimize its life-saving potential. Such a patient should have only temporary closure of all the perforations and ligation or shunting of the major bleeding sites. Then, the patient should be packed and returned with an open abdomen to the Intensive Care Unit for resuscitation. The definitive repairs can be done in follow-up procedures, as described above.

42.3 Conclusions

DI are rather infrequent injuries which may prove to be particularly challenging in terms of intra-operative selection of the correct procedure according to the extent of the injury and the patient's hemodynamic status. The existing evidence does not elevate above Level III and, therefore, universally accepted guidelines are hard to find. In general, the following recommendations can be considered, even if not applicable to all patients:

1. Grade I injuries are almost always managed non-operatively. Be patient if there is obstruction from a hematoma. Most will open up with time and nasogastric tube decompression.
2. Grade II injuries are almost always managed by simple repair. Debride the edges of the wound and close it primarily.
3. Grades III and IV injuries require careful intra-operative evaluation. Most grade III injuries are amenable to simple repair. Most grade IV injuries require a more complex procedure, which usually is a pyloric exclusion.
4. Grade V injuries fall under the "all or nothing" rule. You will either need to do a Whipple procedure after suspecting major pancreatic duct injury on a

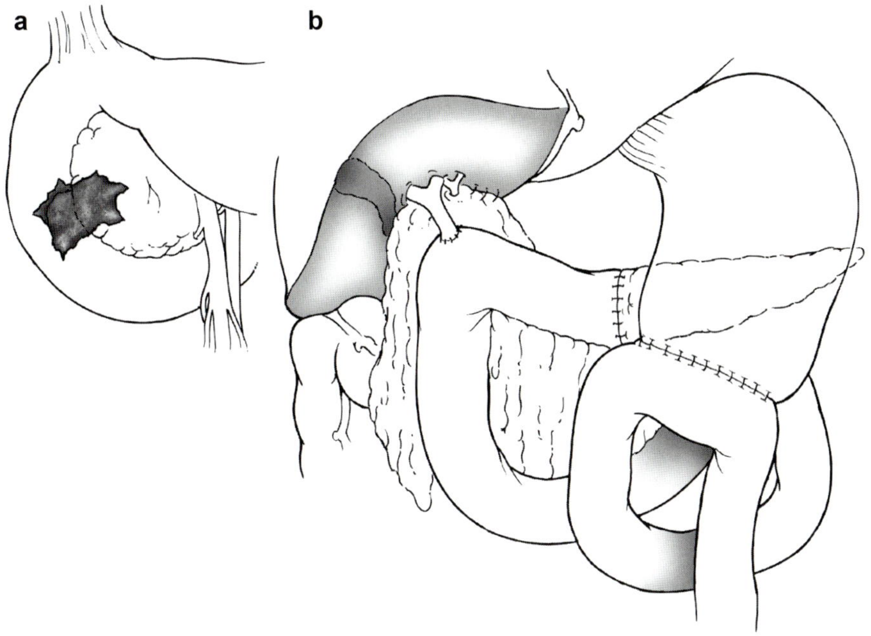

Fig. 42.14 Pancreatoduodenectomy

hemodynamically stable patient or a damage-control procedure on an unstable patient. If in doubt, prefer to do the minimal required. You can then re-evaluate the patient under more controlled conditions and offer the definitive operation at a later stage.

Important Points

1. The majority of duodenal injuries can be sufficiently managed by primary repair only
2. Always put drains at the area of repair
3. Concommittant injury to the head of the pancreas increases morbidity and mortality
4. Pyloric exclusion can be considered in high grade injuries
5. Grade V duodenal injuries usually require damage control or pancreatoduodenectomy or both

Recommended Reading

Degiannis E, Krawczykowski D, Velmahos GC, Levy RD, Souter I, Saadia R (1993) Pyloric exclusion in severe penetrating injuries of the duodenum. World J Surg 17(6):751–4

Degiannis E, Boffard K (2000) Duodenal injuries. Br J Surg 87(11):1473–9

Velmahos GC, Kamel E, Chan LS, Hanpeter D, Asensio JA, Murray JA, Berne TV, Demetriades D (1999) Complex repair for the management of duodenal injuries. Am Surg 65(10): 972–5

Seamon MJ, Pieri PG, Fisher CA, Gaughan J, Santora TA, Pathak AS, Bradley KM, Goldberg AJ (2007) A 10-year retrospective review: does pyloric exclusion improve outcome after penetrating duodenal and combined pancreatoduodenal injuries? J Trauma 62(4):829–33

Lopez PP, Benjamin R, Cockburn M, Amortegui JD, Schulman CI, Soffer D, Blackbourne L, Habib F, Jerokhimov I, Trankel S, Cohn SM (2005) Recent trends in the management of combined pancreatoduodenal injuries. Am Surg 71(10): 847–52

Penetrating Trauma to the Pancreas

43

Martin D. Smith and Elias Degiannis

The pancreas is likened to the base player in a band; no one ever knows the name of the base player but when he is not there the band falls terribly flat. This rather innocuous gland situated posteriorly in the retroperitoneum is only really taken seriously when it gives trouble and when it gives trouble it requires experience and a good knowledge of anatomy and surgical techniques to solve the problems. Penetrating trauma to the pancreas is not very common. Due to its anatomical location and relationship to major vessels, isolated injury to the pancreas is even more rare and it is usually the associated injuries, often aggravated by the consequences of the pancreatic injury, that result in the fairly high morbidity and mortality associated with pancreatic trauma [1, 2].

Blunt pancreatic trauma is more often isolated and due to the often insidious nature of the clinical picture is difficult to diagnose. Much has been written about the role of biochemical markers and imaging studies to diagnose pancreatic trauma in the absence of an acute abdomen or in the hemodynamically unstable patient. In penetrating trauma, the diagnosis is often only made intra-operatively and it is therefore very important to recognize the subtle intra-operative findings.

Identification often requires extensive mobilization of the pancreas but in general the management requires less aggressive surgery. There are two guiding principles; identify the extent of the parenchymal injury and secondly the injury to the pancreatic duct needs to be identified and quantified.

The general rules that apply to the management of penetrating trauma to the abdomen apply. Full resuscitation including the primary and secondary survey is followed and the decision to proceed to surgery is based on the accepted criteria and protocols. In essence there are those patients who remain unstable who require urgent transport to the OR. In the stable patient with an acute abdomen, they require surgery and should be fully resuscitated and taken to the OR. The patient who has limited abdominal signs should be investigated further and observed as per accepted protocols.

Once in theater a midline laparotomy is performed and again the usual guidelines as to how to manage penetrating trauma to the abdomen is followed. Often following the tract of the bullet or knife may indicate an injury to the pancreas. This is not always the case and as such certain features may suggest the presence of a pancreatic injury. Bile staining in the retroperitoneum, midline hematoma around the "c" loop of the duodenum can indicate a vascular injury to the IVC or aorta but can also suggest a pancreatic injury. Saponification of fat in the upper abdomen may be present in those cases when there has been a delay in getting the patient to the OR.

If a pancreatic injury is suspected, the next thing to establish is the site of the injury. To do this the pancreas should be fully exposed depending on the site. The body

M.D. Smith
Department of Surgery, Chris Hani Baragwanath Hospital, University of the Witwatersrand, Johannesburg, South Africa

Hepatopancreaticobilary Unit, Chris Hani Baragwanath Hospital, University of the Witwatersrand, Johannesburg, South Africa
e-mail: martin.smith@wits.ac.za

E. Degiannis (✉)
University of the Witwatersrand Medical School, Chris Hani Baragwanath Academic Hospital, Trauma Directorate, 7 York Road, Parktown, 2193 Johannesburg, South Africa (RSA)
e-mail: degiannis@yebo.co.za

G.C. Velmahos et al. (eds.), *Penetrating Trauma*,
DOI 10.1007/978-3-642-20453-1_43, © Springer-Verlag Berlin Heidelberg 2012

and tail are exposed by dividing the gastrocolic omentum. Identify an appropriate site through which to enter the lesser sac, this is often done for you by the bullet of knife. Open the lesser sac as far to the left as possible staying outside the gastroepiploic vascular arcade. If the injury is far laterally you may need to divide the inferior couple of short gastric vessels. Be careful not to tear the insertion of the spleno-colic attachments because this can cause irritating bleeding to the spleen and on some occasions may even require a splenectomy to control the bleeding. If the injury is more medial, then the lesser sac will need to be opened onto the head of the pancreas. In patients with significant amounts of intraperitoneal fat and a short thickened transverse mesocolon, this can be somewhat difficult because as the middle colic vein enters the superior mesenteric vein this can be avulsed by too vigorous traction on the transverse colon. In addition, the right gastrocolic vein passed inferiorly and posteriorly to enter the Superior Mesenteric vein at the same point, and as you try to expose the head of the pancreas you can also damage this vein causing unnecessary bleeding and aggravation.

Exposure of the head of the pancreas requires kocherization of the head of the pancreas. Retract the inferior surface of the liver superiorly, retract the transverse colon including the hepatic flexure inferiorly. Your assistant should place his/her hand over the head of the pancreas and second part of the duodenum and retract the head toward the left. The role of the assistance retracting the duodenum to the left cannot be underestimated, because it is this maneuver that exposes the correct dissection plane. This maneuver exposes the lateral aspect of the retroperitoneal portion of the duodenum. Incise the peritoneal reflection being careful not to damage the serosa of the duodenum. The IVC is identified posterior to this plane. Using a combination of blunt and sharp dissection, I use the diathermy knife to achieve this dissection, the duodenum is freed to the left until the aorta is identified. There is a vein that runs inferiorly to the right of the IVC that is easily torn in this maneuver. The duodenum is freed from the retroperitoneum as far superiorly as the foramen of Winslow that identifies the tunnel that passes behind the portal triad. Inferiorly the duodenum is mobilized distally by carefully identifying the tissue that holds the transverse mesocolon and the lateral aspect of the junction between the second and third parts of the duodenum. This plane is identified by the surgeon holding the head of the pancreas and duodenum in his left hand while the assistant holds the transverse colon and mesentery upward and into the incision. Dividing this tissue opens up the head of the pancreas and mobilizes the uncinate process up to the right lateral edge of the superior mesenteric vein. Be prepared to mobiles the head of the pancreas as far medially as the aorta. At this point the head of the pancreas is easily examined both anteriorly and posteriorly.

Vascular injuries are common associated injuries and are the highest cause of mortality in pancreatic injuries. Bleeding in the lesser sac can either be coming from the splenic artery or vein but can also from the left renal pedicle which lies just posterior to the neck of the pancreas. Injuries to the head of the pancreas can penetrate and pass through the IVC or aorta and may require further management which is beyond the scope of this chapter.

Mobilization of the pancreatic body and tail is fairly easy. The peritoneum at the base of the transverse mesocolon is divided using sharp dissection as it takes root from the anterior inferior surface of the pancreas. I usually start just to the left of the superior mesenteric vein. This avascular plane is easily developed lifting the pancreas up and gently retracting it superiorly. This plane should pass posterior to the splenic vein and can be developed to the left and right as far as is required, determined by the site of the injury.

Once the pancreas is mobilized and the site of the injury fully defined, it is important to classify the extent of the injury. There are numerous classification systems and they all have in common a measure of the extent of the parenchymal and main ductal injury. We prefer the American Association for the Surgery of Trauma (AAST) Committee on Organ Injury Scaling classification. See Table 43.1 [3].

For minor parenchymal injuries without ductal disruption, we do not suture the gland but would leave a drain onto the site of the injury. We use soft silicone suction drains [4, 5].

If the parenchyma is significantly divided or the main pancreatic duct (MPD) disrupted, for injuries to the left of the PV/SMV we advocate a distal pancreatectomy. In most patients, a splenectomy would also be performed [6, 7]. However, in skilled hands and in a stable patient, one can consider a splenic preserving distal pancreatectomy. The basis for this is the unproven benefit of splenic preservation in HIV- and Malaria-infested communities.

I find it easier to do a retrograde distal pancreatectomy in the trauma setting. The ligaments around the

Table 43.1 The organ injury scaling (OIS) Committee of the American Association for the Surgery of Trauma (AAST) for pancreatic trauma [3]

Grade	Criteria
I	Simple contusion of the pancreas
II	Major contusion or laceration without tissue loss or involvement of the main pancreatic duct
III	Complete transection of the pancreas or a parenchymal injury with involvement of the major duct to the left of the SMV
IV	Ductal transection or a major parenchymal injury to the right of the SMV
V	Massive disruption of the head of the pancreas

spleen are divided by sharp dissection starting at the inferior pole of the spleen. The operator's left hand is then placed behind the spleen retracting it anteriorly and to the patient's right. As the lienorenal, lienophrenic ligaments are divided, the spleen mobilizes easily. The tail of the pancreas is mobilized from the left to the right with ease. The retroperitoneal attachment of the pancreas is relatively avascular as long as you stay anterior to gerotas fascia over the left kidney. This is done with a combination of diathermy dissection and sharp dissection. The pancreas is mobilized for up to 2 cm beyond the injury or your elected site of transection. The short gastric vessels need to be divided and this can be done rapidly between tissue clamps. If the patient is stable, a hemostatic devise or electrocautery sealing devise can be used for this fiddly dissection. Be careful to avoid including the gastric wall in the artery clamps when dividing the short gastric vessels; this can result in a delayed gastric leak. The next stage is to divide the splenic artery and vein. Toward the right of the patient they do not lie together and should be individually identified and suture ligated.

Post-operative pancreatic fistula is the most significant post-operative complication and much has been written about the management of the pancreatic stump at operation. I am afraid there is no magic bullet. In the trauma setting the pancreas is soft, the duct is small and often there is already significant edema of the cut end of the pancreas making the tissue handling of sutures even more difficult. Staples with or without some form of tissue re-inforcement have been reported to have some benefit in the non-trauma setting. We prefer a hand divided technique where we use diathermy to cut the pancreas. The pancreatic duct can usually be identified and remember it lies more to the posterior aspect of the pancreas. When found the duct is suture ligated with a fine 5/0 monofilament suture using a figure of eight suture over the duct. When dividing the gland I always keep in mind the intention to approximate the cut end and so slightly angulate the cut edge anteriorly inward and posteriorly outward to facilitate a fish mouth closure. Unless there is significant edema this is usually possible. I use a 4/0 or 3/0 monofilament suture and run a continuous suture along the pancreatic edge. I always leave a drain in situ and usually only remove it when the volume is less than 50 mL/day and the patient's pancreas has been stimulated by appropriate oral intake.

If a splenectomy is performed, remember to give the patient pneumococcal vaccine soon after the procedure to help reduce the incidence of overwhelming post-splenectomy sepsis. If you are intending to do a splenectomy, pneumococcal vaccine given preoperatively is more effective if administered with spleen in situ.

A parenchymal injury to the head without major duct disruption requires good suction drainage alone. If one is unable to classify the ductal injury in the head, then our recommendation is to err on the conservative side and only drain the head. Should a MPD injury be missed and a pancreatic fistula develop, endoscopic intervention with ERCP and MPD stenting works well in our experience to stop the leak. We do not advocate major resections of the head unless there is a defined major injury to the duodenal-ampullary complex or the missile has essentially divided the pancreas for you. When the head of the pancreas is shattered and there is a significant duodenal injury and minimal dissection is required to remove the head, a pancreaticoduodenectomy is performed. When dividing the pancreas as it runs posterior to the PV/SMV, it is important to identify by palpation where the superior Mesenteric artery runs to the left of the veins. Traction on the pancreas head during the process of dividing the uncinate process can tent up the artery and injury to the SMA is possible at this point.

The remaining issue is the timing of the reconstruction. In experienced hands and with a stable patient without the need for damage control, an immediate reconstruction can be performed. However this is the exception. We advocate that the reconstruction is performed at a second procedure, delayed for 48–72 h to address the patient's general condition as per damage control guidelines [8]. Again it is the pancreatic reconstruction that is difficult due to the normal pancreas and small duct. We make no recommendation as to the type of pancreatic reconstruction that should be employed. Our own practice is to perform a posterior pancreaticogastrostomy. A proximal gastrojejunostomy followed about 10 cm distally with a side-to-side hepaticojejunostomy. There is some suggestion that the gallbladder can be used as a conduit for biliary reconstruction. We think this is unnecessary and unwise and recommend routine cholecystectomy. In addition, the bile duct is also usually not dilated and care and experience should be employed to prevent post-operative strictures of the bile duct anastomosis. Should the bile duct be small, mobilize the common bile duct proximally and identify the left hepatic duct. Open the anterior wall of the common hepatic duct onto the left hepatic duct for at least 2 cm. During this dissection a small branch of the hepatic artery crosses the left hepatic duct and is often divided at this point. This vessel is hard to identify before you cut it and can be controlled with a small suture or diathermy. A note of caution at this point is important, preservation of the blood supply to the biliary tree is very important. Excessive mobilization can devascularize the bile ducts resulting in late ischemic strictures. A side-to-side hepaticojejunostomy using a 4/0 or 5/0 monofilament absorbable, as originally described by Hepp and Couninard, is then performed. The bowel loop is brought antecolic based on the recent evidence that this reduces the incidence of delayed gastric emptying.

The challenge in the patient without a shattered head of pancreas is to identify the major injury to the ampulla. If the ampulla is not accessible through the duodenal injury, some recommend an on-table cholangiogram to identify the injury. In our experience this is usually not required and can be very difficult from a logistics point of view in the middle of the night. The damage control approach is very valuable in this setting and allows one to revisit the decision making in the cold light of day with all the resources available. This may include MRCP.

With the growing evidence that minimally invasive interventions such as ERCP and EUS can assist in managing post-trauma complications to the pancreas, especially in the blunt trauma setting, if at operation a borderline indication for a pancreaticoduodenectomy exists we would recommend drainage and referral to a center where endoscopic and interventional radiological expertise exist. The role of duodenal exclusion procedures is again gaining popularity [9]. In the situation where there is a significant injury to the duodenum with a borderline injury to the pancreas with an intact ampulla, we believe that a well-placed purse string suture, using an absorbable suture, occluding the pylorus and placed from inside the stomach in addition to a gastrojejunostomy using the same gastric incision made to insert the above purse string should be performed. The duodenal injury should be closed with meticulous interrupted monofilament sutures. If there is a concomitant biliary injury, a cholecystectomy and placement of a T tube into the common bile duct can be added to divert bile from the duodenum or from the site of injury.

We believe, in general, that with the advent of endoscopic interventions and the progress made in interventional radiology, the aggressive approach to pancreatic injuries should be reviewed. Clearly when there is significant parenchymal and MPD disruption to the left of the PV/SMV, resectional surgery is required. However, in the borderline cases, when the MPD integrity is uncertain or the status of the ampullary complex poorly defined, the value of intraoperative techniques to identify and classify the injury is uncertain and is not reliable enough and is meddlesome and should be avoided. However, what has not been mentioned is the role of intra-operative ultrasound. No studies have been reported defining the role and benefit, if any, from intraoperative ultrasound. This tool is common place in an HPB theater and ultrasound of the pancreas is a very valuable way of looking for small lesions in the pancreas and their relationship to the MPD, which is well seen. As such this investigation needs to be investigated as it may be valuable in the trauma setting.

Post-operative complications are common and are often due to the associated injuries. The complications related to the pancreas are mainly related to surgical site infections, pancreatico-cutaneous fistulae and the development of pancreatic and peripancreatic fluid collections.

Surgical site infections are usually treated using interventional radiological techniques. However, if bowel fistulae resulting in intra-abdominal collections occur and are associated with pancreatic duct leaks, in addition to the radiological interventions, the duct leak must be addressed.

Pancreatic fistulae are the most significant of the primary pancreatic complications. They have a significant associated morbidity if not treated adequately and this may require a number of simultaneously employed techniques. The initial problem is to define a clinically significant fistula. In the literature there are numerous classifications and consensus statements. However, a leak of amylase-rich fluid persisting for a number of days and having clinical implications should be defined as a fistula. The role of the volume of fluid in the definition is unclear. We consider a daily output of between 50 mL and 100 mL to be significant. In such a patient the first step is to exclude a peripancreatic collection that is not adequately addressed by the drain. CT scan is the investigation of choice. If there is a collection, percutaneously placed pigtail drains are inserted. Control of the fistula is the main objective in this situation. Can we avoid the development of fistulae? The role of octreotide in the post-operative period is not well defined. Some work from Heidelberg in Germany suggests a real benefit in reducing the post-operative fistula rate [10]. We do not use it routinely but if there is real concern regarding the risk of a fistula in an individual patient we would use it. In well-established post-operative fistulas we would routinely use octreotide in addition to TPN or semi-elemental enteral feeds. In a low output fistula we would start with enteral semi-elemental oral feeds. If the fistula output does not increase we continue with this regimen. However, if the output is very high or increases with enteral feeding, we convert to TPN as our primary nutritional support. ERCP and MPD stenting does have a role in managing these ductal leaks. The main issue is however timing. If the leak is controlled, then there is no rush and the patient's general condition will determine the timing. In addition, many low-output fistulae will close spontaneously within a few days and do not require endoscopic interventions. It is difficult to move an unstable patient to the ERCP suite and therefore when the patient is stable and the fistula persists longer than 5–7 days we perform ERCP and if a duct disruption is defined a small pancreatic duct sphincterotomy is performed and a 7fr plastic stent inserted. Removal of the stent should be as soon as possible to prevent damage to the duct. We recommend removal within 4–6 weeks of the fistulae clinically closing.

Pancreatic pseudocysts usually present as a delayed presentation. This can be when a minor pancreatic injury was missed or after the removal of the surgically placed drains when the extent of the ductal injury was underestimated. The management of pancreatic pseudocysts is beyond the scope of this chapter. Our primary approach is always endoscopic and today this is usually endoscopic ultrasound guided. However, other endoscopic approaches including ERCP and transpapillary stenting have been shown to work and can be employed. Surgical cystenterostomy should be avoided as minimally invasive approaches are usually successful.

Penetrating injuries to the pancreas are usually diagnosed at operation. The well-established protocols determining damage control and the management of penetrating injuries to the abdomen should be followed. When pancreatic injuries are present, the aim of the surgery is primarily to identify the extent of the parenchymal injury and the degree of duct disruption. All minor injuries and indeterminate injuries should be treated with suction drains. Resection should be reserved for injuries to the left of the PV/SMV and should include a splenectomy. Pancreaticoduodenectomy should be only performed when the injury is of such a nature that the head of the pancreas is already divided or where the injury to the duodenal ampullary complex prevents reconstruction. We recommend a two-stage resection and reconstruction. Duodenal exclusion techniques are again becoming accepted and we certainly believe in the right setting they should be used. A more conservative approach to pancreatic injuries can be justified by the increasing reports of success in treating pancreatic sequelae with endoscopic and radiological interventions. The initial treatment is usually successful in most trauma units. More advanced injuries and complications should be referred to specialized pancreatic units where experience and access to advanced endoscopy usually exist.

Important Points

- Isolated pancreatic injuries are rare and it is the associated injuries that result in the high morbidity and mortality in pancreatic trauma
- Pre-operative diagnosis of pancreatic injuries is difficult
- Guiding principles for operative treatment:
  - Indentify the extent of the parenchymal injury
  - Identify and quantify the injury to the pancreatic duct
- Evaluation of the pancreatic injury requires full mobilization of the affected part of the pancreas
- Major injuries to the left of the portal vein/superior mesenteric vein require resection with splenectomy. Minor injuries should be adequately drained
- Where possible major injuries to the head of the pancreas are treated with drainage alone. Resection is indicated where there is a major injury to the duodenal – ampullary complex or when the resection is almost completed by the mechanism of injury
- The availability of endoscopic techniques to manage post-operative leaks from the pancreas supports a more conservative approach to surgical therapy

References

1. Degiannis E, Glapa M, Loukogeorgakis SP, Smith MD (2008) Management of pancreatic trauma. Injury, Int J Care Injured 39:21–29
2. Krige JE (2004) Pancreatic trauma. In: Nicol AJ, Steyn E (eds) Handbook of trauma. Oxford University Press, Cape Town, pp 258–265
3. Moore EE, Cogbill TH, Malangoni MA, Jurkovich GJ, Champion HR, Gennarelli TA, McAninch JW, Pachter HL, Shackford SR, Trafton PG (1990) Organ injury scaling, II: pancreas, duodenum, small bowel, colon, and rectum. J Trauma 30:1427–1429
4. Degiannis E, Levy RD, Velmahos GC, Potokar T, Florizoone MG, Saadia R (1996) Gunshot injuries of the head of the pancreas: conservative approach. World J Surg 20:68–71
5. Degiannis E, Levy RD, Potokar T, Lennox H, Rowse A, Saadia R (1995) Distal pancreatectomy for gunshot injuries of the distal pancreas. Br J Surg 82:1240–1242
6. Degiannis E, Krawczykowski D, Velmahos GC, Levy RD, Souter I, Saadia R (1993) Pyloric exclusion in severe penetrating injuries of the duodenum. World J Surg 17:751–754
7. Degiannis E, Bowley DM, Smith MD (2003) Non-operative management of splenic injury in adults – current management status and controversies. S Afr J Surg 41:33–34
8. Krige JE, Nicol AJ, Navsaria PH, Jones O, Bornman PC (2005) Emergency pancreatoduodenectomy for complex pancreatic trauma. HPB Surg 7:104
9. Wisner DH, Hoyt DB (1993) Definitive care phase: abdominal injuries. In: Greenfield LJ (ed) Surgery: scientific principles and practice. JP Lippincott, Philadelphia, pp 305–310
10. Buchler M, Friess H, Klempa I, Hermanek P, Sulkowski U, Becker H, Schafmayer A, Baca I, Lorenz D, Meister R (1992) Role of octreotide in the prevention of postoperative complications following pancreatic resection. Am J Surg 163:125–130

Liver and Extrahepatic Bile Ducts

44

Frederick Millham

Penetrating liver injury offers surgeons a wide spectrum of challenges ranging from making a decision for non-operative management to devising strategies to manage complex combined hepatic vascular and biliary injuries. The successful management of complex penetrating liver injuries can require a broad range of skills, from the ability to expose and control bleeding rapidly, to the ability to coordinate care of an unstable patient over a long period. A theme pervading all management of complex liver injuries, though, is the simple notion that, ultimately, the liver is a forgiving organ, if one can keep the patient from bleeding to death on the day of injury or dying of sepsis from leaking bile later on, even the most complex injuries can be managed successfully. Damage control in the face of complex or multiple injury with bleeding arrestable with compression is the standard of care [1, 2]. For ease of discussion, I will discuss management of liver and extrahepatic biliary injuries separately.

44.1 Immediate Considerations

Choosing a management strategy for penetrating liver injury is informed by several factors known immediately on patient presentation. First, and most important, is hemodynamic stability. Patients who are in persistent shock due to penetrating injury always require immediate surgical intervention. More challenging from a decision-making standpoint are patients who may have shown some early signs of shock but who have responded well to either time or resuscitation. For these patients there may be an opportunity to obtain imaging that will support a non-operative strategy. A good general principle is to avoid axial imaging in patients in shock. Critical review of vital signs and patient's acid–base status are important when considering non-operative management of any visceral injury.

A second consideration is the mechanism of injury. Penetrating injuries to the liver can be conveniently divided into three categories: (1) stab and other low-energy wounds, (2) low-energy gunshot wounds, and (3) high-energy gunshot wounds or wounds due to military ordnance. Hemodynamically stable stab wound victims who have no evidence of active or ongoing bleeding can be safely managed by observation. Mortality in this setting is a function of laceration of a named vessel such as the vena cava or hepatic vein. If there is low suspicion for vascular injury, observation is the best strategy. Low-velocity gunshot wound patients who are hemodynamically stable can also be observed provided there is convincing evidence on axial imaging that the liver injury is tangential and not associated with extravasation of blood [3]. High-velocity gunshot wounds, or other wounds caused by military ordnance, create extensive wounds to the liver. The inelastic structure of the liver does not respond well to the physics of high-velocity projectiles, which tend to create complex, shattered, wounds, challenging to even the most skilled trauma surgeon. Patients with high-velocity wounds are essentially never candidates for non-operative management.

F. Millham
Department of Surgery, Harvard Medical School,
Boston, MA, USA

Chair of Surgery, Harvard Medical School,
Green 664, 2014 Washington St, Newton, MA 02462, USA
e-mail: fmillham@partners.org

G.C. Velmahos et al. (eds.), *Penetrating Trauma*,
DOI 10.1007/978-3-642-20453-1_44, © Springer-Verlag Berlin Heidelberg 2012

44.2 Non-operative Management

Patients who arrive with normal vital signs and who do not appear to be in shock or to be actively bleeding are good candidates for non-operative management [3]. CT scanning done with dynamic contrast injection, and delayed imaging, can exclude active liver bleeding and support a strategy of observation alone in such patients. Should CT scanning show arterial extravasation, angio-embolization is an excellent intervention. Simple tangential stab or low-velocity gunshot wounds rarely require aggressive operative intervention. In some cases, drainage of the perihepatic space may be necessary to control bile leakage. When bile collections occur subsequent to admission, these drains can be placed laparoscopically [4].

Injuries to the retro-hepatic vena cava, if not bleeding, may also be managed non-operatively [5]. Here a good rule of thumb is "don't poke a skunk." Stable non-expanding pericaval hematomas only become problems when surgeons expose them. The careful trauma surgeon is willing to observe these injuries carefully from a far. Some authorities have recently demonstrated excellent outcomes with endovascular stenting of vena caval injuries [6], though in the absence of active bleeding doing nothing may be best.

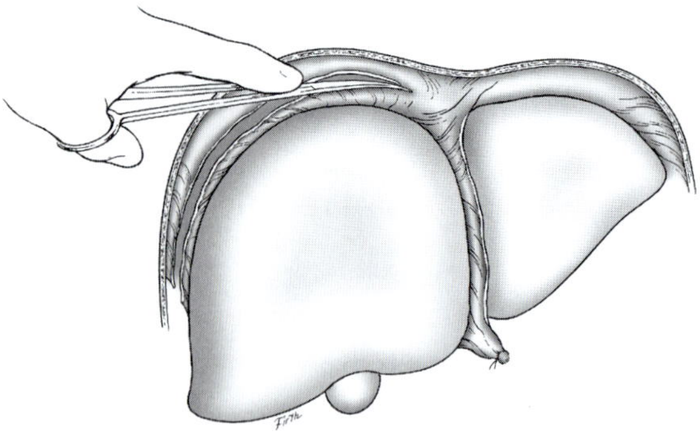

Fig. 44.1 First step in controlling liver bleeding: completely mobilize the liver from the diaphragm

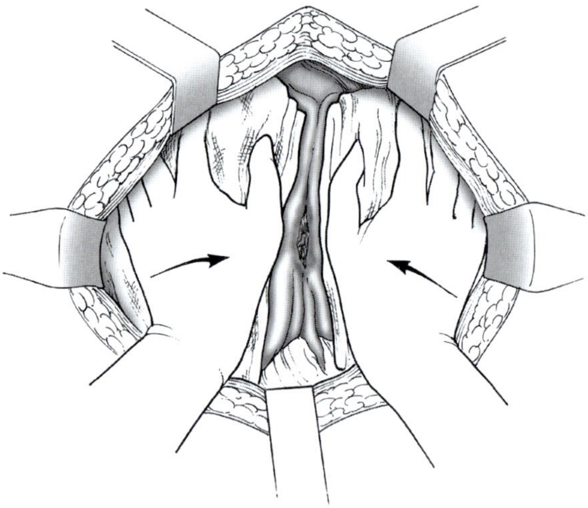

Fig. 44.2 Second step in controlling liver bleeding: manual compression with hands compressing both lobes toward the hepatic hilum

44.3 Operative Management

As a rule, you should manage penetrating abdominal injury through a midline incision. There is always enough uncertainty regarding projectile trajectory to make the midline the safest route of approach. As with any trauma laparotomy prep and expose the patient from the neck to the mid thighs.

There are several keys to the operative management of penetrating liver injuries. First, you must fully mobilize the liver by taking down all of its ligamentous attachments to the diaphragm. Using a Metzenbaum scissor, divide completely the falciform and coronary ligaments (Fig. 44.1). This is necessary to expose the liver entirely for inspection but more importantly, to facilitate compression of the liver as a means of hemostasis. If the liver is fractured to any extent by the injury, attempting compression without full mobilization risks extending the existing injury. In the case where there is active bleeding from the liver substance, following mobilization of the liver the surgeon or assistant should manually compress the liver by placing your left hand over the right lateral portion of the liver and the right hand over the left lobe and pressing the liver together (Fig. 44.2). In most cases, this will slow or stop bleeding from the liver substance and allow a chance both for resuscitation and assessment of the extent of injury.

The next key step is to distinguish between arterial and venous injury. A surgical truism states: "Arterial bleeding scares the amateurs, venous bleeding scares the professionals". The Pringle maneuver is useful to distinguish amateur from professional bleeding from a penetrating liver injury. You can accomplish it in a matter of seconds by passing your left index finger through the Foramen of Winslow and directing it anteriorly

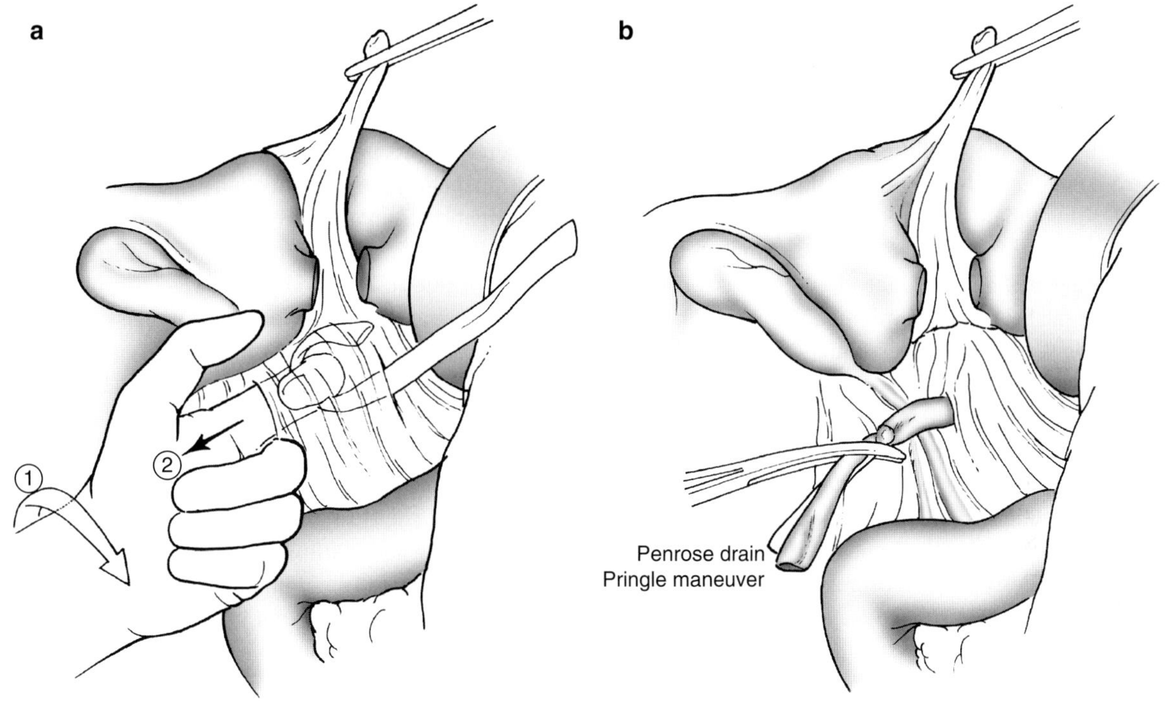

Fig. 44.3 (**a**) Pringle maneuver step A: insert left index finger into the foramen of Winslow, then push the finger tip through the lesser omentum (aka: gastro-hepatic ligament). (**b**) Pringle maneuver step B: encircle the porta hepatis with a ¾″ Penrose drain hooked around the index finger, then tourniquet the porta by twisting the drain and securing with a Kelly clamp

through the lesser omentum (gastrohepatic ligament). You do this bluntly. Once the fingertip appears, sweep a three quarter inch penrose drain around the porta hepaits in the same manner one encircles the spermatic cord during a hernia repair. The Penrose can then be tightened with a Kelly clamp to occlude all inflow to the liver (Fig. 44.3a, b). The time inflow occlusion starts should be recorded. Ideally, hepatic ischemia should be limited to 30 min or less. If this arrests the bleeding, then arterial hemorrhage is almost always the problem. If bleeding persists, then injury to a hepatic vein or adjacent vena cava should be suspected.

In the case of brisk arterial bleeding, threatening immediate exsanguination, ligation of the common hepatic artery or the right or left hepatic artery is an alternative. With the Penrose drain – Pringle tourniquet on downward traction, you can find the hepatic artery by first identifying the common bile duct and looking medially.

Prior to closing the abdomen with towel clips, packs are applied anteriorly across the surface of the liver. If you have ligated or embolized the right hepatic artery, the gallbladder will be devascularized and should be removed.

If the Pringle maneuver does not arrest the bleeding, then assume venous injury. At this point it is important to evaluate the vena cava for injury. Many times the real source from liver injuries is in fact the vena cava or the junction of the vena cava and hepatic veins. Vena caval injuries can be classified into three types: supra-hepatic, retrohepatic, and infrahepatic.

If a suprahepatic injury is suspected, proceed directly to a thoracoabdominal approach. While a "hockey-stick" incision into the costal cartilages from the superior pole of the midline wound is possible, I prefer to perform median sternotomy in cases where injury to the cava appears to be in the "no man's land" between the liver and heart. These wounds have a very high mortality. Successful management requires rapid control which is best gained by dividing the sternum and diaphragm. The sternum is best divided with a power driven sternal saw. Finger dissection in the suprasternal notch to keep the innominate veins away from the saw blade is a good first step. Next, with the saw guard introduced through the sternal notch and on upward traction the sternum can be opened in a matter of seconds. A Finochietto retractor or similar rib spreader can provide access to the heart and mediastinum. Take quickly down the pericardium and anterior attachments of the mediastinum with scissors. Divide the diaphragm with the cautery down onto the caval hiatus. This should expose the injured segment. A side biting vascular clamp is usually the simplest tool for controlling the injury. Once the clamp is on blood return to the heart will be minimal. Mortality for these injuries is very high. It is essential that one work with alacrity in the setting [7].

Retro-hepatic caval injuries are among the most challenging injuries the trauma surgeon faces. In the setting of penetrating trauma, where bleeding is not contained within a soft tissue space, the vena cava must be exposed rapidly. In patients where the liver is relatively large or the exposure is difficult, access to the chest as described above may be useful. Generally, however, it is not necessary to open the chest to approach the retro-hepatic vena cava. Having already mobilized the ligamentous attachments, it is possible to rotate the liver medially exposing the retro-hepatic cava. If the injury involves the intra-hepatic portion of the cava, it may be necessary to take down the small veins draining directly from the substance of the liver into the vena cava. These usually number between 7 and 14 and in an emergency can be well managed with small clips. Failure to control these veins will result in creation of an additional source of bleeding. Inflow and outflow occlusion of the cava above and below the injury can be usually achieved with direct compression using sponge sticks. As in the supra-hepatic vena cava injury, there is a high premium on efficiency. Having 3-0 or 4-0 vascular nylon suture ready on a long needle driver prior to diving in to the retro-hepatic space is a good idea.

Injuries to the infra-hepatic cava can be exposed by the so-called Brasch-Cattell maneuver, where you should open the white line of Toldt in the right paracolic gutter and sweep the right colon medially on its mesentery. Mobilize the duodenum medially in a similar way. Sponge sticks are useful here too for proximal and distal control in a hurry. Traditionally, it has been thought that it is necessary to preserve at least 25% of the lumen of the vena cava above the kidneys [8]. Recent experience indicates less lumen may be acceptable, it is certainly better to leave a conduit of diminished diameter than ligate the cava or, worse, have a patient expire while performing an interposition graft. Endovascular stenting is emerging as an option for management of penetrating injures infrahepatic vena cava [9].

Where patients are unstable and complex injury of the infrahepatic vena cava precludes a simple vascular repair, ligation is an acceptable option [10].

Patient suffering from multiple gunshot wounds to the liver or injuries caused by high-velocity rounds or military ordinance may have complex, massive, liver fractures, difficult to control by packing. These wounds are fortunately rare in civilian practice. Bleeding uncontrollable by packing disqualifies the patient for a damage control procedure. It is in this setting that maneuvers such as hepatic exclusion may be the only option. With the Pringle tourniquet engaged, the hepatic inflow and outflow controlled with sponge sticks, one looks for the dominant sources of hemorrhage and clips or ligates them. In limited cases formal lobectomy may be preferable if the injury is limited to an anatomic lobe or segment.

More advanced techniques such as veno-venous bypass for hepatic exclusion have been used by some centers to manage complex liver injuries [11]. These methods usually require existing experience and rapid access to extracorporeal circulation technology and expertise. These techniques are difficult to improvise or implement without planning ahead of time.

If bleeding is indeed uncontrollable with packing, and a transplant program is available, a last effort at salvage may include hepatectomy with hope for an emergency transplant. This option is obviously limited to a small number of centers and even then unlikely to succeed.

44.4 Extrahepatic Biliary Injury

Penetrating injury of the extra patent bile ducts is relatively uncommon, and usually occurs in conjunction with a more serious injury to a vascular or other visceral structure. Injuries to the extrahepatic biliary system are far more common in the setting of cholecystectomy. Experience managing misadventures in this setting is useful in informing our approach to penetrating injury of the common bile duct [12].

Isolated injury of the common bile duct can be repaired primarily if caused by an edged weapon. However, most penetrating trauma victims are young people with no pre-existing biliary pathology. The common duct in such patients is a small, more delicate structure with a diameter of 5 mm or less. Therefore, a better plan is to repair injuries of the common bile duct over a T-tube or stent. Biliary stents can be placed operatively through the injury and passed down through the ampulla Vater for later endoscopic recovery. My preference is to close simple wounds in small ducts over an appropriately sized T-tube. The T-tube can be removed 4–6 weeks postoperatively following a normal cholangiogram.

Complex injuries of the extrahepatic biliary tree, involving loss of a segment of the common bile duct or significant injury of the origin of the common bile duct from the right and left hepatic duct, require more complex management. Injuries of this type occurring in isolation can be managed in one step with a choledocho or hepato-jejunostomy, best constructed as a Roux-en-Y limb. Ureteral stents are a useful adjunct that one can place through the anastomotic region and bring out through the anterior abdominal wall downstream. Tack the mid portion of the Roux limb to the anterior abdominal wall, and bring the stents out as one might a feeding jejunostomy tube.

In the face of aggressive hemorrhage or injuries to other vital organs, it is not necessary to repair the common bile duct at the first operative encounter. The management principles are simple: control bile leakage and prevent or manage sepsis. Damage control in this setting may be as simple as tying the end of the hepatic or common duct around ureteral stents, brought out with ample additional closed suction drainage. If the ducts are not identifiable, provide adequate drainage by placing ample closed suction drains as adequate. If bile leakage and sepsis are controlled, biliary enteric continuity can be re-established weeks or even months later when other problems have been settled.

44.5 Conclusion

Penetrating liver and extrahepatic biliary injury represents a wide spectrum of disease, from the mundane to the lethal. Patients with non-bleeding injuries do not require surgical intervention. Successful management of complex hepatobiliary injury frequently requires a damage control philosophy. The initial approach to such patients may involve "simply" stopping the bleeding and draining the bile, leaving definitive restoration of biliary enteric drainage for another day. Endovascular techniques such as embolization and stenting represent important methods that are part of a multi-disciplinary approach these injuries may demand.

Important Points

- Don't poke a skunk: Non-bleeding injuries can usually be watched
- In a crisis: Damage Control is the path to success
- Stop the bleeding today, fix the biliary anatomy tomorrow
- Mobilize the liver before attempting compression or packing
- If the Pringle maneuver arrests life-threatening bleeding, ligate, or embolize
- If the Pringle maneuver does not control life-threatening bleeding look to the vena cava

References

1. Richardson JD (2005) Changes in the management of injuries to the liver and spleen. J Am Coll Surg 200(5):648–669
2. Christmas AB et al (2005) Selective management of blunt hepatic injuries including nonoperative management is a safe and effective strategy. Surgery 138(4):606–611
3. Demetrios D et al (1999) Gunshot injuries to the liver: the role of selective nonoperative management. J Am Coll Surg 188(4):343–348
4. Franklin GA et al (2007) Prevention of bile peritonitis by laparoscopic evacuation and lavage after nonoperative treatment of liver injuries. Am Surg 73(6):611–617
5. Buckman RF, Miraliakbari R, Badellino MM (2000) Juxtahepatic venous injuries: a critical review of reported management strategies. J Trauma 48(5):978–984
6. Angeles APMD, Agarwal NMD, Lynd CJMD (2004) Repair of a juxtahepatic inferior vena cava injury using a simple endovascular technique. J Trauma Inj Infect Crit Care 56(4):918–921
7. Asensio JAMD et al (2000) Approach to the management of complex hepatic injuries. J Trauma Inj Infect Crit Care 48(1):66
8. Burch JM et al (1988) Injuries of the inferior vena cava. Am J Surg 156(6):548–552
9. de Naeyer G, Degrieck I (2005) Emergent infrahepatic vena cava stenting for life-threatening perforation. J Vasc Surg 41(3):552–554

10. Degiannis E et al (1996) Penetrating injuries of the abdominal inferior vena cava. Ann R Coll Surg Engl 78(6): 485–489
11. Biffl WL, Moore EE, Franciose RJ (1998) Venovenous bypass and hepatic vascular isolation as adjuncts in the repair of destructive wounds to the retrohepatic inferior vena cava. J Trauma 45(2):400–403
12. Kapoor VK (2007) Bile duct injury repair: when? what? who? J Hepatobiliary Pancreat Surg 14(5):476–479

Large and Small Bowel

45

Herb A. Phelan

When discussing penetrating hollow viscus injuries, it is best to think of their management as consisting of two distinct phases. The first stage consists of the initial pass through the patient's abdomen and centers around the temporary control of spill from perforated bowel. The second phase is the remainder of the operation and focuses on the specific management goal for the involved viscus at the time of that operation. In this chapter, we will focus on technical tricks for identifying these injuries, the options available to deal with them, and (most importantly in my view) the factors influencing the smart trauma surgeon's choice of procedure to perform for injuries occurring between the Ligament of Treitz and the sacral promontory. So let's dive in…

45.1 The First Pass Through the Abdomen

While circumstances dictate the pace of the first stage, the exploratory techniques should always be the same for the first minutes of any trauma laparotomy after a gunshot or stab wound. While the techniques for rapidly getting into the peritoneal cavity are covered well in another chapter of this book, I want to emphasize that one should strive to do it the same way every time. If I close my eyes, I can rapidly run through my own personal sequence: rapid clot and hemoperitoneum evacuation; run a hand over the right lobe of the liver, palpate the right diaphragm, fast inspection of the portal triad, anterior stomach, left lobe, and gastroesophageal junction; over to the spleen and left diaphragm for a quick palpation and inspection; take the transverse colon cephalad and eviscerate the small bowel to the patient's right to look at the retroperitoneum overlying the root of the mesentery, aorta, and left kidney; flip the viscera back to the patient's left to look at the retroperitoneum overlying the cava, right kidney, and pancreaticoduodenal complex; eviscerate all of the small bowel cephalad to look at the contents of the pelvis; and finally take the stomach cephalad while distracting the transverse colon caudally to put the gastrocolonic ligament under tension where an avascular plane can be quickly identified and opened to inspect the lesser sac. If exsanguinating hemorrhage is encountered during these maneuvers, it should be rapidly controlled at that time. If the bleeding is not audible or contained hematomas are found, they are best dealt with by packing the area until the entire abdomen has been assessed.

Once this sequence is complete, then and only then should one run the bowel. This is performed as a philosophical extension of the first portion of the exploration in which the overall approach is fast, fast, fast. Remember, all that you are doing at this point in the operation is looking for sites of frank perforation or bleeding. Start at the Ligament of Treitz, and run the entire small and large intestine by hand-over-handing it to your assistant, making sure to visualize the entire mesentery all the way down to its root. Nonbleeding partial thickness injuries to the bowel

H.A. Phelan
Division of Burns/Trauma/Critical Care,
Department of Surgery,
University of Texas-Southwestern Medical Center,
5323 Harry Hines Blvd, E5.508A, Dallas
75390-9158, TX, USA
e-mail: herb.phelan@utsouthwestern.edu

G.C. Velmahos et al. (eds.), *Penetrating Trauma*,
DOI 10.1007/978-3-642-20453-1_45, © Springer-Verlag Berlin Heidelberg 2012

wall or mesentery should be noted but not addressed on this initial pass through the abdomen. The time will come soon enough to contend with those injuries on a slower, more thorough inspection later. If a site of frank perforation or bleeding is found, one should just place a quick figure-of-eight stitch at the serosal edges to control the spill of succus/stool or quickly clamp and tie a discrete "pumper" to get rapid hemostasis. Cut the tails of your stitch long to make the site easier to find in a little while. Do this to the bowel in its entirety.

At the completion of these maneuvers, one should sit back for a moment and take stock of the situation. You have completely inspected the abdomen, temporized the spill of bowel contents, and gotten an idea of the magnitude of injuries with which you are contending. Is your patient dying? Do you expect them to rapidly start getting sicker or better? What are the number and complexity of their associated injuries, both known and suspected? Are you dealing with an isolated hollow viscus injury? How much peritoneal soilage and blood loss has occurred? The answers to these questions will dictate how you manage that fluted segment of small bowel and blown-out sigmoid that you just finished whip-stitching. This is a good time to take a moment, catch your breath, and come up with a plan before you just start fixing things. One should start by resisting the urge to overthink things and just ask, "How sick is the patient?"

45.2 The Second Pass Through the Abdomen: The Stable Patient

Few operations for trauma are as enjoyable as the isolated hollow viscus injury in the hemodynamically stable patient after penetrating trauma, as they are straightforward in nature and yield immensely satisfying results. The pace of the case is relaxed, and glances up at the telemetry monitors are reassuring. There are some traps that one should still be aware of, however, which can turn a nice case into a delayed horror show.

When dealing with mesentery bleeding that is adjacent to the bowel but not involving the viscus itself, a simple whip stitch will frequently be all that is needed. Once hemostasis is secured, however, you will need to watch the bowel downstream for ischemia. Typically, if this is going to be a problem it will declare itself within several minutes. In my experience this is unusual

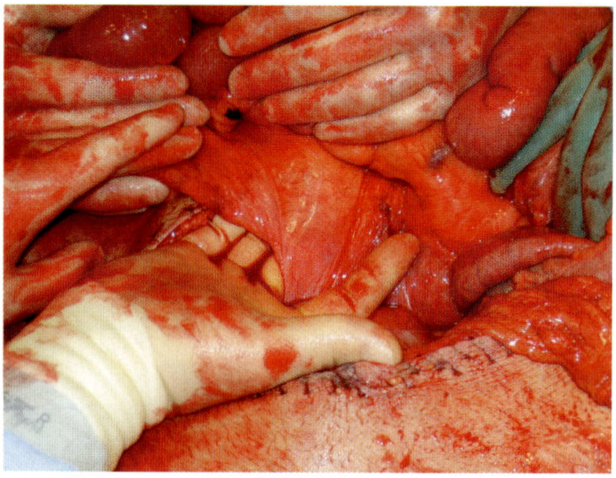

Fig. 45.1 To control injuries at the base of the mesentery, begin by placing the root of the mesentery between the index and middle fingers of the non-dominant hand

for the peripheral mesenteric defects that result after penetrating injury, as they are typically smaller than the larger, ragged mesenteric injuries that are commonly seen after blunt trauma. Injuries close to the root of the mesentery are much more problematic. These frequently present with an expanding hematoma within the sheets of the mesentery, and efforts to address them are fraught with the potential for iatrogenic injury to the superior mesenteric artery (SMA) or vein (SMV). Usually the injured vessel has retracted back into the mesentery making life difficult for all involved. Begin by placing the root of the mesentery between the index and middle fingers of the nondominant hand (Fig. 45.1). Then place your index finger and thumb on opposite sides of the injury (Fig. 45.2). By tenting the injury across the middle finger in this fashion, one can quickly get a significant degree of proximal and distal control of most injuries in this area. Once the field is dry, open up the sheets of the mesentery to precisely define the bleeding vessels and address them. It is wise to avoid blind clamping and figure-of-eight stitches in the high-priced real estate adjacent to the SMA and SMV.

If the injury is to the bowel itself, at this point in the operation you should be looking at several rapidly closed holes with long silk tags, or areas of hematoma adjacent to the colon or at the bowel/mesentery junction without frank spill. The first step is to avoid the temptation to start contending with the holes that you know you have and instead fully define all of the injuries with which you are dealing. This may save you

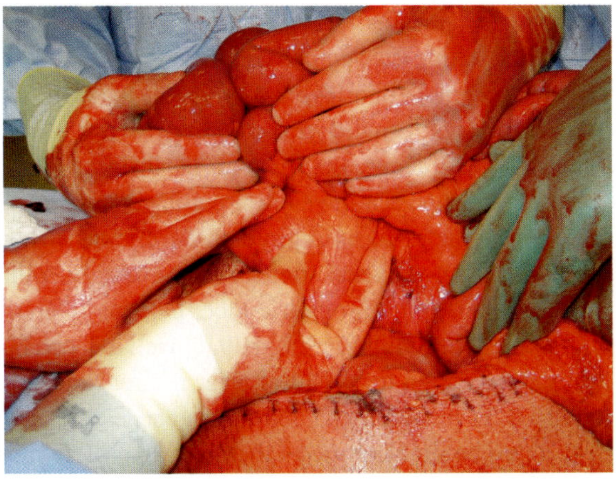

Fig. 45.2 Next, place the thumb and index finger on opposite sides of the injury. By squeezing the area of injury in this fashion, effective hemostasis is quickly achieved. The sheets of mesentery can then be incised and the points of bleeding accurately identified and addressed

from wasting time on primary repairs that will later wind up in a resected piece of bowel after other injuries are discovered. While this is frequently straightforward, a few particulars are worth mentioning. First, any pericolonic hematoma needs to be completely inspected. This means rolling the colon and dissecting all other tissues away until only the colonic serosa remains. If a subserosal hematoma is found, unroof it. Similarly, any hematoma at the junction of the bowel wall and mesentery should be considered to be an injury until proven otherwise by direct visual inspection of the serosa of the involved area. Do not let the fear of an iatrogenic injury stop you from completely inspecting the area of concern. Occasionally, for injuries close to the root of the mesentery, it will be necessary to actually take the ligament down. The important thing to remember is to never look at a hematoma immediately adjacent to a viscus and leave it thinking that it is probably OK. In the words of the esteemed surgeon Benton DuPont, "That works about as well as ball bearing book ends." Similarly, an odd number of holes in the bowel should trigger fears for a missed injury. While tangential wounds can occur, the finding of an odd number of holes should cause one to spend extra time looking for a missed perforation. Keep in mind the mobility of the small bowel, that people get shot in all manner of bodily positions, and that bullets do not travel in straight lines. In short, when looking for bowel injuries, paranoia is a healthy attitude.

Once an injury to the bowel wall is located, debriding the edges to healthy tissue and a transversely oriented primary repair should be the default first choice. Personally, I prefer a single layer running suture. If I have a relatively short segment of small bowel that has been fluted, I will resect it in order to minimize the number of suture lines. When making the decision about whether or not to resect an intervening piece of small bowel between two injured segments in order to save an anastomosis, I will check to see if I am leaving the patient with at least 250 cm of small bowel if a resection is performed as short bowel syndrome should not be a concern with that length. In adults, particularly those lacking a functional colon, lifelong TPN dependence is likely to occur in those who have 100 cm or less. While the presence of a functional ileocecal valve is thought to increase this length to an unknown degree, trauma patients are clearly at higher risk for subsequent bowel resections at their initial admission as well as over their lifetime (trauma recidivism rates are significant, proving the old saying, "Trauma is a chronic disease with acute exacerbations"). Given that, it is smart to leave them with plenty of bowel to spare. When dealing with two enterotomies that are within a centimeter or so of each other, the bridging wall of bowel separating them can become devascularized and slowly necrose over the course of a few days. Avoid the temptation to perform two primary repairs in this setting, as it is prudent to debride this segment and convert them into one larger enterotomy which can then be closed easily.

If a resection is required, the decision to perform an anastomosis versus diversion has vexed generations of surgeons. During World War II, failure to treat a penetrating colon injury with diversion was a court martial offense. With time, as it came to be realized that civilian injuries are not necessarily equivalent to military injuries and that ostomy reversal carried its own morbidity, the pendulum began to swing toward a lower threshold for anastomosis at the time of first operation [1]. In the stable, previously healthy penetrating trauma patient who is exhibiting no signs of shock and has received no blood products, I will always perform a primary anastomosis regardless of the location of the injury or the amount of peritoneal soilage from stool. This includes left colon injuries. The one exception to this general rule is the elderly patient with minimal physiologic reserve. In that setting, I will still perform enteroenterostomy and enterocolostomy. When considering the higher risks of colocolostomy in conjunction with the fact that an anastomotic leak in this specific population is often a death sentence, I will generally opt to perform resection and diversion in those patients. One should realize, though, that frequently means these will become permanent ostomies.

Typically the stable patient has relatively normal caliber bowel, and if this is the case either hand-sewing or stapling the anastomosis should be fine [2].

45.3 The Second Pass Through the Abdomen: Damage Control

Now let us consider a different situation. You have just finished a fast right nephrectomy and packing the liver; a quick glance up shows you multiple units of blood products hanging on the IV pole and on the floor around anesthesia's side of the drapes. Despite your best efforts, anesthesia tells you that the patient's core temperature is 33.9°C. You need to be getting out of this patient's abdomen ASAP. Having temporized the patient's enterotomies on the first pass with whip stitches, what do you do now?

For the patient who is in extremis, the answer is simple: nothing. Leaving the injuries alone with figure-of-eight closures is not something about which you should be cavalier, because this suboptimal technical closure is prone to breaking down (particularly in the setting of bowel edema and splanchnic vasoconstriction from shock and pressors). In the patient who is actively dying, however, the risk posed by this strategy may be balanced out by the benefit of saving a few minutes in a setting where time is critical. If one elects to leave the whip-stitches in place, it is important that you take the patient back at or around 24 h post-injury as longer delays begin to make the risks of breakdown with renewed spill of stool prohibitive. While I realize that the plural of anecdote is not data, I can say that I have resorted to this strategy a handful of times, and have yet to have a whip-stitch closure break down in this time frame.

If a damage control approach is being utilized but the patient is not in extremis, a different approach is used for hollow viscus injuries temporized on the first pass through the abdomen. If it is a matter of dealing with three or fewer small, discrete perforations, I will take the time necessary to perform simple, running, single-layer closures. These definitive repairs are quick, and a time-consuming second layer is unnecessary. If many more injuries exist, or a destructive injury is present, one should resect the involved piece of bowel and leave the patient in discontinuity. Alternatively, one can fire a linear cutting stapler adjacent to both sides of an injury, effectively excluding the injury from the fecal stream and preventing spill. With a functioning nasogastric tube, patients tolerate being left in discontinuity surprisingly well and can be left in this fashion for 48 h or longer if circumstances require it. Diversion in this setting is unnecessary, and in fact can be problematic as the abdominal wall frequently becomes quite edematous in damage control patients. This can put an ostomy that initially looked good under significant tension and predispose it to ischemia.

45.4 The Planned Re-operation After Successful Resuscitation

The first thing worth mentioning is that this operation does not necessarily need to take place in the operating room [3, 4]. When your patient has a pulmonary artery catheter in, is on very high levels of positive end expiratory pressure, and has a high pressor requirement, a "road trip" to the operating room can be a perilous undertaking. For the patient in whom ongoing bleeding is not a concern, a bedside re-exploration may be appropriate (Fig. 45.3). The only thing that should be different from the usual performance of the operation is its geographic location and the lack of an anesthesiologist. Laparotomy trays and electrocautery should be brought in, the abdomen should be prepped and draped in the usual fashion, and a scrub nurse and circulator should be present. Bowel resections and ostomies can be performed in a relatively straightforward manner. Typically, patients this ill are not candidates for a bowel anastomosis, but one can be performed if necessary. I would strongly advise against taking packing out at the bedside in the intensive care unit as renewed bleeding is difficult to deal with in this setting. The lighting is typically suboptimal, access to the head of the bed is usually difficult, and a strong ICU nurse is still not a match for an anesthesiologist if trouble is encountered. Having said that, I have become more and more comfortable with doing larger caliber procedures at the bedside as my career has progressed

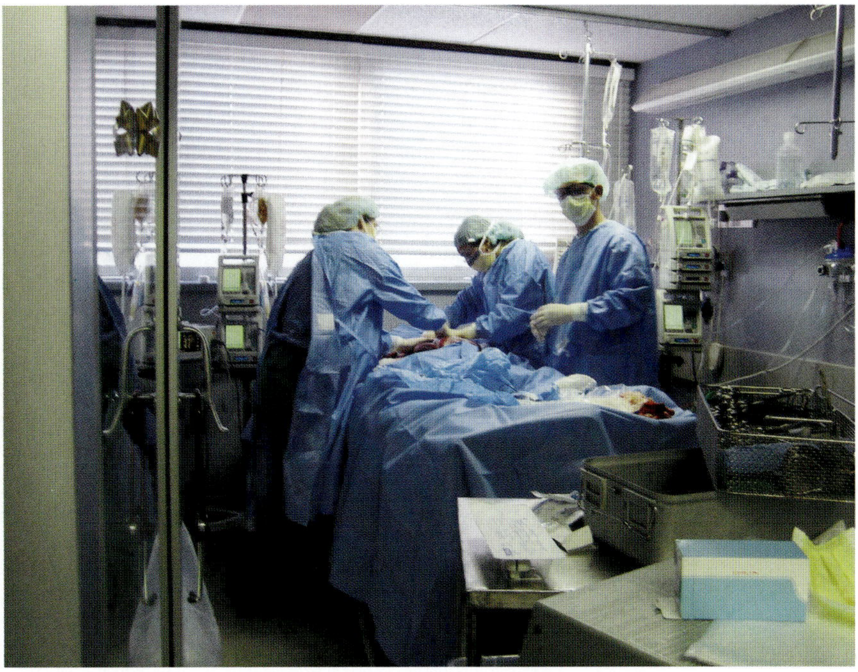

Fig. 45.3 Bedside re-exploration. In the severely ill patient in whom intrahospital transport is problematic, re-exploration at the bedside in the intensive care unit is a legitimate option. Bowel can be resected, ostomies matured, and fascial closure can be safely performed

and can recommend the technique without hesitation when dealing with the very, very sick patient.

At the time of reoperation, the first thing that one should do is to sit back and take a look at exactly what you are dealing with in terms of resected bowel, and small perforations that have been either whip-stitched or definitively addressed. Then one should develop a plan based on the general principle of balancing the number of suture lines versus the length of bowel remaining. As previously mentioned, there is a significant chance that this will not be the patient's last resection over their lifetime: anastomotic leaks, fistulae, bowel obstructions, and trauma recidivism all conspire to make this patient population high risk for future operations on their GI tract. In general, I will not leave a patient with more than three anastomoses total.

At the time of reoperation, injuries that were whip-stitched at the time of a damage control procedure should have the suture cut out, the edges of the wound trimmed to get back to healthy, bleeding bowel wall, and a primary repair performed. This should be done in either the small bowel or the colon. If you are dealing with a segment of bowel that has been left in discontinuity, the situation gets more complicated as you have to take other factors into account when making the decision as to whether to perform a high-risk anastomosis or commit the patient to an ostomy and all of its sequelae. In my practice, I follow the management strategy promulgated by the Eastern Association for the Surgery of Trauma (EAST) for colon injuries. The evidence-based guidelines which they put forth [5] essentially suggest that for a destructive colonic injury, diversion should be performed if the patient had sustained pre- or intraoperative hypotension or ongoing shock; or has significant underlying disease, associated injuries, or peritonitis. While useful as a general philosophy, one can see that there is still considerable room for interpretation and individual judgment. What about the 19-year-old patient who initially got 4 units of blood at the time of first operation, and now looks good with no pressor requirement and a plan for extubation after the OR? What about 6 units? Or 8? What constitutes significant pre-existing disease? These gray areas have been the cause of significant dyspepsia for me through my career. While categorical statements cannot be made about these situations, it is important to remember that generally speaking patients who are sick enough to require damage control procedures are ones in whom diversion should be the default plan (this is particularly true with colocolonic anastomoses). To contemplate an anastomosis of any kind in the setting of a pressor requirement is to be mentioned only to be condemned as the patient's natural splanchnic vasoconstriction from a hypotensive state is magnified by the pressor effect. Together, these serve to doom any reconstruction. In the very proximal small bowel where the nutritional and physiologic consequences of a high output ostomy are serious enough that the risk/benefit ratio begins to tilt in favor of reestablishing gastrointestinal continuity, I will lower my threshold for reanastomosis (albeit at the expense of some sleepless nights). If the patient is off pressors and is completely resuscitated, I will consider a proximal small bowel anastomosis in a young patient regardless of transfusion requirement. In this setting, however, the anastomosis should be handsewn as staples frequently cannot accommodate the extra bowel wall thickness. For more distal small bowel resections, I will perform an anastomosis in a patient who received as many as 8–10 units of blood if the patient resuscitated easily, is relatively young, and has a promising clinical trajectory. If any of these caveats are violated, or if a higher blood volume was administered, I will perform an ileostomy. The morbidly obese patient with superimposed abdominal wall edema can make exteriorization of an ischemia-free ostomy difficult. When faced with a patient who mandates diversion but in whom an ostomy was not technically possible, a former colleague would place a large-caliber Malincott catheter into the afferent limb of bowel and exteriorize the catheter. This would theoretically convert it into a controlled fistula, and he reported good results with that technique.

Important Points

- On the first pass through the abdomen, just whip stitch enterotomies and colotomies.
- Beware of an odd number of holes in the bowel.
- Avoid blind whip stitching at the root of the mesentery.
- Paranoia is a healthy attitude when looking for bowel injuries.
- Leaving patients in discontinuity during a damage control procedure is safe and well-tolerated for up to 48 h.
- Planned re-explorations in which bleeding is not a concern can be safely done at the ICU bedside.
- Injuries less than 50% of the circumference of the bowel wall need only a primary repair.
- Colocolostomy should be your first choice after resection in young patients with no shock.
- For the patient who has had a damage control procedure, diversion should be the default choice.

References

1. Demetriades D, Murray JA, Chan LS et al (2001) Penetrating colon injuries requiring resection: diversion or primary anastomosis? An AAST prospective multicenter study. J Trauma 50:765–775
2. Demetriades D, Murray JA, Chan LS et al (2002) Handsewn versus stapled anastomosis in penetrating colon injuries requiring resection: a multicenter study. J Trauma 52: 117–121
3. Diaz JJ Jr, Mauer A, May AK et al (2004) Bedside laparotomy for trauma: are there risks? Surg Infect 5:15–20
4. Diaz JJ Jr, Mejia V, Subhawong AP et al (2005) Protocol for bedside laparotomy in trauma and emergency general surgery: a low return to the operating room. Am Surg 71:986–991
5. Cayten CG, Fabian TC, Garcia VF et al (1998) EAST patient management guidelines for penetrating intraperitoneal colon injuries. http://www.east.org/tpg/chap4.pdf Accessed 2010. (online only)

Injury of the Kidney, Ureter, and Bladder

46

Dorothy W. Bird and Suresh Agarwal

When a urologic injury is suspected in the context of penetrating trauma to the flank, abdomen or low chest, imaging of the upper urinary system is crucial for diagnosis. CT scan with IV contrast and delayed films at 10 min is the imaging modality of choice for hemodynamically stable patients. Images from CT scan should permit accurate injury staging based on the AAST criteria, which is highly predictive for operative management. Medial hematoma, with or without extravasation, on early films suggests renal vascular injury while that on delayed films is usually indicative of renal pelvic injury or proximal ureteral injury. Any part of the renal parenchyma that fails to show contrast on early phase images suggests arterial injury [1].

CT cystogram should be included in initial imaging if bladder injury is suspected as a result of penetrating trauma to the lower abdomen or pelvis. If this modality denies evidence of bladder injury despite clinical suspicion, retrograde cystography with full bladder distension and post-drainage images should also be performed [2, 3]. Importantly, retrograde cystogram should be performed only in the absence of uretheral injury.

In the hemodynamically unstable patient who proceeds immediately to surgery, bypassing CT scan, an on-table one-shot intravenous pyelogram (IVP) should be performed by giving a 2 mg/kg IV contrast bolus followed by flat plate x-ray 10 min later. The main purpose of the IVP is to demonstrate two functioning kidneys and an intact drainage system [2, 4, 5]. The presence of an injured solitary kidney should prompt more aggressive measures to spare nephrectomy that would otherwise commit the victim to a lifetime of dialysis or future transplantation.

D.W. Bird • S. Agarwal (✉)
Surgical Critical Care, Boston Medical Center, Boston, MA 02118, USA

Department of Surgery, Boston Medical Center, Boston University School of Medicine, 850 Harrison Avenue, Dowling 2 South, Boston, MA 02118, USA
e-mail: suresh.agarwal@bmc.org

46.1 Committing to Operative Management

With the broadening criteria for nonoperative management of renal injury, even in penetrating trauma including some gunshots, the only *absolute* indications for operative management are hemodynamic instability, expanding or pulsatile perirenal hematoma, incomplete renal injury staging, renal pelvic injury [6], or non-visualization of the injured kidney on IVP [7]. AAST stage I–III renal injuries are usually hemodynamically stable and are managed nonoperatively. Isolated stage IV renal injuries *may* be managed nonoperatively when hemodynamically stable but must be continually re-assessed and re-imaged by CT scan at 48 h or sooner depending upon clinical decompensation [7]. Superselective embolization may be attempted for certain patients with stage IV renal injuries who fail conservative management due to persistent bleeding from segmental arteries [4, 8]. Stage V renal injuries nearly always require operative intervention. This in mind, renal injuries suffered from penetrating trauma are almost always associated with other injuries that dictate the decision to operate.

All ureteral injuries require immediate operative repair. All bladder neck and intraperitoneal bladder

G.C. Velmahos et al. (eds.), *Penetrating Trauma*,
DOI 10.1007/978-3-642-20453-1_46,

injuries mandate repair, while most extraperitoneal injuries can be observed unless the victim undergoes laparotomy for other injuries.

46.2 Operative Technique

Once committed to operative management, a standard transabdominal midline incision is best for assessing renal injury as both kidneys can be inspected through this single approach and it allows for standard access to the remainder of the abdominal cavity [3, 9]. Abdominal packing, in typical trauma laparotomy fashion, will help control bleeding. Attention should first be turned to the destabilizing injury, urologic or otherwise [4].

46.3 Vascular Control

When the time comes to assess the bleeding kidney, vascular exposure is the first priority. Lift the transverse colon with a moist lap pad to the chest and move the small bowel to the right in order to expose the retroperitoneum. Carefully incise the retroperitoneum over the aorta at the inferior mesenteric artery and extend superiorly to the ligament to Treitz (Fig. 46.1). The left renal vein can be identified where it crosses the aorta anteriorly, noting that it rarely crosses posteriorly and when it does it may be duplicated. Sometimes a large retroperitoneal hematoma will distort endogenous anatomy. In this case, make the incision just medial to the inferior mesenteric vein and proceed to identify the left renal vein. Wrap a vessel loop around the vein without occluding it, unless bleeding from this vessel is heavy. The remaining renal vessels should be identified in order: left renal artery, right renal vein, right renal artery. The left and right renal arteries are posterior and superior to the left renal vein on either side of the aorta. Apply vessel loops to the renal arteries and veins, but ONLY occlude the vessels if severe bleeding must be controlled (Fig. 46.2) [3, 9].

Renal occlusion must be minimized to preserve function. Generally, arterial occlusion alone is enough to control hemorrhage. If occlusion is necessary for more than 60 min and patient stability permits, then ice slush may be used to cool the kidney to minimize warm ischemia time [3].

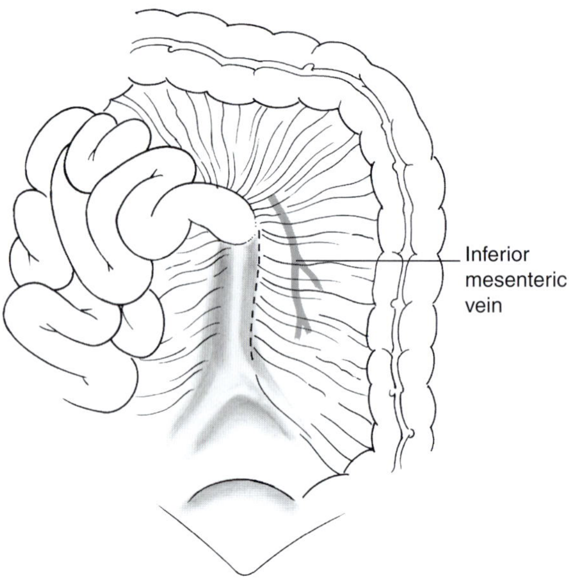

Fig. 46.1 Carefully incise the retroperitoneum over the aorta at the inferior mesenteric artery and extend superiorly to the ligament to Treitz (*dotted line*)

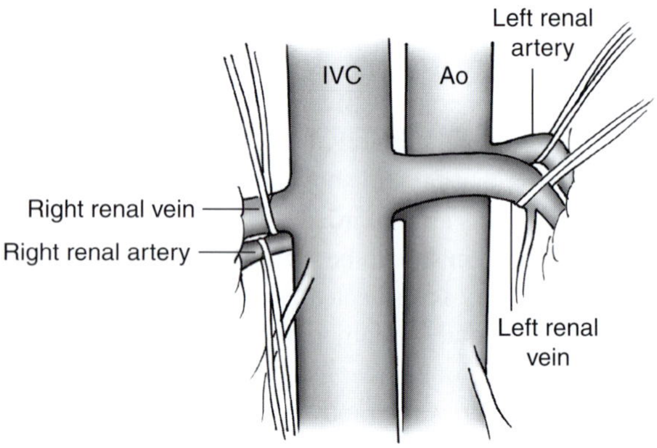

Fig. 46.2 Apply vessel loops to the renal arteries and veins but ONLY occlude the vessels if severe bleeding must be controlled

Anatomic variation of the renal vasculature is not uncommon with a high frequency of multiple renal arteries and veins making vascular control potentially difficult. Most notable are the prevalence of renal arteries originating below the IMA, multiple right renal veins, and less frequently retroaortic or circumaortic left renal vein [10]. When bleeding is not controlled through occlusion of standard renal vessels, thought must be paid to these anatomic variants.

When more urgent hemostasis is required or if the source of bleeding is unclear, then proximal control may be gained via the aorta at the GE junction or in the chest.

46.4 Vascular Repair

Vascular injuries to renal vessels are rare in the context of trauma and their repair is successful less than half of the time. You should only attempt renal artery salvage in the case of a solitary kidney, bilateral injuries, and if the injury is less than 6 h old [9].

Arterial and venous injuries should be repaired with running or interrupted vascular sutures. You can ligate segmental veins given extensive collateral blood flow. On the other hand, ligation of segmental arteries is problematic because they are end-organ vessels. If their sacrifice is necessary, distal parenchyma will become ischemic and subsequent evaluation and debridement must follow [3, 11].

Complete renal artery disruption will require debridement and excision of damaged vessel tissue followed by end-to-end tension-free anastomosis. Use saphenous vein or internal iliac artery graft to augment arterial repairs that may result in severe narrowing, usually defects greater than 2 cm. Try and avoid synthetic graft material due to the contaminated nature of the trauma laparotomy [3].

Renal autotransplantation may be considered if the renal artery pedicle is severely injured but the kidney itself is salvageable, especially if the patient has multiple injuries and damage control is the priority. The removed kidney may be re-implanted up to 48 h later when it is appropriately preserved.

Complete renal vein disruption may result in nephrectomy unless it is the left main renal vein at its origin with the vena cava, in which case you may ligate it as the kidney will benefit from the collateral drainage of the gonadal and adrenal veins [3].

46.5 Renal Exposure

Attention may be turned to renal exposure once renal vascular identification and control has been established. These techniques may also be applied to renal vascular exposure, especially in case of a large retroperitoneal hematoma.

Incise the retroperitoneum lateral to the colon at the white line of Toldt and reflect medially. On the left side, division of the splenorenal ligament followed by medial reflection of the spleen and colon will completely expose the left kidney and associated vasculature. When exploring the right side, incise the hepatic flexure in addition to the retroperitoneum lateral to the colon. Once the duodenum and pancreatic head are mobilized medially, the right renal artery and vein can be identified along with the origin of the left renal vein. Gerota's fascia may be incised along its lateral aspect for complete renal exposure. Preserve as much of the renal capsule as possible as it will likely be used for closure of the reconstruction [3, 9, 11].

46.6 Partial Nephrectomy

Partial nephrectomy is required when either pole of the kidney is severely damaged. You must be generously debride nonviable renal tissue down to active bleeding parenchyma noting that only 30% of a single normal kidney is needed to avoid dialysis. Suture-ligate individual bleeding vessels with 4-0 chromic sutures. Do not use nonabsorbable suture material in the parenchyma or collecting system. Parenchymal hemostasis may be achieved with direct pressure. Alternatively, a Keith needle with absorbable suture can be passed through the full thickness of the parenchyma, from capsule to capsule and back, with supporting pledgets to help achieve hemostasis. This should not be attempted if the collecting system is involved. Diffuse oozing can be managed with direct compression while electrocauterizing the denuded surface [4].

Close the collecting system with a watertight running 4-0 chromic suture. Integrity of the closure may be tested by injecting methylene blue dye into the renal pelvis while compressing the ureter and inspecting for extravasation. Thrombin-soaked gelfoam may be placed between cut parenchymal edges to improve hemostasis. Gently pull the capsule directly over the defect and secure. If sufficient capsule is unavailable, an omental pedicle flap may be used to cover the defect (Fig. 46.3) [3, 9].

46.7 Renorrhaphy

Renorrhaphy is necessary for middle kidney damage. As for partial nephrectomy, debride nonviable tissue to bleeding parenchyma. Ligate vessels and close the collecting system with 4-0 chromic suture as above.

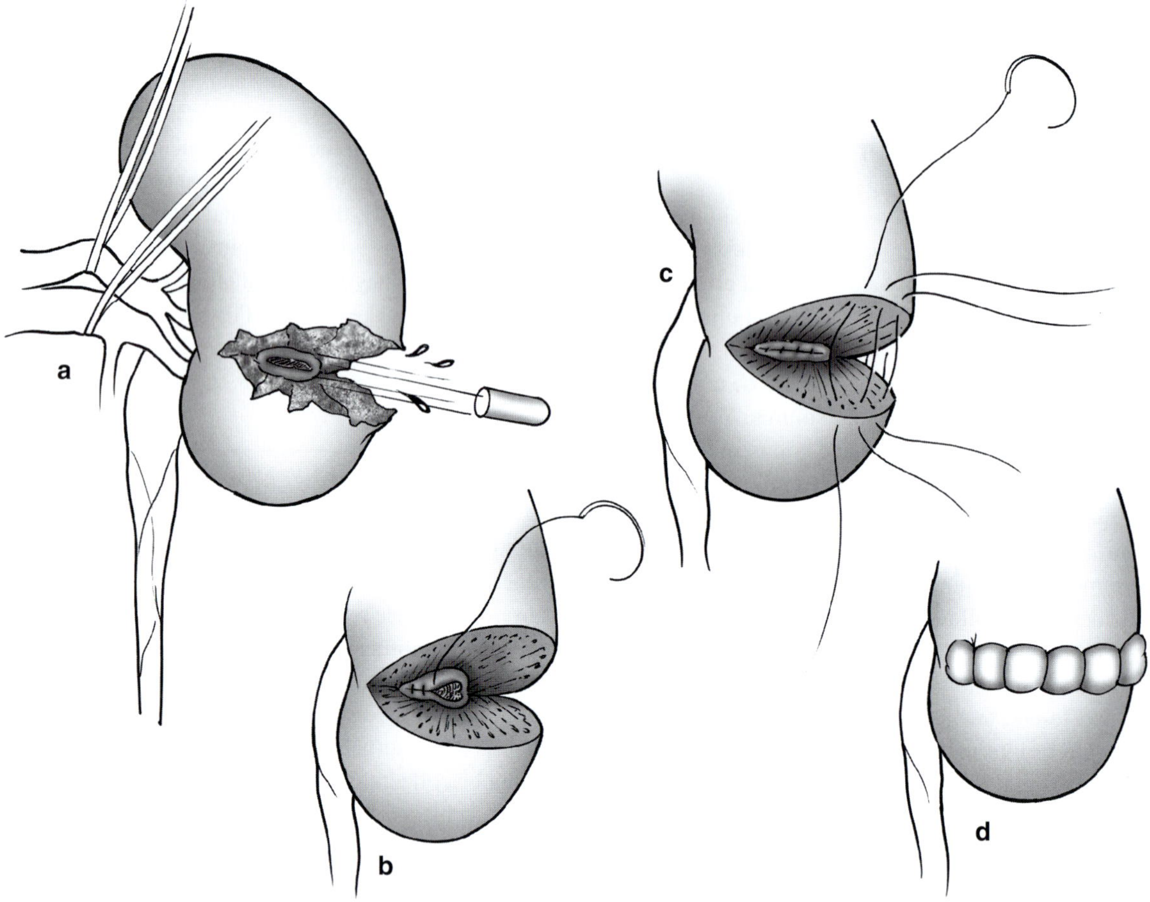

Fig. 46.3 The injured kidney is debrided sparsely (**a**). Gently pull the capsule directly over the defect and secure (**c**) after closure of the collecting system (**b**). If sufficient capsule is unavailable, an omental pedicle flap may be used to cover the defect (**d**)

Approximate parenchymal edges and secure with interrupted 3-0 absorbable sutures anchored to the capsule for support, tied over an absorbable gelatin bolster. As for partial nephrectomy, an omental pedicle flap can be used to close the defect if capsule quantity is inadequate. Similarly, absorbable mesh can help stabilize the extensively repaired kidney [3, 9].

Following partial nephrectomy or renorrhaphy, a retroperitoneal drain should be placed WITHOUT suction and left in place for 2–3 days, or longer if output is high or creatinine from the drainage is elevated.

46.8 Nephrectomy

When the kidney is shattered or in the context of damage control laparotomy, nephrectomy may be inevitable. Perform ligation of the renal artery first with long-lasting absorbable suture. Double suture ligation is necessary only in the presence of severe atherosclerosis. Follow with ligation of the renal vein. Complete renal isolation by ligating the ureter in two places close to the bladder [11].

46.9 Ureteral Repair

A high index of suspicion is required to diagnose ureteral injury. Although CT scan, IVP, or retrograde pyelography may diagnose this injury, intraoperative diagnosis via direct inspection with or without intravenous or intra-ureteral injection of indigo carmine or methylene blue to confirm the integrity of the collecting system may be required to diagnose ureteral disruption. Ureteral blast injury from nearby intra-abdominal gunshot is more difficult to diagnose as the delayed necrosis that occurs as a result of intimal disruption is often not apparent immediately, although sometimes may appear as bruising on the ureteral wall [3, 12].

Immediate repair is needed when ureteral injury or devascularization is identified. Debride nonviable tissue to healthy bleeding tissue and perform a watertight tension-free repair. During damage control laparotomy, tying off the injured ureteral segment with a long silk suture is preferred until the patient is stable for delayed ureteral reconstruction, usually several months later. Urinary diversion via percutaneous nephrostomy drain can be undertaken postoperatively [3, 12, 13]. Alternatively, drainage of the proximal end of the disrupted ureter with a ureteral stent or pediatric feeding tube brought out through the skin with spatulated ureteral edges sewn to skin, forming a stoma, is another option [14].

Partial ureteral transection may be closed primarily with interrupted 4-0 or 5-0 absorbable monofilament suture, unless the injury is caused by gunshot, in which case more extensive debridement plus ureteroureterostomy is recommended. Handling of the ureters during mobilization should always be minimized as blood supply is easily disrupted. Approximate the lumen with absorbable 4-0 or 5-0 monofilament suture and place a double J stent when the defect is greater than 50% of the lumen and complete the repair with interrupted sutures as above. Remove the stent after 6 weeks. A guidewire will facilitate stent placement when placed through a side hole of the double J stent and directing one end of the stent upward to the renal pelvis and the other end to the bladder. Use an omental flap to isolate the segment if the repair is tenuous or if significant contamination is present in the peritoneal cavity. A retroperitoneal gravity drain is strongly encouraged as it will permit early diagnosis of urinary leakage should it occur and will help small anastomostic gaps heal [3, 12, 13].

46.10 Ureteroureterostomy

Middle and upper ureteral injuries are best repaired with ureteroureterostomy. Mobilization of proximal and distal segments should be performed gingerly to avoid devascularization. As above, debride nonviable tissue to healthy bleeding and spatulate the ends. Tack the apices of each spatulation through the opposite ureter with 4-0 or 5-0 absorbable suture, ensuring that knots are exterior. Clamps applied to the tails of these sutures will help stabilize the field to minimize handling. Insert a double J sent and complete the anastomosis with interrupted 4-0 or 5-0 absorbable suture; anterior side first, posterior side second (Fig. 46.4). Consider an omental flap if contamination is high or infection likely. Drain retroperitoneally without suction [3, 12, 13].

If a tension-free anastomosis cannot be achieved through direct re-approximation of proximal and distal segments, then end-to-side transureteroureterostomy should be considered. The proximal segment of the injured ureter can be brought through the mesentery either above or below the IMA (depending on degree of loss), always being mindful of the potential for ureteral devascularization. Spatulate the end of the mobilized ureter before incising the contralateral ureter with a 2-cm longitudinal medial ureterotomy. Tack the apices of the spatulated end to the inferior and superior poles of the ureterotomy with a 4-0 or 5-0 absorbable suture. Start the stitch from the ureterotomy, then bring through spatulated end. Insert a double J stent and close the anastomosis with 4-0 or 5-0 absorbable interrupted suture. Apply an omental flap as needed and always insert a retroperitoneal drain [3].

46.11 Ureteroneocystostomy

Distal ureteral injuries in the stable patient are best repaired with ureteroneocystostomy. Debride the proximal ureteral end to healthy, bleeding tissue and spatulate the end. A tunnel should be created for its insertion superior and medial to the original distal ureteral opening at a length of three times the ureteral diameter. Anastomose the ureter to the interior aspect of the bladder using 5-0 absorbable sutures and place an internal stent (Fig. 46.5). Ligation of the original distal ureteral stump is needed only if reflux is suspected [12].

Other alternatives to help achieve a tension-free anastomosis include ureteral re-implantation with psoas hitch and the Boari flap, both of which can provide additional distal length when needed. Both are beyond the scope of this discussion and are well described in the texts referenced at the end of this chapter.

46.12 Autotransplantation

Renal autotransplantation is rarely the best option for the renal trauma patient, but in instances of a damaged solitary kidney or renal artery avulsion or collecting system avulsion in the setting of damage control

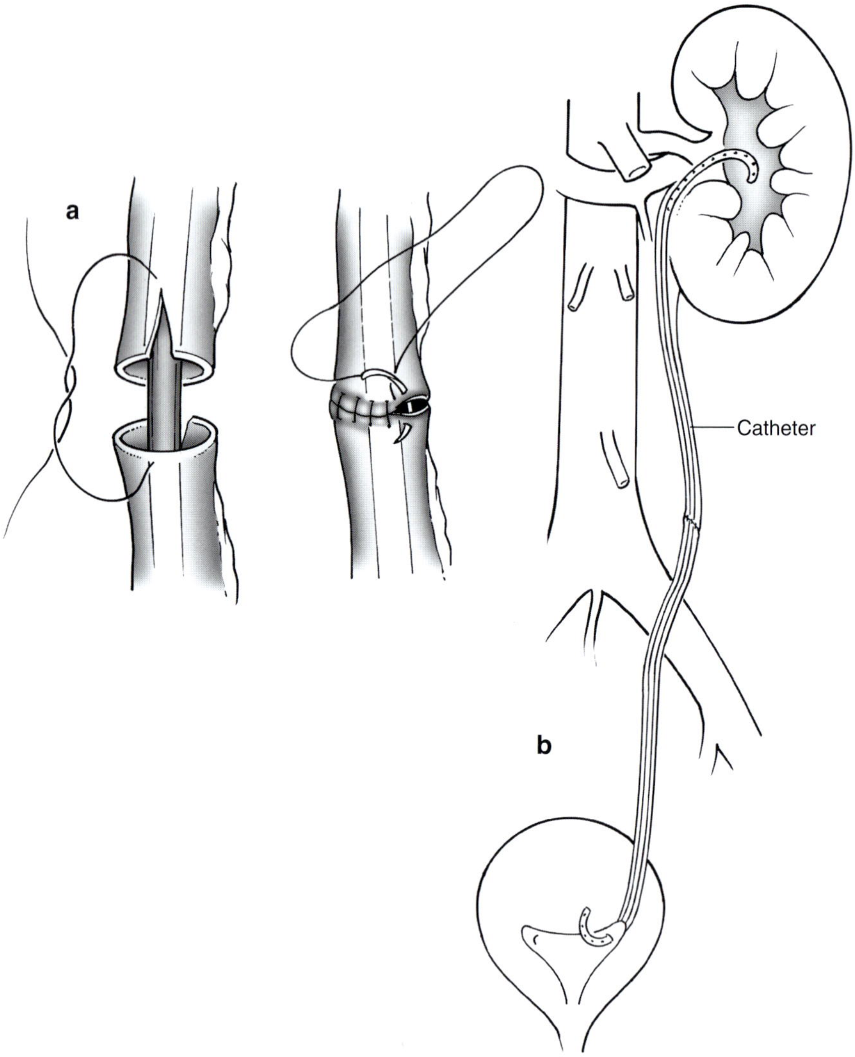

Fig. 46.4 In ureteroureterostomy, insert a double J stent (**a**, **b**) and complete the anastomosis with interrupted 4-0 or 5-0 absorbable suture; anterior side first, posterior side second (**a**)

surgery, renal autotransplantation may potentially save the patient from a lifetime of dialysis or allograft. Once the choice has been made to proceed with autotransplantation, the kidney should be removed rapidly with minimal surgical manipulation. Maximize length of donor vessels and ureter. The removed kidney should be flushed immediately with cold intracellular electrolyte solution (500 mL of Collins or University of Wisconsin solution) intra-arterially and submerged in a basin of ice slush saline solution until transfer to an appropriate cooler if the transplant will take place at another operation.

The renal artery is typically replanted end-to-end to the hypogastric artery or end-to-side to the external or common iliac artery. Depending on the available anatomy, the end-to-end operation is usually performed in the contralateral iliac fossa whereas the ipsilateral iliac fossa is used for end-to-side operations. The iliac fossa should be exposed by reflecting the peritoneum superiorly and medially so that the common iliac artery and bladder can be visualized. A self-retaining ring retractor will help maintain exposure; however, retractor blades must be placed with caution to the lateral femoral cutaneous nerve and inferior common iliac artery. Lymphatic tissue must be meticulously ligated to avoid postoperative lymphatocele, as this region is rich in lymphatic channels.

Dissect the external iliac vein carefully from its origin to the femoral junction. Place vascular clamps proximally and distally on the external iliac vein and

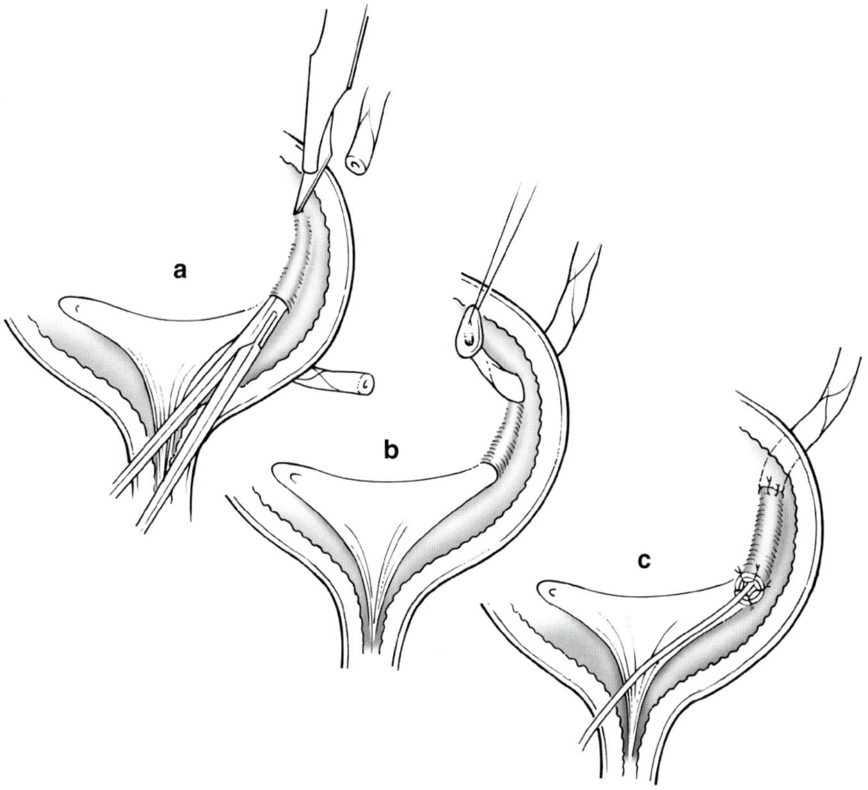

Fig. 46.5 In ureterocystostomy, anastomose the tunneled ureter to the interior aspect of the bladder using 5-0 absorbable sutures and place an internal stent (**a**–**c**)

complete a narrow elliptical venotomy on the vein's anterolateral aspect. If the hypogastric artery is to receive the renal artery, it should be occluded proximally and ligated and divided distally. If the external iliac artery or common iliac artery is to be used, occlude the common iliac, external iliac and hypogastric arteries with vascular clamps before making the arteriotomy. Inject heparin into the recipient vessels and bring the autotransplant into the field.

The end-to-side venous anastomosis is performed first using continuous 5-0 vascular suture. The arterial anastomosis is performed second using interrupted 6-0 vascular suture. At this point, the vascular clamps should be removed to assess for leaks and repairs performed as needed.

Finally the ureteroneocystostomy should be performed. Using the shortest possible length of ureter to avoid kinking and ischemia, spatulate the distal end of the donor ureter. Make a 3-cm incision at the posterolateral aspect of the bladder and incise down the expose the mucosa. Undermine the muscular layer of the bladder, slightly make a small opening into the bladder mucosa at the inferior pole of the incision. Complete a mucosa-to-mucosa anastomosis between the ureter and bladder using 4-0 chromic sutures (continuous or interrupted). The distal-most end of the anastomosis should be anchored through the full thickness of the bladder wall. The 3-0 chromic sutures are then used to close the bladder muscle over the ureter [3].

46.13 Bladder Repair

Repair of intraperitoneal bladder injuries is usually achieved through primary closure of the defect and placement of a urethral catheter. A transperitoneal cystotomy should be made to visualize the entire lumen as unrecognized extraperitoneal ruptures are not uncommon and should be repaired at the time of intraperitoneal bladder repair. If bleeding from pelvic hematoma is encountered (as it frequently is in the context of pelvic fractures), be prepared with sponges and perform suture-ligations as needed [3, 11, 15, 16].

The ureteral orifices should be identified, and after IV indigo carmine injection, blue urine should be observed effluxing from each opening. If the injury is close to or involving the ureteral opening, a ureteral stent should be placed [14].

Debridement of damaged bladder tissue is usually minimal in light of its extensive blood supply. The intraperitoneal bladder injury can be closed with running 3-0 suture in the mucosa and running 2-0 in the muscularis propria. The peritoneum should be closed with a separate 3-0 running absorbable suture [3].

46.14 Bladder Neck Repair

Bladder neck injuries are notoriously difficult to repair, but should be attempted to preserve continence. The injury should be exposed through a cystotomy at the dome and all tears closed with absorbable sutures. Placement of Foley catheter and suprapubic tube, as described above, is recommended. Vaginal lacerations should be repaired at the same time [3, 14, 15].

Important Points

1. On-table one-shot IVP should be used to prove the presence of two functional kidneys and an intact collecting system when CT scan is not possible.
2. Renal vascular exposure and control should be addressed first, occluding vessels only as needed and only for less than 30 min.
3. Partial nephrectomy is indicated for polar injuries, renorrhaphy for middle kidney injuries, and nephrectomy for shattered kidneys and unsalvageable vascular injuries.
4. During damage control laparotomy, nephrectomy is appropriate with consideration for delayed autotransplantation if the kidney is salvageable.
5. Directly inspect the ureters for injury with a low threshold for resection and debridement, especially in the context of intra-abdominal gunshot injury.
6. Ureteral ligation with delayed percutaneous nephrostomy drainage or externalized ureteral stent is acceptable, temporizing measures for ureteral injury during damage control laparotomy.
7. Utilize ureteroureterostomy for proximal and middle ureteral injury and ureteroneocystostomy for distal injury.
8. Always use a retroperitoneal drain following reconstruction WITHOUT suction.
9. Always use absorbable sutures in the genitourinary tract.
10. Operative repair is standard for intraperitoneal bladder injury, whereas nonoperative management with catheter drainage is standard for most extraperitoneal bladder injuries.

References

1. Alskiafi NF, Rosenstein DI (2006) Staging, evaluation, and nonoperative management of renal injuries. Urol Clin North Am 33:13–19
2. Tezval H, Tezval M, von Klot C, Herrmann T, Dresing K, Jonas U, Burchardt M (2007) Urinary tract injuries in patients with multiple trauma. World J Surg 25(2):177–184
3. McAninch J, Carroll P, Jordan G (1996) Traumatic and reconstructive urology. W. B. Saunders Company, Philadelphia
4. Mattox KL, Feliciano DV, Moore EE (2000) Trauma, 4th edn. McGraw-Hill, New York
5. Goldman S, Sandler C (2004) Urogenital trauma: imaging upper GU trauma. Eur J Radiol 50(1):84–95
6. Broghammer JA, Fisher MB, Santucci RA (2007) Conservative management of renal trauma: a review. Urology 70:623–629
7. Buckley JC, McAninch JW (2006) Selective management of isolated and nonisolated grade IV renal injuries. J Urol 176:2498–2502
8. Brewyer BN, McAninch JW, Elliott SP, Master VA (2008) Minimally invasive endovascular techniques to treat acute renal hemorrhage. J Urol 179:2248–2253
9. Master VA, McAninch JW (2006) Operative management of renal injuries: parenchymal and vascular. Urol Clin North Am 33:21–31
10. Kaneko N, Kobaysashi Y, Okada Y (2008) Anatomic variations of the renal vessels pertinent to transperitoneal vascular control in the management of trauma. Surgery 143: 616–622
11. Krane RJ, Siroky MB, Fitzpatrick JM (2000) Operative urology. Churchill Livingstone, New York
12. Elliott SP, McAninch JW (2006) Ureteral injuries: external and iatrogenic. Urol Clin North Am 33:55–66
13. Elliot S, McAninch J (2003) Ureteral injuries from external violence: the 25-year experience at San Francisco General Hospital. J Urol 170:1213–1216
14. Thal ER, Weigelt JA, Carrico CJ (2002) Operative trauma management, 2nd edn. McGraw-Hill, New York
15. Corriere JN, Sandler CM (2006) Diagnosis and management of bladder injuries. Urol Clin North Am 33:67–71
16. Volpe MA, Pachter EM, Scalea TM, Macchio RJ, Mydlo JH (1999) Is there a difference in outcome with treating traumatic intraperitoneal bladder rupture with or without a suprapubic tube? J Urol 161(4):1103–1105

Lower Genitourinary Injuries

47

Donald Hannoun and Charles D. Best

47.1 Acute Scrotal and Testis Injuries

Trauma to the external genitalia can be separated into blunt versus penetrating injury. Differentiating between these two mechanisms will have the immediate benefit of facilitating patient care in the trauma suite. Noting the mechanism of injury will also help you determine the likelihood of need for eventual surgery, the potential length of convalescence, and the possibility of injury to the contralateral testis. Particularly with penetrating injuries, you should have a high index of suspicion of injury to the contralateral testicle. It may also assist in prediction of future fertility.

Several features of the scrotum and testis make these structures relatively resilient to trauma. The mobility of the scrotum allows displacement from inciting injury, and the cremasteric reflex helps move the testis superiorly upon scrotal contact. Additionally, the testis has a relatively tough tunica albuginea, which can help contain a developing hematoma and prevent seminiferous tubule extrusion [1, 2].

The vast majority (between 75% and 85%) of scrotal/testicular injuries results from blunt trauma and are typically unilateral [1, 3]. Penetrating injuries to the scrotum are typically gunshot or stab wounds and are more likely to result in bilateral testicular injury (30%), while only 1.5% of blunt scrotal injuries are bilateral. [1]

D. Hannoun (✉) • C.D. Best
Department of Urology and Surgery,
USC Institute of Urology, USC Keck School of Medicine,
LAC+USC County Medical Center,
Los Angeles, CA, USA
e-mail: dhannoun@usc.edu; cbest@usc.edu

A detailed history and physical exam will usually indicate the likely mechanism and underlying injury, often dictating further workup and management. We will often acquire a testicular ultrasound to determine whether the testicle itself is injured, and assess the contralateral testicle as well. Basic palpation is also a simple but very helpful aspect of the initial physical exam. Inability to palpate the testis may suggest the presence of testicular rupture or testicular displacement (often back towards the superficial or external inguinal ring) by an expanding scrotal hematoma. As always, you should always maintain a high index of suspicion for urethral injury, especially with penetrating trauma. Inability to void and an expanding scrotum with or without scrotal ecchymosis may suggest urinary extravasation, and should proceed to work up with a retrograde urethrogram (RUG) or gentle passage of a urethral catheter.

During initial evaluation and work up of scrotal or testicular injury, you should also take into account the patient's clinical status and hemodynamic stability. Lower genitourinary injuries are not often life threatening. If the patient is clinically stable for transfer, a scrotal ultrasound can help identify the injury (i.e., hypoechoic testicular lesions suggest hematoceles, disruption of the tunica albuginea suggests rupture, lack of blood flows suggests torsion, etc.). Facilitating these diagnostic studies early in a clinically stable patient allows for early diagnosis.

If the patient is physiologically unstable, then a portable study can be performed at the bedside in the intensive care setting. Unfortunately, scrotal ultrasounds can have a high false-negative rate even in the presence of an experienced examiner. For this reason, if the index of suspicion for testicular injury is high,

G.C. Velmahos et al. (eds.), *Penetrating Trauma*,
DOI 10.1007/978-3-642-20453-1_47, © Springer-Verlag Berlin Heidelberg 2012

which is often the case with penetrating injuries of the scrotum, explore the patient if noninvasive diagnostic testing is unavailable or unsafe. Realistically, if the patient is unstable, the scrotal or testicle injury is low on the list of priorities.

The management of scrotal/testicular injury will also often depend on the overall clinical status of the patient. In the face of multiple medical or surgical comorbidities, the patient may not be stable enough for transfer to the operative suite for intervention. Communication between the primary team and consulting services should dictate the appropriate plan of action best suited for the patient's overall improvement.

In the case of multiple injuries requiring exploration, surgical intervention for scrotal or testicular injury should be as rapid as clinically possible. Even when the involved testicle is an isolated injury, we recommend minimizing any delay in repair. Several studies have shown that prompt surgical intervention with testicular rupture, especially if performed within 72 h of the injury, will often prevent superinfection of the scrotal hematoma, lessen the length of convalescence, decrease the potential for chronic pain, and may even improve fertility [4]. Gross et al. reported an improvement in testicular salvage rate from 32% to 80% if surgical exploration was performed within 3 days of the inciting injury [2, 4], and Jeffrey et al. and Lupetin et al. went on to show testicular salvage rates of 90% when surgical intervention was performed within 72 h [2, 5, 6].

Surgical intervention is usually performed transscrotally, with the incision made down the midline raphe of the scrotum to allow bilateral testicular assessment and management. Carry down the dissection through the dartos layer to the tunica vaginalis, which may or may not be intact. Bring the testis, epididymis, and distal spermatic cord onto the field, and examine closely for any evidence of injury. If the testicular injury is severe and salvage is unlikely, then proceed to an orchiectomy. Tunica albuginea violation should be apparent once the testis is delivered from the tunica vaginalis. With tunica albuginea disruption, you should attempt to debride any unviable seminiferous tubule tissue. The presence of active bleeding is a sign that remaining tissue is viable. If there is any question about testicular viability, an intraoperative Doppler study should be performed to guide further intervention. Repair the defect with a running 4-0 suture, prolene being the suture of choice at our institution (Fig. 47.1b). Damage to the vas deferens should be addressed with ligation and delayed reconstruction. Vasovasostomy is not a trivial procedure, and should not be done in an acute setting.

You should always anticipate potential postsurgical complications and should pay strict attention to hemostasis prior to scrotal closure. In the presence of persistent bleeding or an underlying coagulopathy, place a quarter inch penrose drain in the inferior/dependent portion of the scrotum to prevent accumulation of a postoperative hematoma. The dartos closure is carried out with a running 4-0 Vicryl stitch, and the scrotal skin closure with a running or interrupted 3-0 chromic suture with locking of each suture. Leave the penrose drain to gravity drainage into a kerlix roll, which is held closely to the scrotum with a scrotal support for comfort and elevation. Remove the drain 24–48 h postoperatively. Antibiotics are routinely recommended for 7–10 days postoperatively to prevent abscess formation or infections along the incision line [2]. Apply antibiotic ointment to the suture line three times a day for 7–10 days.

Genital avulsion injuries can be considered another form of penetrating trauma to the scrotum. These injuries are sustained during rapid deceleration of the body and concomitant shearing mechanism against the scrotum and perineum, leading to loss of the scrotal skin. In the majority of situations, you can close the scrotal skin primarily at the time of surgery with a running chromic suture as previously described, after copious irrigation. Even with up to 60% of the scrotal skin lost, the skin can still often be closed primarily [7]. Larger amounts of genital skin loss will necessitate wet-to-dry dressings postoperatively with delayed grafting [2]. As always, scrotal avulsion injuries should always be assessed for underlying testicular injury, and you should manage them appropriately.

47.2 Penile Injury

Penetrating penile injuries are relatively rare, and usually take the form of gunshot and stab wounds. However, one can also encounter penile avulsion injuries from motor-vehicle or bicycle accidents as well as the occasional self-mutilating injuries and animal or

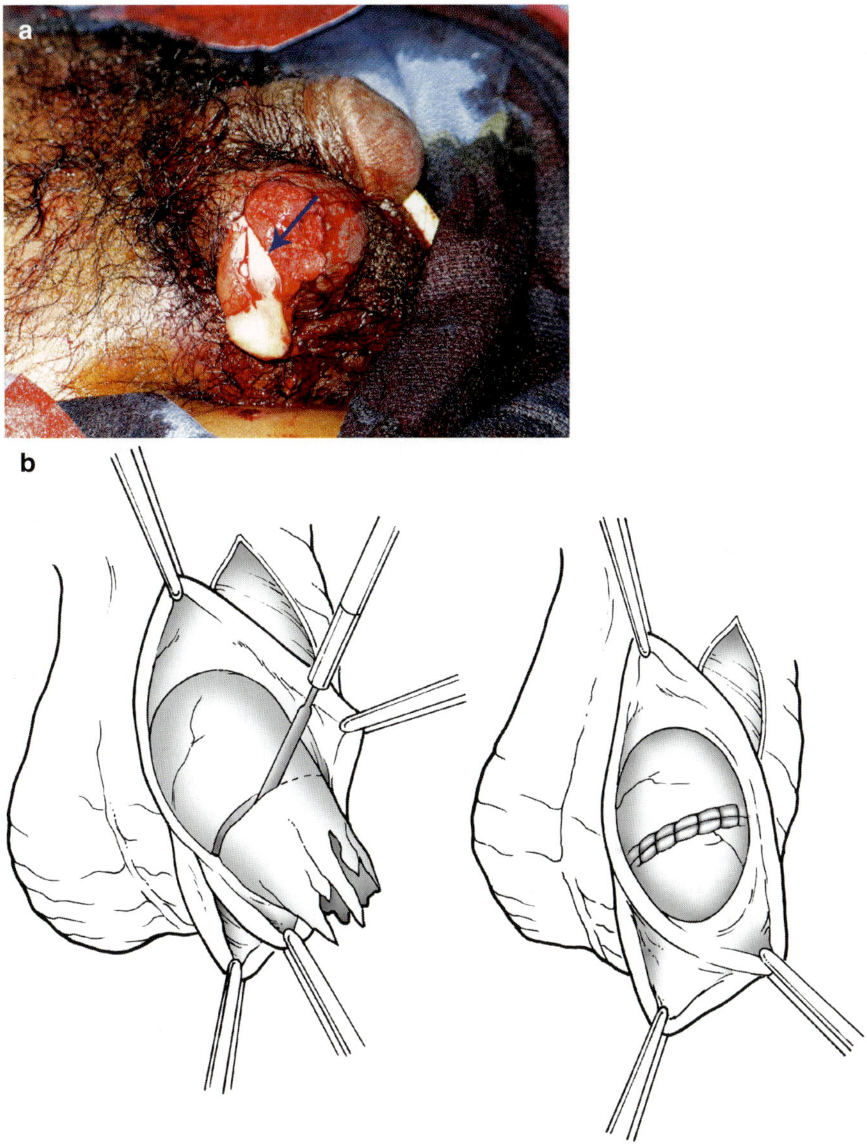

Fig. 47.1 (**a**) Often with penetrating injuries, the testicular injury is obvious, as is seen here where the tunica albuginea has been disrupted (*arrow*). (**b**) Repair the defect with a running 4-0 suture, prolene being the suture of choice at our institution

human bites. Despite the above-mentioned multiple possible mechanisms of penile trauma, significant penile injuries remain rare secondary to the tough tunica albuginea covering of the penis [8]. Penetrating penile injuries may result in a tear of the tunica albuginea encasing the corpora cavernosum, which allows extravasation of blood from the corpora into the penile shaft. Because of the penetrating nature of the injury, blood will exit out of the wound site, typically not extending along fascial lines, as with penile fracture. The penis may swell and have some ecchymosis, but you usually do not see the so-called "eggplant penis" appearance in penetrating injuries.

With penetrating injuries to the penis, you should always suspect compromise of the tunica albuginea. The mechanism alone will almost always mandate surgical exploration. However, if the diagnosis is in question, further imaging studies are available, although with highly variable results and inter-interpreter variations. Cavernosograms can be performed with injection of contrast material into the corpus cavernosum, with serial radiographs taken to identify the site of extravasation [2, 9]. The false-negative rate is unfortunately very high with this modality, as the tear can be too small to see, and often the presence of a clot at the tear site will mask the extravasation. False-positive studies result when the physiologic egress of contrast through emissary veins is misinterpreted as extravasation. Similarly, penile ultrasound cannot consistently identify the site of tear unless in the hands of a very skilled examiner [10, 11]. MRI in the T1 phase, although more sensitive than cavernosography and ultrasound, has a limited role secondary to the time required, the difficulty with transportation, and the frequent clinical instability of the patient [12]. These studies have no role in significant penetrating injuries. They have value in cases of penile fracture, when there is an atypical presentation. You should always suspect underlying urethral injury with any penetrating penile trauma. If the patient has not spontaneously voided clear urine, or has hematuria, either gross or microscopic, a RUG should be performed prior to surgical exploration to assess for urethral injury.

Tunical violation injuries of the penis should ideally be surgically corrected within 36 h of sustaining the injury. Exploration is mandatory to prevent the sequelae of infected hematomas, impotence, and penile curvature that may result without prompt operative intervention [13, 14]. Again, other more life-threatening injuries should be identified and addressed first.

Once the patient has reached the operative suite, the appropriate area is prepped and draped in standard sterile fashion. Insert a urethral catheter at the beginning to ensure ease of passage into the bladder. You can then use this catheter for the retrograde instillation of saline/dye during the procedure to evaluate for any urethral discontinuity [15]. First make a circumferential ("degloving") incision, which allows access to the length of the corpora cavernosum and spongiosum. Place a tourniquet at the base of the penis as it can aid with hemostasis and dissection (Fig. 47.2a). Carry out evacuation of the hematoma, and localize the site of tunical violation after you dissect free Buck's fascia. Once you have identified the defect, debride the wound edges and do copious irrigation, particularly important with gunshot injuries or bites. Carry on primary closure of the defect with 4-0 prolene suture in a figure-of-8 fashion. We prefer to do this with the knots buried, to decrease the chance of the patient potentially feeling the suture under the thin penile skin (Fig 47.2b). Avoid any significant length of running suture, as any cinching of the tissue may result in penile curvature. If there has been any rupture of the tunica albuginea close to one centimeter or larger, perform an artificial erection after the repair. This is necessary to determine if any curvature has resulted from the repair. Do this by applying a tourniquet at the base of the penis, and injecting one of the cavernosal bodies, via a butterfly needle, with normal saline until appropriate turgor is achieved. If there is any notable curvature, a plication of the tunica on the opposite side of the defect may be necessary. Repair any urethral injuries over a urethral catheter as mentioned in the chapter section to follow. After you have reapproximated the skin, place a compressive dressing and remove it the evening of surgery or the following morning. Leave the catheter in place until the following morning unless a urethroplasty is performed. Administer antibiotics for 7–10 days following the repair to prevent penile abscess development.

Surgical exploration may be unnecessary if the penetrating penile injury fails to result in tunical violation. Relatively small penile tears can be locally irrigated, debrided, and repaired with simple, interrupted closure and an absorbable 2-0 or 3-0 suture. With larger defects, initially perform local irrigation and debridement. Evaluate the wounds later for either primary closure with reapproximation, or reconstruction with delayed grafting. These wounds are frequently contaminated, and all patients should be placed on a 10-day antibiotic course with an antibiotic that provides adequate coverage of typical skin flora, such as cephalexin. For penicillin allergic patients, you can use chloramphenicol.

Penile amputation injuries can be accidental or self-inflicted. The timing of the incident and the presence and handling of the severed penis are crucial to the initial management. The severed penis should be wrapped with saline-soaked gauze, placed into a sterile bag (if possible), and immediately placed in ice water. The ice should never be in direct contact with the penis to prevent necrosis [2, 16]. If possible, the amputated penis should be reimplanted within 24 h of the injury. Transfer to a tertiary medical center is usually required for the expertise of microvascular anastomoses that is often necessary. After appropriate medical and psychosocial issues have been addressed and other more life-threatening injuries have been ruled out, the patient is taken to the operating room immediately for reimplantation. It is extremely important to have an experienced team of urologists, plastic surgeons, and OR staff in order to have a good result. Of primary importance is the cavernosal and spongiosum/urethral reanastomoses. A urethral catheter is inserted prior to the urethral anastomosis. Microsurgical techniques can be

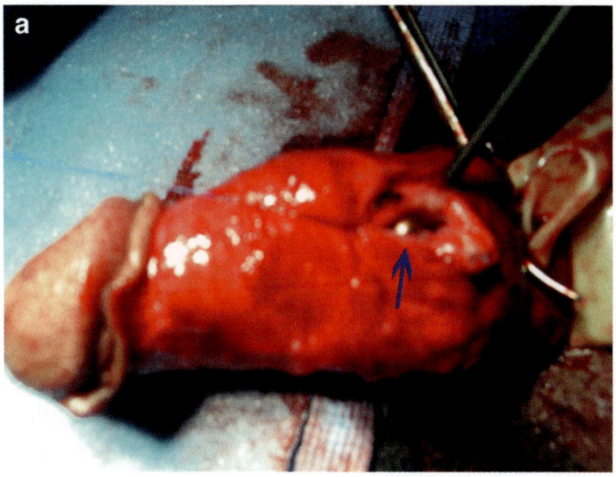

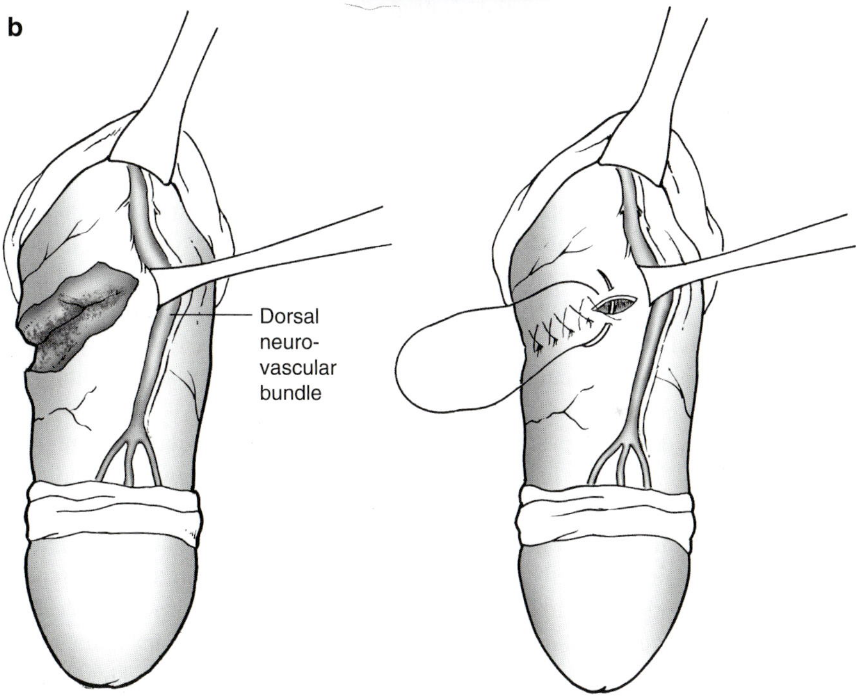

Fig. 47.2 (**a**) Place a tourniquet at the base of the penis as it can aid with hemostasis and dissection. (**b**) Debride the wound edges and do copious irrigation, particularly important with gunshot injuries or bites. Carry on primary closure of the defect with 4-0 prolene suture in a figure-of-8 fashion, and avoid any significant length of running suture, as any cinching of the tissue may result in penile curvature. In this figure, a corporal injury is present with the bullet visible (*arrow*)

used to reapproximate the dorsal arteries and nerve of the penis to improve the recovery of postoperative perfusion and sensation, respectively. Next, the tunica should be reconstructed. Finally, the debrided skin should be sewn together, much like any other superficial anastomosis. It is not unusual to have delayed sloughing of the penile skin. This does not necessarily imply that the reimplant as a whole has not survived. Delayed skin-grafting may be all that is necessary. If the severed penis is not available, then overclosure of the corpus cavernosum with advancement of the urethral stump can be performed to allow voiding while standing. An inadequate distal urethral remnant may obviate the need for perineal urethrostomy, with delayed genital reconstruction pending complete psychosocial evaluation.

47.3 Urethral Injury

As with other traumatic genitourinary injuries, the mechanism of urethral injury can be divided into blunt versus penetrating. Urethral injuries can be further subdivided into posterior (prostatic/membranous urethra) and anterior (bulbar/pendulous urethra) in location. These subdivisions not only classify the location of the injury but also dictate further management. Penetrating anterior and posterior urethral injuries are usually secondary to gunshot and stab wounds. These injuries are much more prevalent in males than females owing to the shorter urethral length, greater urethral mobility, and lesser pubourethral attachments in females.

The diagnosis of urethral injury would ideally be elicited from a detailed history and physical examination. For obvious reasons, this is not always the case. Often, the urologic team becomes involved after prior failed attempts have already been made in the emergency department (ED) to place a urethral catheter. This often culminates in improper catheter placement with possible conversion of a partial urethral tear to a full and circumferential urethral tear. We try to emphasize not attempting blind urethral catheterization if there is any suspicion of urethral injury. The mechanism of injury should prompt the initial suspicion for urethral injury. Failure to void since the incident or suprapubic fullness/distention should be assumed to represent urethral injury until proven otherwise. Gunshot wounds with either an entrance or exit from the perineum or penis should alert any diagnostician to a possible urethral injury.

The classical finding of a urethral injury on examination is the presence of blood at the meatus, though its presence is not definitive evidence and its absence is not exclusionary. Severe or expanding scrotal swelling, with or without ecchymosis, may also suggest urinary extravasation. Perineal hematomas, which can take on the classic "butterfly" hematoma pattern, should also alert the clinician for further urethral workup. Hematoma along the entire penile shaft (so-called sleeve hematoma) can be secondary to penile, urethral, or testicular injury.

With any of the aforementioned history or physical exam findings (suspected mechanism of injury, penetrating injury, blood at the meatus, scrotal/perineal hematoma), one should proceed with a retrograde urethrogram (RUG) or attempt gentle catheter placement [17]. The RUG can be performed in several ways, and can be done either in a formal radiology suite with the combination of fluoroscopy, in the ED, operating room, or at the bedside. A 12–14Fr catheter can be inserted just into the fossa navicularis, with only 1–2 cm^3 instilled into the balloon to tamponade the urethra and prevent the antegrade leakage of contrast. Next, inject about 15–20 cm^3 of contrast, with the radiograph being performed at the end of the injection to ensure adequate urethral distention. Alternatively, the aforementioned procedure can be performed with a 60 cm^3 catheter tip syringe (filled with contrast) inserted very gently into the urethra until a snug fit is obtained. At our institution, the RUG is performed by placing the patient in a slightly lateral (about 30°–45°) decubitus position. The penis is appropriately sterilized with a betadine preparation, and sterile draping placed underneath the penis. Next, about 20 cm of a small Kerlix roll is cut, soaked with water/saline, and then tied to the subcoronal position of the penis with a simple tie. This maneuver will allow penile traction during contrast instillation to help delineate the entire urethra, as well as appropriately shield the examiner's hands/body from the radiation field. A separate catheter tip is then lubricated and placed on a 60 cm^3 Luer-lock syringe pre-filled with contrast, and the injection is performed. The radiograph is taken after 20 cm^3 of contrast has been instilled. Urethral injuries on a RUG will appear as a disruption of the normally concentric urethra from meatus to bladder neck. A partial disruption represents extravasation along the course of the urethra with some contrast instillation into the bladder, whereas a complete disruption will fail to fill the bladder at all, with contrast accumulating in a periurethral or perivesical location.

The management of urethral injuries can be divided simply into immediate open surgical repair versus temporary urinary diversion with suprapubic or urethral catheter placement. With temporary urinary diversion, delayed repair and/or reconstruction would be performed, if necessary, 6–12 weeks following the injury. In any situation, the initial management of urethral injury should proceed first and foremost with prompt bladder decompression and broad-spectrum antibiotics [2]. The controversial aspect of managing penetrating urethral injury, however, is whether immediate open repair versus diversion with delayed repair and reconstruction should be performed. In a recent study and review of posterior urethral injuries with pelvic fractures, immediate open repair was associated with a 49% stricture rate, 21% incontinence rate, and 56% impotence rate. When primary realignment was performed, the stricture rate remained at 53%, but the incontinence and impotence rate dropped to 5% and 36%, respectively. If suprapubic urinary diversion was the initial management option, the urethral stricture rate rose to 97%, with a 4% incontinence and 19% impotence rate [18]. In a recent retrospective series by

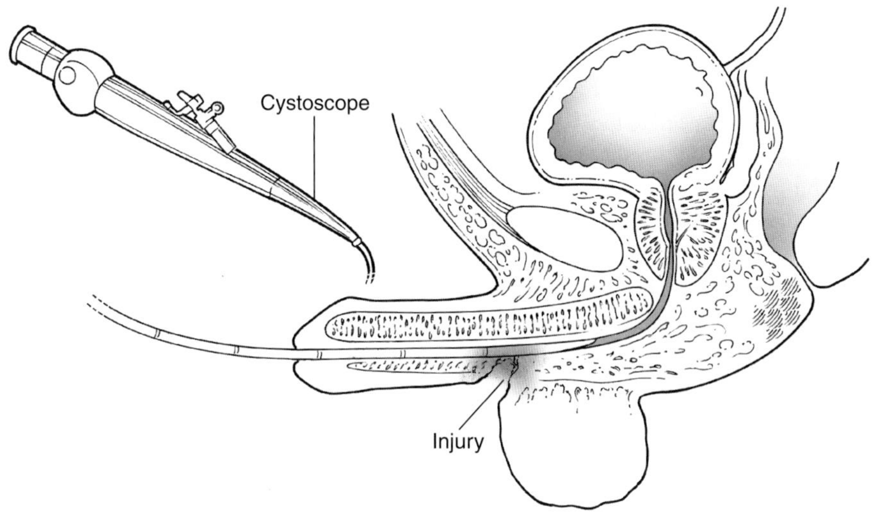

Fig. 47.3 Once you reach the site of urethral injury, the cystoscope is often successful in identifying some normal mucosa or the other side of the defect

Hadjizacharia et al., 14 patients presenting with an acute urethral injury were managed with immediate endoscopic realignment, compared to 7 patients treated with delayed (open) therapy. The outcomes of the study showed the immediate realignment group to have a lower rate of stricture formation (14%) compared to the delayed therapy group (100%). In addition, the authors found a shorter time to spontaneous voiding in the immediate realignment group (35 ± 23 days) compared to the delayed therapy group (229 ± 79 days) [19]. In general, no single treatment protocol will fit each patient perfectly. Therefore, the overall clinical status of the patient as well as concomitant injuries should be taken into account before final management decisions are made. These same complications do not apply to penetrating injuries, with the exception of stricture rates. The high impotence and incontinence rates are more specific to the nature of the pelvic fracture injury. Penetrating injuries are more commonly in the anterior urethra, with less disruption of the surrounding neurovascular bundles.

Immediate surgical repair of posterior urethral injuries is indicated in the presence of a concurrent bladder neck or rectal injury to prevent subsequent urinary incontinence, fistula formation, or persistent leak. Urinary continence is a function of both the internal and external sphincter mechanisms. Posterior urethral injuries are usually associated with damage to the external sphincter mechanism for urinary continence. This would leave the internal sphincter, located at the bladder neck, as the only remaining source of urinary continence. For this reason, any bladder neck injuries should be explored and repaired immediately; without proper repair and reapproximation of the sphincter, eventual urinary incontinence is almost guaranteed. In the absence of a bladder neck or rectal injury, posterior urethral injuries should be managed with temporary urinary diversion via suprapubic or urethral catheter placement. The placement of a urethral catheter in the presence of a urethral injury is called immediate endoscopic (or primary) realignment (IER). Regardless of mechanism, posterior urethral injuries are initially managed with an attempt at immediate endoscopic realignment. Traverse the normal urethral mucosa by using flexible cystoscopy with low flow irrigation. Once you reach the site of injury, the cystoscope is often successful in identifying some normal mucosa or the other side of the defect (Fig. 47.3). Once across the defect and into the bladder with the cystoscope, advance a guide wire into the bladder. Then remove the cystoscope and place a Council tip Foley catheter over the wire and into the bladder. This allows urethral drainage without necessitating surgery. The majority will heal without significant stricture. If attempts at IER are unsuccessful, a suprapubic tube can be placed, followed by delayed definitive repair.

Anterior urethral injuries can also be repaired early on with open surgery, especially in the setting of low-velocity penetrating injuries where major tissue destruction has not occurred [20]. In the presence of major tissue destruction, excessive and often inadvertent tissue debridement may take place, which can further the risk of ischemic stricture development. In cases of anterior urethral repair for pendulous urethral injuries, approach with a circumcision/degloving penile incision, and proceed to local debridement of nonviable tissue, spatulation of the two urethral ends, and a tension-free anastomosis of the lacerated corpus spongiosum and urethra with interrupted absorbable sutures over a 14–16Fr urethral catheter [21]. For bulbar urethral injuries, place the patient in the dorsal lithotomy position, and make a vertical perineal incision to gain access to the bulbar urethra [20]. Carry a tension-free urethral anastomosis; perform it over a 16–18Fr catheter in this relatively dilated portion of the urethra. Keep the catheter in place for a minimum of 10–14 days, and perform a pericatheter RUG prior to removal to ensure no further extravasation. The presence of extravasation warrants continued catheter drainage.

Urinary diversion with delayed repair is another management option, especially when the patient is too unstable for surgery or if the injury is very posterior. If IER fails, urinary diversion can be performed with suprapubic cystostomy tube placement (percutaneous versus open). Open suprapubic cystostomy placement will guarantee placement into the bladder, allow concomitant bladder repair if present, and allow bladder neck reconstruction if an injury is found. Open tube placement will also allow antegrade urethral endoscopy and urethral catheter placement if initial catheter placement or retrograde urethroscopy failed to reach the bladder. The other option for suprapubic cystostomy tube placement is a percutaneous kit, which is less invasive than the open suprapubic tube placement and can be performed under mild sedation. Blind urethral catheter placement, on the other hand, can be attempted in the setting of small, partial lacerations, and in general should be avoided because of the risk of transforming a partial laceration to a full circumferential transection. Again, we emphasize obtaining a RUG if any index of suspicion for urethral injury is present. However, the catheter can be safely placed under direct visualization with retrograde urethroscopy and catheter placement over a wire. As an alternative, antegrade urethroscopy can be performed at the time of open pelvic surgery or during repair of a concomitant bladder rupture with passage of the scope down the urethra and out of the meatus. This will allow tying of a catheter to the cystoscope with a silk suture or over a wire and retrograde passage of the catheter into the bladder as the cystoscope is withdrawn.

In summary, penetrating injuries to the urethra, testicles, and external genitalia usually take the form of gunshot and stab wounds. The importance of the mechanism of injury cannot be overemphasized, and combined with a very thorough and detailed physical examination, will lead the diagnostician to the correct diagnosis. If ever in doubt, or the mechanism does not seem correct, perform radiological studies to further delineate any underlying injuries, which may of course change the course of management. Other life-threatening injuries should always maintain a higher priority, but it is the responsibility of the trauma and urology team to work together and maintain effective communication to deliver the best possible care.

Important Points

- An IVP or CT alone are not always reliable to demonstrate bladder rupture. This requires a high-pressure cystogram.
- Undiagnosed bladder rupture in the presence of pelvic fracture can lead to serious complications.
- Urethral injury can be associated with rupture of the bladder.

References

1. Cass AS et al (1991) Testicular injuries. Urology 37:528–530
2. Morey AF et al (2004) Consensus on genitourinary trauma: external genitalia. BJU Int 94:507–515
3. McAninch JW et al (1984) Major traumatic and septic genital injuries. J Trauma 24:291–298
4. Gross M et al (1969) Rupture of the testicle: the importance of early surgical treatment. J Urol 101:196–197
5. Jeffrey RB et al (1983) Sonography of testicular trauma. Am J Roentgenol 141:993–995
6. Lupetin AR et al (1983) The traumatized scrotum: ultrasound evaluation. Radiology 148:203–207
7. McAninch JW et al (1989) Management of genital skin loss. Urol Clin North Am 16:387–397
8. Wein et al. Campbell-Walsh urology. 9th edn. Saunders-Elsevier, Chapter 83, pp. 2649–2673
9. Pliskow RJ et al (1979) Corpus cavernosography in active fracture of the penis. Am J Roentgenol 133:331–332
10. Dierks PR et al (1983) Sonography and penile trauma. J Ultrasound Med 2:417–419

11. Koga S et al (1993) Sonography in fracture of the penis. Br J Urol 72:228–229
12. Fedel M et al (1996) The value of magnetic resonance imaging in the diagnosis of suspected penile fracture with atypical clinical findings. J Urol 155:1924–1927
13. Nicolaisen GS et al (1983) Rupture of the corpus cavernosum: surgical management. J Urol 130:917–919
14. Tan LB et al (1991) Traumatic rupture of the corpus cavernosum. Br J Urol 68:626–628
15. Mydlo JH (2001) Surgeon experience with penile fracture. J Urol 166:528–529
16. Jezior JR et al (2001) Management of penile amputation injuries. World J Surg 25:1602–1609
17. Sandler CM et al (1998) Lower urinary tract trauma. World J Urol 16:69–75
18. Koraitim MM (1996) Pelvic fracture urethral injuries: evaluation of various methods of management. J Urol 156:1288–1291
19. Hadjizacharia P et al (2008) Evaluation of immediate endoscopic realignment as a treatment modality for traumatic urethral injuries. J Trauma 64(6):1443–1449
20. Chapple C et al (2004) Consensus statement on urethral trauma. BJU Int 93:1195–1202
21. McAninch JW et al (1996) Traumatic and reconstructive urology. W.B. Saunders Company, Philadelphia, pp 347–355, 543–550

Major Abdominal Veins

48

Peep Talving and Kenji Inaba

Abdominal vascular insults are among the most lethal injuries caused by penetrating trauma [1, 2]. Not infrequently, multiple concomitant vascular injuries are encountered in addition to several associated visceral injuries for every injured vessel. The incidence of major abdominal veins injured in descending order includes the inferior vena cava (IVC), iliac veins, renal veins, superior mesenteric vein (SMV), portal vein, hepatic veins, and retrohepatic vena cava [1].

Victims of penetrating vascular trauma may present with complete or relative hemodynamic stability due to a contained retroperitoneal vascular injury. If however, the vascular lesion is freely bleeding into the peritoneal cavity, the patient will present unstable. Most often, a combination of free hemorrhage and partial containment is seen. The presence of shock mandates immediate exploratory laparotomy after obtaining baseline labs. A plain radiograph in the emergency department (ED) can be quickly obtained and sent to the operating room (OR) when processed to help to delineate the trajectory of the offending missile and structures at risk. When a vascular injury is suspected, time is of paramount importance and surgeon's experience is reflected in the speed at which the patient is rushed to the OR. Besides hypotension, peritonitis also mandates an emergent trip to the operating room. A study from one of the largest Level 1 trauma centers in the US noted that a hemodynamically stable cohort of patients sustaining a penetrating abdominal injury presenting with peritonitis had an intra-abdominal vascular injury rate of 11%, with subsequent intraoperative hypotension and a transfusion requirement seen in 25% and 39%, respectively [3].

Finally, patients presenting in extremis or in cardiac arrest will be subjected to resuscitative thoracotomy in the ED as described in Chap. 16. The need for thoracotomy, however, reflects a dire physiological state and very few patients subjected to resuscitative thoracotomy for a subdiaphragmatic vascular injury are expected to survive [1, 4].

Do not spend excessive time inserting intravenous lines in the ED if not necessary. Do not induce anesthesia in the ED as this will result in a pharmacological sympathectomy, and your patient may arrest before entering the OR. Do notify the blood bank about a possible massive transfusion while rushing the patient to the OR. From the ED, alert the OR that an emergency laparotomy is on its way, allowing preparation of both a vascular and sternotomy/thoracotomy tray, fixed retractor to optimize exposure, headlights, two suction devices, lots of laparotomy pads, and a primed autotransfusion device. Large bore venous access above the diaphragm must be obtained in the OR. With the potential of iliac vein or IVC injury obtaining venous access in the groin may result in your transfusion efforts ending up in the abdominal cavity or in the retroperitoneal space. Infuse blood products early with blood loss because excessive administration of crystalloids will dilute clotting factors resulting in coagulopathy and rebleeding, in addition to predisposing your patient to a systemic inflammatory response as well as subsequent abdominal compartment syndrome [5–8]. Ensure that the first blood draw for typing is sent to the lab as soon as possible in order to

P. Talving (✉) • K. Inaba
Division of Trauma and Surgical Critical Care,
Department of Surgery, Keck School of Medicine, University of Southern California, LAC+USC Medical Center,
1200 North State Street, IPT-C5L100 Los Angeles, USA
e-mail: peep.talving@surgery.usc.edu; kinaba@surgery.usc.edu

G.C. Velmahos et al. (eds.), *Penetrating Trauma*,
DOI 10.1007/978-3-642-20453-1_48, © Springer-Verlag Berlin Heidelberg 2012

expedite the release of type specific or ideally fully matched blood. This will allow conservation of uncrossmatched blood. We maintain a ready supply of prethawed liquid plasma, which is dispensed as type specific. As soon as this is dispensed, more is thawed to replace the units removed from the blood bank. They are sent in a cooler to prevent wastage of those units not used. One OR nurse is designated as the blood coordinator to ensure that accurate 2-way communication occurs, facilitating delivery while decreasing wastage. When massive transfusion protocol is required, i.e., more than 6 units of red blood cells within 24 h of admission, the transfusion practice should aim for a 1:1:1 ratio of red blood cells, plasma, and platelets, respectively [9].

In the OR, the patient should be prepared with their arms abducted at 90° and the skin cleaned from chin to knees to allow maximal flexibility in access. The skin and fascia is divided along its full length from xiphoid process to symphysis, also called as "from Cape to Cairo." Once anesthesia is prepared for hypotension, you can go ahead and decompress the hemoperitoneum, which may induce significant bleeding and hypotension. You should at this point eviscerate the small bowel, scoop the blood and clots out of the peritoneal cavity and apply direct pressure on the site of hemorrhage with laparotomy pads. If not localizable, four quadrant packing may be used. In severe hypotension, consider aortic inflow control by compressing the aorta with your thumb and index finger at the aortic hiatus below the left hepatic lobe. To apply a vascular clamp at the hiatus is quite ineffective due to the diffuse neuronal tissue around the aorta causing the clamp to slide off the aorta. Dividing the left diaphragmatic crus allows clamp placement to the very distal thoracic aorta that has no surrounding neurofibrous tissue. Try not attempt to achieve aortic inflow control by making an additional incision into the left chest as these patients are already cold and coagulopathic. If resuscitative thoracotomy was performed in the ED, the aortic clamp should already be controlling inflow. Autotransfusion of shed blood from the peritoneal cavity is controversial with a concomitant hollow viscus injury; however, for vascular injuries, if cell-saving is available, this should be utilized [10].

Your next step is to identify injuries with vascular lesions taking precedence. The retroperitoneum is broken into functional zones (Fig. 48.1). With a few exceptions that will be discussed in this chapter, for penetrating injuries, all retroperitoneal hematomas are explored. Zone I is the central zone extending from aortic hiatus to sacral promontory containing the aorta and major branches, IVC with its major tributaries, portal vein, SMV, and central renal vessels. Zone II contains the renal hilum and parenchyma, and zone III the iliac vessels. A sophisticated trauma surgeon may also define a Zone IV in the retrohepatic space behind the liver containing the retrohepatic IVC and hepatic veins. This is an area you should avoid exploring unless your patient is exsanguinating from a decompressed retrohepatic venous injury. A series of sequenced, rehearsed actions are required to save the patient. These injuries are associated with a very high mortality rate and there are no series available to convincingly support any recommendation over avoiding the exposure of these structures if at all possible. If contained, it is best to do nothing. If uncontained, the goal should be to pack and institute damage control. If packing does not prevent exsanguination, try repacking. If this does not work, desperate alternatives such as total hepatic exclusion with atrio-caval shunting

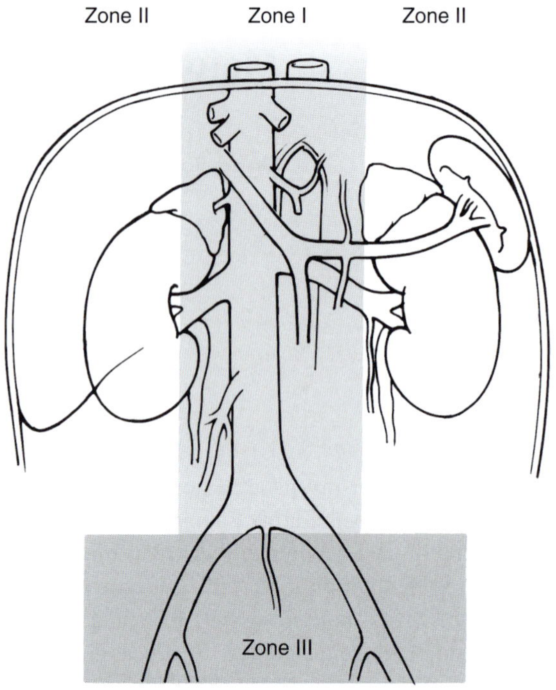

Fig. 48.1 Functional zones of the retroperitoneum

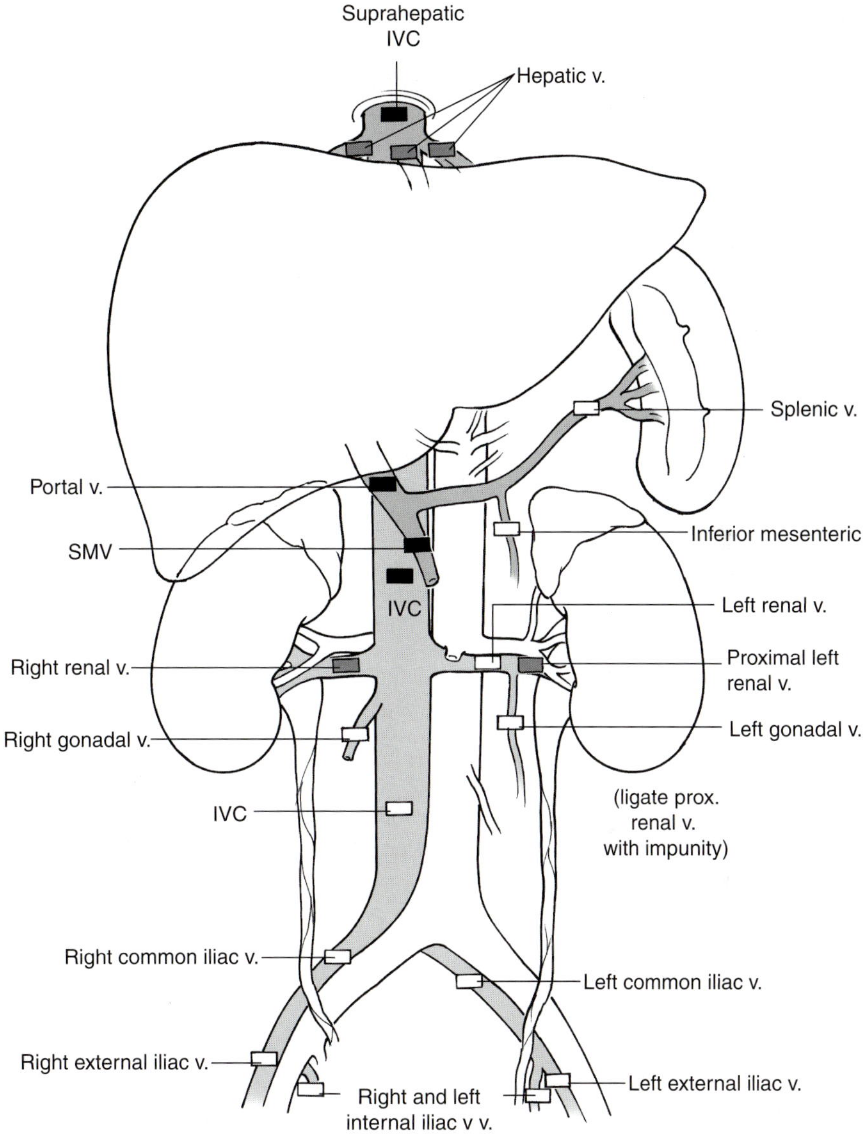

Fig. 48.2 Ligatable (*white*), potentially ligatable (*gray*), and preferably non-ligatable abdominal veins (*black*)

may be considered. Although there are multiple case reports describing atrio-caval shunting, very few survivors attest to the devastating nature of this injury.

Once an intra-abdominal venous injury is identified, you should immediately be planning out your potential operative strategies: to ligate the injured vessel, to shunt it, or attempt to repair. All major abdominal veins are depicted in Fig. 48.2/Table 48.1 and marked as amenable for ligation with relative impunity, ligate with consideration, and ligate in life-threatening scenarios only. All treatment decisions must be made in the context of the patients' physiological condition at the time of laparotomy.

48.1 IVC Injury

Approximately 1 out of every 50 patients with a GSW to the abdomen will have an *IVC injury*. Prehospital mortality is close to 50% and survival of those who

Table 48.1 Quick overview of management options while dealing with abdominal veins

Ligate with impunity	Recommendation
Infrarenal IVC	Wrap and elevate lower extremities
Common iliac vein	Wrap and elevate lower extremity
External iliac vein	Wrap and elevate lower extremity
Internal iliac vein	
Inferior mesenteric vein	
Splenic vein	
Ligate with the following considerations	
Right renal vein	Right nephrectomy
Left renal vein, distal to gonadal vein	Left nephrectomy
Hepatic veins	Follow up liver ischemia
Ligate only in life saving scenario	
Suprarenal/perirenal IVC	Consider renal replacement therapy
Superior mesenteric vein	Second look for gut ischemia
Portal vein	Second look for gut ischemia

reach hospital alive is reported to range between 20% and 40% [11]. As a rule, injury to IVC will be associated with multiple visceral injuries [12].

48.1.1 Exposure

Injury to the IVC presents at laparotomy with a hematoma or hemorrhage from zone I, most commonly to the right of midline. After evacuating blood from the abdominal cavity and direct control of the hemorrhage with compression, consider aortic inflow control. The next step is a right medial visceral rotation, which along with a Kocher maneuver will expose the entire infrahepatic IVC. Before visceral rotation, ensure that you have multiple sponges on sticks, vessel loops, vascular clips, laparotomy pads, intravascular occlusion catheters, vascular instruments, and 4–0 vascular sutures on a large needle. Place a fixed retractor to maximize exposure and warn your anesthesia colleagues that in short order, major hemorrhage may occur. Start the exposure by dividing the avascular colonic peritoneal attachments at the line of Toldt from the ileocecal region up to the hepatic flexure (Fig. 48.3). With an IVC injury, the blood will have tracked out laterally completing the majority of the dissection. The Kocher maneuver reflects the duodenum and the head of pancreas to the left facilitating the exposure of injuries of the suprarenal IVC. Multiple options exist for controlling the IVC hemorrhage. The immediate goal is directed digital control of the injury or proximal and distal pressure on the IVC using sponges on a stick. With local control, vessel loops or vascular clamps can be used for more definitive control. With vascular clamps, one must be careful not to cause iatrogenic injuries when dealing with veins. If the injury is small, a side-biting Satinsky clamp may cover the entire length of the injury. Rapid control will minimize further blood loss and decrease the chance of air embolism. If tolerated, the Trendelenburg position prior to definitive repair may also obviate venous air embolism. If bleeding from the IVC continues after proximal and distal occlusion, the cause of bleeding is the lumbar veins. There are 4–5 pairs of lumbar veins entering the infrarenal IVC from the posterior aspect of the vessel. To access them, you need to rotate the IVC slightly and apply vascular clips, vessel loops, or ligatures on the lumbar veins. Dividing the lumbar veins after ligation improves exposure of the posterior aspect of the IVC if necessary for repair. In repairing a wound of the perirenal IVC, you will also need to occlude the renal veins with vessel loops or vascular clamps.

48.1.2 Repair

There are numerous options for repairing the IVC (Fig. 48.4). Lateral repair is your first-line therapy. When using the side-biting Satinsky clamp, you may run a suture line along the clamp. If control was obtained with a laparotomy sponge, roll your compressive pads along the IVC and as soon as you identify the vessel edges, apply a Babcock clamp to close the visualized segment. Continue rolling your pad followed by application of additional Babcocks until the wound is entirely clamped. The suture line can then run under the Babcock clamps removing each as the suture line progresses. In some instances, a missile will blow a larger hole into the IVC and lateral repair will cause significant stenosis of the vessel. If this stenosis approaches 50%, consider repairing with a PTFE

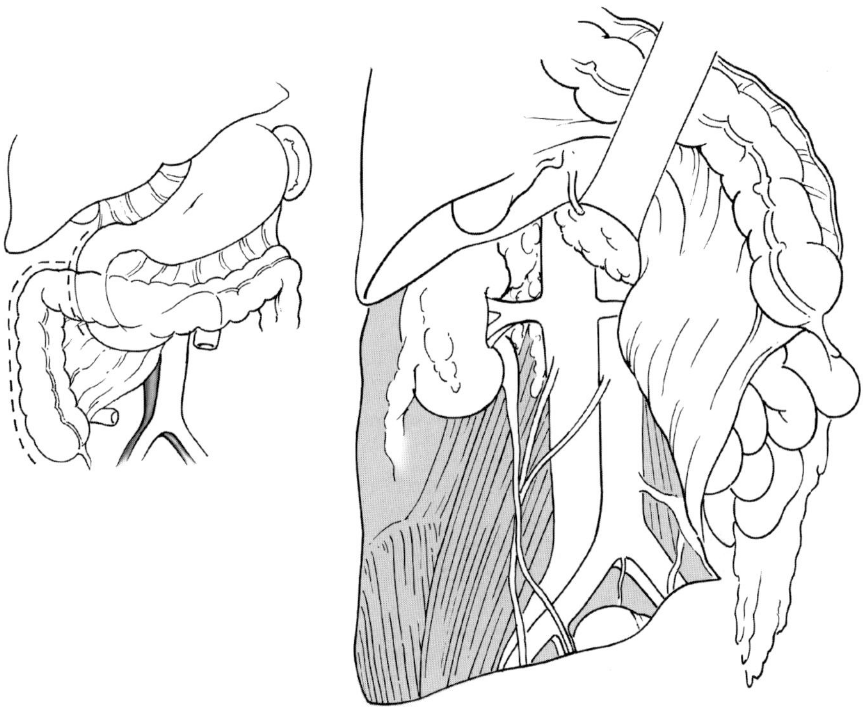

Fig. 48.3 Access to the infrahepatic inferior vena cava

(polytetrafluoroethylene) patch. Always look for a through-and-through injury. Attempt to close this by rotating the vessel, ligating and dividing the lumbar veins if required. If this is not possible, another option is to extend the anterior wound. You should make every attempt to repair the suprarenal and perirenal IVC as ligation is associated with a high rate of renal failure. You may consider shunting the vessel if repair is not feasible as in a damage control setting. For infra-renal injuries, if the repair is highly complex, or the patient is physiologically compromised, proceed with ligation.

48.1.3 Complications

The morbidity associated with IVC repair is due to venous stasis below the repair or ligation site. Elevation and wrapping of the lower extremities with elastic bandage alleviates the edema in the lower extremities. Long-term outcomes are very ill defined. If there was visible stenosis at the time of repair, you may consider prophylaxis when patient is stabilized in ICU with low molecular weight heparin.

48.2 Portal Vein Injuries

Portal vein injuries are associated with an extremely high mortality ranging between 40% and 70% among victims who arrive to the ED alive. Associated with the portal vein injury may be injury to the SMV, renal vessels, suprarenal IVC, liver, biliary tree, or bowel.

48.2.1 Exposure

The portal vein starts at the confluence of the SMV and splenic vein behind the neck of the pancreas. After coursing behind the first portion of the duodenum, it enters the posterior aspect of the hepatoduodenal ligament. When dealing with a portal vein injury, you will notice either a hematoma or brisk dark hemorrhage in the upper central retroperitoneum either at the mesenteric root or in the hepatoduodenal ligament. Also, there may be massive bleeding from the wound in the pancreatic neck or head. Such venous bleeding can originate either from

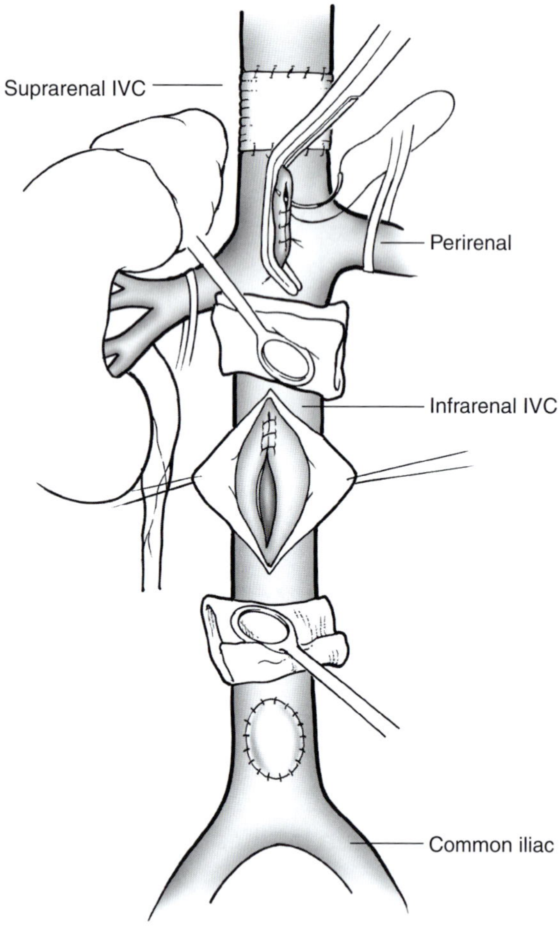

Fig. 48.4 Inferior vena cava repair options

the suprarenal IVC or portal vein. Most commonly, portal vein injuries are combined with an injury to the suprarenal IVC. Again, you must be ready to obtain rapid local control of the vascular injury. The vast majority of those who reach the OR alive will exsanguinate during the exploration while unroofing the hematoma. Your primary aim is to arrest the bleeding by applying local compression and if required controlling the aortic inflow at the hiatus. Parallel to this, volume restoration with blood products requires constant communication with the anesthesia team. To approach the portal vein for suprapancreatic or retropancreatic injuries, the same exposure principles apply. Start with a right medial visceral rotation followed by a Kocher maneuver, which exposes the posterior and lateral aspects of suprapancreatic portal vein (Fig. 48.5). Divide the cystic duct and attempt to obtain vascular control by identifying the injury and applying vascular clamps proximal and distal. Avoid iatrogenic injuries to the hepatic artery and common bile duct. Whereas many experienced trauma surgeons would discourage pancreatic division unless the injury has already done so, if exposure does not allow visualization of the injury, stapled pancreatic division may be required.

48.2.2 Repair Versus Ligation

Always stay in damage control mode while dealing with these potentially lethal injuries. The goal is lateral venorrhaphy or if this is not possible, ligate immediately. Clinical evidence is available that survival rates are reasonable when the ligation is done in very early stages of intervention [11]. Ligation of the portal vein requires that the hepatic artery is intact. If not, options include for the stable patient an interposition graft of saphenous vein and if not, shunting with delayed reconstruction.

48.2.3 Complications

Ligation of the portal vein is compatible with survival; however, this requires a patent hepatic artery. Portal vein ligation results in transient hypotension from splanchnic pooling of intravascular volume. Fluid requirements must be vigorously addressed. Use a temporary abdominal closure and do not close the abdominal fascia after portal vein ligation as massive bowel edema is expected within 24–72 h post-ligation. By default, you should plan on a "second look" to evaluate for bowel ischemia and to reassess the fascia for closure.

48.3 SMV Injuries

SMV injuries are associated with injury to their arterial counterparts in 34% of cases [13]. Patients sustaining SMV injury also sustain 3–4 associated visceral injuries per vascular injury. The mortality associated with SMV injuries ranges from 29% to 57% over the last decade [2].

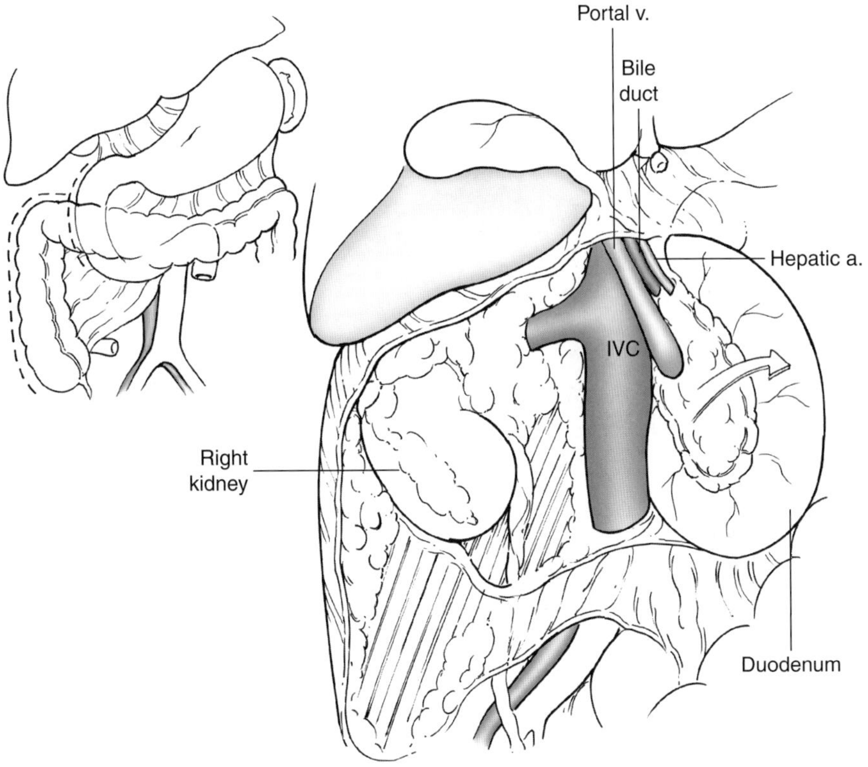

Fig. 48.5 Access to the portal vein

48.3.1 Exposure

The main trunk of the SMV passes anterior to the third segment of the duodenum and in front of the uncinate process of the pancreas. The SMV joins the splenic vein to form the portal vein behind the neck of the pancreas. Intraoperatively, the injury presents as a hematoma either at the base of the transverse mesocolon or as a supramesocolic hematoma in the lesser sac at the neck of the pancreas. Dividing the avascular ligament of Treitz between the base of transverse mesocolon and fourth portion of the duodenum accesses the proximal SMV. Start dividing the ligament horizontally from left to right with Metzenbaum scissors. The first vessel encountered is the SMA. The SMV is located just right to the SMA. Reflect the transverse mesocolon cranially and the small bowel caudally which will expose the SMV at the root of the mesentery. You will note the middle colic vein confluencing with the SMV at the base of the transverse mesocolon. Control the bleeding with compression or pinch the root of the mesentery. As soon as an injury is identified, while exposing the injury, start thinking about your plan for repair, shunting, or ligation depending of the extent of the injury and patient's overall condition. Further exposure of the SMV becomes more difficult as the vessel courses behind the neck of the pancreas and is frequently embedded in the pancreatic tissue. You may try to access it from the lesser sac. Open the retroperitoneum just below the neck of the pancreas and isolate the proximal and distal ends of the vessel. By careful traction of the pancreatic neck cranially, you will achieve more distal access to the SMV (Fig. 48.6). As discussed above, if this is not sufficient, stapled transection of the pancreas is an acceptable option.

48.3.2 Repair Versus Ligation

If lateral repair is feasible, this is the best option. If the patient is physiologically unstable, you may at this point insert a vascular shunt. When anchoring the shunt, care must be taken to tie the shunt as close as possible to the wound to spare the vessel length for subsequent reconstruction at secondary intervention.

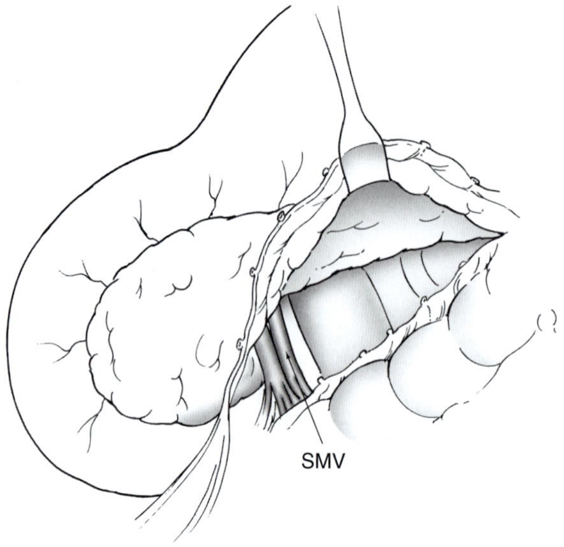

Fig. 48.6 Access to the superior mesenteric vein

If the patient is in extremis, ligation is required and is compatible with survival.

48.3.3 Complications

Complications of the SMV ligation are similar to ligation of the portal vein.

48.4 Renovascular Injuries

Renovascular injuries occur in 5–7% of penetrating abdominal trauma. However, a renal vein is the third most common venous injury in the abdominal cavity and an isolated injury carries a mortality rate of approximately 10%. Renal salvage is expected in approximately 50% in isolated renal vein injuries. Mortality is linked to the associated vascular and visceral injuries. At laparotomy, you will find a hematoma overlapping the transition of zones I and II. A peripheral non-expanding zone II hematoma does not mandate exploration.

48.4.1 Exposure

For renal trauma, the nephrectomy rate is not significantly decreased by obtaining vascular control prior to renal mobilization [14]. This is only an option for hemodynamically stable patients and may be tedious. The simplest approach on both sides is to proceed laterally with a medial visceral rotation. Open Gerota's fascia and mobilize the kidney gently by inserting your fingers below the kidney and bringing the kidney up into the wound. This provides excellent exposure to vascular injuries on both sides. On the left, if you decide to obtain vascular control first, retract the transverse mesocolon superiorly and eviscerate the small bowel. Division of the ligament of Treitz exposes the left renal vein crossing over the aorta. Loop it and retract it gently in a caudal direction. The short segment of renal artery is visualized behind the vein slightly superior, taking off from the aorta. In the setting of bleeding or hemodynamic instability however, as on the right, mobilize the left colon, open the perirenal fascia, and bring the kidney into the midline to access the vessels.

48.4.2 Repair Versus Ligation

Your options on the right side are either lateral repair or ligation. Avoid complex repairs, especially if the patient requires damage control. Ligation equals nephrectomy on the right side. On the left, ligation of the renal vein close to the IVC, distal to the gonadal vein, is compatible with renal salvage as the venous outflow will be rerouted through the gonadal, adrenal, and lumbar veins.

48.4.3 Complications

Even if the injury is repairable, preoperative and intraoperative hypotension along with renal inflow occlusion results in ischemic damage. Despite the anecdotal successes with ischemia times in excess of 3–5 h, function starts to decline after even 1 h of warm ischemia time. These patients are therefore at high risk of acute renal failure postoperatively.

48.5 Iliac Vein Injuries

Mortality is in excess of 35% for isolated *iliac vein injuries* [13]. Penetrating injuries to the lower abdomen, pelvis, or buttocks in the presence of hypotension are suspicious for iliac vascular injury. The incidence of penetrating iliac vessel injury in the civilian arena ranges from 10% to 22%, and in 70% of those instances, a combined arteriovenous injury is identified. The most frequent segment injured is the common iliac vessel. At laparotomy, the intra-abdominal finding of iliac vessel injury is a hematoma in Zone III [15]. These hematomas must be explored in conjunction with penetrating trauma.

48.5.1 Exposure

Iliac vein injuries are often more challenging than arterial injuries due to the difficult surgical exposure and the risk of air embolism. The distal right common iliac vein is particularly cumbersome to expose. Similarly, the confluence of the iliac veins behind the right common iliac artery is a real challenge. Local hemostatic control is obtained initially by direct compression. The left iliac vein is exposed by mobilizing the lateral peritoneal attachments of the sigmoid colon and rotating the bowel medially. On the right, the cecum should be mobilized and displaced cranially exposing both the proximal IVC and right iliac vessels. Apply vessel loops on the common, external, and internal iliac arteries to expose the vein behind. Difficulty in exposure has led many authors to advocate transection of the overlying artery while many experienced trauma surgeons would argue strongly against it. Ligation and division of the internal iliac artery, however, may further facilitate mobilization of the artery to allow access to the venous injury behind. For distal injuries, the midline incision can be continued obliquely through the inguinal ligament on the appropriate side. Exposure is crucial for these injuries and will facilitate distal control.

48.5.2 Repair Versus Ligation

You should consider repair whenever it is simply feasible with lateral repair. If repair is difficult or if the patient is unstable, simply ligate! This is well tolerated by most patients. Be cautious to avoid injury to the ureter, which rides over the iliac artery at the bifurcation.

48.5.3 Complications

The mortality associated with isolated iliac vein injuries is 10%. However, the injury very infrequently occurs in isolation. Repair of the iliac vein with subsequent stenosis is associated with the risk of venous thrombosis and pulmonary embolism. In cases where repair would result in stenosis, we advocate ligation. Significant edema and postphlebitic syndrome will be decreased by wrapping the extremity and elevation postoperatively [15]. You may consider anticoagulation if the vessel was repaired, with significant stenosis.

Important Points

- Vascular injuries must be ruled out in hypotensive penetrating abdominal trauma.
- Spare no time for investigations if the patient is hypotensive: Run to the OR.
- Hemostatic resuscitation should be started promptly and continued through the OR and into the SICU.
- Have a complete vascular tray in your OR before you start.
- Your mind should be attuned to the need for damage control even prior to laparotomy.
- Divide the skin and fascia fully prior to decompressing the hemoperitoneum.
- Right medial visceral rotation exposes most of the abdominal veins.
- Attempt lateral repair or shunt the suprarenal IVC, portal vein, and SMV if feasible.
- In a life-threatening scenario, there is no role for complex repair, just ligate.
- Abdominal compartment syndrome will follow ligation of the SMV or portal vein.
- Wrap the legs on patients with a ligated IVC or iliac veins.
- Consider the risk of venous thromboembolism in venous repair.

References

1. Asensio JA, Chahwan S, Hanpeter D et al (2000) Operative management and outcome of 302 abdominal vascular injuries. Am J Surg 180(6):528–533
2. Asensio JA, Forno W, Roldan G et al (2002) Visceral vascular injuries. Surg Clin North Am 82(1):1–20
3. Brown CV, Velmahos GC, Neville AL et al (2005) Hemodynamically "stable" patients with peritonitis after penetrating abdominal trauma: identifying those who are bleeding. Arch Surg 140(8):767–772

4. Davis TP, Feliciano DV, Rozycki GS et al (2001) Results with abdominal vascular trauma in the modern era. Am Surg 67(6):565–570
5. Balogh Z, McKinley BA, Cocanour CS et al (2003) Supranormal trauma resuscitation causes more cases abdominal compartment syndrome. Arch Surg 138(6):637–642
6. Bulger EM, Jurkovich GJ, Nathens AB et al (2008) Hypertonic resuscitation of hypovolemic shock after blunt trauma: a randomized controlled trial. Arch Surg 143(2):139–148
7. Koustova E, Stanton K, Gushchin V et al (2002) Effects of lactated Ringer's solutions on human leukocytes. J Trauma 52(5):872–878
8. Sondeen JL, Coppes VG, Holcomb JB (2003) Blood pressure at which rebleeding occurs after resuscitation in swine with aortic injury. J Trauma 54(5):110–117
9. Holcomb JB, Wade CE, Michalek JE et al (2008) Increased plasma and platelet to red blood cell ratios improves outcome in 466 massively transfused civilian trauma patients. Ann Surg 248(3):447–458
10. Bowley DM, Barker P, Boffard KD (2006) Intraoperative blood salvage in penetrating abdominal trauma: a randomised, controlled trial. World J Surg 30(6):1074–1080
11. Buckman RF, Pathak AS, Badellino MM, Bradley KM (2004) Portal vein injuries. In: Rich NM, Mattox KL, Hirshberg A (eds) Vascular trauma, 2nd edn. Elsevier Saunders, Philadelphia
12. Navsaria PH, de Bruyn P, Nicol AJ (2005) Penetrating abdominal vena cava injuries. Eur J Vasc Endovasc Surg 30(5):499–503
13. Asensio JA, Britt LD, Borzotta A et al (2001) Multiinstitutional experience with the management of superior mesenteric artery injuries. J Am Coll Surg 193(4):354–365
14. Gonzalez RP, Falimirski M, Holevar MR et al (1999) Surgical management of renal trauma: is vascular control necessary? J Trauma 47(6):1039–1042
15. Asensio JA, Petrone P, Roldan G et al (2003) Analysis of 185 iliac vessel injuries: risk factors and predictors of outcome. Arch Surg 138(11):1187–1193

Major Abdominal Arteries

49

Lydia Lam and Kenji Inaba

Vascular injuries are the most common cause of death after penetrating abdominal trauma. Any penetrating injury to the abdomen should be considered a potential vascular injury until proven otherwise. This is critical for understanding that this is a true emergency and requires running the patient to the operating room before they exsanguinate. Only a novice would saunter over. In this chapter, we will address how to quickly access and manage injuries to the major arteries in the abdomen. We will begin with key features that include staying calm, rapid exposure, obtaining temporary control until further decisions can be made, and various approaches to treatment.

Abdominal arteries can range from small, inconsequential branches to major trunks that, when injured, can commonly determine whether life or death results after penetrating trauma. Vascular injuries are found in 10–20% of patients undergoing laparotomy for penetrating injury. Mortality rates of up to 70% have been documented for major abdominal arterial injury; the treatment of which, despite many advances in medical technology, has not changed since Debakey's initial description in 1946. The general approach to penetrating abdominal trauma can be found in Chap. 39. For these patients, quick indicators that a vascular injury may be present are hypotension, peritonitis, mental status changes, diminished lower pulses, and a distended abdomen. It is important to recognize that hypotension can be your friend! Relative hypotension will decrease the amount of hemorrhage and theoretically not dislodge any clot that may have formed. It is ok to maintain relative hypotension until you reach the operating room.

In patients meeting criteria for a laparotomy after penetrating trauma, there is always the chance that there may be a vascular injury and an experienced trauma surgeon will understand that the patient's best shot at survival is to control the bleeding STAT! This has been documented in several studies looking at factors affecting mortality in major abdominal vascular trauma. The underlying message is the same: Rapid identification and control of bleeding will allow for adequate resuscitation and improved survival [1, 2]. It is a race for time if vascular injury is suspected. Never walk to the OR; always run!

While running to the OR, the first vessel that comes to mind is the aorta. However, there are a few others that can challenge your skills, requiring rapid identification and control. These arteries include the superior mesenteric artery, splenic artery, iliac arteries, and renal arteries. These are the vessels that are at the root of the dreaded "expanding hematoma" in the retroperitoneum. When injured, these vessels appear chaotic and messy when seen for the first time, very different from the clean drawings of textbooks or the careful cadaver dissections during medical school. Get as much experience as you can while training and if you are not experienced, get help as soon as you realize

L. Lam (✉) • K. Inaba
Division of Trauma and Surgical Critical Care,
Department of Surgery, LAC+USC Medical Center,
1200 North State Street, IPT-C5L100 Los Angeles, CA, USA
e-mail: lydialam2@gmail.com; kinaba@surgery.usc.edu

G.C. Velmahos et al. (eds.), *Penetrating Trauma*,
DOI 10.1007/978-3-642-20453-1_49, © Springer-Verlag Berlin Heidelberg 2012

what the injury is. Ensure that blood and plasma are ordered and a rapid infuser is prepared while the patient is intubated, prepped, and draped. Prepare the area from sternal notch to knees. This will be important in the event that you have to cross-clamp above the diaphragm for hypotension or requires saphenous vein to bypass. In addition, have vascular instruments opened or in the room, you may need them on a seconds notice; you are now ready.

49.1 Stay Calm

It is imperative that when you see the expanding hematoma, pulsatile bleeding, or bright red blood welling up in your field, you stay calm. As the captain of the ship, if you panic, everyone else will panic. Panic prevents clear decision making, stalls rapid treatment, and decreases the efficiency of the entire surgical team. Keep your senses in check and let anesthesia know that you have arterial bleeding. Make sure that they have enough help and that blood products are on the way. Additionally, anticipate and secure all of the tools you may need including vascular sutures, vascular clamps, vessel loops, shunts, and retractors that may not normally be available but needed emergently to gain immediate control of a vessel.

49.2 Get Temporary Control

While anesthesia is preparing for war and the surgical scrub is loading up your "emergent" prolene 2-0 to 5-0 noncutting sutures, it is critical for you to obtain temporary control.

Remember your hands; these are some of the best tools you have! They are accurate, allow highly variable pressure application, quick and easy to apply, and (usually) atraumatic to the vessel wall. A finger with direct pressure on the injured vessel is the best way to obtain control while you regroup and allow the others in the operating room to catch up to the torrential bleeding.

Recognizing when your patient is in trouble is key to a good outcome. Major vascular injury is in fact one of the most common triggers for initiating damage control. The concept of damage control will be covered in detail in Chap. 2.4.3. For arterial injuries, the damage control options include ligation and shunting (Table. 49.1).

Table 49.1 Options of repair, graft, and ligation in selected vessels

Artery	Primary repair	Graft or vein	Ligate?	Recommendations
Aorta	3-0 or 4-0 prolene	Dacron 14–20 mm	No	❑ Prefer left medial visceral rotation exposure
Splenic	N/A	N/A	Yes	❑ Splenectomy
Common hepatic	5-0 or 6-0 prolene	Saphenous vein graft	Yes	❑ Need intact portal vein ❑ Cholecystectomy
Celiac axis	5-0 or 6-0 prolene	N/A	Yes	❑ Ligate
SMA	5-0 or 6-0 prolene	Vein preferred	No	❑ Ligate in life-saving scenario only ❑ Shunt whenever possible for damage control
IMA	6-0 prolene	N/A	Yes	❑ Ligate
Common iliac	4-0 or 5-0 prolene	PTFE $\geq$ 6 mm	No	❑ Shunt or immediate bypass ❑ Watch for need of leg fasciotomy
External iliac	4-0 or 5-0 prolene	Vein or PTFE$\geq$6 mm	No	❑ Shunt or immediate bypass
Internal iliac	4-0 or 5-0 prolene	N/A	Yes	❑ Ligate
Renal	5-0 or 6-0 prolene	Vein or PTFE	No	❑ Nephrectomy if ligation required ❑ Ensure contralateral kidney function prior to ligation
Mesentery (unnamed)	No	N/A	Yes	❑ Ligate with impunity ❑ Explore all hematomas for arteries in spasm that need ligation

The shunt is an important tool to keep in your back pocket. It is a rapid, inexpensive, technically simple tool that allows you to follow the underlying principle in vascular trauma which is to restore blood flow and reperfuse ischemic tissue or organs. If the patient begins that downward spiral of the lethal triad and the vessel that is bleeding can be ligated, ligate. If not, get a shunt into the vessel, restore flow, and proceed to the ICU. A shunt can be anything from a feeding tube for smaller vessels to a chest tube for a large vessel such as the aorta. Typically, we use commercially available and purpose designed vascular shunts at our institution; however, any hollow tube is acceptable, ensuring it is slightly smaller than the vessel lumen so as to not damage the endothelium. A silk tie is secured to the center of the shunt to mark the middle and prevent shunt migration. After placing the middle silk tie, slip the proximal and distal ends of the shunt into the respective ends of the injured vessel. Keep in mind that the segment of the vessel that is tied down to hold in the shunt will be damaged and will have to be removed during definitive repair. Therefore, do not trim or debride the injured vessel prior to shunt insertion to maximally preserve native vessel length. In addition, secure the shunt as close as possible to the end of the injured vessel so as to preserve length. In general, the flow drives shunt patency and anticoagulation is not used, as patients requiring damage control shunting often have diffuse nonsurgical bleeding which may be exacerbated by this. You have now restored flow and can bring the patient safely to the ICU for further resuscitation.

After the patient is adequately resuscitated, acidosis corrected, and hypothermia eradicated, you are now ready to return for definitive repair of this vessel which can be a simple primary repair, or more involved with an interposition graft comprising of saphenous vein or a synthetic graft.

49.3 Retroperitoneal Hematomas: Plan of Action

When discussing abdominal bleeding and the trauma exploratory laparotomy, it is common to refer to the areas of hematoma that will help you plan your exploration. The retroperitoneum is divided into 4 areas: zone 1–3 and zone 4, the retrohepatic area (Fig. 49.1). The retrohepatic area is comprised of the hepatic veins

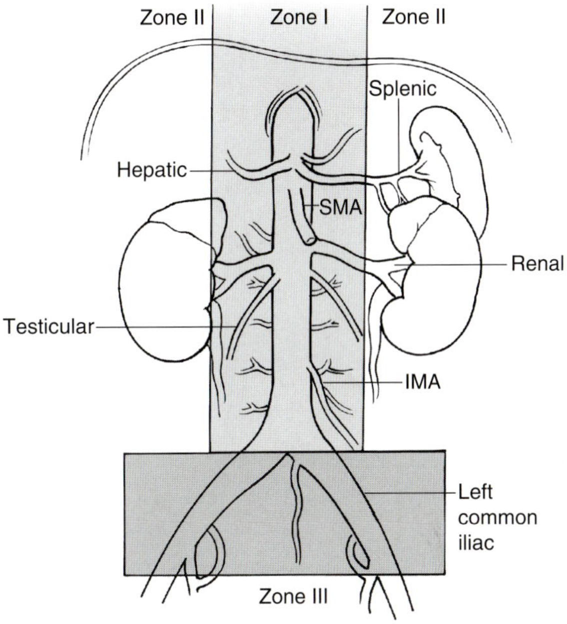

Fig. 49.1 Anatomical vascular regions

and retrohepatic IVC and thus will not be discussed in this chapter.

49.3.1 Zone I

Zone 1 refers to a central retroperitoneal hematoma. A hematoma in the supramesocolic location suggests that the suprarenal aorta, celiac, or superior mesenteric artery (SMA) may have been injured, while an inframesocolic location would suggest injury to the distal SMA or infrarenal aorta.

49.3.1.1 Aorta

The suprarenal aorta can be accessed by a left medial visceral rotation also known as a Mattox maneuver. This can expose the entire length of the aorta and its branches to include the celiac axis, superior mesenteric artery, and inferior mesenteric artery. After making your midline incision from xiphoid to pubis, take down the falciform ligament posteriorly making sure to stop short of the hepatic veins. The Balfour retractor is a simple instrument for retracting the abdominal wall. For larger patients or for areas such as the iliac vessels, a large fixed retractor may be required. Reflect the omentum and transverse colon superiorly, eviscerate the small bowel to the right, and find the sigmoid

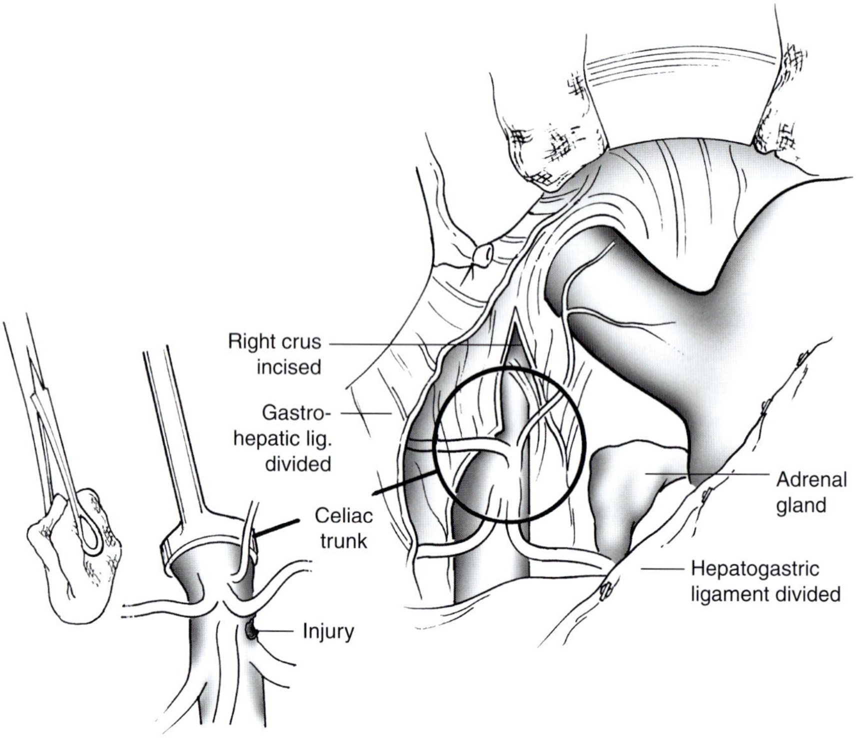

Fig. 49.2 Supraceliac aortic control

colon. Lift the sigmoid colon up into the field and start your dissection on the White Line of Toldt (aka the peritoneal reflection). Once the peritoneum is taken down, your hand can easily dissect through the loose areolar tissue in the retroperitoneal space, especially if blood has dissected through the soft tissue planes. Continue this dissection superiorly keeping on top of the psoas muscle to include the descending colon, splenic flexure, stomach, spleen, and pancreatic tail. This will allow you to bluntly lift up these structures and mobilize them into the midline. At this point, the aorta and its branches can be visualized.

If bleeding is not adequately controlled with direct pressure and cross-clamping of the aorta is your next move, the supraceliac aorta should be accessed. Keep in mind that inflow control will cause ischemia to all structures distal; thus, the time the cross-clamp remains on the aorta needs to be kept as short as possible. The longer the clamp remains in place, the more difficult removal becomes and the more profound the reperfusion effect. For intra-abdominal supraceliac control, direct compression manually is best, especially if there is sufficient blood pressure to allow for easy palpation of the aorta as it exits the chest. If dissection is required or if you are going to attempt clamp placement, cutting the left crus of the diaphragm (at 2 o'clock to avoid bleeding) will facilitate exposure. Using your fingers, bluntly dissect away the dense neural and fibrous tissue over the aorta and create a space on either side. You may attempt to place a large vascular clamp across the aorta. If successful, secure the clamp so that it cannot fall off or be knocked off inadvertently. Practically however, it is usually very difficult to keep the clamp in place because it slips off easily. What we recommend for better control of the aorta is direct compression of the aorta against the vertebral bodies. This can be achieved by a compression device, a sponge stick, or your assistant's hand (Fig. 49.2). In rare instances with high supramesocolic injuries, the safest way to achieve proximal aortic control is through a left thoracotomy.

Any repair of the aorta will need to be done with a nonabsorbable monofilament suture, usually a 4-0. If possible, try a lateral aortorrhaphy or PTFE patching. Unfortunately, if it is a gunshot wound, quite a bit of damage may result requiring resection of that portion. Direct primary repair is difficult due to limited mobility. Therefore, after obtaining exposure and proximal and distal control, insert a short interposition graft of

14–20 mm Dacron and perform an end-to-end anastomosis. When size matching, remember that the acutely injured aorta is likely vasoconstricted; so, if trying to decide between two sizes, choose the larger size. Although the vast majority of penetrating aortic injuries will be accompanied by other injuries, commonly hollow viscus, enteric spillage is not a strict contraindication to prosthetic graft placement and all gross spillage should be washed out. In addition, after you have achieved blood flow back to the lower part of the body, omental covering over the anastomotic site is strongly encouraged; this will protect your graft and help prevent aorto-enteric fistula formation. Find an avascular line in the omentum and take down a portion to adequately cover up the repair.

49.3.1.2 Celiac Axis

The celiac artery is a rare injury but can become deadly fast. Because it is tucked behind the stomach, there is usually an associated stomach or liver injury. In one review, over a 10-year period of celiac artery injuries at a single institution, the majority (92%) were, not surprisingly, due to penetrating injury with a mortality rate of 38%. The majority of these patients underwent ligation of the artery [3].

When a hematoma is found in the lesser sac, it can take a while to perform a Mattox maneuver to attain proximal control. In this case, supraceliac aortic control may be helpful. If there is massive bleeding, although in general blind clamping or suturing is not encouraged, directed ligation can be useful since it is acceptable to ligate the celiac trunk.

If this does not stop the bleeding, medially rotate the spleen and pancreas to expose the root of the celiac artery while leaving the kidney down. This should allow access to the celiac takeoff. Although direct dissection through the lesser sac is possible, it is often difficult while holding direct pressure on the injury. Once the injury is exposed, then either ligation or reconstruction can begin. Again, keeping in mind the patient's physiological state, ligation in almost all cases is the easiest and safest way to proceed. However, if the patient is rock solid and the burden of associated injury is low, reconstruction may be attempted using autologous graft.

Transection of the stomach has also been described to access the vessel. This is not routinely performed, nor is it recommended. If it is done in the face of a concomitant gastric injury, ligation will be your only option.

49.3.1.3 Superior Mesenteric Artery

An expanding hematoma in the region of the base of the mesentery or the lesser sac is concerning for an SMA injury and must be explored. The mortality associated with injury to the SMA can approach 70% [4]. The SMA has been described using the Fullen classification:

Zone I– beneath pancreas
Zone II–between the pancreaticoduodenal and middle colic branches of the SMA
Zone III–beyond the middle colic branch
Zone IV–enteric branches

As expected, the more proximal the injury, the higher the mortality rate because more of the bowel will be affected. This injury is usually associated with multiple other injuries and the patient is often in profound hypovolemic shock on presentation to the hospital [5].

After direct compression, the most important thing is adequate exposure. A key maneuver for temporary control of the SMA is to rapidly perform a Kocher maneuver and place your hand behind the head of the pancreas to the root of the mesentery and grasp the vessels between your thumb and fingers. Your assistant can be doing this while you continue the dissection for better exposure and control. Start with the Mattox maneuver which will give you good access to the aorta, which can then be clamped superior and inferior to the SMA takeoff. Once proximal control is achieved, Fullen zones I and II can be exposed anteriorly by using a retractor to reflect the inferior edge of the pancreas upward; however, this can be awkward (Fig. 49.3). If this still proves inadequate, stapled transection of the pancreas neck to give full exposure of the artery is indicated. Bluntly dissect anterior to the CBD with your finger, much like a Whipple, and lift up the pancreatic neck for stapling. Alternatively, use either a knife or cautery to transect the pancreas over your finger to allow you to access the SMA.

Fullen zones III and IV hematomas are below the pancreas and are exposed by reflecting the transverse mesocolon cephalad and taking down the ligament of Treitz. Behind this lies the SMA and it can be dissected out for direct visualization of the injury. A Cattell-Brasch maneuver (see figure in Chap. 48) for this part

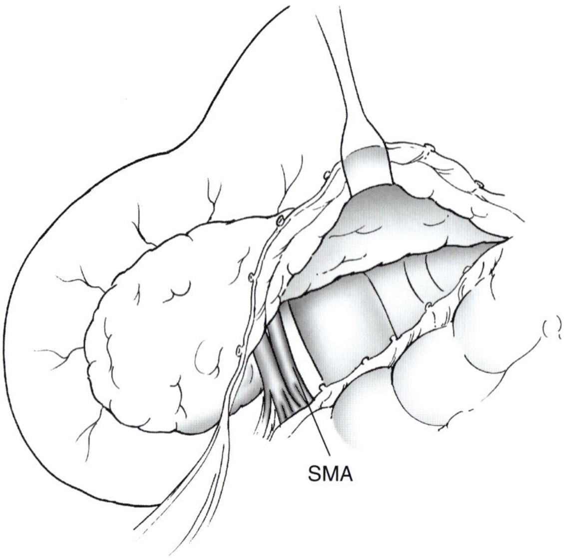

Fig. 49.3 Superior mesenteric artery exposure

of the SMA is also possible as it will allow good exposure to the posterior vessel.

Ligation of the SMA, despite the theoretical collateral flow that may allow gut viability with the proximal ligation, should be avoided. Patients sustaining SMA injuries have compromised distribution of blood flow through all organ beds and there is no guarantee of gut viability even if intraoperative ischemia is not seen. The best damage control maneuver is shunting. If stable, definitive repair to any part of the SMA can include primary repair (preferable if possible without narrowing), patch angioplasty, or reconstruction. Ideally, autologous grafts would be preferred for reconstruction but a ringed synthetic graft would be acceptable. If damage control shunting is performed, delayed reconstruction can be done from the right common iliac artery or the infrarenal aorta to the SMA using autologous graft. Do this as a staged operation to maximize your chance of success. Position the reconstruction as far away from any pancreatic leak as possible to avoid any anastomotic breakdown or arterio-enteric fistula formation. Always remember the omentum; place some omentum around your anastomosis to protect it. Even in the best hands, postoperative bowel ischemia is a risk and must be carefully watched for. Most of these patients will have an open abdomen post reconstruction, facilitating a second-look operation.

49.3.2 Zone 2

The major arteries in this zone include the renal arteries and adrenal arteries, with the renal arteries being of significant concern. Virtually all penetrating renal injuries are diagnosed intraoperatively and usually close to the time of injury. This is important as the kidneys do not tolerate ischemia well. Most surgeons avoid revascularization after 6 h as renal function is affected after even 90 minutes of ischemia. The results of revascularization are poor, and postoperative hypertension is a problem that may require nephrectomy. Therefore, it is not commonly done but depends on the extent of injury burden, patient status, and contralateral kidney. If the injured kidney is the only kidney, we are much more aggressive about attempting revascularization with the caveat that you do not want to end up with a well-perfused kidney in a dead patient.

There are two approaches to the renal arteries – laterally and medially. In general, all zone 2 hematomas after penetrating trauma are explored. Small lateral hematomas away from the hilum that are not expanding may be left alone by some surgeons.

The medial method approaches the renal vessels directly. The advantage of this approach is that you can obtain proximal control of the renal vessels and the kidney in the face of bleeding. The disadvantage is that this can be a difficult dissection. The advantage to the lateral approach is that the majority of the dissection has been done by the expanding hematoma, and is therefore very fast. Start by performing a left lateral medial visceral rotation as discussed in the exposure of the aorta for the left kidney and a right medial visceral rotation for the right kidney (Fig. 49.4a, b). As the dissection moves cephalad, keep your hand on top of the psoas muscle as the kidney is lifted up bluntly. Once that kidney is in your hand, vascular control can be obtained by pinching the hilum in your fingers to allow you time to carefully place a clamp across the vessels. Another advantage to this approach is that, at this point, you have the injured kidney mobilized and up into the field of the operation. Again, rarely will there be an isolated renal artery injury. With the kidney mobilized and bleeding controlled, the extent of the damage can be rapidly assessed.

Once the lesion has been identified, you have some choices to make. A simple injury can be repaired with

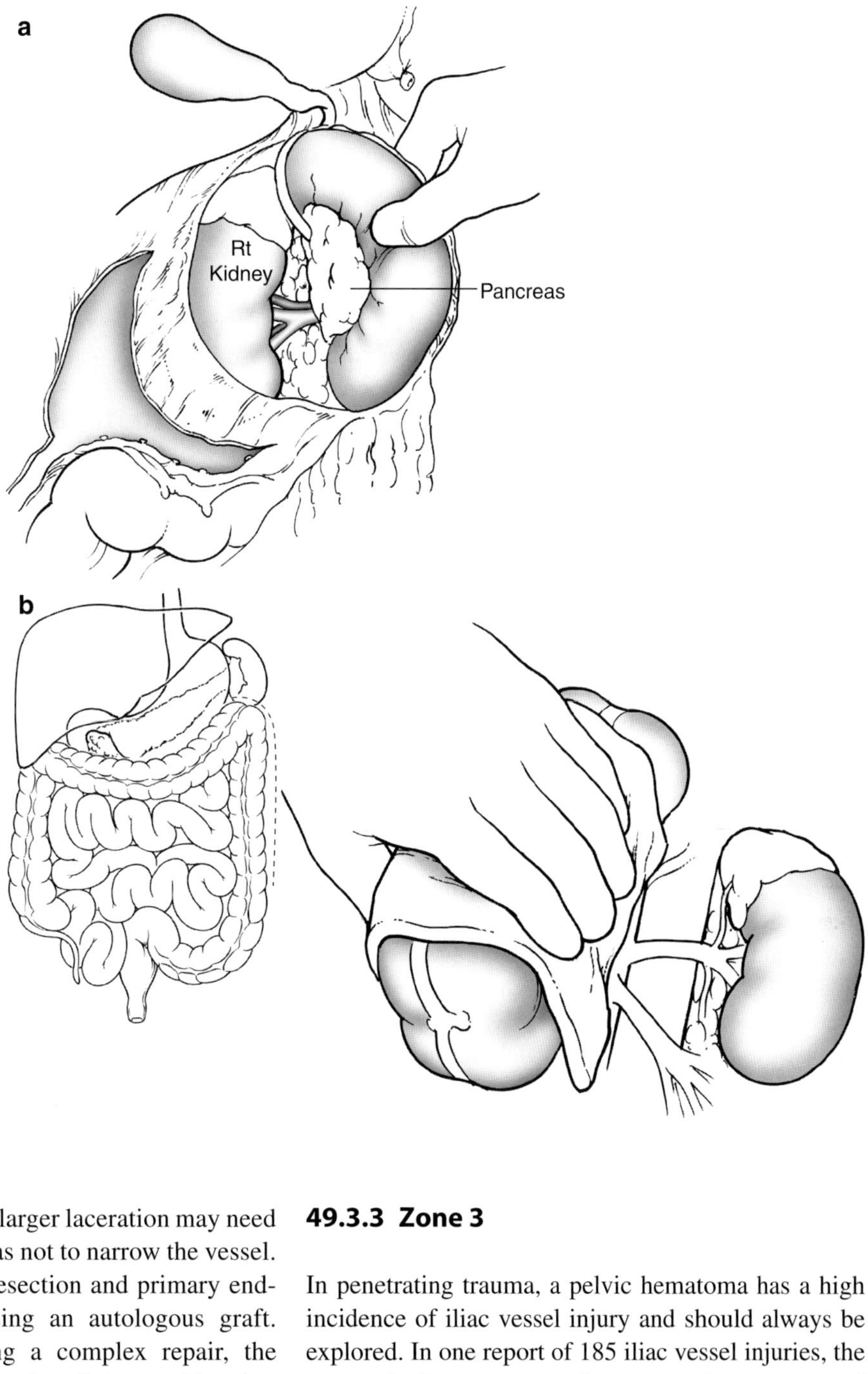

Fig. 49.4 (**a**) Right renal artery exposure. (**b**) Left renal artery exposure

interrupted sutures while a larger laceration may need a saphenous vein patch so as not to narrow the vessel. Complex repairs include resection and primary end-to-end anastomosis or using an autologous graft. Again, prior to attempting a complex repair, the patient condition must be taken into consideration along with the ischemia time and predicted chance of success. In most cases, as the arterial injury will be associated with a concurrent venous injury, the damage control procedure would be a nephrectomy rather than shunting.

49.3.3 Zone 3

In penetrating trauma, a pelvic hematoma has a high incidence of iliac vessel injury and should always be explored. In one report of 185 iliac vessel injuries, the vast majority were seen after penetrating trauma and the mortality rate was seen to be high at 43%, and 62% if combined with an iliac vein injury [6].

These patients may present with evidence of intra-abdominal bleeding or may present with a unilateral pulse discrepancy in the lower extremity on the injured side. To expose a right-sided zone 3 hematoma, start at the cecum and dissect along the peritoneal reflection. Mobilize the entire cecum and reflect it toward the head. At this point, you are looking into the retroperitoneal area and should be able to see the psoas muscle. Place your finger on the psoas muscle and move medially and toward the feet to find the pulse that will be the iliac artery. With a major hematoma, the anatomy may become distorted and you may need to go toward the head to identify the aorto-bifurcation and then each common iliac trunk. Remember that the ureter comes across anteriorly at the bifurcation of the common iliacs; so look out for it and do not transect it. Similarly, if the hematoma is on the left side, take down the peritoneal reflection along the sigmoid colon, reflect it medially, and identify the psoas muscle. Again, palpate along the muscle until you feel a pulse and that will be the iliac artery. Bluntly dissect, using your fingers, the loose areolar tissue around the vessel (see Cattell Brasch maneuver in Chap. 39). Remember to stay anterior to the artery and you will not encounter any branches. At this point, you should have a pretty good idea of where the bleeding is coming from and your goal is to obtain local control with direct compression using your finger. Carefully dissect an area proximally and distally to place a vessel loop around the iliac artery. This will help with proximal and distal control. Remember, if the injury is distal, exposure is critical and the incision should be continued across the inguinal ligament and into the groin. Next, identify the internal iliac arteries which are easy to recognize because they take a direction straight down toward the back of the patient. If the injury is localized to the internal iliac artery, you can ligate it. Although the proximal segment is easy to manage, distal segment gunshot injuries within a tight hole that is bleeding can be difficult to control. In the unstable patient requiring damage control, packing or balloon occlusion may be used.

Contrary to the internal iliac arteries, ligation of the external iliac arteries is associated with a significant amputation rate. If the injury is located at the external iliac artery, then a decision will have to be made about your next step: Repair primarily, shunt, or proceed with graft. When the injury requires a resection with an interposition graft, autologous graft is preferred if suitably size matched. However, a synthetic graft of at least 6 mm is quite acceptable as this is a large caliber, high-flow vessel. Often the size match is better and insertion of PTFE is much quicker with good results. As discussed earlier, concomitant hollow viscus injury is not a contraindication to synthetic graft placement.

For the external iliac artery, if the patient meets criteria for damage control, be prepared to shunt. We have had excellent success with this technique for temporizing with a delayed repair once the patient is stabilized. We do not advocate prophylactic fasciotomies but have a high index of suspicion postoperatively for intervening.

49.4 Afterthoughts

Almost all patients with an abdominal vascular injury will have sustained a major physiologic stress and many will have associated injuries. Once the patient has made it through the operation, it is important to continuously re-assess their physiological status as it normalizes. Adequate resuscitation and careful monitoring of their hemoglobin will be important over the next 24–72 h. If there are no contraindications, consider starting a platelet inhibitor for up to 3 months for specific injuries where there is high concern for thrombosis.

Important Points

- Never walk to the OR– always run!
- Hypotension can be your friend.
- Stay calm. Be in control.
- Temporary control can start with your hands.
- Recognize when the patient is or will become physiologically impaired – these patients need damage control.
- Lateral repair is preferable but only if there is minimal to no stenosis.
- Shunt common and external iliacs and SMA. Repair aorta.
- Ligate celiac and internal iliacs.
- Compress supraceliac aorta for global control of abdomen.
- Transection of the pancreas to access the SMA is ok.
- Keep SMA anastomosis away from pancreas with omental covering.
- Nephrectomy is acceptable to save a life.

References

1. Deree J, Shenvi E, Fortlage D et al (2007) Patient factors and operating room resuscitation predict mortality in traumatic abdominal aortic injury: a 20-year analysis. J Vasc Surg 45:493–497
2. Tyburski JG, Wilson RF, Dente C et al (2001) Factors affecting mortality rates in patients with abdominal vascular injuries. J Trauma 50:1020–1026
3. Asensio JA, Petrone P, Kimbrell B et al (2005) Lessons learned in the management of thirteen celiac axis injuries. South Med J 98:462–466
4. Asensio JA, Chahwan S, Hanpeter D et al (2000) Operative management and outcome of 302 abdominal vascular injuries. Am J Surg 180:528–533; discussion 533–534
5. Asensio JA, Britt LD, Borzotta A et al (2001) Multiinstitutional experience with the management of superior mesenteric artery injuries. J Am Coll Surg 193:354–365; discussion 365–366
6. Asensio JA, Petrone P, Roldan G et al (2003) Analysis of 185 iliac vessel injuries: risk factors and predictors of outcome. Arch Surg 138:1187–1193; discussion 1193–1194

Spleen

50

Heena P. Santry

In past decades, as many as 25–50% of patients with splenic injury were victims of penetrating trauma [1–3]. Today, while the majority of patients presenting with splenic injury are victims of blunt trauma, up to 14% are still victims of penetrating trauma [4]. Conversely, for victims of penetrating trauma, the spleen has been reported to be one of the most infrequently injured organs, ranging from 7% to 9% [5, 6].

In recent years, due to an increase in nonoperative management of splenic injuries through a combination of observation and endovascular approaches, fewer and fewer patients have been brought to the operating room for splenic injury. Once in the OR, fewer splenectomies overall have been performed due to concerns regarding the infectious risks of asplenia, new modes of splenorrhaphy with topical hemostatic agents and artificial mesh, and advances in techniques of partial splenectomy. Thus, overall, fewer and fewer splenectomies have been performed for penetrating trauma. Still, severe penetrating injuries to the spleen can result in uncontrolled bleeding and death if not rapidly addressed with splenectomy.

Assessing the severity of splenic injuries has been standardized over the years. Currently, most surgeons use the 1994 modification of the AAST organ injury scale which relies on intraoperative and/or CT findings [7] (see Table 50.1 and Fig. 50.1). Importantly, however, due to the relative rarity of penetrating splenic injuries, these grading systems have been based largely, if not exclusively, on data from victims of blunt trauma. Typically, grade I–III injuries can be managed nonoperatively or with a splenic salvage procedure. However, more extensive injuries to the spleen will require splenectomy. Approximately 50% of patients with penetrating injury to the spleen go directly to the operating room [8]. Of these, 15% represent a grade IV or V injury that will likely require rapid mobilization and removal of the spleen [8].

Table 50.1 An illustrated guide to grading penetrating splenic injuries

Grade	Description	Figure
I	Capsular tear, <1 cm parenchymal depth	1a
II	Capsular tear, 1–3 cm parenchymal depth that does not involve a trabecular vessel	1b
III	>3 cm parenchymal depth or involving trabecular vessels	1c
IV	Laceration involving segmental or hilar vessels causing major devascularization (>25% of spleen)	1d
V	Completely shattered spleen or hilar vascular injury with devascularizes spleen	1e

50.1 Exposure

As with most cases of traumatic hemorrhage, a generous midline incision is the best approach for trauma splenectomy. If further exposure of the left upper quadrant is needed, as in the case of obese patients or those with unusually narrow costal angle, you can extend the incision the left hypochondrium – although it is rarely needed.

H.P. Santry
Trauma, Critical Care, University of Massachusetts Medical School, UMassMemorial Medical Center,
55 Lake Avenue North, Worcester, MA 01655, USA
e-mail: heena.santry@umassmemorial.org

G.C. Velmahos et al. (eds.), *Penetrating Trauma*,
DOI 10.1007/978-3-642-20453-1_50, © Springer-Verlag Berlin Heidelberg 2012

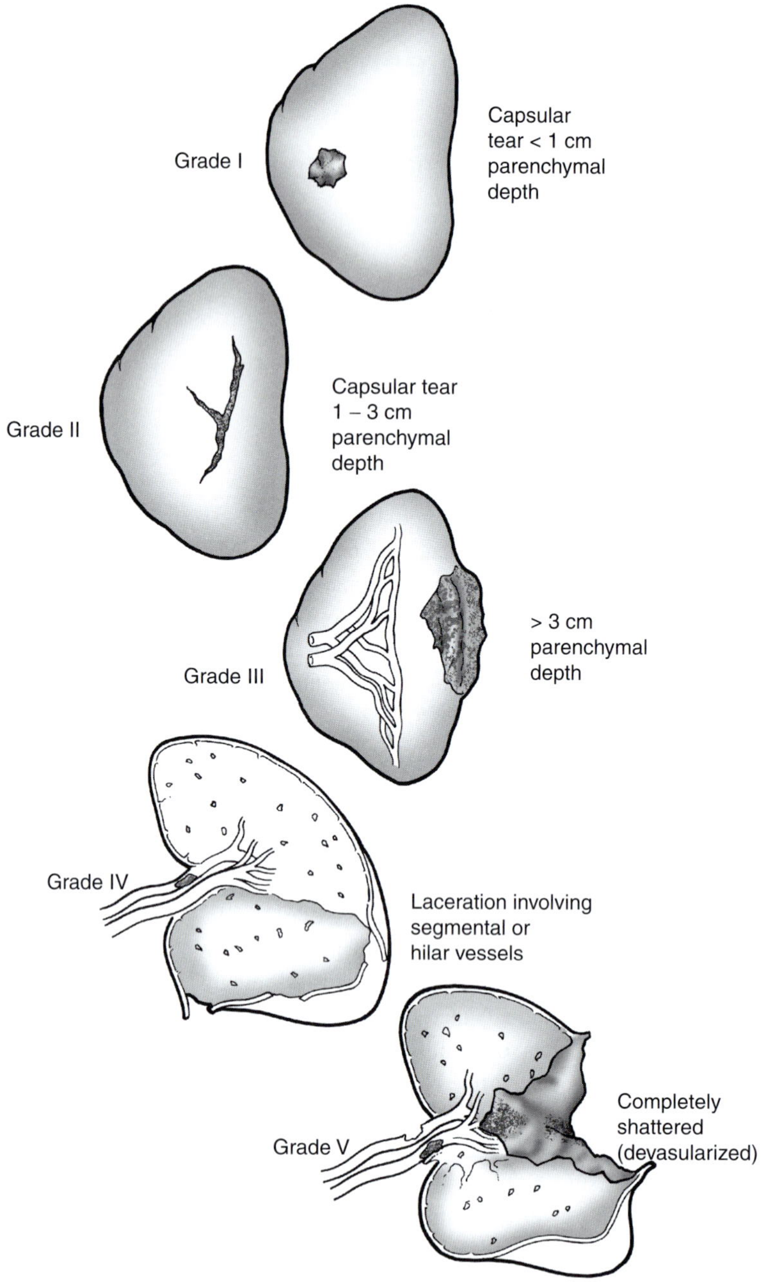

Fig. 50.1 Severity of splenic injuries has been standardized with the 1994 modification of the AAST organ injury scale

In most cases of multiple injuries, you should address the spleen first, as continued bleeding from the organ can harm the patient due to both ongoing blood loss and due to obscuring the operative field. Further, if you are having difficulty identifying the source of bleeding in a particularly bloody abdomen despite packing and suctioning, you will identify the main source of bleeding by turning to the site of clot formation. Defibrinated blood tends to spread freely throughout the peritoneal cavity whether or not the spleen is the source.

Thus, after opening the abdomen, you should pack all four quadrants or suction to clear hemoperitoneum and rapidly identify obvious injuries. If you identify more pressing injuries to address than that of the spleen, you should quickly address them; in most

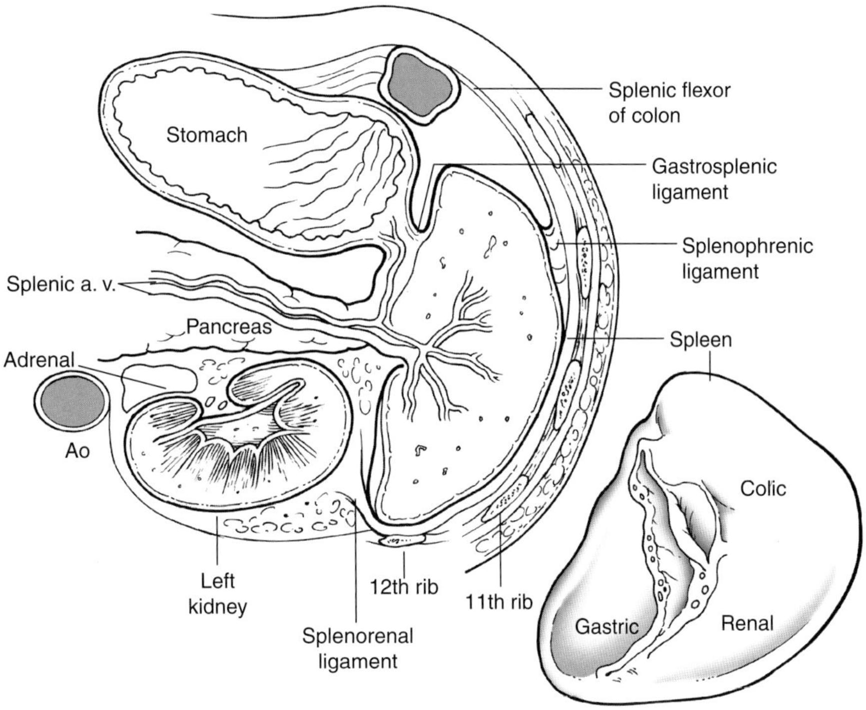

Fig. 50.2 Splenic ligaments and attachments. Division of these attachments may be facilitated by placing a clamp or finger under these attachments prior to division to develop a plane

cases, you can delay definitive repair of most injuries until you have completed the splenectomy. Pack the small bowel inferiorly into the lower abdomen and pelvis. Then, you deliver the spleen into the operative field with gentle inferior and medial traction so as to not exacerbate the underlying injury. Depending on the length and density of the splenic attachments to surrounding structures, you may not be able to fully deliver the organ without mobilization.

50.2 Mobilization

Start mobilizing the spleen by sharply dividing its superolateral attachment, the spleno-phrenic ligament, to the level of the esophageal hiatus, followed by its inferolateral attachment, the spleno-renal ligament. Take care during this maneuver not to injure the left adrenal gland which is characteristically located in an anti-hilar position. Division of these attachments may be facilitated by placing a clamp or finger under these attachments prior to division to develop a plane (see Fig. 50.2).

Once the lateral and inferior attachments are divided (Fig. 50.4), you rotate the spleen medially by cupping the palm of the right hand around the anti-hilar side of the spleen and engaging the fingers of your non-dominant hand around the posterior aspect of the organ in the plane between itself and the retroperitoneal lining of the kidney. It will then be possible to bluntly dissect behind the tail of the pancreas and deliver the spleen and pancreatic tail as a unit into the midline wound. The degree of dissection required behind the tail will be determined by the length of the patient's pancreas with shorter organs requiring less mobilization (see Fig. 50.3).

The final step in mobilization is division of the spleno-colic ligament. You may encounter sizable vessels traversing this ligament, and they should be appropriately controlled with the clamp and tie method using 3-0 silk sutures or a hemostatic device such as the Ligasure device or Harmonic scalpel (see Fig. 50.3).

50.3 Vascular Control

You can control excessive hemorrhage during the course of the mobilization by digital pressure on the hilum and gastrosplenic ligament with an assistant's hand, or in extreme circumstances with a clamp across

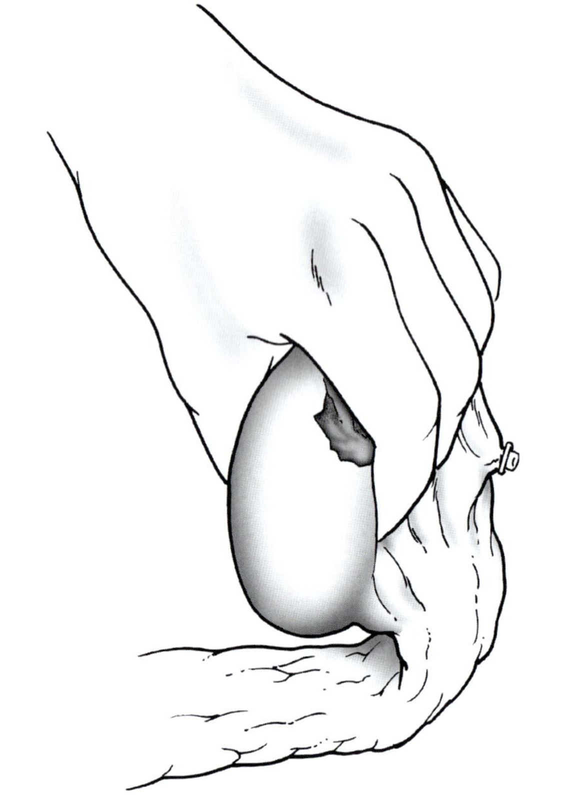

Fig. 50.3 Mobilize the spleen and pancreatic tail gently after it has been freed of all attachments

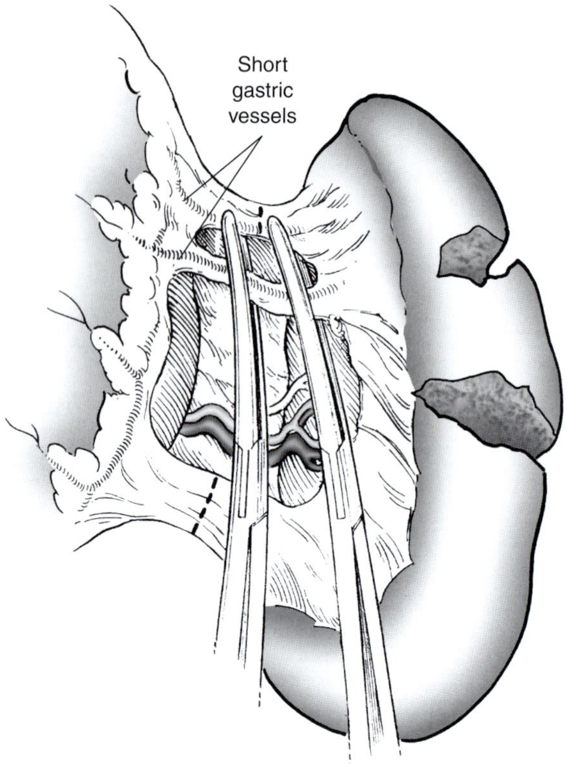

Fig. 50.5 Control the short gastric vessels by taking the vessels closer to the specimen to avoid inadvertent gastric wall ischemia. If a vessel must be taken close to the gastric wall, consider inverting the area with a Lembert suture

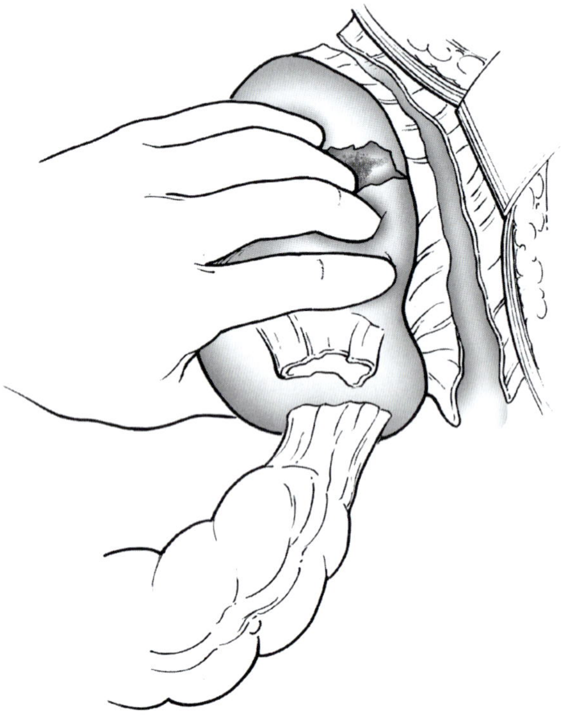

Fig. 50.4 Gently pull the spleen to easily detach the ligaments

the hilum. In general, the latter maneuver should be avoided prior to full mobilization as it puts the tail of the pancreas at risk for injury. After you have fully mobilized the spleen, as described above, you should address its dual blood source supply.

With the spleen rotated inferiorly and medially into the field in your assistant's hand, you should control the short gastrics within the gastrosplenic ligament with the clamp and tie method with 3-0 silk ties or with the Ligasure device or Harmonic scalpel (see Fig. 50.5). Standard electrocautery should not be used as the vessels will rebleed if simply cauterized. You should divide and ligate the vessels along the greater curvature proximally to distally. If ties are used and encompass a small area of the gastric wall, this poses a risk for later necrosis and leak from that area. In such instances, over sew the tied-off area along the greater curvature with 3-0 silk Lembert sutures to bury the potentially compromised area.

Finally, you address the hilar vessels. You serially dissect and individually divide the main arterial and

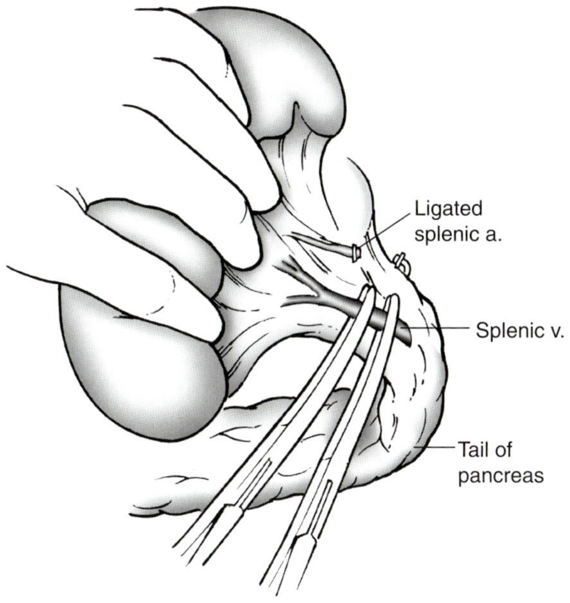

Fig. 50.6 Control of the hilar splenic vessels

venous branches heading into the hilum. Mass division must be avoided as it may result in later arterio-venous fistula formation. The individual branches into the splenic parenchyma from the main splenic artery and vein are variable in anatomy. You should divide each of these branches on the side of the pancreas with a suture ligature of 0-0 silk followed by a similar tie or with a vascular stapler. While the division should take place as close to the spleen side of the vessels as possible to avoid injury to the tail of the pancreas, do not waste time tying the side of the vessels that are to become part of the specimen (see Fig. 50.6).

50.4 Specimen Removal and Final Inspection

After you divide the hilar vessels, the specimen will be free to pass off the table. You should reinspect the left upper quadrant at this point, or after addressing other injuries noted upon entry into the abdomen, for any missed injuries. In particular, the left kidney and the diaphragm are at risk when penetrating trauma has also injured the spleen severely enough to require splenectomy. Operative treatment of these injuries is discussed elsewhere in the text. You must also re-examine the tail of the pancreas closely. If injured by the original mechanism or by the splenectomy, leave a closed suction drain in place. Otherwise, the spleen bed does not require drain placement. Consider vaccinating the patient for *Pneumococcus, Meningococcus, and H. influenza* 2-3 weeks after the splenectomy.

Important Points

- Extend the midline laparotomy incision superiorly to the left of the xiphoid if exposure is inadequate.
- Look for clotting to find the bleeding source.
- Develop a plane under the lateral attachments using a clamp or finger under these to ease the sharp division of these attachments.
- Mobilize the spleen medially with the tail of the pancreas by getting into the plane between the retroperitoneal lining over the kidney and the posterior aspect of the spleen.
- Bury short gastric ties that may compromise the stomach wall with Lembert sutures to prevent future necrosis and leak.
- Avoid mass ligation of the hilar vessel as this will result in AVF formation.
- Clamp close to the spleen and tie on the pancreas side to complete division of hilar vessels.
- Rule out diaphragm and left kidney injury for all splenic injuries.
- Leave a closed suction drain in place for injuries to the tail of the pancreas.
- Do not drain the splenic bed otherwise.

References

1. Clancy TV, Ramshaw DG, Maxwell JG, Covington DL, Churchill MP, Rutledge R et al (1997) Management outcomes in splenic injury: a statewide trauma center review. Ann Surg 226(1):17–24
2. Feliciano DV, Bitondo CG, Mattox KL, Rumisek JD, Burch JM, Jordan GL Jr (1985) A four-year experience with splenectomy versus splenorrhaphy. Ann Surg 201(5): 568–575
3. Carlin AM, Tyburski JG, Wilson RF, Steffes C (2002) Factors affecting the outcome of patients with splenic trauma. Am Surg 68(3):232–239
4. Brady RR, Bandari M, Kerssens JJ, Paterson-Brown S, Parks RW (2007) Splenic trauma in Scotland: demographics and outcomes. World J Surg 31(11):2111–2116
5. Feliciano DV, Burch JM, Spjut-Patrinely V, Mattox KL, Jordan GL Jr (1988) Abdominal gunshot wounds. An urban

trauma center's experience with 300 consecutive patients. Ann Surg 208(3):362–370
6. Nicholas JM, Rix EP, Easley KA, Feliciano DV, Cava RA, Ingram WL et al (2003) Changing patterns in the management of penetrating abdominal trauma: the more things change, the more they stay the same. J Trauma 55(6):1095–1108; discussion 108–110
7. Moore EE, Cogbill TH, Jurkovich GJ, Shackford SR, Malangoni MA, Champion HR (1995) Organ injury scaling: spleen and liver (1994 revision). J Trauma 38(3):323–324
8. Demetriades D, Hadjizacharia P, Constantinou C, Brown C, Inaba K, Rhee P et al (2006) Selective nonoperative management of penetrating abdominal solid organ injuries. Ann Surg 244(4):620–628

Penetrating Rectal Injuries

51

Andrew John Nicol and Pradeep Navsaria

The management of penetrating rectal trauma has been evolving over the last century. There has more recently been a shift in policy from the mandatory colostomy suggested from the military experience to the realisation that civilian low-velocity *intra-peritoneal* rectal injuries can be managed similar to other colonic injuries. The introduction of laparoscopy in trauma has provided screening for and the identification of the trans-pelvic gunshot wound that has not breached the peritoneal cavity. This has allowed for a far more conservative but safe approach to the management of the extra-peritoneal rectal injury. Debate has also arisen about the need for distal rectal washout and the effectiveness of pre-sacral drainage.

51.1 Historical Perspective

The mortality rate from rectal injuries was in the order of 90% at the turn of the twentieth century. This rate dropped to 60% during the First World War due to debridement and primary repair of rectal wounds. Mandatory proximal faecal diversion and pre-sacral drainage during the Second World War saw a further decrease in mortality to 30%. Irrigation of the distal rectal stump was introduced during the Vietnam and Korean conflicts, and the wide availability of antibiotics, intensive care management and blood products saw a further decline in mortality to 15%.

A.J. Nicol (✉) • P. Navsaria
Trauma Centre, Ward C14, Groote Schuur Hospital, University of Cape Town, Observatory, Cape Town, South Africa
e-mail: andrew.nicol@uct.ac.za; pradeep.navsaria@uct.ac.za

There is no universal consensus on the application of this military surgical experience in the field of civilian low-velocity penetrating rectal trauma, but the following are presented as guidelines that have been effective and safe in the management of these injuries at our own institution [1].

51.2 Surgical Anatomy

The surgical management of the penetrating rectal injury is dependent on the part of the rectum that is injured and whether this is extra- or intra-peritoneal.

The rectum is around 12-cm long and is divided into thirds according to the peritoneal attachments. The peritoneal covers the upper one-third of the rectum on the front and sides and this is the intra-peritoneal rectum. The middle third is only covered on the anterior aspect by peritoneum. The lower third is completely extra-peritoneal as the peritoneum is reflected on to the upper part of the bladder in the male (to form the rectovesical pouch) or on to the upper vagina in the female (to create the recto-uterine pouch).

Injuries to the lower one-third of the rectum and to the entire posterior wall are considered to be extra-peritoneal.

51.3 Incidence

Penetrating rectal injuries occur infrequently but the majority (>80%) that do occur are secondary to gunshot wounds as reported from most trauma centres. Our own experience has shown low-velocity gunshot injuries to be responsible for 99% of rectal trauma [1].

G.C. Velmahos et al. (eds.), *Penetrating Trauma*,
DOI 10.1007/978-3-642-20453-1_51, © Springer-Verlag Berlin Heidelberg 2012

Stab wounds and impalements are uncommon but do occur.

51.4 Special Investigations

The presence of blood on the rectal should alert the surgeon to the presence of a colonic injury. If there is suspicion of a potential rectal injury from the tract of the gunshot wound or the knife, then a sigmoidoscopy must be carried out to exclude this even in the absence of blood on rectal examination. Genito-urinary tract injuries are commonly associated with rectal injuries and indeed, concomitant bladder injuries have been present in up to one-third of patients with rectal trauma. Ensure that a CT scan (with rectal contrast) and CT cystogram have been performed pre-operatively in the haemodynamically stable patient. This will provide information with respect to the tract of the bullet and allow you to plan the most appropriate form of intervention.

51.5 Surgical Strategies

51.5.1 Patient Position

The patient should be positioned in Lloyd-Davies position. This provides the best access into the pelvis particularly if bleeding is encountered and the extra-peritoneal rectum requires mobilisation. A sigmoidoscopy should be performed in the haemodynamically stable patient in order to diagnose and locate the position of the rectal injury. A urinary catheter should already be in situ.

51.5.2 Laparotomy

A midline laparotomy is performed in haemodynamically unstable patients or in those with an acute abdomen. Ensure that your skin incision reaches the pubic symphysis. Do not injure the bladder on entering the peritoneal cavity. The principles of abdominal trauma surgery apply; control any haemorrhage and prevent contamination.

Intra-peritoneal rectal injuries are dealt with in a similar fashion to other colonic trauma. Ensure that the wound edges have been debrided and are bleeding. Simple holes are closed with a single layer absorbable suture. No drains are required.

In the event of a high-velocity gunshot wound to the rectum, the surgeon should be in a damage control frame of mind, and the sigmoid should be ligated and the distal rectal stump transfixed with a TA stapler. Identify the ureters bilaterally or follow them down from the bifurcation of the common iliac artery to ensure that they are not ligated. We find a silk is superior to linen in the ligation of bowel. Simply pass an artery forceps through the mesentery and then pull the silk suture through and tie off the colon. A single suture usually suffices. At the subsequent relook laparotomy, the sigmoid colon is brought out as an end stoma and the injured rectum removed.

In stab wounds and in low-velocity gunshot wounds, the site of the injury needs to be identified. If there is a single hole, ensure that you are not missing the second hole. Place a finger in the hole and palpate the colon for any further holes. It can be easy to miss a hole where the mesentery attaches to the rectum. If there is any doubt, then the hole in the intra-peritoneal rectum can be enlarged and looked at under direct vision. If there is a second hole but this is extra-peritoneal, then this second hole can be left unsutured and a proximal defunctioning loop sigmoid colostomy performed.

The extra-peritoneal rectum only needs to be mobilised if there is massive haemorrhage adjacent and looking as if there is involvement of the vessels in the mesorectum (superior and middle rectal arteries). This may also depend on the experience of the surgeon involved as these can also be packed with abdominal swabs into the pelvis for haemostasis. If the injury to the rectum is entirely extra-peritoneal, then these holes do not need to be sutured. There is no advantage to repair, and in many cases, it is technically difficult to do so. A defunctioning sigmoid loop colostomy should be the mainstay in the management of these extra-peritoneal injuries.

Look also for any bladder involvement. The bladder may even be opened in the anterior midline if necessary to exclude an injury. Another option is to have an unscrubbed assistant fill the bladder with a mixture of sterile water and methylene blue via the urinary catheter. Traumatic rectovesical fistulas need to be recognised and dealt with. The bladder must always

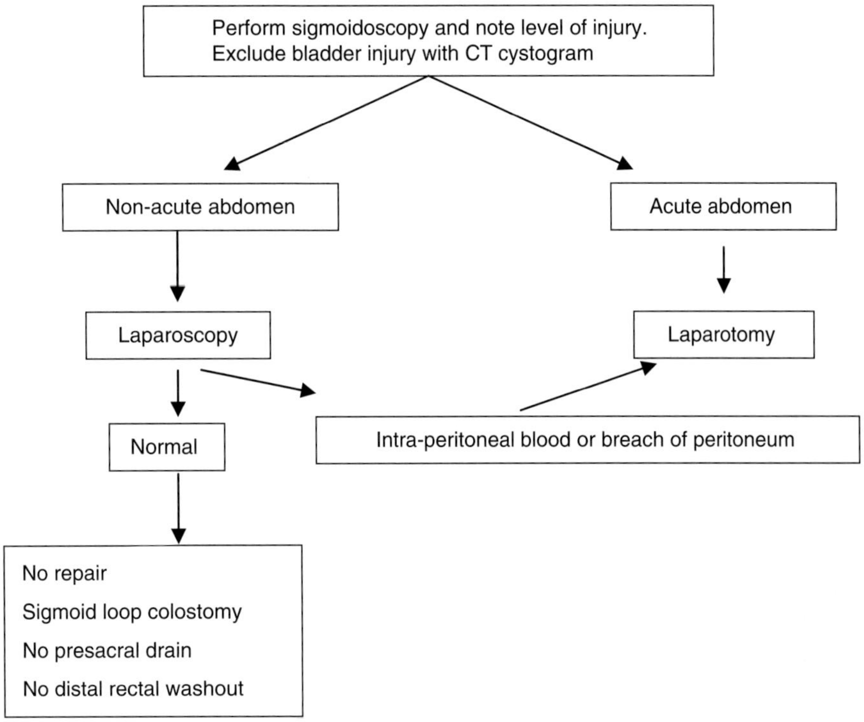

Fig. 51.1 Management strategy for an extra-peritoneal gunshot wound of the rectum

be repaired and then an omental pedicle placed between the bladder and the rectum in order to reduce the high incidence of rectovesical fistulae from combined rectal and genito-urinary trauma [2].

51.5.3 Laparoscopy and a Trephine Loop Colostomy

A laparoscopy is indicated in the haemodynamically stable patient with a transpelvic gunshot wound who presents with blood per rectum but no abdominal peritoneal signs. If there is no blood or urine in the peritoneal cavity, then the patient can be safely managed with a trephine loop sigmoid colostomy in the left iliac fossa without the need for a laparotomy [3, 4] (Fig. 51.1).

51.5.4 Distal Rectal Washout

The value of distal rectal washout in civilian injuries has been questioned. Present day experience with low-velocity gunshot wounds tends to show no benefit from distal rectal washout and it is considered to be associated with a high risk of infection because of spillage from the unrepaired extra-peritoneal rectal perforation [5]. This has resulted in most trauma surgeons abandoning this procedure.

51.5.5 Pre-sacral Drainage

The placement of a drain in the pre-sacral space through an incision in the anococcygeal raphe was advocated in the military experience, but the only randomised clinical trial in the civilian setting has shown that this did not reduce septic complications and is currently not recommended [6].

51.5.6 Antibiotic Treatment

Broad-spectrum antibiotics should be administered for a full period of 7 days in the event of an extra-peritoneal injury that has been purely managed with a loop colostomy and no laparotomy and the patient should be monitored closely for the development of pelvic sepsis. If this does occur, then the collection is usually amenable to percutaneous drainage under ultrasound guidance.

Important Points

- Always place the patient in the Lloyd-Davies position as the surgical access into the pelvis is improved.
- Identify and sling both ureters early in the dissection. This avoids an iatrogenic injury and helps exclude any traumatic injury to the ureter.
- Follow the tract of the bullet and ensure that any bone or joint involvement is extensively washed out.

References

1. Navsaria PH, Edu S, Nicol AJ (2007) Civilian extraperitoneal rectal gunshot wounds: surgical management made simpler. World J Surg 31:1345–1351
2. Franko ER, Ivatury RR, Schwalb DM (1993) Combined penetrating rectal and genitourinary injuries: a challenge in management. J Trauma 34:347–353
3. Navsaria PH, Graham R, Nicol A (2001) A new approach to extraperitoneal rectal injuries: laparoscopy and diverting loop sigmoid colostomy. J Trauma 51:532–535
4. Navsaria PH, Shaw JM, Zellweger R, Nicol AJ, Kahn D (2004) Diagnostic laparoscopy and diverting sigmoid loop colostomy in the management of civilian extra-peritoneal rectal gunshot injuries. Br J Surg 91:460–464
5. Velmahos GC, Gomez H, Falabella A, Demetriades D (2000) Operative management of civilian rectal gunshot wounds: simpler is better. World J Surg 24:114–118
6. Gonzales RP, Falimirski M, Holevar R (1998) The role of presacral drainage in the management of penetrating rectal trauma. J Trauma 45:656–661

Abdominal Compartment Syndrome

52

Zsolt J. Balogh, Osamu Yoshino, and Michael Sugrue

The application of damage control surgery (DCS) principles and aggressive fluid resuscitation makes it possible to save critically injured penetrating trauma patients. These survivors suffer whole body ischemia/reperfusion injury (hemorrhagic shock followed by resuscitation), which is associated with bowel edema, abdominal wall swelling, retroperitoncal swelling, and ascites formation. The abdominal packing and the formal closure of the abdomen together with the increased volume of the abdominal content can cause increased abdominal pressure, which compromises the function of vital organs (kidneys, liver, lung, heart, and intestines). Abdominal compartment syndrome (ACS, increased intra-abdominal pressure with organ dysfunction/failure) has emerged as a life-threatening complication among survivors of DCS. Prevention of ACS is a solution, but when it is attempted, the abdominal decompression and use of temporary abdominal closure is required. The liberal use of open abdomen strategy decreases the incidence of ACS and mortality from ACS but creates a new challenge: The management of the open abdomen is a condition with significant morbidity and potential mortality.

Z.J. Balogh (✉) • O. Yoshino
John Hunter Hospital and Hunter New England Area Health Service, University of Newcastle, Newcastle, NSW, Australia
e-mail: zsolt.balogh@hnehealth.nsw.gov.au

M. Sugrue
Letterkenny General Hospital, Letterkenny, Ireland

52.1 Definitions

Abdominal compartment syndrome (ACS) is defined as sustained increased intra-abdominal pressure (IAP > 20 mmHg), also known as intra-abdominal hypertension (IAH), and is associated with newly developed organ dysfunctions [1]. While IAH is graded [from Grade I (12–15 mmHg) to Grade IV (over 25 mmHg)], ACS is considered as an "all or nothing" phenomenon. ACS can be classified based on the etiology (for example, postinjury, postburn, after abdominal aortic surgery, pancreatitis, septic patients) and the acuity of the syndrome (acute, subacute, and chronic). This chapter focuses on acute postinjury abdominal compartment syndrome, which can be further classified as primary (injury to the abdomen) or secondary (extra-abdominal trauma only) ACS (Table 52.1).

52.2 When to Expect ACS in Penetrating Trauma?

ACS as a severe complication of penetrating trauma can develop in both abdominal and extra-abdominal penetrating trauma. ACS typically develops in patients who present in shock and requires urgent hemostasis and fluid resuscitation [2, 3].

Typical presentations of ACS after penetrating trauma are listed in Table 52.1 and described below.

1. Penetrating abdominal trauma with shock (Figs. 52.1 and 52.2): This is the classic pattern; patients with major abdominal injuries, especially with abdominal vascular trauma, are at high risk of developing primary ACS [4]. Hemorrhagic shock and subsequent

G.C. Velmahos et al. (eds.), *Penetrating Trauma*,
DOI 10.1007/978-3-642-20453-1_52, © Springer-Verlag Berlin Heidelberg 2012

Table 52.1 Causes of abdominal compartment syndrome in penetrating trauma

Primary abdominal compartment syndrome	Secondary abdominal compartment syndrome
• Severe penetrating abdominal trauma + shock	• Severe extra-abdominal bleeding requiring massive resuscitation.
• Aortic cross-clamping	• Extra-abdominal sepsis requiring massive resuscitation
• Abdominal sepsis as late complication	

resuscitation is whole body ischemia reperfusion injury to the body, which is associated with generalized and localized (intestinal) edema [5]. The venous return from abdominal organs is further compromised by the space occupying nature of the packs used for hemorrhage control. Open abdomen strategy is a proven approach to prevent ACS, in most of the cases [2, 6–8]. Fascial closure of the abdomen after damage control surgery (DCS) is not feasible because it can cause ACS and in any case, a second look is necessary to remove the packs and any potential necrotic tissue and to restore the continuity of the intestinal tract. Urgent need to go to the operating room and the presence of damage control physiology (acidosis, coagulopathy and hypothermia) are independent predictors of the primary ACS [9].

2. Penetrating chest or extremity trauma with shock: This is the classic example of secondary ACS, as there is no abdominal injury or pathology but the whole body ischemia reperfusion injury is present and driving the pathophysiology [3]. The intestinal tract has a significantly lower antiedema capacity than other vital organs like brain, lung, or heart. Secondary ACS has the same symptoms (increased airway pressures, decreased urine, and cardiac output) like primary ACS, but secondary ACS is much more elusive since there is no obvious abdominal cause [10]. Massive resuscitation is always present as a major independent predictor. Secondary ACS can be present at the time of the initial surgery on extra-abdominal bleeding sources. Reassessment on the table for potential ACS is important, and while a distending non-injured abdomen with high airway pressures could be a clue, measuring the intra-abdominal pressure is always helpful in the differential diagnosis [3].
3. After closure of the open abdomen: Premature closure of the open abdomen at the time of the second look laparotomy can result in recurrent ACS. Intraoperative measurement of the IAP during closure and reassessment on the table are advisable when the desired level of closure is achieved. It is important to remember that the IAP is most likely to be at its lowest while the patient is on the operating table (anesthetized, paralyzed, flat, and supine) and it will be higher in the intensive care unit (elevation of the head of bed, avoidance of neuromuscular

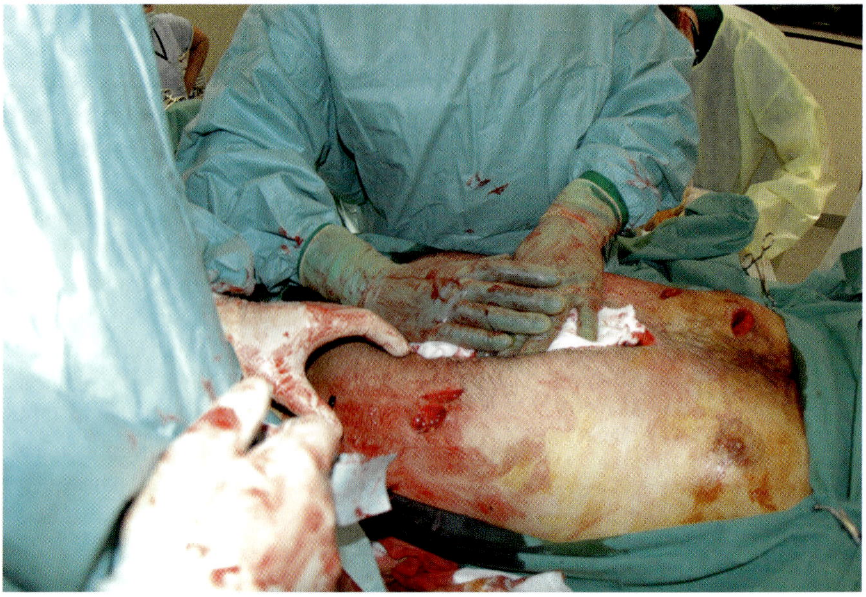

Fig. 52.1 Multiple stab wounds requiring damage control surgery, high risk for abdominal compartment syndrome

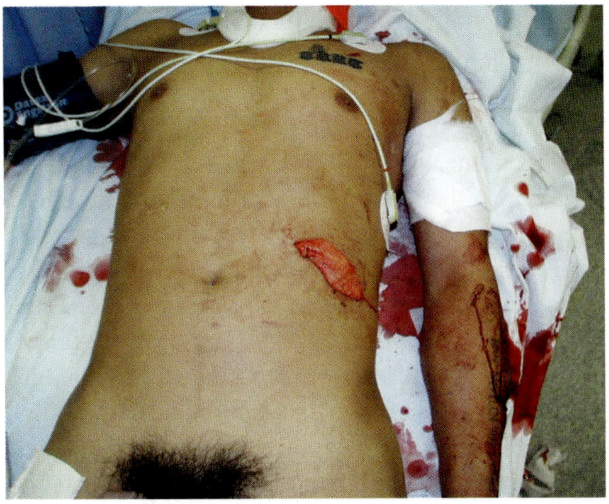

Fig. 52.2 Isolated stab wound without hemodynamic compromise, suitable for definitive surgery, low risk for abdominal compartment syndrome

paralysis, nursing) [11]. It is hard to measure IAP at the end of surgery unless there is an IVC line or a urinary catheter that is connected to the OR monitor. If there is no IAP measure available when you close the abdomen, airway pressures should be discussed with the anesthesiologist.

4. Late presentation compounded with sepsis: ACS can present in penetrating trauma patients later as a complication of uncontrolled abdominal (primary ACS) or extra-abdominal (secondary ACS) sepsis. Remember that treating the sepsis will also treat the ACS.

52.3 Diagnosis

The presentation of ACS after penetrating trauma with shock is very rapid; most of the cases develop with 12 h of hospital admission representing a second life-threatening insult after the exsanguination [12]. In some extreme cases, ACS can develop on the operating table while thoracic or skeletal life-/limb-saving operation is performed [13]. However, there are some ways to reduce the incidence of ACS, as shown in Table 52.2.

The diagnosis of ACS involves the measurement of the IAP. Clinical examination is unreliable in estimating the IAP [14]. The most feasible method is the intravesical route, originally described by Kron and modified by others [15, 16]. The measurement can be done with improvised devices, but today there are several reliable proprietary devices available. All these techniques require saline instillation into the bladder before measurement. Historically, the recommended instilled volume was 50 mL and above. However, recent research has shown that there is no need for more than 25 mL of saline through a safe closed system [11]. The limitation of the technique is the intermittent nature and the 5–8 min required to perform each measurement. The IAP can be monitored continuously via a three-way urinary catheter in the most critical patients where the timely recognition of increased IAP is crucial.

The other component of the diagnosis is the organ dysfunction related to the increased IAP [17]. The differentiation of the IAP-related organ dysfunctions can be difficult from the ongoing circulatory, respiratory, and renal dysfunction of an acute penetrating trauma patient. Acute penetrating trauma patients are

Table 52.2 The common avoidable mistakes, which can cause abdominal compartment syndrome in penetrating trauma

Prehospital	Delay to definitive care
	Poor control of external hemorrhage
	Uncontrolled crystalloid resuscitation
Emergency department	Delay to hemorrhage control
	Uncontrolled large volume crystalloid resuscitation
	Extensive imaging with uncontrolled resuscitation
	Underestimation of non-cavity bleeders
	Poor control of the environment (hypothermia)
Operating room	The need for aortic cross-clamping
	Delay to hemorrhage control
	Uncontrolled resuscitation
	Inability to improve hypothermia, acidosis, and coagulopathy
	Tight packing with fascial closure
	Inadequate temporary abdominal closure
	Poor control of abdominal bleeding
	Long surgery
Intensive care unit	Chasing supra-normal resuscitation endpoints
	Crystalloid boluses to maintain filling pressures or for Starling curve assessment
	Not measuring IAP
	Inability to recognize re-bleeding

not necessarily anuric or oliguric when they develop ACS. The urine output has to be judged in the context of the magnitude of the fluid resuscitation (100 mL/h in a patient who is in 10 L positive balance does not necessarily indicate adequate urine output). Young healthy trauma patients are expected to have a hyperdynamic response after major trauma and resuscitation. Close to normal cardiac output in these scenarios can mean compromised circulation. The filling pressures (Central venous pressure and pulmonary capillary wedge pressure) can be falsely normal or elevated in patients with increased IAP [18]. Many factors can directly and/or indirectly effect ventilation during the initial phase of shock resuscitation. If no significant lung or intrapleural injury/pathology exists, high airway pressures and low compliance associated with increased IAP can be diagnostic as well.

52.4 Treatment

The treatment of a compartment syndrome is decompression; in postinjury ACS, this involves a full midline laparotomy. The nonoperative measures, which are more frequently described in acute general surgical and medical literature, are unlikely to be helpful in critically ill penetrating trauma patients where the syndrome is evident within a few hours of ICU admission. In this scenario, there is no time for you to wait and see the potential modest decreases of IAP due to nonoperative measures (positioning, neuromuscular paralysis, evacuation of gastric, and intestinal intraluminal contents). These patients are dying. Your immediate efficient action is required. In obvious secondary ACS cases (no intra-abdominal injury), bedside ultrasound-guided drainage of the acutely developed ascites might be a solution, but in most cases not only the peritoneal fluid but rather the intestinal edema which is the main component of the increased IAP [11]. If intra-abdominal injury is excluded, you can even perform decompression in the ICU by using sterile technique (ICU procedure team) [19]. In primary ACS cases, usually re-bleeding is present, which requires you to perform further formal exploration of the abdomen and control of the hemorrhage preferably after transfer of the patient to the operating room.

After decompression or re-exploration, you need to apply a temporary abdominal closure to prevent evisceration and contamination but allow space for potential progressive swelling. Historically, this was done with skin-only closure with running stitch, towel clips, or with the "Bogota-bag." This latter is a large sterile infusion bag (arthroscopic or cystoscopic 3 L normal saline bag) fashioned and stitched into the fascia or to the skin of the abdominal wound edges. The skin-only closures do not provide enough room for swelling during the acute resuscitation. These measures can be utilized in the operating room after quick packing to gain hemostasis and prevent further heat loss while allowing time to the anesthesiologist to "catch up" with the blood loss and coagulation factors. The patient abdomen should be reassessed (repacked as required) and temporary abdominal closure applied. The Bogota-bag allows room for swelling but its control of the peritoneal fluids is poor and potentially ruins the skin/fascia, which could prevent future fascial closure. Most of the centers prefer to use some elastic self-adhesive coverage with abundant drainage. This can be performed with commercial vacuum-assisted devices or with a homemade (hand towel, adhesive foil, and suction drains) vacuum pack method. For first dressing after DCS, probably, a homemade technique is fine (cheaper and readily available) and less likely to cause ongoing blood loss due to low suction. Commercial devices are definitively beneficial from the first re-look laparotomy and dressing change, but many institutions use them successfully from day one. If stomas are indicated at the time of the re-look laparotomy, you should place them as lateral (further away from the midline) as possible, to prevent potential interference with fascial closure.

52.5 Open Abdomen

The open abdomen is the recognized preventive and therapeutic measure of postinjury ACS. The liberal application of the open abdomen strategy has led to a decrease in the incidence of lethal ACS but has created significant morbidity and resource utilization [2, 7]. Temporary abdominal closure is efficient in preventing ACS, but in low-risk patients, it leads to unnecessary morbidity and cost. From the first re-look laparotomy, the goal should be to achieve fascial closure or at least minimize the size of the hernia. Most preventive open abdomens can be closed with one or two extra trips to the operating room. Vacuum-assisted techniques are very effective in controlling the local edema and preventing the retraction of the abdominal wall [20, 21]. Fascial closure should occur within less than 10 days. Dynamic closure systems may help with this. The earlier that closure or cover is achieved, the less the risk of fistula formation. Since the areas above the costal margin and below the iliac crests are difficult to cover with component separation, extra attention must be given to close the fascia as soon as it is safe. If the fascial edges are retracted, the options for short term are insertion of a mesh, or skin grafting over the granulating bowel or skin-only closure. The closure over the intestines is important to prevent further protein loss, fistula formation, peritonitis, or anastomosis breakdown [22]. The quality of life with open abdomen patients is generally poor, and the continued restoration of the abdominal wall significantly improves it [23]. Late reconstruction is usually not considered before 6 months and component separation, non-resorbable mesh, or pedicled muscle flaps are the main options.

Important Points

- Abdominal compartment syndrome only develops in live patients, so at first, you need to save them from imminent exsanguination.
- It is imperative to think about it even before the patients come to the ER-never mind the OR!
- Abdominal compartment syndrome is defined by elevated intra-abdominal pressure and organ dysfunction/failure associated with it.
- Abdominal compartment syndrome can develop in penetrating trauma without penetration to the abdomen (secondary abdominal compartment syndrome).
- Abdominal compartment syndrome after major penetrating trauma usually develops within a few hours after ICU admission.
- Do not be fooled and try to overcome the abdominal compartment syndrome–related organ dysfunctions/failures with fluid resuscitation and with the ventilator. Preload-driven resuscitation in impending abdominal compartment syndrome is the recipe for making the situation worse. As a surgeon, use a scalpel rather than salty water.
- The damage control physiology (hypothermia, acidosis, coagulopathy): The urgent need for operative hemorrhage control and the amount of crystalloids used (>3 L until the operating room and more than 7 L until ICU admission) are independent predictors of postinjury abdominal compartment syndrome. Remember to watch out for polycompartment syndromes.
- The open abdomen is one efficient method for prevention of abdominal compartment syndrome. Most important is to stop the bleeding and avoid excess resuscitation.
- After the first damage control laparotomy, fancy temporary abdominal closures are not necessary. The main principles to follow are: ensuring plenty of room for swelling, good seal, control of the peritoneal fluids, and abdominal wall friendliness.
- Abdominal compartment syndrome can develop in patients with open abdomen.
- Saving a patient with abdominal decompression is a satisfying experience but managing the subsequent open abdomen can be challenging and less rewarding.
- While the decompression of the abdominal compartment syndrome is an urgent life-saving intervention, the management of the open abdomen is a quality of life restoring activity where consultation with experts should occur in a timely fashion.
- A strategy which ensures the timely and safe (fistula, abscess, peritonitis, and hernia-free) management of the open abdomen at your institution with the aim of fascial closure within 7–10 days should be developed.

References

1. Malbrain ML, Cheatham ML, Kirkpatrick A et al (2006) Results from the international conference of experts on intra-abdominal hypertension and abdominal compartment syndrome. I. Definitions. Intensive Care Med 32:1722–1732
2. Ivatury RR, Porter JM, Simon RJ, Islam S, John R, Stahl WM (1998) Intra-abdominal hypertension after life-threatening penetrating abdominal trauma: prophylaxis, incidence, and clinical relevance to gastric mucosal pH and abdominal compartment syndrome. J Trauma 44:1016–1021; discussion 21–23

3. Balogh Z, Moore FA, Moore EE, Biffl WL (2007) Secondary abdominal compartment syndrome: a potential threat for all trauma clinicians. Injury 38:272–279
4. Raeburn CD, Moore EE, Biffl WL et al (2001) The abdominal compartment syndrome is a morbid complication of postinjury damage control surgery. Am J Surg 182:542–546
5. Moore EE (1996) Thomas G. Orr Memorial Lecture. Staged laparotomy for the hypothermia, acidosis, and coagulopathy syndrome. Am J Surg 172:405–410
6. Mayberry JC, Mullins RJ, Crass RA, Trunkey DD (1997) Prevention of abdominal compartment syndrome by absorbable mesh prosthesis closure. Arch Surg 132:957–961; discussion 61–62
7. Offner PJ, de Souza AL, Moore EE et al (2001) Avoidance of abdominal compartment syndrome in damage-control laparotomy after trauma. Arch Surg 136:676–681
8. Hirshberg A, Wall MJ Jr, Mattox KL (1994) Planned reoperation for trauma: a two year experience with 124 consecutive patients. J Trauma 37:365–369
9. Balogh Z, McKinley BA, Holcomb JB et al (2003) Both primary and secondary abdominal compartment syndrome can be predicted early and are harbingers of multiple organ failure. J Trauma 54:848–859
10. Balogh Z, McKinley BA, Cocanour CS et al (2002) Secondary abdominal compartment syndrome is an elusive early complication of traumatic shock resuscitation. Am J Surg 184:538–543
11. Cheatham ML, Malbrain ML, Kirkpatrick A et al (2007) Results from the international conference of experts on intra-abdominal hypertension and abdominal compartment syndrome. II. Recommendations. Intensive Care Med 33:951–962
12. Balogh Z, McKinley BA, Cox CS Jr et al (2003) Abdominal compartment syndrome: the cause or effect of postinjury multiple organ failure. Shock 20:483–492
13. Rodas EB, Malhotra AK, Chhitwal R, Aboutanos MB, Duane TM, Ivatury RR (2005) Hyperacute abdominal compartment syndrome: an unrecognized complication of massive intraoperative resuscitation for extra-abdominal injuries. Am Surg 71:977–981
14. Sugrue M, Bauman A, Jones F et al (2002) Clinical examination is an inaccurate predictor of intraabdominal pressure. World J Surg 26:1428–1431
15. Balogh Z, Jones F, D'Amours S, Parr M, Sugrue M (2004) Continuous intra-abdominal pressure measurement technique. Am J Surg 188:679–684
16. Kron IL, Harman PK, Nolan SP (1984) The measurement of intra-abdominal pressure as a criterion for abdominal re-exploration. Ann Surg 199:28–30
17. Sugrue M (2000) Intra-abdominal pressure and intensive care: current concepts and future implications. Intensivmed 37:529–535
18. Balogh Z, McKinley BA, Cocanour CS, Kozar RA, Cox CS, Moore FA (2003) Patients with impending abdominal compartment syndrome do not respond to early volume loading. Am J Surg 186:602–607
19. Diaz JJ Jr, Mejia V, Subhawong AP et al (2005) Protocol for bedside laparotomy in trauma and emergency general surgery: a low return to the operating room. Am Surg 71:986–991
20. Miller PR, Meredith JW, Johnson JC, Chang MC (2004) Prospective evaluation of vacuum-assisted fascial closure after open abdomen: planned ventral hernia rate is substantially reduced. Ann Surg 239:608–614; discussion 14–16
21. Subramonia S, Pankhurst S, Rowlands BJ, Lobo DN (2009) Vacuum-assisted closure of postoperative abdominal wounds: a prospective study. World J Surg 33:931–937
22. Ivatury RR (2009) Update on open abdomen management: achievements and challenges. World J Surg 33:1150–1153
23. Cheatham ML, Safcsak K, Llerena LE, Morrow CE Jr, Block EF (2004) Long-term physical, mental, and functional consequences of abdominal decompression. J Trauma 56:237–241; discussion 41–42

SNOM: Conservative Management of Solid Viscera

53

Pradeep H. Navsaria

The selective nonoperative management (SNOM) of hemodynamically stable, clinically evaluable patients with abdominal stab and low-velocity gunshot wounds without an intra-abdominal injury is safe. The high success rates of the nonoperative management of patients with blunt solid organ injuries have been extended to select patients with documented penetrating liver, kidney, and spleen injuries. While this is not a universally accepted mode of treatment, there is a small, but growing body of evidence to support the SNOM of penetrating solid organs [1–3].

The concept of the NOM of penetrating solid organs is one that deals with patients who have sustained a penetrating abdominal injury, who do not have an emergent indication for laparotomy (hemodynamic instability or peritonitis), who are neurologically (centrally and peripherally) intact, who have undergone computerized (CT) tomography documenting a solid organ injury, and who are then managed *nonoperatively, without a laparotomy.*

53.1 SNOM: Liver

Patients with penetrating injury to the right thoraco-abdomen and right upper quadrant with injury to the right lung, right diaphragm, and liver may be safely observed in the presence of stable vital signs, minimal or no abdominal tenderness, and reliable clinical examination.

53.1.1 The Patient

- Right thoracoabdominal/right upper quadrant penetrating injury

53.1.2 Clinical Findings

- Stable vital signs
- No central or spinal cord neurological deficit
- Minimal or no abdominal tenderness

53.1.3 Plain Chest Radiograph

- Normal
- Right pneumothorax
- Right hemothorax
- Right hemo/pneumothorax
- Right-sided pulmonary opacity signifying lung contusion and/or intrapulmonary hematoma

53.1.4 Special Investigation

Contrasted computerized axial tomography essential (lower chest and upper abdomen)

- CT scan confirms lung and liver injury (diaphragm injury by inference)
- Grades liver injury
- Determines the amount of pleural fluid and degree of lung contusion

P.H. Navsaria
Trauma Centre, Ward C14, Groote Schuur Hospital, Observatory, Cape Town, South Africa
e-mail: pradeep.navsaria@uct.ac.za

G.C. Velmahos et al. (eds.), *Penetrating Trauma*,
DOI 10.1007/978-3-642-20453-1_53, © Springer-Verlag Berlin Heidelberg 2012

- Any contrast "blush" on CT scan is considered a finding of bleeding or false aneurysm and must be followed up immediately by angiography and angioembolization, if the patient remains hemodynamically stable
- Free air, free fluid with no solid organ involvement, localized bowel wall thickening, mesentery stranding, hematoma/free air surrounding hollow viscus suggests hollow viscus injury – proceed to laparotomy

53.1.5 Management

- Admit to high-observation unit for at least 48–72 h.
- Single dose second-generation cephalosporin prophylactic antibiotic.
- Two-hourly blood pressure and hemoglobin estimation for 24 h, then 4-hourly.
- Four-hourly serial abdominal examination.
- Nil per mouth for 24 h, then feed; if tolerated hollow visceral injury unlikely.
- Transfer to general surgical ward.

53.1.6 Complications

Failed abdominal observation: Development of peritonitis and hypotension warrants immediate surgery. Pyrexia and raised leukocyte count must be taken in context of clinical abdominal findings and not necessarily implies failure of nonoperative management.

Infected fluid (bile and/or blood) collections: Infected subphrenic, subhepatic, and intra-hepatic collections usually manifest 3–5 days post-injury. Patients are usually generally well, but have a swinging pyrexia, elevated leukocyte count, and maybe some increase in localized tenderness to the right upper quadrant. Repeat CT scan is essential for diagnosis, and treatment consists of percutaneous drainage and broad-spectrum antibiotic cover (anti-Staphylococcal agent and anaerobic cover is essential). Patients without drainable collections should be empirically commenced on broad-spectrum antibiotics for suspected infected liver "tract hematoma."

53.2 Thoracobiliary Fistulae

All patients with a liver gunshot traversing the diaphragm treated nonoperatively are at risk of thoracobiliary (pleurobiliary and bronchobiliary) fistulae. Diagnosis usually suspected with bilious drainage from tube thoracostomy or reaccummulation of pleural fluid collections that are bile-stained, and bile-stained sputum. Management consists of adequate pleural drainage, percutaneous drainage of any peri/intra-hepatic collections, endoscopic retrograde cholangiography with sphincterotomy and placement of a biliary stent.

53.3 The Evidence

The first reported prospective study by Renz and Feliciano [4] on the NOM of liver gunshot injuries included 13 patients with right-sided thoracoabdominal gunshot wounds, seven of whom had CT-confirmed liver injuries, with a 100% nonoperative management success rate. Similarly, Chmielewski et al. [5], in a series of 12 patients with lower right chest gunshot wounds, confirmed eight hepatic injuries (Grades II–III) in those undergoing ultrasound or CT. One patient required delayed laparotomy without any adverse outcome. Ginzburg et al. [6] managed four patients with liver gunshot injuries successfully nonoperatively. In their retrospective series, Demetriades et al. [7] proposed the notion that only selected patients with Grade I–III injuries should be managed nonoperatively. In a prospective study of SNOM of liver gunshot injuries, Omoshoro-Jones et al. [8] showed that increasing injury severity was associated with an increasing rate of complications; however, injury grade itself was not shown to be an independent predictor of nonoperative management failure. Overall, of the 188 cases of nonoperatively managed liver gunshot injuries identified in the English literature, a success rate of greater than 90% has been reported. This high success rate could be attributed to the fact that most gunshot injuries to the liver require no treatment. In a prospective study by Navsaria et al., [2] of 195 liver gunshot injuries, 81/195 (41.5%) liver injuries required no treatment at laparotomy, and 63/195 (32.3%) patients were considered for nonoperative management without laparotomy. Hence, a total of 144/195 (73.8%) of all liver gunshot injuries in their series were managed conservatively. The Surgeon, however, must recognize the risks of NOM of penetrating liver injuries and have the resources (angiography with angioembolization, percutaneous interventional techniques, endoscopic interventional cholangiography) available to address potential complications.

SNOM of penetrating abdominal wounds, with or without liver injury, with or without advanced CT technology, is still based largely on the findings from *serial clinical examinations.*

53.4 SNOM: Kidney

The mandatory exploration of all patients with penetrating renal trauma is not necessary.

53.4.1 The Patient

- Penetrating abdominal trauma; particularly to the flank and posterior abdomen

53.4.2 Clinical Findings

- Stable vital signs
- No central or spinal cord neurological deficit
- Minimal or no abdominal tenderness
- Hematuria (microscopic/macroscopic)

53.4.3 Special Investigation

Contrasted computerized axial tomography is essential.

- CT scan confirms renal injury.
- CT grades renal injury.
- Ureteric injuries require surgical intervention.
- Nonperfusing kidneys require nephrectomy. Note that parenchymal contrast extravasation is not an absolute contraindication to nonoperative treatment.
- Any contrast "blush' on CT scan is considered a finding of bleeding or false aneurysm and must be followed up immediately by angiography and angioembolization, if the patient remains hemodynamically stable.

Free air, free fluid with no solid organ involvement, localized bowel wall thickening, mesentery stranding, and hematoma/free air surrounding hollow viscus suggest hollow viscus injury – proceed to laparotomy.

53.4.4 Management

- Admit to high-observation unit for at least 48–72 h.
- Single dose second-generation cephalosporin prophylactic antibiotic.
- Two-hourly blood pressure and hemoglobin estimation for 24 h, then 4-hourly.
- Four-hourly serial abdominal examination and daily urine dipstick.
- Nil per mouth for 24 h, then feed; if tolerated hollow visceral injury unlikely.
- Transfer to general surgical ward.

53.4.5 Complications

1. Failed abdominal observation: Development of peritonitis and hypotension warrants immediate surgery.
2. Pyrexia and raised leukocyte count must be taken in context of clinical abdominal findings and not necessarily implies failure of nonoperative management.
3. Perinephric infected hematoma/urinoma: Infected perinephric collections usually manifest 3–5 days post-injury. Patients are usually generally well, but have a swinging pyrexia, elevated leukocyte count and some flank and/or renal angle tenderness. Repeat CT scan is essential for diagnosis, and treatment consists of percutaneous drainage and broad-spectrum antibiotic cover. Persistent urinary leaks can be managed by retrograde ureterogram and endoscopic stent placement.
4. Persistent hematuria/recurrent macroscopic hematuria. Persistent macroscopic hematuria (>72 h) and those who present with delayed-onset macroscopic hematuria (usually 10–14 days post-injury) is an indication for renal angiography and embolization of intra renal arteriovenous fistulae or false aneurysms.
5. Blocked urinary catheters: Usually occurs in the presence of macroscopic hematuria and blood clots in the bladder. An ultrasound of the bladder will confirm blood clots in the bladder and bladder irrigation should be commenced using a three-way hematuria catheter.

53.4.6 The Evidence

The only absolute criteria for emergency surgery in kidney trauma is hemodynamic instability. Patients with vascular pedicle, and renal pelvis and ureter injuries require immediate exploration. The percentage of kidney stab wounds amenable to nonoperative management ranges between 51% and 77% with success rates of greater than 95% [9–11]. It has been reported though that gunshot wounds are significantly more likely to result in severe kidney injuries than stab wounds [12] and thence the reluctance maybe to manage gunshot wounds to the kidney nonoperatively. It has also been suggested that the threshold for exploring urinary extravasation for gunshot wounds should be lower than that for stab wounds because of the increased risk of delayed complications because of extensive tissue damage from the projectile's blast effect. Most studies on conservatively managed gunshot wounds have been retrospective in nature. While there is some evidence to support that with accurate preoperative imaging and grading of the kidney injury, grades I to III need not be explored at the time of laparotomy for other injuries. The evidence to support the nonoperative management of isolated kidney gunshot injuries are few. Overall, of the 63 cases of nonoperatively managed kidney gunshot injuries identified in the English literature, a success rate of almost 95% has been reported [3]. McAninch and colleagues [13] reported a series 87 gunshot kidney units, of which 10 were not explored at laparotomy for associated injuries and 8 (9.2%) patients were managed with a 100% success rate without a laparotomy. Similarly, Velmahos et al. managed 4 patients in a series of 52 consecutive kidney gunshot injuries successfully nonoperatively without laparotomy [14]. Complications that may occur with expectant management are ongoing bleeding or rebleeding (increase in perinephric hematoma or appearance of macroscopic hematuria or persistent microscopic hematuria), infected perinephric fluid collections, and persistent urinary leaks. Therefore, the surgeon must recognize the risks of NOM of penetrating kidney injuries and have the resources (angiography with angioembolization and percutaneous radiological interventional techniques) available to address potential complications. However, NOM of penetrating abdominal wounds, with or without kidney injury, with or without advanced CT technology, is still based largely on the findings from *serial clinical examinations.*

53.5 SNOM: Spleen

Presently, there is very little evidence to support the nonoperative management of splenic injuries.

Important Points

- NOM is for hemodynamically stable, clinically evaluable patients without an intra-abdominal injury.
- NOM is still based largely on the findings from *serial clinical examinations.*
- With or without advanced CT technology, you need to see your patient regularly.
- It takes time to see your patient regularly.
- Clinical serial examination is best done by the same person.

References

1. Demetriades D, Hadjizacharia P, Constantinou C, Brown C, Inaba K, Rhee P, Salim A (2006) Selective nonoperative management of penetrating abdominal solid organ injuries. Ann Surg 244:620–628
2. Navsaria PH, Nicol AJ, Krige JE, Edu S (2009) Selective nonoperative management of liver gunshot injuries. Ann Surg 249:653–656
3. Navsaria PH, Nicol AJ (2009) Selective nonoperative management of kidney gunshot injuries. World J Surg 33: 553–557
4. Renz BM, Feliciano DV (1994) Gunshot wounds to the right thoracoabdomen: a prospective study of nonoperative management. J Trauma 37:737–744
5. Chmielewski GW, Nicholas JM, Dulchavsky SA, Diebel LN (1995) Nonoperative management of gunshot wounds of the abdomen. Am Surg 61:665–668
6. Ginzburg E, Carrillo EH, Kopelman T, McKenney MG, Kirton OC, Shatz DV, Sleeman D, Martin LC (1998) The role of computed tomography in selective management of gunshot wounds to the abdomen and flank. J Trauma 45: 1005–1009
7. Demetriades D, Gomez H, Chahwan S, Charalambides K, Velmahos G, Murray J, Asensio J, Berne TV (1999) Gunshot injuries to the liver: the role of selective nonoperative management. J Am Coll Surg 188:343–348
8. Omoshoro-Jones JA, Nicol AJ, Navsaria PH, Zellweger R, Krige JEJ, Kahn DH (2005) Selective non-operative management of liver gunshot injuries. Br J Surg 92: 890–895
9. Armenakas NA, Duckett CP, McAninch JW (1999) Indications for nonoperative management of renal stab wounds. J Urol 161:768–771
10. Thall EH, Stone NN, Cheng DL, Cohen EL, Fine EM (1996) Conservative management of penetrating and blunt type III renal injuries. J Urol 77:512–517
11. Wessels H, McAninch JW, Meyer A, Bruce J (1997) Criteria for nonoperative treatment of significant penetrating renal lacerations. J Urol 157:24–27

12. Heyns CF (2004) Renal trauma: indications for imaging and renal exploration. BJU Int 93:1165–1170
13. McAninch JW, Carroll PR, Armenakas NA, Lee P (1993) Renal gunshot wounds: methods of salvage and reconstruction. J Trauma 35:279–283
14. Velmahos GC, Demetriades D, Cornwell EE, Belzberg H, Murray J, Asensio J, Berne TV (1998) Selective management of renal gunshot wounds. Br J Surg 85:1121–1124

Bleeding in the Pelvis

54

Edward Kelly

Penetrating injuries to the pelvis often cause complex multi-organ injuries due the crowded space of the pelvic cavity, which contains the rectum, the bladder and ureters, the iliac arteries and veins and the boney pelvis. The trauma surgeon's urgent goals are hemostasis and control of contamination; restoration of continuity of hollow organs should only be undertaken after the urgent goals are met. In this chapter, we will focus on rapid control of bleeding and briefly discuss reconstruction options.

Due to the unpredictable nature of penetrating trauma, bleeding from the pelvis can be encountered unexpectedly, for example, in a patient with a bullet entry wound in the chest or lower extremity. Therefore, in every operation for penetrating trauma, it is best to have long vascular instruments ready and to have a self-retaining retractor system to expose the pelvis. Likewise, have the appropriate sutures (4-0 Prolene for iliac artery, 3-0 for the aorta, and 6-0 for iliac vein), grafts and vascular shunts available. Have balloon occlusion catheters ready to control bleeding from vessels that are hard to reach (distal external iliac, internal iliac). Have at least two suction lines available, and cell-saving equipment may also be useful.

Midline laparotomy is the exposure of choice for penetrating injuries to the pelvis, as it offers the best access to the crowded space and enables proximal vascular control in the abdomen, outside of the field of injury. The pelvis also borders the extremities, and injuries to the pelvis can also involve the groins or more distal structures. When more distal control is indicated, a vertical incision in the groin can be used to expose the femoral arteries and vein. Therefore, the skin prep should include chest, abdomen, both groins, and extremities down to the knees.

Begin with a long vertical midline laparotomy. Liquid blood, bowel contents and clots should be removed quickly to enable exposure. Four quadrant packing can be used to control abdominal sources of bleeding. Evisceration of the small intestine out of the abdomen will facilitate exposure, as will wide retraction with a Bookwalter retractor.

First we will discuss hematomas. Unlike blunt trauma, pelvic hematomas from penetrating trauma should always be explored, as they are strongly associated with injury to the iliac vessels. Obtain proximal control outside of the hematoma at the origin of the iliac artery or at the distal aorta. For a hematoma on either side of the pelvis, perform a right-sided medial visceral rotation, taking care not to disrupt the hematoma, in order to expose the inferior vena cava and distal aorta. If the origin of the iliac artery is free, clamp it with an angled vascular clamp; if the origin is not free, cross clamp the aorta with a large straight vascular clamp. For rapid distal control, direct pressure on the external iliac vessels in the groin will suffice, or compression with a sponge-on-a-stick applied to the distal vessel within the pelvis, if not involved with hematoma. Rapid proximal control of the IVC can also be achieved with simple compression.

Once proximal and distal control is obtained, open the hematoma and identify the injury. Keep in mind that the internal iliac vessels are not controlled with this approach, and may bleed copiously. Keep in mind that the ureter may be inside the hematoma, or compressed,

E. Kelly
Department of Surgery, Brigham Women's Hospital,
75 Francis St., Boston, MA 02115, USA
e-mail: ekelly1@partners.org

G.C. Velmahos et al. (eds.), *Penetrating Trauma*,
DOI 10.1007/978-3-642-20453-1_54,

or distorted, or injured. After the vascular injury is dealt with, it is necessary to expose the ureter and determine if it is injured. When the hematoma is entered, there may be ongoing bleeding from the uncontrolled internal iliac artery or vein. These may be rapidly controlled with a balloon occlusion catheter, or if the exposure is sufficient, vessel loops or vascular clamps.

The surgeon then is faced with the decision to repair the injury in some fashion, or to ligate the injured vessel and manage the consequences. This decision is challenging, as the patient may have other injuries that require urgent attention, or may be physiologically depleted (in terms of temperature, coagulation and acidosis) and may benefit from the damage control approach. In order to make the best decision, identify the injury completely before committing to a specific approach. That is, do not decide on placing an interposition graft until you have seen both ends of the vessel you plan to repair, and do not ligate vessels until you know you have all bleeding ends identified. Damage control surgery only works if the damage is actually controlled!

Proximal iliac vein injury deserves special attention. Anatomically the confluence of the IVC lies behind the aortic bifurcation, immediately posterior to the right common iliac artery. Rapid control can be achieved with compression as outlined above, but to ligate or repair the vein requires more exposure. Division of the right common iliac artery between vascular clamps will enable exposure of the IVC and proximal common iliac veins. Once the vein injury has been addressed, the artery can be repaired with 4-0 Prolene suture, or temporized with a shunt.

Iliac vein injuries have a high rate of thrombosis, even if the injury is limited and a good technical repair is achieved. It is therefore not reasonable to expend valuable time to achieve a perfect venous repair via paneled vein patch or venous interposition graft when the patient has multiple injuries that require intervention.

Destructive complex injuries with profuse bleeding call for lifesaving interventions to stop the hemorrhage. These injuries require a damage control approach, using suture ligation, compression with packing, and topical hemostatic agents (such as Bio-glue) to achieve control.

By comparison, injuries to the iliac or femoral arteries are more forgiving. The higher flows in these vessels make them more resistant to thrombosis, and thus the results of repair are much better. Single layer repair with 3-0 or 4-0 Prolene yields a reliable long-term outcome for simple arterial lacerations. Transections with no loss of length can be managed with primary anastomosis, again with good results. Destructive injuries to the arteries, characterized by loss of length that is too great to allow straightforward primary anastomosis, should be controlled in one of three ways: (1) Reconstruct immediately with conduit. (2) Insert a shunt and return to the operating room when the patient is more stable for definitive reconstruction. (3) Ligate the ends and reconstruct extra-anatomically as soon as possible.

Immediate reconstruction with conduit should only be undertaken when the patient is hemodynamically stable and does not have a high burden of other injuries. Time spent on a definitive repair should not be time taken away from controlling bleeding from the mesenteric vein or liver injury. However, when the patient is stable and has minimal other injuries, reconstruction with conduit yields a reliable long-term result.

In the setting of gross spillage of bowel contents, there is a high rate of infection for both arterial and venous graft reconstruction. When bioprosthetic conduits such as reversed saphenous vein become infected, there is often severe necrolysis of the conduit, leading to renewed hemorrhage in the necrotic infected field. This observation has prompted the author to use non-biological conduits such as ePTFE or Dacron.

Irrespective of the strategy for managing penetrating injury of the pelvis, the risks of deep vein thrombosis, venous hypertension, and pulmonary embolism are very high and should be considered as part of the treatment of all such patients. The author advocates early lower extremity fasciotomy for patients with combined arterial and venous injury, and liberal use of vena cava filters for prevention of pulmonary embolism.

Important Points

- Be prepared! Have the deep vascular instruments you use ready every time you explore a penetrating injury that may include the pelvis.
- Trap the external iliac artery against the boney pelvis for rapid control.
- Remember vascular shunts for the bail out option.
- It is OK to divide the common iliac artery to expose the confluence of the IVC.
- Fasciotomy is indicated for complex injury.

Suggested Reading

Burch J, Richardson RJ, Martin RR, Mattox KL (1990) Penetrating iliac vascular injuries: recent experience with 233 consecutive patients. J Trauma 30:1450–1459

Carillo E, Spain DA, Wilson MA, Miller FB, Richardson DJ (1998) Alternatives in the management of penetrating injuries to the iliac vessels. J Trauma 44:1024–1030

Mattox KL, Rea J, Coyness LE, Beall AC, DeBakey ME (1978) Penetrating injuries to the iliac arteries. Am J Surg 136:663–667

Ryan W, Snyder W, Bell T, Hunt J (1982) Penetrating injuries to the iliac vessels. Am J Surg 144:642–645

Part V

Surgical Strategies in Penetrating Trauma and Orthopedic Injuries

Introduction to Orthopedic Injuries

55

Thomas Scalea

The relationship between bony injury and multiple trauma seems very well defined in patients after blunt trauma. Blunt trauma usually involves diffuse energy transfer. Fractures are common and many of them require operative fixation. Issues such as optimal timing of fracture fixation require close collaboration between the orthopedic surgeon, the general surgeon, anesthesiologist, and intensivist. While this relationship may seem less important in penetrating trauma, in fact, those same relationships do exist and all are important.

Penetrating injury is a disease where blood loss predominates. Soft-tissue injury is less important than it is in blunt trauma. However, missile trajectories still often injure bony structures. Important vascular and neurologic structures run immediately adjacent to the bones, thus injury to multiple structures is not only possible, it is relatively frequent. While strategies may differ from blunt trauma, the priorities of initial evaluation remain the same. Identification of immediately life-threatening injuries is followed by resuscitation, rapid identification of all injuries and then concomitant stabilization and injury repair.

Penetrating injuries to bone can bleed from a variety of sources. While injury to the major vascular structures is more common then following blunt trauma, bleeding from other sources also occurs. The combination of bleeding from the medullary canal, soft-tissue bleeding in the missile track and small vessel bleeding from muscular branch vessels can still produce a clinically important hemorrhage. For instance, a gunshot wound to the thigh that fractures the femur also will injure major branches of the profunda femoris artery and the concomitant soft-tissue producing significant hemorrhage. Penetrating injury to the torso certainly requires emergent evaluation, yet the skilled clinician must keep extremity injury in mind when gauging blood loss as well as planning resuscitation and operative approaches.

T. Scalea
R Adams Cowley Shock Trauma Center, University of Maryland, 22 S Greene St, Baltimore 21201, MD, USA
e-mail: tscalea@umm.edu

55.1 Diagnostics

The vast majority of bone injuries should be suspected by physical exam following penetrating trauma. Similar to blunt trauma, fractures produce soft-tissue swelling and hematoma, as well as significant pain. Pulsatile bleeding from the wound is generally considered a hard sign of vascular injury and should prompt early exploration. Extremities in which fractures are suspected should be splinted for comfort and to reduce bleeding during the remainder of the investigation and resuscitation. Early in the secondary survey, the extremities should be examined for adequacy of distal perfusion. If there is any concern about concomitant vascular injury, measuring an ankle brachial index (ABI) will be helpful. Bony injury can produce spasm in the adjacent blood vessels. However, any degree of impaired perfusion should be assumed to be a named vascular injury until proven otherwise. The generally accepted threshold is an ABI of .9. Injuries to the upper extremities may make measuring an ABI difficult. In that case, using an uninjured lower extremity as a reference point is equally effective.

Plain films of the extremity are usually adequate to make the diagnosis of the bony injury. As with blunt

G.C. Velmahos et al. (eds.), *Penetrating Trauma*,
DOI 10.1007/978-3-642-20453-1_55, © Springer-Verlag Berlin Heidelberg 2012

trauma, all fractures are not created equal. Radiographs should be examined for fracture location, as well as degree of angulation, displacement and comminution. In some locations, plain films may underestimate the degree of bony injury. This is most common around the knee and pelvis. Pelvic fractures secondary to gunshot wounds may not be visible on a screening pelvic x-ray. In addition, fractures of the proximal tibia, particularly the tibial plateau, may not be easily discerned on a plain x-ray. In most cases, a CT scan without IV contrast can be quite helpful in defining injury anatomy. This is fortuitous as many of these patients will undergo CT scanning for other reasons. For instance, double or triple contrast CT is commonly used to rule out both intraabdominal and retroperitoneal visceral injuries in the abdomen and pelvis. Therefore, the possibility of a pelvic fracture can also be investigated. In addition, popliteal vascular injuries are relatively common with penetrating injury around the knee. CT angiography is commonly used as an investigation. Fractures of the proximal tibia can then be diagnosed concurrent with the vascular evaluation.

While all fractures following penetrating injury are technically open, they usually do not have the same degree of soft-tissue injury and exposed bone, as do open fractures following blunt trauma. Thus, a short course of antibiotic prophylaxis is probably wise and all that is needed. The urgency to stabilize open fractures or at least to perform an incision for drainage is not the same as it exists with blunt injuries. An injury from a high-velocity rifle may be an exception.

55.2 Combination Vascular and Bony Injuries

Patients with the combination of vascular and bony injuries are a special subset. Revascularization is an extremely high priority to prevent muscle ischemia and/or limb necrosis. However, bony stabilization is likewise important. A number of characteristics of injury anatomy should be taken into account when planning an operative strategy. Patients with a threatened extremity require urgent revascularization. However, those with some degree of distal perfusion do not have the same risks of muscle ischemia. This is most often determined by physical exam and/or examination with a Doppler.

The bony anatomy is likewise important. Patients with nondisplaced fractures are different than those with badly comminuted and angulated fractures in which the extremity is shortened. While it may make sense to do definitive revascularization first to prevent distal ischemia, the vascular anastomosis and/or bypass graft may then be at risk when the fracture is brought out to length. This can create tension on the anastomosis, causing thrombosis and/or complete disruption.

A detailed conversation between the orthopedic surgeon and the general surgeon is necessary in order to make the best decisions. In patients with a non-threatened extremity, definitive fracture fixation first will allow revascularization to proceed safely. On the other hand, in patients with nondisplaced fractures, vascular repair first often makes some sense. This is particularly true in patients with limited distal perfusion.

Some sets of patients, such as those with both displaced fractures and critical ischemia, or those with multiple competing priorities, may best be served by temporizing measures. These principles are similar to using damage control in the torso. Patients with critical ischemia may be best served by temporary intraluminal shunting. This restores perfusion to the extremity, preventing ischemia. The bone can then be stabilized and vascular repair can occur after bony stabilization.

Temporary bony stability can be achieved by placing an external fixator, so-called Damage Control Orthopedics. The patient can then undergo definitive vascular repair. The more definitive fracture fixation can be delayed for 3–5 days without substantial increased risk of fracture-related complications.

Finally, some patients may benefit from both intraluminal shunting and temporary fracture fixation. This would be useful in patients with multiple competing priorities such as fracture or vascular injury or an important torso injury, or patients with multiple fracture and/or vascular injuries. Care must be individualized to injury anatomy and patient physiology.

55.3 Compartment Syndrome

While the particulars of compartment syndrome will be addressed in a separate chapter, some general comments may be helpful. Compartment syndrome from blunt trauma usually involves all of the compartments in the injured extremity. The diffuse energy transmission puts all of the compartments at equal risk. While not absolute, that degree of energy transfer usually also results in a fracture.

The more specific energy transfer that accompanies penetrating trauma means that fractures are not always present. In addition, not all compartments may be at equal risk. For instance, a gunshot wound or a stab wound through the anterior compartment of a lower extremity can produce anterior compartment syndrome, but the uninjured lateral and posterior compartments will remain normal. Patients with penetrating injury through a muscle compartment should undergo a period of observation to be sure the compartment syndrome is not going to develop.

Patients who develop isolated compartment syndrome come with a very high risk of named vascular injury. In the lower extremity, there may not be signs of distal ischemia. For instance, if the anterior tibial artery is injured, flow may well be preserved via the posterior tibial and peritoneal arteries. The patient may very well have normal pulses and normal ABIs. If possible, preoperative imaging, particularly CT angiography, can be very helpful in making the diagnosis of named vascular injuries in these types of patients. If the vascular injury is diagnosed, transcatheter embolization before fasciotomy may well reduce intraoperative blood loss. It would be important not to delay fasciotomy for this procedure. Alternately, vascular injuries uncovered at the time of fasciotomy can be dealt with directly in the operating room.

55.4 Spinal Injury

Patients with penetrating injury to the torso have some risks of spinal column and spinal cord injuries. Conventional wisdom in the field is to immobilize all such patients on a backboard and in a rigid cervical collar to avoid secondary spinal injury. However, while all injuries are time related, penetrating torso injury is especially best served by utilizing a "scoop and run" philosophy and not "stay and play."

The actual risks of bony instability of the vertebral bodies following penetrating injury are actually quite low, being well under 1%. This is true even if patients have neurologic deficits. In civilian practice, even a gunshot wound spinal column fracture is rarely unstable and very rarely requires operative stabilization.

Placing spinal embolization devices requires EMS providers to spend extra time at the scene, which may not be wise. In addition, these devices limit vascular access and resuscitative maneuvers once the patient presents to the hospital. EMS systems need to carefully evaluate field protocols. Once the patient presents, clinicians should rapidly determine the real risk of spinal instability. In patients who are not at high risk for spinal instability, restraint devices should not be allowed to limit resuscitation and can be removed in the Emergency Department without imaging studies.

55.5 Conclusion

The relationship between bony injury and injury elsewhere in the body remains relevant in patients following penetrating injury. The multidisciplinary team caring for the badly injured patient after penetrating trauma should use standard trauma principles to determine relative treatment priorities. Most often with bony injuries, this will involve anesthesiologists, general surgeons and orthopedic surgeons. Resuscitation and operative strategies must be tailored to injury anatomy and patient physiology. One size never fits all and that is certainly true in these patients, particularly those with more than one trajectory and multiple injuries.

Important Points

1. Recognize that bony injury can be a source of significant blood loss following penetrating trauma.
2. Remember that there is a relatively strong association between bony injury and vascular injury.
3. Suspect bony injury in any patient with a concerning trajectory and any deformity of the extremity.
4. Careful physical exam in essential to investigate the possibility of concomitant vascular and bony injury.
5. CT scan can be helpful in diagnosing occult fractures in a small subset of patients.
6. The principles of damage control are often helpful in treating patients with the combination of bony and vascular injury.
7. Compartment syndrome in the extremity is different in penetrating trauma when compared to blunt trauma.

8. Wise operative strategies in patients with bony and vascular injury are determined by fracture anatomy and degree of distal perfusion.
9. Unstable spinal column injuries following penetrating trauma are quite rare. Spinal restraint devices should not interfere with patient evaluation or resuscitation.

Recommended Literature

Chiu WC, Shanmuganathan K, Mirvis SE, Scalea TM (2001) Determining the need for laparotomy in penetrating torso trauma: a prospective study using triple-contrast enhanced abdominopelvic computed tomography. J Trauma 51: 860–869

Cornwell EE, Chang D, Bonar J, Scalea TM, Bass R (2001) Thoraco-lumbar immobilization for trauma patients with torso gunshot wounds – is it necessary? Arch Surg 136:324–327

Haut ER, Kalish BT, Efron D, Haider AH, Stevens KA, Kieninger AN, Cornwell ED, Chang DC (2010) Spine immobilization in penetrating trauma: More harm than good? J Trauma 68:115–121

Peng PD, Spain DA, Tataria M, Hellinger JC, Rubin GD, Brundage SI (2008) CT angiography effectively evaluates extremity vascular trauma. Am Surg 74:103–107

Scalea TM, Pollak AW, Scott JD et al (2000) External fixation as a bridge to intramedullary nailing for patients with multiple injuries and femur fractures and damage control orthopedics. J Trauma 48:613–621

Subramanian A, Vercruysse G, Dente C, Wyrzykowski A, King E, Feliciano DV (2008) A decade's experience with temporary intravascular shunts at a civilian level I trauma center. J Trauma 65:316–326

Extremity Fractures

56

Jeffrey Ustin

Extremity fracture with penetrating injury occurs in several settings. In the military environment, shrapnel wounds are common. In the civilian setting, gunshot wounds and shotgun wounds prevail. Some areas of the world are plagued with machete wounds, which are a cross between a sharp cut and a blunt crush. Likewise, certain industrial injuries are hybrid. Finally, blunt injuries can act with a penetrating mechanism when the sharp ends of the fractured bone lacerate from within. The particular mechanism can help dictate the approach to evaluating the exact injuries, as described below. It also helps to direct your thinking about the overall trauma burden of the patient.

56.1 Priorities

All anatomic structures are in jeopardy and it is encumbent upon you to prove that there is no injury. Vascular injuries are the most immediately life and limb threatening. In the short term, integrity of the soft tissue envelope will help determine how well any repair heals whereas long-term functionality depends on neurologic injury.

Your priority is to rapidly revascularize the extremity to optimize the patient's functional outcome and to minimize tissue loss and amputation rates. Once blood flow has been returned, limb stability must be regained. Then, turn your attention to the soft tissues, debriding as necessary. Finally, evaluate and consider repairing any nerve injury. The specifics concerning this generic approach are described later.

The above priorities are balanced with considerations of the trauma burden. From the time the patient presents start asking yourself how he or she is doing. Are there multiple other injuries? Has there been large volume blood loss? Is the lethal triad of hypothermia, hypocoaguability, and acidemia present or incipient? Extremity injuries offer many different damage control alternatives to definitive treatment. Putting yourself and your team in a damage control mindset early on is essential.

56.2 The Decision to Operate

The decision to operate can be based on the need to repair the vasculature, bones, soft tissue or nerves. In terms of vascular injury, your physical exam is the gatekeeper to the operating room. Focus on the hard signs. As a reminder, the hard signs include an expanding or pulsatile hematoma, a thrill or bruit, loss of distal pulses, or distal ischemia. Also, measure an ankle-brachial or brachio-brachial index (ABI, BBI). If hard signs are not present and the ABI or BBI is >0.9, the patient does not have a surgically significant lesion and requires neither the operating room nor further workup. Most of the time, the hard signs indicate an operative vascular lesion. The exceptions to this rule are complex soft tissue injuries or blunt mechanism, which have an elevated false-positive rate on physical exam, shotgun or shrapnel wounds, which can present with multiple injuries, chronic vascular

J. Ustin
Division of Trauma, Burns and Critical Care, MetroHealth Medical Center, Case Western Reserve University, 2500 MetroHealth Dr, Cleveland, OH 02114, USA
e-mail: justin@partners.org, jeffustin@gmail.com

G.C. Velmahos et al. (eds.), *Penetrating Trauma*,
DOI 10.1007/978-3-642-20453-1_56, © Springer-Verlag Berlin Heidelberg 2012

disease, in which there may be absent pulses to begin with, or thoracic outlet lesions, in which the hard signs can be hidden around the shoulder girdle. If you find hard signs of vascular injury in the setting of one of these exceptions, obtain an angiogram.

Stabilize the fractures as early as possible. A stable fracture decreases tissue damage, bleeding, inflammation, and pain. It facilitates the patient's mobility with all the associated benefits of getting out of bed and moving such as decreased DVT rates, improved respiratory function, better skin care, less delirium, and improved mood. Earlier stabilization accelerates rehabilitation too.

Likewise, early debridement is helpful for similar reasons. Removing devitalized tissue decreases inflammation and infection. A clean, healthy tissue bed is critical for wound closure and definitive fracture fixation in many circumstances.

Finally, the timing of peripheral nerve repair depends upon the injury. A penetrating low-energy mechanism, such as a stab wound, should be repaired early, preferably within 1 week of injury. Higher energy injuries, such as gun shot wounds, are better repaired in a delayed fashion, to allow better delineation of a zone of injury.

56.3 Preparation for Operation

Control bleeding in the trauma resuscitation room. Start with digital pressure. Avoid blind clamping of bleeding vessels and make an attempt for focused placement of a hemostatic clamp. If needed, place a well-padded tourniquet. Consider allowing the patient to remain hypotensive until the source of bleeding is controlled. Initiate the massive transfusion protocol. If none exists, transfuse 1 unit of fresh frozen plasma (FFP) for every 2 units of packed red blood cells (PRBCs) and a pack of platelets for every 10 units of FFP and PRBCs transfused. Ask the blood bank to stay ahead 6 units of PRBCs and 2 units of FFP.

Use an arm table for upper extremity injuries and prep the thorax into the field allow for proximal control and maximum ability to extend the incision. Partially frog leg an injured lower extremity with a bump under the knee and consider using a fracture table. Prep the abdomen into the field. Prep the affected extremity circumferentially and always prep an uninjured extremity as well for possible vein graft harvest. Try to utilize an angiography compatible table to permit on table angiograms.

In terms of special equipment, request a sterile tourniquet be available, but do not routinely use it. Make sure a full complement of vascular clamps, vascular suture, and embolectomy catheters are available.

56.4 Operative Strategies

The first order of business is to control active hemorrhage. Once temporary control has been achieved, as described above, obtain proximal vascular control. For very proximal extremity injuries, extend the incision into the adjacent body cavity. For example, proximal control for high brachial artery injuries is the axillary artery and for the femoral artery is the external iliac above the inguinal ligament.

Unless there is a simple penetrating injury, perform an on-table angiogram if not done pre-operatively. To do this, place an 18-guage angiocatheter under direct visualization proximally and attach a three-way stopcock. Flush all components with saline prior to placement. Place a clamp proximal to the angiocath and inject 30 cc of contrast. Wait 3 s and take an xray. Alternatively, use fluoroscopy if you have a c-arm available.

Shunt the artery. If you have commercially made shunts available, use these. Otherwise, sterile IV tubing works as well. Prior to shunting, perform balloon embolectomy if needed and flush with heparinized saline. Place the proximal end of the shunt first, flush, and then place the distal end. Consider shunting the vein. Perform a fasciotomy in the following circumstances: (1) popliteal artery injury; (2) greater than 4 h ischemia; (3) patient in shock; (4) ligation of major vein or artery. The method for fasciotomy of each extremity is described in its respective chapter.

Next, stabilize the skeleton. The decision whether to perform temporary or definitive, internal or external fracture repair depends upon the patient's overall trauma burden, whether or not coagulopathy, hypothermia, or acidemia is developing, and the extent of damage to the soft tissue envelope. Additionally, consider the expertise available at your institution. If the patient is in extremis, an external splint may be the only alternative. An external fixator is obviously superior. For example, a patient with multiple shrapnel wounds who needs further chest and abdominal exploration should not undergo internal fixation. Or, a patient with a large tissue defect should undergo external fixation. Multiple fractures in a single extremity can be spanned with an external fixator for rapid stabilization, a technique referred to as damage control orthopedics.

A further discussion of the techniques of internal fixation is beyond the scope of this book. For external fixation, start by choosing a safe area of anatomy. Pay careful attention to the radial nerve distribution in the distal half of the arm and proximal half of the forearm. Also, be careful of the sensory branch of the radial nerve at the wrist. In the leg, the anterior tibial artery and deep peroneal nerve are vulnerable distally. Additionally, try to place the external fixators such that they will not interfere with wound care including debriding and any reconstructive procedures which may be necessary. If possible, plan the placement of the device to allow for further imaging.

Make a small skin incision and gently bluntly dissect. Place a drill sheath and remove the trocar. Slowly drill to minimize heat generation. Use fluoroscopy to follow progress. Tap the hole if not using self-tapping screws. Check depth and place a new pin.

In general, pins placed further apart are more stable. Placement of cross-members close to the extremity adds stability as does utilizing two cross-members.

Again consider the patient's status. If he or she is doing well and the trauma burden is limited, proceed with definitive vascular repair. If not, complete your operation and take the patient to the ICU. You can always return at a later time to remove the shunt and regain vascular integrity. Once the definitive repair has been accomplished, perform a completion angiogram.

At very least irrigate and clean all wounds. If able, debride devitalized tissue. Examine the nerves in the wound. If there is a clean laceration, reapproximate the perineurium with 7-0 or 8-0 prolene. If there is a clean transection, consider tacking the perineurium to a fixed structure near the point of injury. With higher energy mechanisms in which there may be a crush or blast component, examine the nerve for laceration and do no more. Repair of these more complex injuries should be delayed. Examine the nerve sheath and make sure there is no hematoma applying pressure.

Finally, any tendon repairs can be delayed for definitive orthopedic repair.

The decision to amputate a mangled extremity is very difficult and requires experience and clinical judgment. It should be made in consultation with the various teams involved including trauma surgery, orthopedic surgery, and plastic surgery. Certainly there are circumstances when the decision is obvious such as a traumatic amputation and a patient who is doing poorly or truly mangled extremity with loss of nerve, artery and extensive soft tissue defects. However, it is often much less obvious. Avoid making the decision to amputate at initial operation if at all possible.

Important Points

1. Pad appropriately the entire length of the plaster of paris.
2. A patient complaining of pain with a plaster is always right.
3. If the plaster is maybe too tight, release the entire length of plaster and padding.
4. Check the plaster the next day if it is still too tight.
5. Check after a week to see if the plaster is too loose.
6. Do not rely on pulse status if you want to exclude compartment syndrome.

Compartment Syndrome of the Extremities

57

Mark W. Bowyer

Compartment syndrome (CS) is a limb-threatening and potentially life-threatening condition. Long bone fractures and vascular injuries are the most frequent antecedent events. Burns, crush injury, bleeding in enclosed spaces, external compression of the limb, small thrombotic or embolic events, envenomation, allergy, intravenous infiltration, muscle overuse, nephritic syndrome, and intramuscular injection have all been implicated. Current knowledge unequivocally reflects that if you fail to identify and treat compartment syndrome properly, you will have a patient with tissue necrosis, permanent functional impairment, and potentially renal failure and death. CS has been found wherever a compartment is present: hand, forearm, upper arm, abdomen, buttock and the entire lower extremity. The leg (calf) is the area that is most commonly affected, followed by the forearm, and the thigh. As a well-trained surgeon who wants to do the best for each patient, you must become intimately familiar with this topic and the techniques to treat it.

57.1 Pathophysiology

The pathophysiology of CS is relatively straightforward. Groups of muscles and their associated nerves and vessels are surrounded by thick fascial layers that define the various compartments of the extremities which are of relatively fixed volume. As the compartment is filled with fluid from hemorrhage secondary to fracture, blunt or penetrating trauma, coagulopathy, intravenous infiltration, or swelling after reperfusion the pressure within the compartment increases. Likewise, compression from constrictive dressings/casts or improper positioning reduces the volume in the compartment with resultant increase in pressure.

It is not exactly rocket science to understand that as the pressure within the compartment increases, the tissue perfusion decreases and cellular metabolism is impaired, leading to cellular death if prolonged (4–6 h). As nerves are the most susceptible to ischemic insult, the earliest symptoms are neurologic. You must keep in mind that polytrauma patients with low blood pressures can sustain irreversible injury at lower compartment pressures than patients with normal blood pressures, and a very high index of suspicion should be maintained in this group.

57.2 Diagnosis

The diagnosis of compartment syndrome is a clinical diagnosis. The classically described five "Ps" – *pain*, pallor, paresthesias, paralysis, and pulselessness – are pathognomonic of compartment syndrome. However, *these are usually late signs and extensive and irreversible injuries may have taken place by the time they are manifested.* In the earliest stages of CS, patients may report some tingling and an uncomfortable feeling in their extremity followed closely by pain with passive stretching of the muscles of the affected compartment. The most important symptom of CS is *pain greater*

M.W. Bowyer
Division of Combat and Trauma Surgery,
Uniformed Services University of the Health
Services (USUHS), 4031 Jones Road,
Bethesda 20814-4172, USA
e-mail: mbowyer@usuhs.mil

G.C. Velmahos et al. (eds.), *Penetrating Trauma*,
DOI 10.1007/978-3-642-20453-1_57,

than expected due to the injury alone. In the anterior compartment of the lower leg, the superficial peroneal nerve is usually affected early with loss of sensation in the web space between the first two toes. *The presence of pulses and normal capillary refill does NOT exclude CS.* You might be tempted to try to "rule-out" CS in a patient with severe pain that has normal pulses. DON'T be tempted – unless you really have a thing for lawyers. Remember that the loss of pulse is a late finding, and the presence of pulses does not rule-out CS! *The presence of open wounds does* not *exclude CS.* In fact, the worst open fractures are actually more likely to have a CS. In one study, the incidence of CS was found to be directly proportional to the degree of injury to soft tissue and bone, and CS occurred most often in association with comminuted, type-III open fractures.

Tissue pressure (compartment pressure) measurements have a limited role in making the diagnosis of compartment syndrome. You should always remember that compartment syndrome is a clinical diagnosis, and a patient manifesting with signs and symptoms of a compartment syndrome should be operated on expeditiously. However, in polytrauma patients with associated head injury, drug and alcohol intoxication, intubation, spinal injuries, use of paralyzing drugs, extremes of age, unconsciousness, or low diastolic pressures, measuring compartment pressures may be of use in determining the need for fasciotomy.

The pressure threshold for making the diagnosis of CS is controversial. A number of authors recommend 30 mmHg, and others cite pressures as high as 45 mmHg. Many surgeons use the "Delta-P" system. The compartment pressure is subtracted from the patient's diastolic blood pressure. If this value is less than 30, the surgeon should be concerned that a compartment syndrome may be present. For instance, if the diastolic blood pressure was 60 and the measured compartment pressure was 42 ($60 - 42 = 18$), the "Delta-P" would be 18 and the patient is likely to have CS. Other factors to consider when considering fasciotomy are length of time of transport to definitive care and ability to do serial exams. Pressures can be measured using commercially available monitors or by using a needle attached to a side-port arterial line set-up. It is important to keep in mind that the pressure in one compartment can be normal whilst that in the compartment immediately adjacent can be elevated. It is therefore essential that you have a thorough understanding of the anatomy of the compartments and the confidence that you have measured the pressure of all of the compartments of the suspicious extremity prior to making any conclusions about a normal pressure. The bottom line, no bull, keep you out of trouble, take home message here is if you think your patient is at risk for CS you should be on the straight and narrow path to the operating room to perform a fasciotomy.

57.3 Treatment

The definitive treatment of compartment syndrome is *early and aggressive fasciotomy.* In patients with vascular injury in whom you plan to do a fasciotomy in conjunction with a vascular repair, it makes great sense to perform the fasciotomy *before* doing the repair. The rationale for this is that the ischemic compartment is likely to already be tight and thus will create inflow resistance to your vascular repair, making it susceptible to early thrombosis. If you are going to care for traumatically injured patients, it is imperative that you fully understand the anatomy of the extremity compartments and the technique of fasciotomy for each. It is extremely embarrassing for you, and life altering for your patient if you do not do an adequate or timely fasciotomy and the patient loses the limb as a result. In one large series reported by Feliciano et al., 75% of amputations of the lower extremity were related to a delay in performing, or performing an incomplete fasciotomy. In a recent large review of combat patients, Ritenour et al. reported that patients who had incomplete or delayed fasciotomy had twice the rate of major amputation and three times the rate of mortality. In spite of these alarming numbers, many otherwise well-trained surgeons continue to make these mistakes. Do you want to be one of them? Of course not! You want to do the best for your patient and you want to commit to memory the proper steps for fasciotomy which follow.

57.4 Lower Leg Compartment Syndrome and Fasciotomy

The leg (calf) is the most common site for compartment syndrome requiring fasciotomy. The leg has four major tissue compartments bounded by investing muscle fascia (see Fig. 57.1).

It is important that you understand the anatomical arrangement of these compartments as well as some

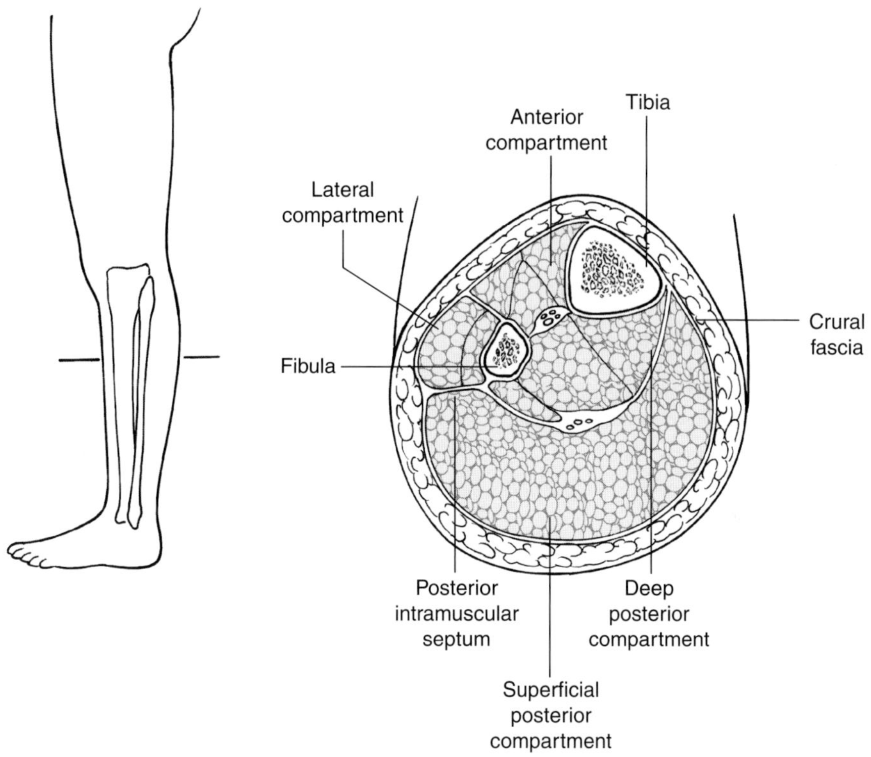

Fig. 57.1 Cross-sectional anatomy of the mid-portion of the right lower leg depicting the four compartments that must be released when performing a lower leg fasciotomy

key structures within each compartment in order to perform a proper four-compartment fasciotomy. It is not necessary for you to remember the names of all the muscles in each compartment, but it is useful for you to remember – that the anterior compartment contains the anterior tibial artery and vein and the deep peroneal nerve; the lateral compartment the superficial peroneal nerve (which must not be injured); the superficial posterior compartment the soleus and gastrocnemius muscles; and the deep posterior compartment the posterior tibial and peroneal vessels and the tibial nerve.

There is absolutely no role for getting fancy when doing fasciotomy of the lower extremity. The use of a single incision for four-compartment fasciotomy of the lower extremity is mentioned to condemn it, and now that it has been mentioned you should promptly forget it. Attempts to make cosmetic incisions should also be condemned and your mantra should be "bigger is better." Compartment syndrome of the lower extremity dictates two incision four-compartment fasciotomy with *generous* skin incisions and you should accept no substitute.

There are several key features that will enable you to perform a successful two incision four-compartment fasciotomy. The most commonly missed compartments are the anterior and the deep posterior. One of the key steps is proper placement of the incisions. As extremities needing fasciotomy are often grossly swollen or deformed, marking the key landmarks will aid in placement of the incisions. The tibial spine serves as a reliable midpoint between the incisions and the lateral malleous and fibular head are used to identify the course of the fibula on the lateral portion of the leg (Fig. 57.2). The lateral incision is usually made just anterior (~1 fingerbreadth) to the line of the fibula, or *A FINGER IN FRONT OF THE FIBULA*. It is important to stay anterior to the fibula as this minimizes the chance of damaging the superficial peroneal nerve. The medial incision is made one thumb-breadth below the palpable medial edge of the tibia, or *A THUMB BELOW THE TIBIA* (Fig. 57.3). The extent of the skin incision should be to a point approximately three fingerbreadths below the tibial tuberosity and above the malleolus on either side.

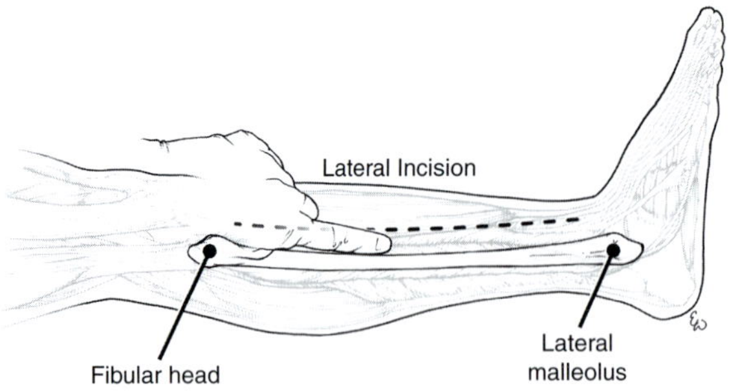

Fig. 57.2 The fibular head and lateral malleolus are used reference points to mark the edge of the fibula and the lateral incision (*dotted line*) is made one finger in front of this. The tibial spine serves as a midpoint reference between the two skin incisions

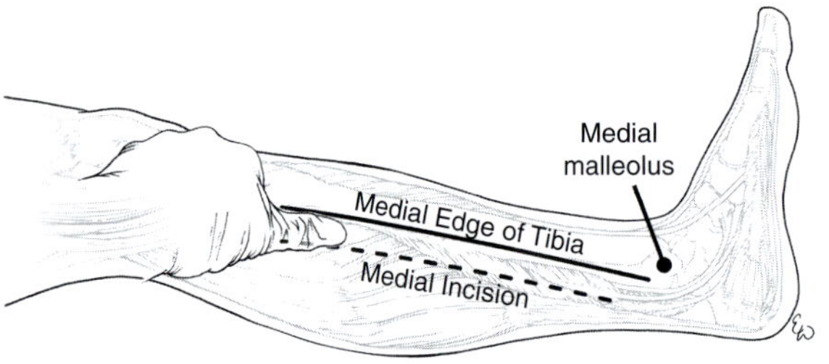

Fig. 57.3 The medial incision (*dotted line*) is made one thumb breadth below the palpable medial edge of the tibia (*solid line*)

It is very important that you mark the incisions on both sides prior to opening them, as the landmarks of the swollen extremity will become rapidly distorted once the incision is made.

57.4.1 The Lateral Incision of the Lower Leg

The lateral incision (Figs. 57.2 and 57.4) overlies is made one finger in front of the fibula and should in general extend from three fingerbreadths below the head of the fibula down to three fingerbreadths above the lateral malleolus. The exact length of the skin incision will depend on the clinical setting. Care must be taken to make sure that it is long enough so that the skin does not serve as a constricting band. The skin and subcutaneous tissue are incised to expose the fascia encasing the lateral and anterior compartments.

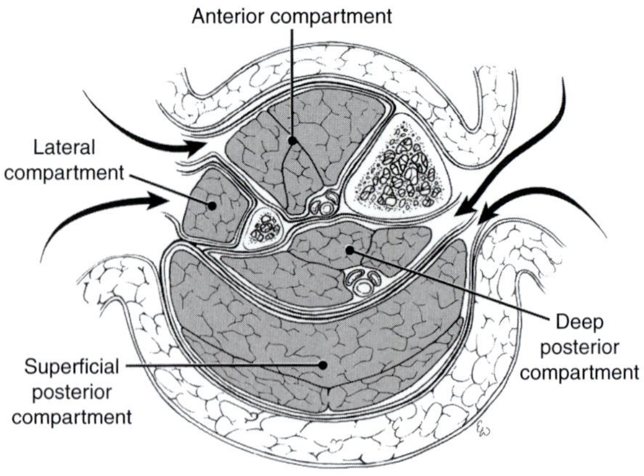

Fig. 57.4 Two incision four-compartment fasciotomy. The lateral incision provides access to the lateral and anterior compartments. The medial incision traverses the superficial compartment allowing entry into both the superficial and deep posterior compartments

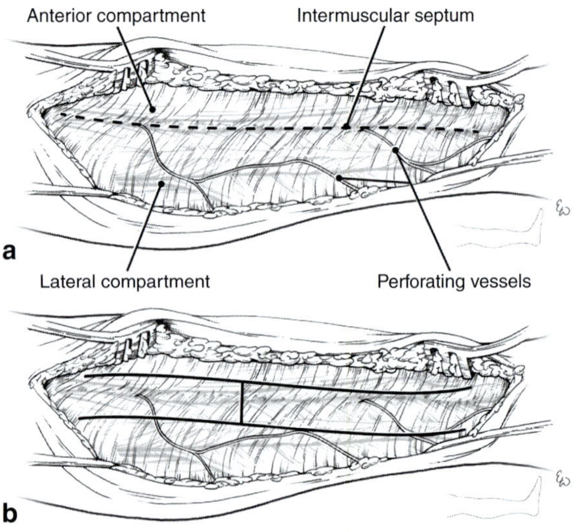

Fig. 57.5 (**a**) The intermuscular septum separates the anterior and lateral compartments and is where the perforating vessels exit. (**b**) The fascia overlying the anterior and lateral compartments is opened in a "H"-shaped fashion

Care should be taken to avoid the lesser saphenous vein and peroneal nerve when making these skin incisions.

Once the skin flap is raised the intermuscular septum is identified. This is the structure that divides the anterior and lateral compartments. In the swollen or

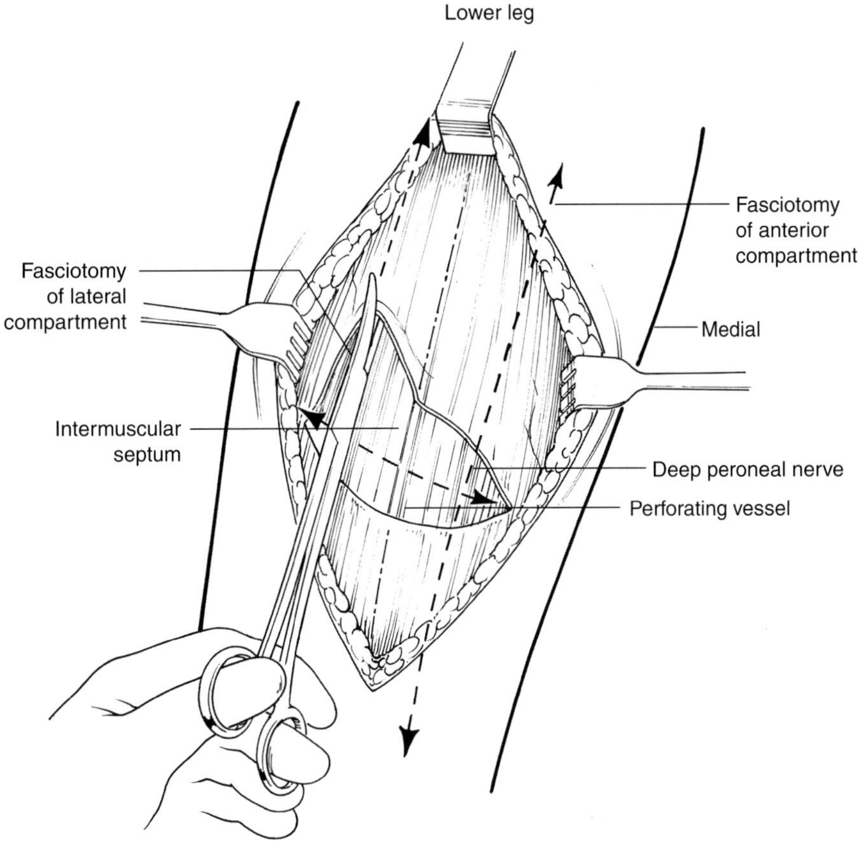

Fig. 57.6 The fascia overlying the anterior and lateral compartments is opened using scissors in a "H"-shaped fashion with the scissor tips turned away from the septum

injured extremity, you may have difficulty finding the intermuscular septum. Often you can find the septum by following the perforating vessels down to it (Fig. 57.5a). Classically the fascia of the lower leg is opened using an "H"-shaped incision. To do this you will make the cross piece of the "H" using a scalpel which will expose both compartments and the septum. You will then construct the legs of the "H" with curved scissors using just the tips which are turned away from the septum to avoid injury to the peroneal nerve (Figs. 57.5b and 57.6). The fascia should be opened by pushing the partially opened scissor tips in both directions on either side of the septum opening the fascia from the head of the fibula down to the lateral malleolus. Inspection of the septum and identification of the deep peroneal nerve and/or the anterior tibial vessels confirms entry into the anterior compartment. The skin incision should be closely inspected and extended as needed to ensure that the ends do not serve as a point of constriction.

57.4.2 The Medial Incision of the Lower Leg

The medial incision (Figs. 57.3 and 57.4) is made one fingerbreadth below the palpable medial edge of the tibia. As you make this incision, it is important to both identify and preserve the greater saphenous vein, as well ligate any perforators to it. In most individuals, the fascia that you will next encounter will be that which overlies the superficial posterior compartment which contains the soleus and gastrocnemius muscle. If you open this fascia from the tibial tuberosity to the medial malleolus, you will have effectively decompressed this compartment (Fig. 57.7). The key to entering the deep posterior compartment is the soleus muscle. The soleus muscle attaches to the medial edge of the tibia, and dissecting these fibers completely free from and exposing the underside of the tibia ensures entry into the deep posterior compartment (Fig. 57.8). Identification of the posterior tibial neurovascular bundle confirms that the compartment

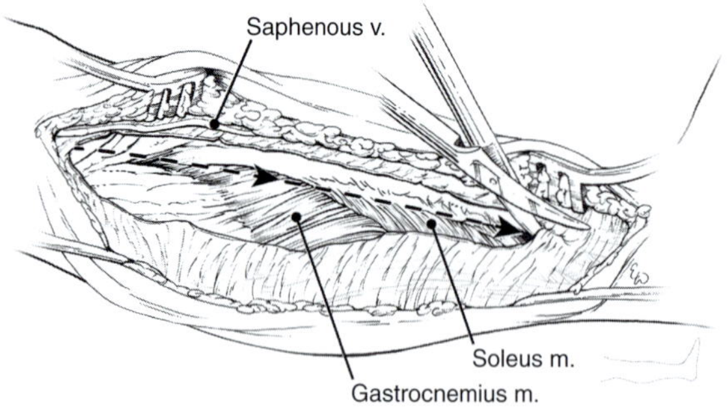

Fig. 57.7 The medial incision is placed such that the saphenous vein can be identified and preserved and the fascia is opened to expose the soleus and gastrocnemius muscles in the superficial posterior compartment

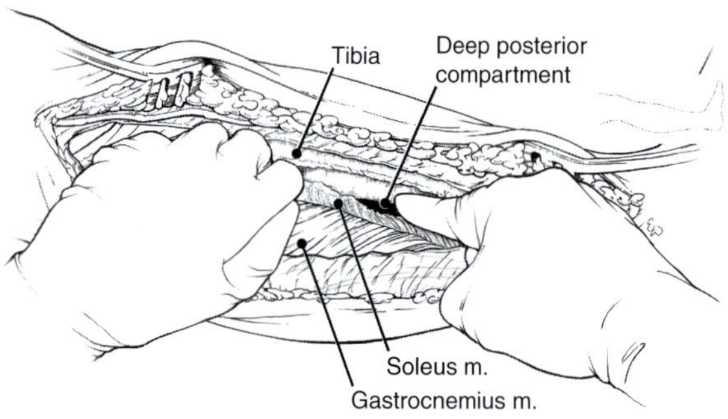

Fig. 57.8 The soleus muscle is dissected off of the inferior border of the tibia allowing entry into the deep posterior compartment

has been entered. The muscle in each compartment should be assessed for viability. Viable muscle is pink, contracts when stimulated, and bleeds when cut. Dead muscle should be debrided back to healthy viable tissue. The skin incision is left open and either covered with gauze or a vacuum-assisted wound closure device which have been shown in recent studies to speed up and improve the chances definitive closure of these wounds.

57.5 Compartment Syndrome of the Foot

You may be asking yourself: Why do I need to know about the foot? The obvious answer to this is that occasionally patients you take care of will develop compartment syndromes of the foot and it is your duty to first make the diagnosis and secondly ensure that they receive appropriate care. Patients in whom you need to worry are those who have crush injuries to the foot (up to a 40% occurrence of CS) and those with calcaneal fractures (up to 10%). Unfortunately, there may be no classic signs in the foot as pain on passive stretch and diminished pulses are not consistent physical findings. Tense tissue bulging may be the most reliable physical finding, and the use of pressure measurements may be of more use than in the leg to assist decision making. As even very experienced trauma surgeons have little experience with the foot, it is a sign of mature judgment to call for reinforcements, namely your friendly orthopedic or podiatric colleague. However, it is important to know how to perform fasciotomies on the foot yourself, in case the Calvary is not readily available. The foot contains four compartments (Intraosseous or Intrinsic, Medial, Lateral, and Central) which all must be released. This is accomplished with two incisions on the dorsum of the foot and one medial (Fig. 57.9).

57.6 Compartment Syndrome of the Thigh

Compartment syndrome is uncommon in the thigh because of the large volume that the thigh requires to cause an increase in interstitial pressure. In addition, the compartments of the thigh blend anatomically with the hip allowing for extravisation of blood or fluid outside the compartment. Risk factors for thigh compartment syndrome include: severe femoral fractures, severe blunt trauma/crush or blast injury to thigh, vascular injury, Iliofemoral Deep Venous Thrombosis, and the use of military anti-shock trousers or other external compression of the thigh. The thigh contains three compartments: anterior, posterior and medial. If compartment syndrome of the thigh exists, you should start with a lateral incision first as this enables decompression of both the anterior and posterior compartments (Fig. 57.10). Often, the lateral incision is all that is needed, though on occasion with a severely swollen extremity a medial incision will be needed as well (Fig. 57.10).

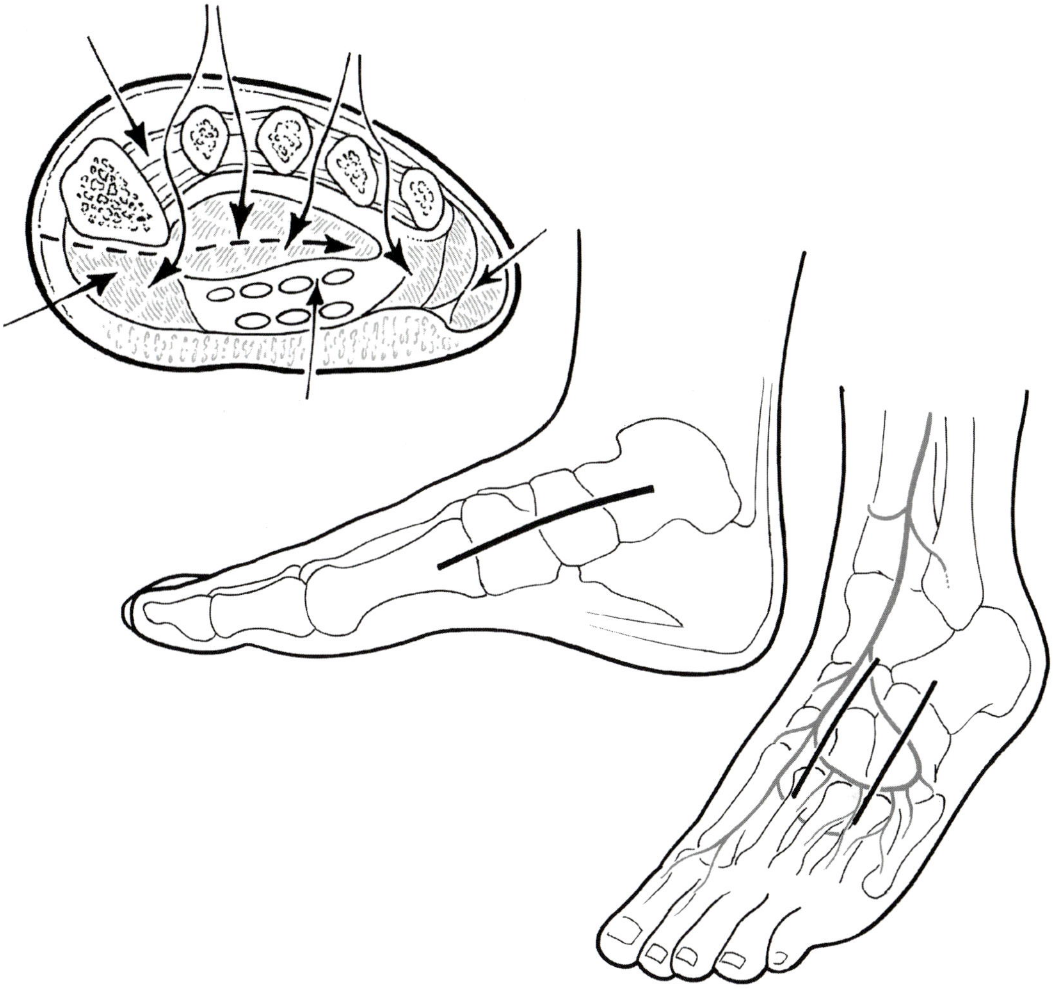

Fig. 57.9 The four-compartment fasciotomy of the foot requires two dorsal and one medial skin incision allowing entry into the intrinsic compartment on either side of each metatarsal bone as well as the medial, central, and lateral compartments as depicted

57.7 Compartment Syndrome of the Forearm and Hand

Compartment syndromes of the hand and forearm are much less common than in the lower extremity, but it is equally vital that you be able to recognize and treat it should it occur. Compartment syndrome of the upper arm is very unusual, but may follow supracondylar fracture of the humerus. Compartment syndrome of the forearm may be associated with fractures, crush or blast injury, burns or vascular injury. CS of the hand can occur from trauma but is more commonly associated with infiltration of intravenous fluids. As there are no sensory nerves in the hand compartments, physical findings do not include sensory abnormalities, and the pressure threshold is much less than in the legs (15–20 mmHg is indication for release).

The classic fasciotomy of the forearm is performed though a curvilinear incision on the volar surface (to release the anterior compartment) which is extended to the hand to release the carpal tunnel (Fig. 57.11). The posterior compartment of the forearm is released

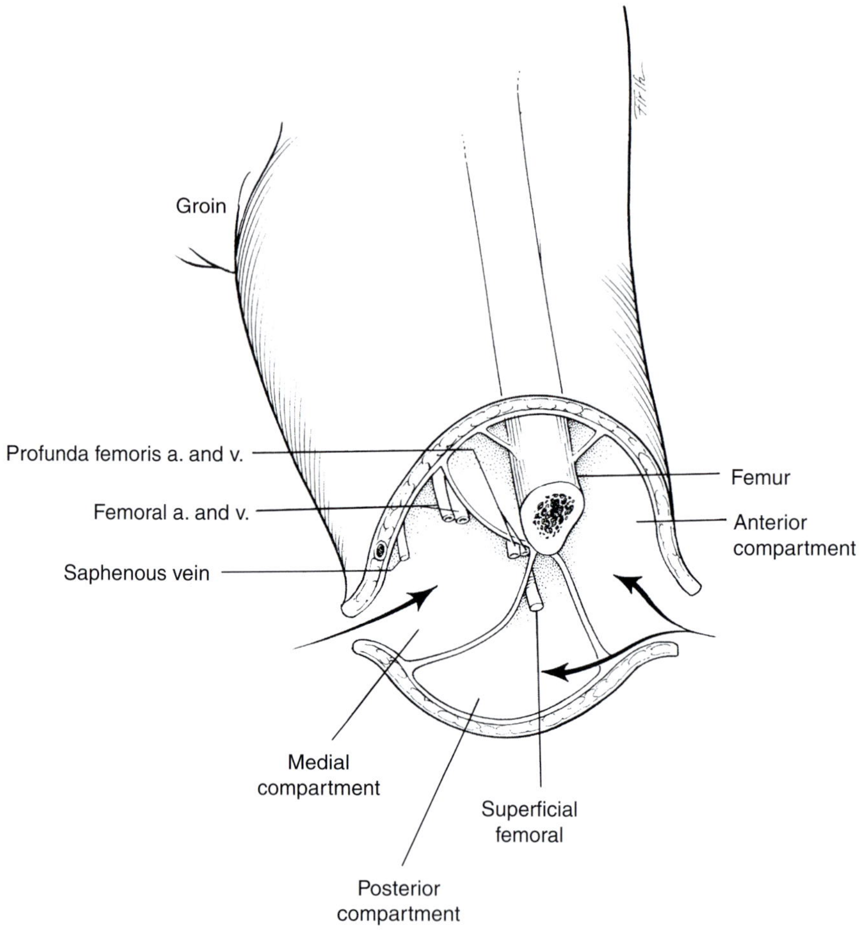

Fig. 57.10 The anterior and posterior compartments of the thigh can be decompressed through a single lateral incision. On occasion, the medial compartment will need decompression through a separate medial incision

through a linear dorsal incision, with two additional incisions on the dorsum of the hand to release the hand (Fig. 57.11). As with the foot, there is no shame in calling in appropriate help (hand surgeon) to optimally care for the patient with CS of the hand.

57.8 Aftercare and Complications

The last thing you want to see when you do a fasciotomy is necrotic muscle, because it means that you waited too long to take the patient to the operating room. But having read this book obviously the necrotic muscle is the result of the patient not being transferred to you in a timely fashion and now you must take care of the problem. If necrotic muscle is present, it should be debrided at the time of original fasciotomy. Having paid attention to the preceding tips and tricks you have made large incisions that will need care. The open wounds should be covered with non-adherent dressing or moist gauze. If you have access to a vacuum-assisted wound closure device, application to the wound will help to protect the tissue and may speed time to wound closure. The wound should be re-evaluated 24–48 h after the initial fasciotomy with further debridement as indicated. After the acute process subsides, delayed primary closure or split-thickness skin grafting may be performed. Patients with open fasciotomy wounds are at risk for infection and incomplete or delayed fasciotomies can lead to permanent nerve damage, loss of limb, multi-system organ failure, rhabdomyolysis and death. Early recognition and aggressive fasciotomy will help to minimize these adverse outcomes.

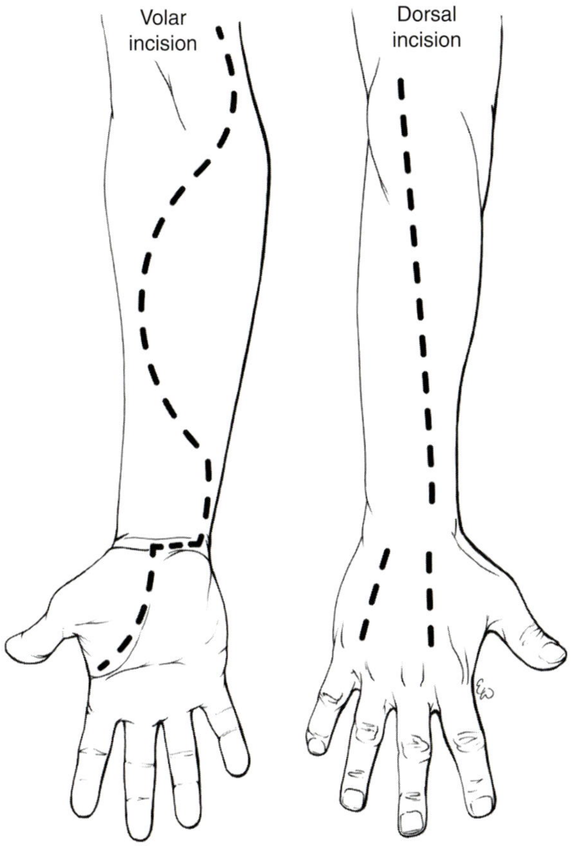

Fig. 57.11 The volar incision enables decompression of the anterior compartment of the forearm and is carried down onto the hand to release the carpal tunnel. The dorsal incision allows for decompression of the posterior compartment and the two dorsal hand incisions enable release of the intraosseous compartments

Important Points

1. Compartment syndrome must be suspected in all polytrauma patients especially if they are hypotensive.
2. Compartment syndrome is a clinical diagnosis. There is a very limited role for measuring compartment pressures (unconscious, paralyzed, hand and foot, etc.).
3. The earliest and most important symptom of compartment syndrome is pain greater than expected due to the injury alone.
4. The presence of pulses and normal capillary refill does not exclude compartment syndrome.
5. If you wait for the five "Ps" to make a diagnosis of compartment syndrome, your patient will be left with the sixth "P" – a Peg leg.
6. The presence of an open fracture does not exclude compartment syndrome and in fact may make it more likely.
7. The lower leg is the most common site of compartment syndrome followed by the forearm and thigh.
8. Fasciotomies performed for trauma must include generous skin incisions and complete release of the fascia. The skin can act as a constricting band even if the fascia is fully opened.
9. Lower extremity four-compartment fasciotomy must be done through two skin incisions. There is no role for the one skin incision fasciotomy in the lower leg.
10. The lateral incision is made a *finger in front of the fibula.*
11. The medial incision is made a *thumb* below the *tibia.*
12. A cosmetic incision for compartment syndrome equals an improper fasciotomy. Cosmetic surgery is best left to the plastic surgeon.
13. In the swollen lower leg, the lateral intermuscular septum can be difficult to find and the perforating vessels will help you find it.
14. Taking the time to mark all the landmarks and proposed incisions prior to cutting will improve your chances of successful fasciotomy.
15. The anterior and deep posterior compartments of the lower extremity are the most commonly missed. Identifying the respective neurovascular structures in each compartment confirms you have entered them.
16. Necrotic muscle does not contract when electrocautery is applied. It must be debrided at the time of the initial fasciotomy.
17. Compartment syndrome of the foot and hand are infrequent and best outcomes are obtained in conjunction with subspecialty input.

Suggested Literature

Dente CJ, Feliciano DV, Rozycki GS et al (2004) A review of upper extremity fasciotomies in a level 1 trauma center. Am Surg 70:1088–1093

Feliciano DV, Cruse PA, Spjut-Patrinely V (1988) Fasciotomy after trauma to the extremities. Am J Surg 156:533–536

Harris IA, Kadir A, Donald G (2006) Continuous compartment pressure monitoring for tibia fractures: does it influence outcome? J Trauma 60:1330–1335

Kakar S, Firoozabadi R, McKean J, Tornetta P III (2007) Diastolic blood pressure in patients with tibia fractures under anaesthesia: implications for the diagnosis of compartment syndrome. J Orthop Trauma 21:99–103

Myerson M, Manoli A (1993) Compartment syndromes of the foot after calcaneal fractures. Clin Orthop Relat Res 290:142–150

Ritenour AE, Dorlac WC, Fang R et al (2008) Complications after fasciotomy revision and delayed compartment release in combat patients. J Trauma 64(2S):S153–S162

Schwartz JT, Brumback RJ, Lakatos R et al (1989) Acute compartment syndrome of the thigh. A spectrum of injury. J Bone Joint Surg Am 71:392–400

Shadgan B, Menon M, O'Brien PJ, Reid WD (2008) Diagnostic techniques in acute compartment syndrome of the leg. J Orthop Trauma 22:581–587

Zannis J, Angobaldo J, Marks M et al (2009) Comparison of fasciotomy wound closures using traditional dressing changes and vacuum-assisted closure device. Ann Plast Surg 62:407–409

Anterior Exposure of the Thoracic and Lumbar Spine

58

Hani Seoudi

Injuries to the thoracic and lumbar spine occur in 6.3% of all trauma patients [1]. The great majority of those injuries are due to blunt trauma. Spinal cord injury occurs in 1.3% of trauma patients [1]. Fractures occur most commonly in the thoracolumbar region (T10-L2) as it is the most mobile part of the thoracic and lumbar spine. Severe burst-type fractures of the vertebral body can render the spine unstable and puts the cord at risk for injury by the protruding fragments.

Patients complain of pain at the level of the fracture and may also have varying degrees of neurological deficits if there is a spinal cord injury. Once a fracture is identified, the remainder of the vertebral column should be imaged to rule out concomitant injuries which are not uncommon [2]. Patients who suffered a high-energy mechanism of injury and cannot be assessed clinically due to altered mental status should have their entire spine imaged. CT scan with three dimensional reconstruction is the preferred imaging method of the spine [3]. The spinal cord ends about the level of the L1 vertebra; injuries below that level may, therefore, present with a cauda equina syndrome characterized by neurological deficits in one or both lower extremities as well as disturbance of bowel and urinary bladder function. High thoracic spinal cord injuries interrupt the sympathetic outflow and may be associated with neurogenic shock characterized by hypotension, bradycardia, and warm skin. If a spine surgeon is not available, the patient should be transferred to a higher level of care expeditiously. Keep the patient flat in the supine position with reverse Trendelenburg position as needed if there is respiratory distress. Avoid using a hard backboard for a long time as it is uncomfortable and does not provide protection to the spine more than keeping the patient in the supine position; a well-padded stretcher is sufficient.

The decision to perform a vertebral corpectomy (excision of the vertebral body) and anterior spine fixation is made by the spine surgeon based on the extent of damage to the vertebra, degree of neural canal narrowing, clinical and radiologic evidence of cord injury, as well as the likelihood of the patient to comply with non-operative management. Complete loss of motor function and sensation below the level of injury carries a dismal prognosis. This could be the result of a severe spinal cord contusion in which case early surgical stabilization of the spine can make a great difference in outcome. Patients who have radiologic evidence of complete spinal cord transaction will not regain neurologic function; however, spine instrumentation may be required to maintain stability and allow mobilization of the patient. Most spine surgeons seek the assistance of a general, vascular, or thoracic surgeon to provide anterior exposure of the spine. A trauma surgeon in a busy center should be able to perform those procedures. When a relationship is established between the trauma and spine surgery services, trauma surgeons will also be called upon to provide anterior spine exposure for non-trauma-related conditions such as disc disease, osteomyelitis, and tumors. The techniques of anterior exposure of the spine at different levels are described below.

H. Seoudi
Trauma Services, Inova Fairfax Hospital,
Virginia Commonwealth University
3300 Gallows Road, Falls Church, 22042, VA, USA
e-mail: hani.seoudi@inova.org

G.C. Velmahos et al. (eds.), *Penetrating Trauma*,
DOI 10.1007/978-3-642-20453-1_58, © Springer-Verlag Berlin Heidelberg 2012

58.1 General Principles

- For corpectomy procedures, the diseased/fractured vertebra as well as the one above and the one below need to be fully exposed. This allows the spine surgeon to adequately place fixation screws.
- For disc excision procedures, the spine surgeon may or may not place anterior plates and screws. If a plate and screws are not needed, only the disc space, the inferior end plate of the vertebra above and the superior end plate of the vertebra below need to be exposed.
- The level of the incision is chosen based on preoperative radiologic localization of the desired spine segment rather than empiric incisions for certain vertebral levels. Use a Kelly clamp and fluoroscopy to place a skin mark corresponding to the spine level in question. Use this mark as the center of your incision.
- The spine should always be in the neutral position throughout the procedure. "Cracking" the table for presumed better exposure is not helpful and may result in improper alignment of the spine.
- For vertebral levels T10 to L4, the patient should be in the right lateral decubitus (right side down) position. It is easier to deal with the aorta than to deal with the inferior vena cava.
- For vertebral levels proximal to T10, a right posterolateral thoracotomy is used. The azygos vein and the esophagus are relatively easier to negotiate than the aorta. On the left side, the proximal descending aorta is in a more lateral position relative to the spine and interferes with adequate anterolateral exposure of the vertebral bodies.
- In exposures requiring a thoracic incision for vertebral corpectomy, the rib should be excised and preserved for the spine surgeon to use as a bone graft.
- For anterior lumbar inter-body fusion (ALIF) of L4-L5 and L5-S1, the patient is placed in the supine position and a left paramedian incision is used.

58.2 Anterior Exposure of T10-L2

This is the most common level to be exposed as it is where most injuries occur. As mentioned above, the patient should be in the right lateral decubitus position and fluoroscopy is used to place a mark on the skin corresponding to the location of the disease. The mark is placed in the posterior axillary line and is used as the center of an oblique incision overlying the rib. The 10th rib tends to correspond to the T12-L1 disc (Fig. 58.1a). The serratus anterior muscle fibers are divided over the rib throughout the length of the incision. Latissimus dorsi fibers typically do not need to be divided at that level. The periosteum of the rib is elevated circumferentially using Doyen's periosteal elevators, taking care not to injure the neurovascular bundle under the inferior margin of the rib. Using a rib cutter, the segment of the rib spanning the length of the incision is now removed and preserved to be used as a bone graft.

The periosteum of the posterior wall of the rib and the parietal pleura are now divided as a single layer to enter the chest cavity. There is no need to deflate the lung for this level of exposure. The lung, instead, is retracted cephalad with a laparotomy pad. The diaphragm is now in view. A curvilinear incision of the diaphragm leaving a 2-cm rim of diaphragmatic insertion into the costal margin is made (Fig. 58.1b). The anterior extent of the diaphragmatic incision varies from one patient to another but can be extended to the costal margin if needed. The posterior extent of the diaphragmatic incision is to the medial arcuate ligament (lumbo-costal arch) over the psoas muscle (Fig. 58.2a, b). The plane between the diaphragm and the peritoneum is developed. The plane is gradually extended using blunt dissection, taking care not to injure the peritoneum or the underlying spleen. This is best achieved by staying away from the proximal aspect of the diaphragm where there is not enough extraperitoneal fat. Instead, you should dissect caudad to the inferior margin of the diaphragmatic incision where abundant extraperitoneal fat allows for safe blunt dissection. Extending the diaphragmatic incision and developing the extraperitoneal plane are done simultaneously.

Once the posterior extent (the medial arcuate ligament) of the diaphragmatic incision has been reached, a radiolucent self-retaining retractor blade is used to retract the diaphragm medially. This blade should be carefully applied as it may injure the spleen, kidney, or their blood supply. Dissection is now carried out between the left crus of the diaphragm and the psoas muscle fibers both of which take origin from the anterolateral aspect of the lumbar vertebral bodies (Fig. 58.2a, b). A combination of blunt dissection and electrosurgery is used to free those fibers from their

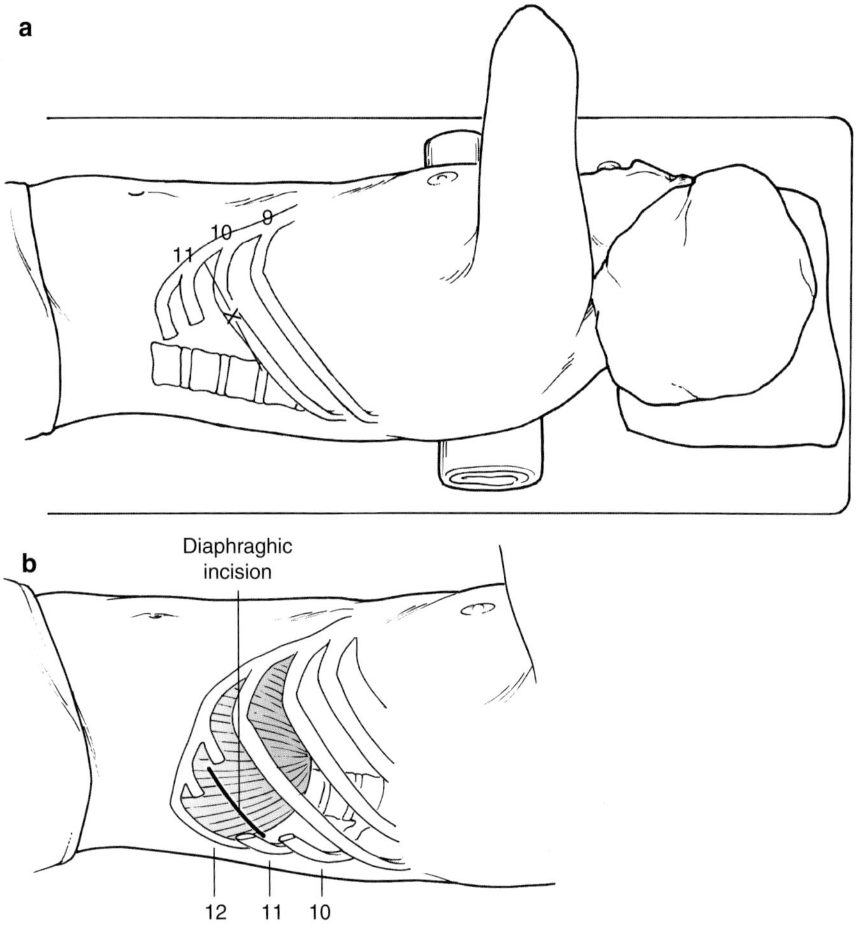

Fig. 58.1 (**a**) An oblique incision (parallel to the underlying rib) is centered over the mark corresponding to the desired vertebral level. (**b**) The 10th and 11th ribs are removed from the diagram to show the posterolateral diaphragmatic incision (*black line*)

attachment to the anterior longitudinal ligament of the spine. Above the level of the diaphragm, the pleura covering the spine is incised vertically (Fig. 58.2a, b). Intercostal vessels are usually preserved. The greater splanchnic nerve is usually encountered immediately beneath the pleura overlying the spine and is easily retracted away from the vertebra in question.

The upper part of the psoas muscle is bulky, and it obscures the entire lateral aspect of the vertebral bodies. Gradually divide as much psoas fibers as needed in order to adequately expose the spine. As the psoas muscle fibers are being divided, care should be taken to identify and control segmental vessels going to the diseased vertebra. Bipolar electrosurgery should suffice to control those vessels. Remember that you will continue to look for and deal with those vessels as you extend your dissection laterally toward the vertebral pedicle. Other segmental vessels should be preserved. The radiculo-medullary artery of Adamkiewicz originates from the intercostal and/or lumbar arteries on the left side in 70% of patients, frequently at the T8-L1 vertebral level [4]. Injury to this artery can result in spinal cord ischemia. Your dissection does not need to reach the midline anteriorly. The spine surgeon is only interested in the anterolateral aspect and the pedicle of the vertebral body. Too much medial dissection is unnecessary and is associated with the risk of injuring the aorta and its branches.

As the psoas muscle fibers are gradually shaved off of the spine, the diseased vertebra begins to emerge. Remember that discs are convex and vertebral bodies are concave. In case of a fracture, the vertebral height is diminished and there is an associated hematoma. Use two 18-gauge spinal needles to mark what you believe is the body of the vertebra above and the body of the vertebra below. Those needles should fit in the operative

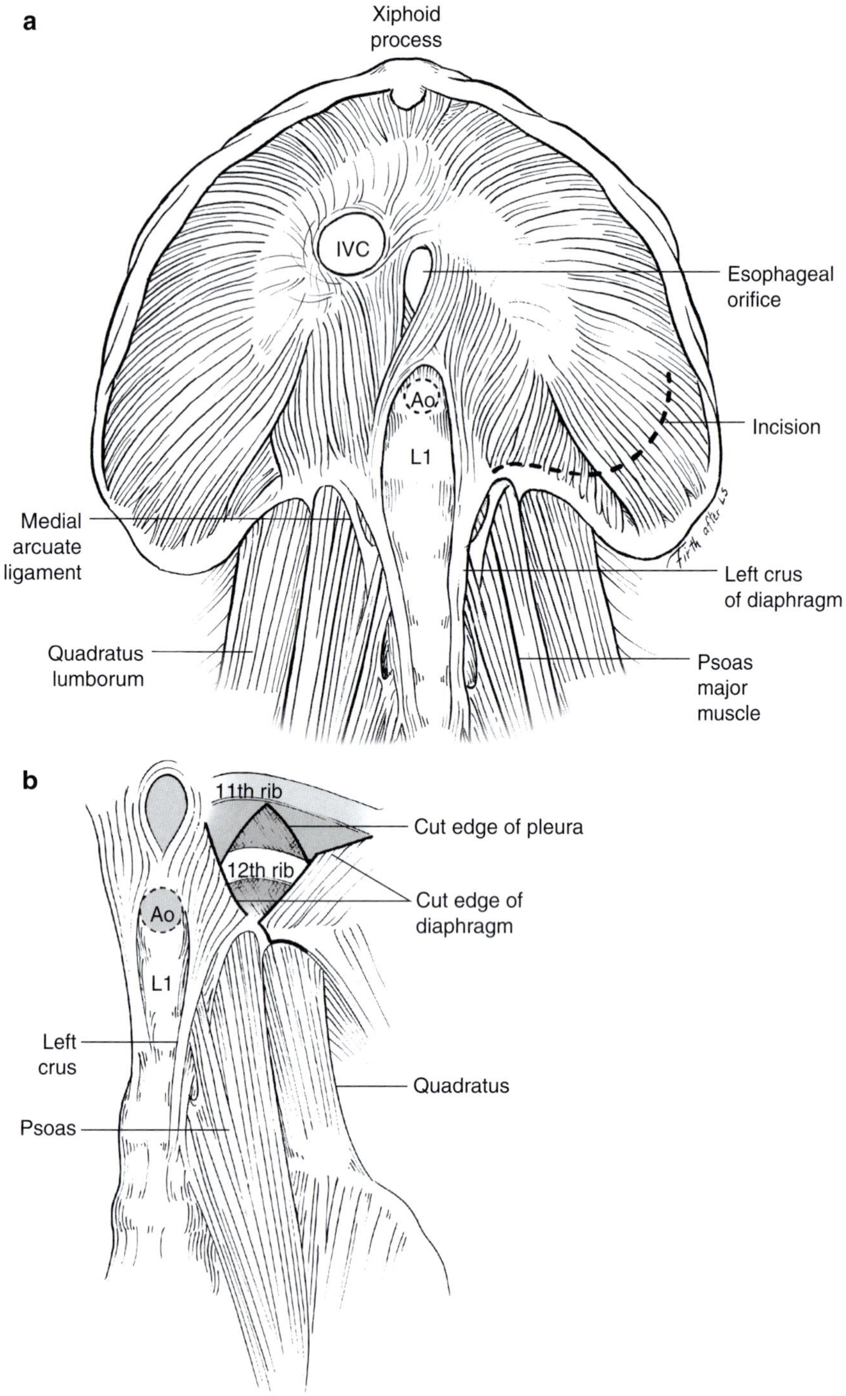

Fig. 58.2 (**a**, **b**) Inferior view of the diaphragm showing the posterior extent of the diaphragmatic incision with the divided medial arcuate ligament over the psoas muscle. The pleura over the anterolateral aspect of T12 has been incised

field perpendicular to the waist of the vertebral body as this is how the screws will need to be positioned. Use fluoroscopy to confirm the level of exposure. At this point, the spine surgeon begins his/her part of the procedure.

Upon completion of the spine surgeon's part, the exposure surgeon places a chest tube through a separate stab incision in the intercostal space above the main incision. This allows the lung to re-expand fully and also helps to drain blood. The tube can be removed if there is no residual pneumothorax and the fluid output is less than 150 cc/day. The medial arcuate ligament is now approximated with a 0-PDS suture which is continued as a running suture to reapproximate the diaphragm. The intercostal muscles and serratus anterior are repaired with 0-Vicryl running sutures. The skin is closed with either staples or subcuticular suture.

58.3 Anterior Exposure of L3-L5

For this level of exposure, no ribs need to be resected and the diaphragm is not divided. The patient is placed in the right lateral decubitus position. A mark corresponding to the diseased vertebra is placed in the posterior axillary line as mentioned above. An oblique flank incision centered over the mark is made. The external oblique aponeurosis and its more lateral fleshy fibers are divided. The fibers of the internal oblique and transversus abdominis are now bluntly split to expose the transversalis fascia which is incised to expose the extraperitoneal plane. Blunt dissection is done from a lateral to a medial direction until the quadratus lumborum muscle is seen. Further medial dissection brings the psoas muscle into view. Remember that the aorta and inferior vena cava bifurcate at the L4 level and that you should be careful not to injure the iliac vessels as you carry your dissection down toward the L5 vertebra. In order to retract the iliac vessels medially to expose L5, the iliolumbar vessels (the segmental equivalents to the 5th lumbar vertebra) [5] will need to be ligated and divided. Screws placed by the spine surgeon into the L5 vertebra will have to come from an anterolateral direction because the iliac bone will prevent instruments from coming at a straight lateral direction. The psoas muscle and segmental vessels to L3 and L4 are dealt with as described above (Fig. 58.3a, b).

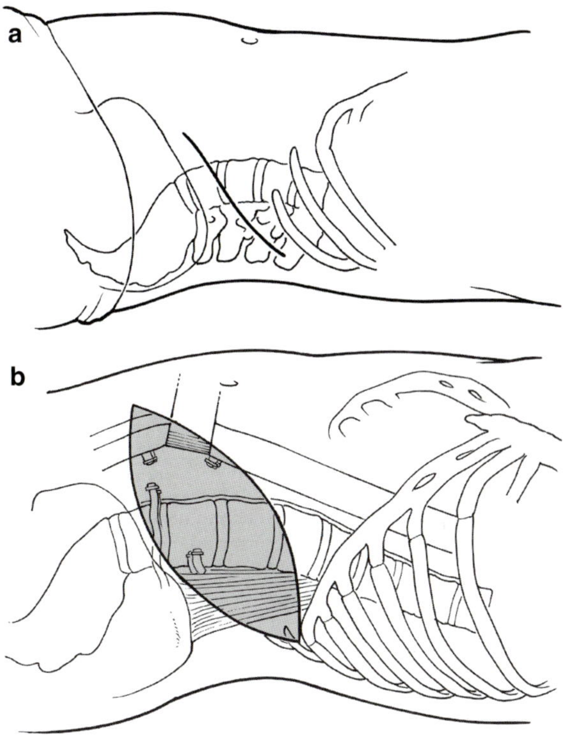

Fig. 58.3 (**a**, **b**) An oblique flank incision between the costal margin and the iliac crest has been made. The left common iliac vessels are retracted medially after the segmental vessels to L4 and L5 have been divided

58.4 Anterior Exposure of the Thoracic Spine Proximal to T10

The patient is placed in the left lateral decubitus position. A double lumen endotracheal tube is used in case the lung needs to be deflated; this is usually not required. The chest cavity is entered using the same steps described above. The latissimus dorsi muscle fibers will need to be divided. For higher levels, the trapezius muscle and rhomboids will also need to be divided and the scapula retracted laterally. The lung is retracted medially and anteriorly. The inferior pulmonary ligament may need to be divided when dealing with the lower thoracic vertebrae. The pleura over the spine is incised vertically. Tributaries to the azygos vein are divided as needed to expose the desired level. The intercostal artery overlying the diseased vertebra will need to be divided. Other intercostal arteries are preserved when possible especially in the lower levels where the artery of Adamkiewicz may take origin. The esophagus is typically far enough medially that it does not require any mobilization to expose the anterolateral aspect of the spine. The azygos vein, although in a posterolateral position to the esophagus,

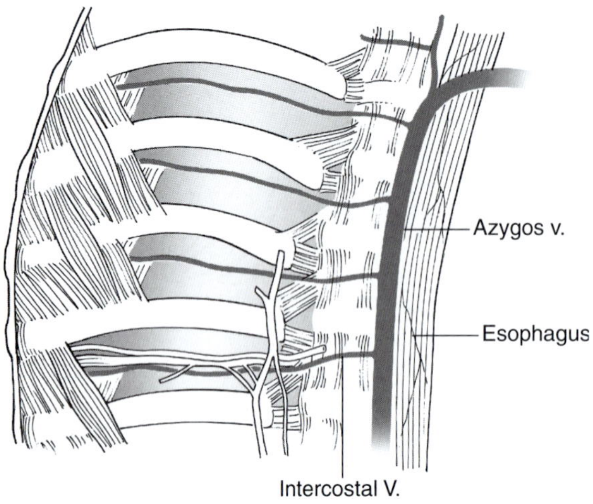

Fig. 58.4 Lateral view of the thoracic spine showing the azygos and intercostal veins. The esophagus is medial to the azygos vein

also does not require mobilization except maybe at T4 where it arches forward to drain in the SVC (Fig. 58.4).

58.5 Anterior Lumbar Interbody Fusion (ALIF) at the L4/L5 and L5/S1 Levels

This exposure is done for non-trauma-related conditions. The typical patient is one who has chronic discogenic pain or motor deficit. The spine surgeon excises the disc fully and places an implant in the disc space. The spine surgeon may or may not place a plate and screws anteriorly. In order to perform an adequate discectomy, the spine surgeon needs good exposure of the midline anteriorly. The incision is therefore quite different from that done for the above-mentioned exposures. A 3–4 in. left paramedian incision is made starting at the level of the umbilicus. The anterior rectus sheath is incised vertically. There is typically a rectus muscle inscription at the level of the umbilicus which needs to be divided carefully without injuring the muscle. Once the muscle has been freed from its attachment to anterior sheath, it is retracted laterally to expose the posterior sheath. Do not retract the muscle medially as this will injure its nerve supply (the lower intercostal nerves) which enters the muscle at its lateral border. Now look for the linea semilunaris and begin a blunt dissection between the posterior rectus sheath and the peritoneum. Stay as far laterally as you can where there is more extraperitoneal fat to allow for dissection without injuring the peritoneum (Fig. 58.5a, b).

As the extraperitoneal space begins to develop, place a laparotomy pad over the peritoneum and push it medially to maintain retraction and to help further develop the plane. The lateral aspect of the posterior rectus sheath may be vertically divided to help develop the upper extent of the plane. More laparotomy pads can be used to maintain medial and superior retraction of the peritoneum with the help of radiolucent self-retaining retractor blades. As the psoas muscle begins to emerge, look for the iliac vessels. The common and external iliac arteries are seen first since they lie lateral to their corresponding veins. The iliac vessels are left in place and blunt dissection is continued medially until the aortic bifurcation is reached. The left common iliac vein (LCIV) lies posterior and partially inferior to the aortic bifurcation and the proximal part of the left common iliac artery. By this time, you should have identified the ureter which crosses the bifurcation of the left common iliac artery. The ureter is retracted medially along with the peritoneum to which it is typically adherent.

Continue medial retraction of the peritoneum until the proximal part of the right common iliac artery is reached. A Kitner dissector is now used to mobilize the fat below the aortic bifurcation. This will further expose the proximal part of the LCIV which should be dealt with very carefully as it is very difficult to control given its posterior location. The middle sacral vessels are identified and divided using bipolar electrosurgery. Try to minimize the use of electrosurgery in this area to avoid injury to the lumbosacral plexus which can result in retrograde ejaculation. As you mobilize the fat inferior to the LCIV, the L5/S1 disc appears. Continue the dissection inferiorly until the S1 vertebra is exposed. The superior extent of the dissection is reached by carefully mobilizing the LCIV cephalad

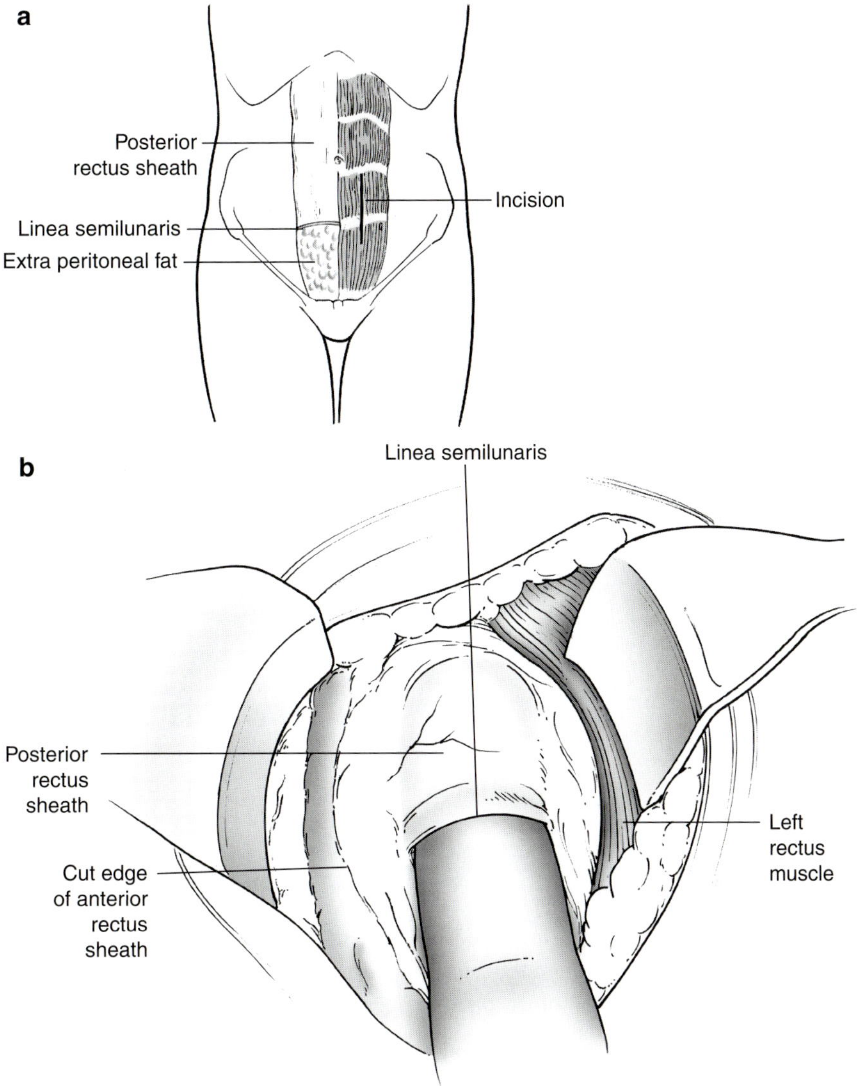

Fig. 58.5 (**a**, **b**) The anterior rectus sheath has been incised and the rectus muscle is retracted laterally. Blunt dissection between the posterior rectus sheath and the peritoneum is being done at the level of the linea semilunaris

until the inferior end plate of L5 is seen (Fig. 58.6). If the spine surgeon is planning on placing screws in L5, the lower third of that vertebra will need to be exposed. This can be achieved by very carefully placing a retractor over the LCIV to maintain cephalad retraction. Instead, a handheld vein retractor can be used.

Exposing the L4/L5 disc is more challenging and usually cannot be achieved by further superior mobilization of the LCIV. Instead, the distal aorta, the proximal left common iliac artery, and proximal LCIV are mobilized medially. The iliolumbar vessels must be divided for this to be achieved.

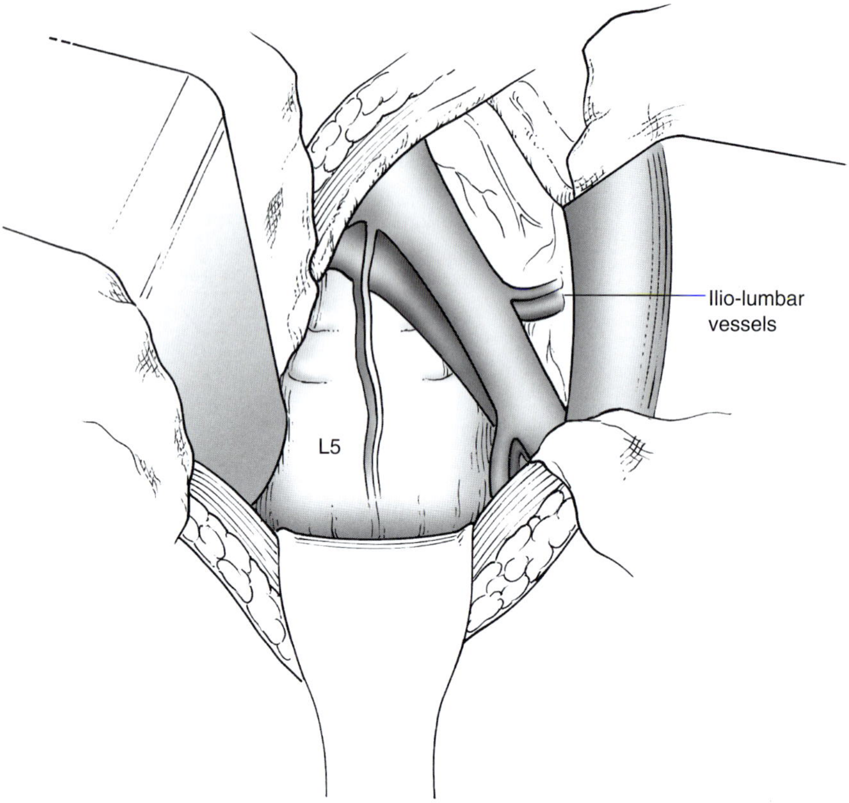

Fig. 58.6 Retroperitoneal dissection has been done and the right common iliac vessels are retracted laterally. The left common iliac, middle sacral, and iliolumbar vessels are shown

Important Points

- Vertebral corpectomy is indicated when there is significant intrusion into the neural canal by fracture fragments, or other pathologic processes, particularly when there is evidence of cord impingement.
- The use of fluoroscopy preoperatively to place the incision at the appropriate level, and intraoperatively to confirm exposure of the diseased vertebra is essential.
- To avoid violating the peritoneum, perform dissection in the extraperitoneal plane as far inferiorly away from the dome of the diaphragm, and as far laterally away from the rectus sheath as possible.
- Retractor blades should be carefully applied to avoid interruption of the blood supply to the spleen and kidney.
- The LCIV should be handled with extreme care. Injury to that vein at the bifurcation of the aorta is hard to repair due to difficulty to obtain proximal and distal control.

References

1. Holmes J, Miller P, Panacek E et al (2001) Epidemiology of thoracolumbar spine injury in blunt trauma. Acad Emerg Med 8:866–872
2. Inaba K, Munera F, McKenney M et al (2006) Visceral torso computed tomography for clearance of the thoracolumbar spine in trauma: a review of the literature. J Trauma 60(4): 915–920
3. Antevil J, Sise M, Sack D et al (2006) Spiral computed tomography for the initial evaluation of spine trauma: A new standard of care? J Trauma 61(2):382–387
4. Koshino T, Murakami G, Morishita K, Mawatari T, Abe T (1999) Does the Adamkiewicz artery originate from the larger segmental arteries? J Thorac Cardiovasc Surg 117(5): 898–905
5. Jasani V, Jaffray D (2002) The anatomy of the iliolumbar vein. A cadaver study. J Bone Joint Surg Br 84-B: 1046–1049

Penetrating Trauma: Amputations

59

Cyrus E. Taghavi, Nelson F. SooHoo, and Areti Tillou

Trauma is the leading indication for amputation in young patients [1]. The incidence is greater in males and steadily increases with age, reaching a peak among individuals 85 years or older [2]. Although blunt trauma is the predominant cause of traumatic amputation, the incidence of penetrating trauma resulting in amputation has steadily increased over the last two decades. These are primarily due to gunshot wounds and stab injuries. When the penetrating trauma results in a combined arterial and skeletal injury, the risk for primary amputation greatly increases secondary to greater disruption of collaterals, soft tissues, and nerves [3].

A trauma surgeon's primary goals in managing such patients are to stabilize the patient, control hemorrhaging, and prevent any concomitant contamination or infection. The most difficult decision you will have to make as a trauma surgeon is to salvage the limb or amputate. In large trauma centers, this is frequently a group decision involving consultation with orthopedic, vascular, and plastic surgeons.

In this chapter, we will primarily focus on the principles of traumatic limb amputation, followed by some of the more common surgical techniques to manage acute, life-threatening traumas that require major limb amputations.

59.1 Principles of Amputation

59.1.1 Initial Wound Evaluation

Some of the most important decisions for patients with traumatic amputation or near amputation are made in the trauma room. Management in the first few minutes is of essence and may severely impact outcome. As in every trauma patient, the priorities of assessment should follow the ATLS protocol and focus on the primary and secondary survey. Injuries such as complete or near amputation of a limp can be very distracting for the trauma team. It is the responsibility of the trauma surgeon to maintain the priorities. The initial evaluation of a penetrating extremity injury should focus on hemostasis. Remember that direct pressure works better than anything else in achieving quick hemostasis in the trauma room. Avoid using clamps and blind sutures as this may result in significant injury to vessels that may hinder reconstruction. Another common mistake is constantly reinforcing a bulky dressing that inefficiently hides the bleeding from the eyes of the trauma team and endangers the patient. Tourniquets may be useful in coagulopathic patients with large profusely bleeding open wounds when applied for a brief period of time until the patient can be transferred to the operating room where better lighting and instruments are available to help with hemostasis. Most of the time

C.E. Taghavi
Department of Orthopaedic Surgery, University of California, Davis 4860 Y Street, Suite 3800, Sacramento, CA 95817, USA

N.F. SooHoo
UCLA Dept. of Orthopaedic Surgery, 10945 Le Conte Ave. 3355, Los Angeles, CA 90095, USA

A. Tillou (✉)
Division of General Surgery, David Geffen School of Medicine, UCLA, 10833 Le Conte Avenue, CHS, Room 72-231, Los Angeles, CA 90095, USA
e-mail: atillou@mednet.ucla.edu

G.C. Velmahos et al. (eds.), *Penetrating Trauma*,
DOI 10.1007/978-3-642-20453-1_59,

Table 59.1 Hard signs of vascular injury [15]

• Active hemorrhage
• Large, expanding, or pulsatile hematoma
• Bruit or thrill over wound
• Absent distal palpable pulses
• Manifestations of distal ischemia (pain, pallor, paralysis, paresthesias, poikilothermy)

even very large wounds are relatively hemostatic and simple pressure is sufficient to temporize bleeding until the initial evaluation is completed and the patient can be transferred to the operating room.

If the extremity or part of an extremity is completely amputated, make sure that the amputated part does not end up in the trash, but is rather preserved properly until at least all possibilities of replantation have been addressed. Orthopedic and plastic surgeons will usually make that decision based on the patient's age, condition, associated injuries, part that is amputated, and available expertise and resources. Additional imaging may be necessary to address other severe associated injuries prior to treating the extremity injury. A prompt diagnosis of vascular involvement is essential due to the well-established relationship between the time interval from injury to treatment and the increasing chance of limb loss. Physical examination, segmental pressures, Doppler or Duplex imaging in the trauma room, or CT angiography may help establish the diagnosis. Depending on your resources, CT angiography might be the most rapid and accessible choice. In critical patients where time is of essence, intraoperative angiography might be necessary. Ask for an angio-compatible table before you go to the operating room. Also request vascular instruments; notify your vascular surgeon if there is one available and you are not comfortable performing vascular reconstructions. Make sure there are blood, FFP, and platelets available. Initiate the massive transfusion protocol if there is one in your facility. After hemostasis, removal of any nonviable tissue and devascularized bone should be preformed, while retaining all viable tissue that may be used in fabricating a residual limb. Once in the operating room, the presence of hard signs of vascular injury necessitates arteriography to confirm or exclude arterial trauma. The absence of hard signs does not always reliably exclude significant arterial injury and additional workup may be necessary if an injury is suspected (Table 59.1). Restoration of blood flow should take priority over skeletal injury management. If necessary, you can use a temporary shunt while stabilizing unstable fractures or dislocations prior to definitive arterial repair [3].

59.1.2 Deciding Primary Amputation Versus Limb Salvage

One of the major challenges that surgeons face with a limb-threatening injury is the decision to perform a primary amputation or limb salvage. The only absolute indication for amputation is irreversible ischemia in the traumatized limb, a diagnosis that is usually difficult to establish in the trauma resuscitation room. Although unattractive as a therapeutic option, amputation should not be viewed as a failure or destructive surgery, but rather as a life-saving and reconstructive alternative. Some studies on long-term functional outcomes of amputation versus limb salvage have shown similar functional outcomes and self-rated disability among both patient groups at a 7-year follow-up, with a high level of disability in both groups [4–6].

Many factors must be taken into account when deciding to amputate or salvage. First, each treatment has its distinct short- and long-term risks. Limb salvage, for example, is associated with a longer rehabilitation time, greater costs, higher rates of rehospitalization, additional surgeries, and complications, such as osteomyelitis, sepsis, failure of wound healing, and rhabdomyolysis [5]. Second, a realistic assessment of functional expectations at the conclusion of treatment is critical. Finally, the performance of the salvaged limb versus that of a prosthetic limb as well as the financial, physiological, and psychosocial burden that the patient will face with each treatment option must be discussed. The significance of these factors will vary between patients; thus, the decision-making process must be individualized. Most patients and families are shaken by the acute situation and certainly emotionally disturbed and unable to think clearly. It is essential to educate the patient and their family so they can adequately make informed decisions. Most people are appalled by the idea of an amputation and the resulting disfigurement; however, this is partly due to the lack of awareness of recent advances in amputation surgery and prosthetic design that offer results paralleling the advances in limb salvage surgery [1]. Situations where patients are unconscious and no family is available may cause challenging dilemmas. Close

Table 59.2 Risk factors for primary amputation [7, 8, 15]

- Gustilo III-C injuries (comminuted, open tibial-fibular fractures with vascular injury)
- Transection of the sciatic or tibial nerve, or 2 of the 3 upper extremity nerves
- Significant wound contamination
- Older age
- Severe comorbidity
- Significant loss of soft tissue that cannot be repaired with a free flap
- Segmental bone loss
- Unrestorable blood supply
- Multiple serious secondary bone or soft tissue injuries involving the ipsilateral limb

collaboration and communication of the surgical subspecialty teams under the oversight of the trauma surgeon is of paramount importance in these situations. Regardless of the approach, primary goal should always be to return the patient as closely as possible to their preinjury functional level.

Although each situation is clearly unique and an individualized plan should be developed, there are certain risk factors that make primary amputation a more appropriate treatment (Table 59.2). Another tool to help with decision making is the mangled extremity severity score (MESS, Table 59.3), which takes into account the level of energy that caused the injury, presence of shock or ischemia, and the patient's age. Studies indicate that a MESS of 6 or less is consistent with a salvageable limb, while a score of 7 or more is close to 100% predictive of amputation [7, 9]. Prospective reliability of the MESS score is not sufficient to permit a firm decision for amputation and should not replace experience and good judgment.

59.1.3 Level of Amputation

The next challenge is usually determining the most distal level for amputation with a reasonable chance of healing. You must consider the tradeoffs between increased function with a more distal level of amputation and a decreased rate of complications with a more proximal level of amputation. The optimal level of amputation is one that will provide a stump length that allows a controlling lever arm for the prosthesis, has a vascular supply sufficient for healing, and an adequate quantity of protective soft tissue coverage for weight bearing [1, 10]. The patient's general medical condition, overall well-being, and rehabilitation potential must be evaluated in this balance. A vascular surgery consultation can aid with this decision. When in doubt and in a relatively stable patient with no other life-threatening injuries, a more conservative initial amputation can be attempted with a plan to revise it later if necessary.

Table 59.3 Mangled extremity severity score

Skeletal/soft tissue injury		Points
Low-energy	Stab wounds, simple closed fractures, small-caliber gunshot wounds	1
Medium-energy	Open or multiple-level fractures, dislocations, moderate crush injuries	2
High-energy	Shotgun blast (close range) high-velocity gunshot wounds	3
Massive crush	Logging, railroad, oil rig accidents	4
Shock		
Normotensive	Blood pressure stable in the field and in the operating room	0
Transiently hypotensive	Blood pressure unstable in field but responsive to intravenous fluids	1
Prolonged hypotension	Systolic blood pressure <90 mmHg in the field; responsive to intravenous fluids only in the operating room	2
Ischemia		
None	A pulsatile limb, no sign of ischemia	0
Mild	Diminished pulses, no signs of ischemia	1
Moderate	No Doppler pulse, sluggish refill, paresthesias, diminished motor activity	2
Advanced	Pulseless, cool, paralyzed, no refill	3
Age		
<30 years		1
30–50 years		2
>50 years		3

59.1.4 Skin and Muscle Flaps

You must handle all soft tissues gently in order to keep tissues viable for a healthy and highly functional amputation stump. A desirable soft tissue envelope distributes the load to the underlying bone and dissipates the forces applied during weight bearing. The use of thick myofasciocutaneous flaps will lead to an optimal soft tissue envelope. Do not dissect tissue planes between muscle and subcutaneous tissue, as this may further devascularize the compromised tissues and lead to skin flap necrosis [1, 10, 11]. The goal is to achieve a mobile, nonadherent muscle mass and a full-thickness, skin and soft tissue envelope that can withstand the direct pressures of weight bearing and shearing forces that occur within a prosthetic. A sufficient muscle mass between the skin and bone will allow the bone to piston within the envelope. If standard flaps are not possible, you may use atypical skin flaps in order to salvage residual limb length [1, 10, 11]. The location of the scar is usually not important as long as the scar is not adherent to the underlying bone, as this can make prosthetic fitting extremely difficult and will most likely break down after prolonged prosthetic use [1, 10].

To create a viable muscle flap, divide the muscles at least 5 cm distal to the intended bone resection, with either a number 10 scalpel or electrocautery. Ligate any bleeding muscular vessels with 2-0 absorbable sutures. A hematoma under the muscle flaps can be detrimental as it may lead to infection and stump breakdown resulting in prolonged healing time and delays in rehabilitation. Stabilize the muscle by myodesis at their normal physiological length, as this will provide a stronger insertion, help maximize strength and function of the residual limb, and minimize atrophy. However, if this is not possible, myoplasty will suffice. Ensure that all muscle repairs are performed at normal resting muscle tensions with the limb in a neutral position to prevent iatrogenic joint flexion contractures.

59.1.5 Hemostasis

To minimize blood loss, elevate and wrap the limb with an elastic bandage prior to the amputation and apply a pneumatic tourniquet in order to exsanguinate it. Isolate and double ligate arteries with 2-0 silk suture ligatures. Veins can be effectively ligated with surgical clips, electrocautery, or 2-0 silk sutures. Remember to deflate the tourniquet prior to closure to check for small bleeders and ensure hemostasis. Most cases warrant a postoperative drain placed deep to the fascia for 48–72 h to prevent fluid collections and hematomas that frequently get infected [1].

59.1.6 Nerves

Never clamp or subject nerves to strong tension, as this may lead to prolonged neurogenic pain, even after the crushed or damaged nerve is removed [11]. To manage nerves in amputation, isolate and gently grasp each nerve with a surgical sponge, pull it distally into the wound, cleanly transect it under gentle tension with a fresh blade, and allow the cut end to retract proximally into the wound. Ensure that the cut end is well padded in the soft tissue and not exposed to pressure bearing areas. Because neuromas develop frequently after nerve division and become painful with repeated trauma, this technique allows the cut end to retract proximally into the wound and embed any resulting neuroma within muscle, protecting it from external pressure. Some larger nerves, such as the sciatic, contain substantial vessels, which should be isolated and ligated.

59.1.7 Bones

Bones can be cut with a Gigli or circular saw. All bone ends should be rasped to achieve a smooth contour, and they should be padded by a thick layer of soft tissue. However, do not excessively strip the periosteum, as this may lead to the formation of ring sequestra or bony overgrowth. Bleeding from the bone surface and bone marrow can be difficult to control in a coagulopathic patient. Direct pressure, electrocautery, and bone wax are usually effective. Copious irrigation will facilitate the removal of any bone dust and residual fragments and decrease the chances of wound infection.

59.1.8 Open Amputations and Wound Closure

Traumatic amputations are frequently completed in multiple stages. Gross contamination, coagulopathy, hemodynamic instability, unclear level of amputation, and severe associated injuries are some of the factors that necessitate a staged approach. An open amputation stump allows the tissues to return to their resting tensions, which avoids further trauma, and also allows serial debridements of a severely destructed and contaminated wound, thus decreasing the chances of wound infection. In cases of hemodynamic instability and in the presence of life-threatening injuries, it also allows time for patient resuscitation and stabilization prior to stump revision. Immediately after the primary debridement, apply a wound vacuum-assisted closure to the stump. If this is not available, cover the wound with moist gauze and wrap with an elastic dressing. Change the dressing once or twice a day until the patient is ready for stump revision or closure. It is critical to ensure complete hemostasis before applying a vacuum-assisted closure. If unrecognized, persistent oozing under continuous suction may result in severe hemorrhage and exsanguination. If the patient is coagulopathic and complete hemostasis is not possible, initial application of a pressure dressing might be necessary. In addition to appropriate antibiotics, repeat debridements every 48–72 h, each time reapplying a new vacuum-assisted closure or dressing until the wound is ready for closure. If the patient's condition permits, definitive reconstruction is best to perform within 5–10 days following the trauma. An open amputation could be the source of persistent hemorrhage and may go unnoticed. Alert your health care team about the open wound and ensure that it is vigilantly monitored for possible bleeding.

When you return to the operating room for wound closure, ensure that there is no devitalized tissue that needs further debridement. Wash out the wound with normal saline. Use a pulse irrigator if available at your institution. You may need to revise the skin flaps or trim the soft tissues for a better functional and cosmetic result. Check for bleeding one last time before starting to close. The closure should be done in layers. Approximate the deep fascia and subcutaneous tissue with interrupted 2-0 absorbable sutures. Consider placing a drain under the skin flaps. Carefully approximate the skin with interrupted mattress sutures with 3-0 nonabsorbable sutures. Handle tissues and most importantly the skin flaps gently. Do not use crushing forceps to retract. The skin flaps should not be closed under tension, as this can lead to delayed healing and skin necrosis. The initial dressings should be placed while still in the operating room. Carefully wrap the stump in a bulky absorbent dressing and protective splint. The wound should be examined frequently, with necrotic tissue debrided and dressings changed accordingly.

59.2 Upper Extremity Amputations

Trauma is the leading cause of upper extremity amputations, with upper extremity amputations including finger injuries accounting for 68.6% of all trauma-related amputations [2]. Frequently the care of such injuries requires involvement of a hand specialist to ensure the best functional and cosmetic result. However, as a trauma surgeon, you will be the first and maybe the only surgeon available to care for these patients. You can use surgical principles described above to guide your management. First ensure that active hemorrhage is controlled and life-threatening injuries are diagnosed and addressed. Prevent further injury and take measures to preserve all possible length, including utilizing all possible soft tissue flaps [1, 12]. These flaps allow coverage of the wound, preservation of functional amputation length, and salvation of a critical joint when possible, without additional donor site morbidity [12]. As a trauma surgeon, your first responsibility is to preserve the patient's life before limbs. A state-of-the-art extremity amputation, especially one of the upper extremities, might be beyond your level of expertise. An imperfectly done amputation can always be revised by an expert as long as the patient fares well and the tissues are viable and well preserved. The brief descriptions of amputation techniques that follow are not a complete guide on how to perform the procedures, but rather focus on basic information on the steps and structures involved that any general surgeon caring for patients with extremity injuries would find useful.

59.2.1 Wrist Amputations

When possible, transcarpal amputation or wrist disarticulation is greatly preferable to amputation through the forearm, as these procedures help preserve pronation and supination. Both of these functions are critical for the successful application of a prosthesis. If you are not familiar with the procedure, you may choose to control hemorrhage and contamination and temporarily close the wound preserving as much length as possible until the patient can be evaluated by a hand specialist.

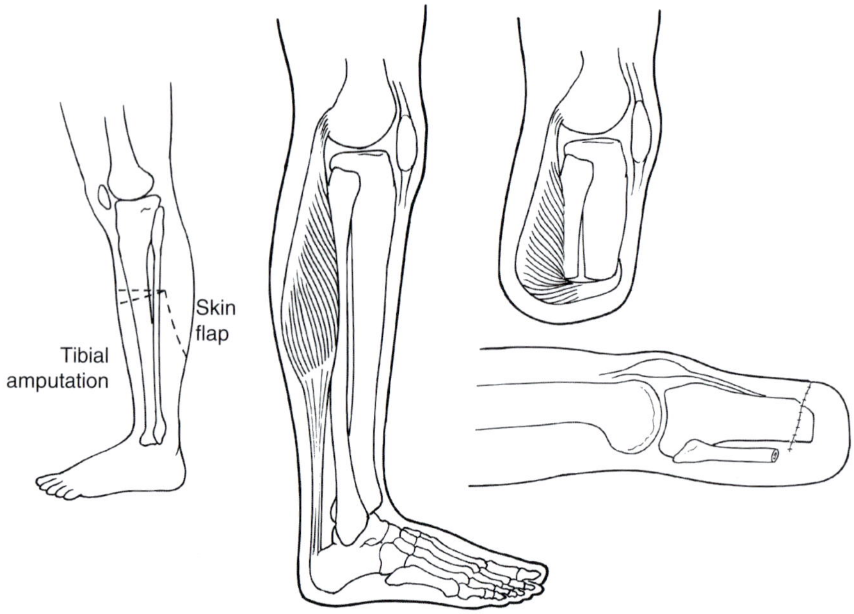

Fig. 59.1 Transtibial amputation

59.2.2 Transradial and Transhumeral Amputations [16]

When possible, equal dorsal and palmar flaps distal to the intended level of bone amputation are desired when performing a transradial amputation. The technique of dividing the structures, soft tissues, and bones is similar to what has been described. Myoplastic closure can be performed by stabilizing the deep muscles with myodesis or tenodesis directly to the bone or periosteum and the more superficial muscles with myoplasty to the fascia of the deeper layers. With very proximal amputations, where the end of the stump is not at least distal to the insertion of the biceps tendon, it may be necessary to detach the tendon from the radius and reattach it to the ulna. The radius should then be removed entirely to functionally lengthen the stump and enhance prosthetic fitting.

When performing a transhumeral amputation, the level of the bone transection should be at least 3.8 cm proximal to the elbow joint in order to allow room for the prosthetic elbow-lock mechanism. If it is necessary to perform a transhumeral amputation at the level of the axillary fold or more proximally, preservation of the most proximal part of the humerus is valuable. Equal anterior and posterior skin flaps are again preferable if you are able to fashion them. Identify, ligate, and divide the brachial vessels proximal to the level of amputation. Then transect the median, ulnar, and radial nerves so that their proximal ends retract proximally. Divide the muscles in the anterior compartment of the arm approximately 1.5 cm distal to the level of intended bone section so that they retract to this level. Preserve the triceps fascia, its insertion to the olecranon and the muscle as a long flap unless you are performing a more proximal amputation. In that case you will need to divide the triceps muscle 3.8–5 cm distal to the level of amputation. Next divide, smoothen, and round the end of the humerus with a rasp. Bevel the triceps tendon to form a long flap, carry it over the end of the bone, and suture it to the anterior muscle fascia. Insert a drain deep to this flap and close the wound in layers (Fig. 59.1).

59.3 Lower Extremity Amputations

59.3.1 Transtibial (Below-Knee) Amputations

A longer residual limb allows more normal gait; however, the distal third of the leg is relatively avascular and has less soft tissue available for weight bearing, rendering stumps at this level suboptimal. A bone length of 12.5–17.5 cm (2.5 cm of bone length for each 30 cm of body height) in transtibial amputations is ideal [1] (Fig. 59.2). As for creating skin flaps, there are advocates for both skew flaps, equal, and long posterior flaps, but in a recent Cochrane review, the choice of technique had no effect on the clinical outcome [8]. Additionally, in the setting of acute trauma, incision

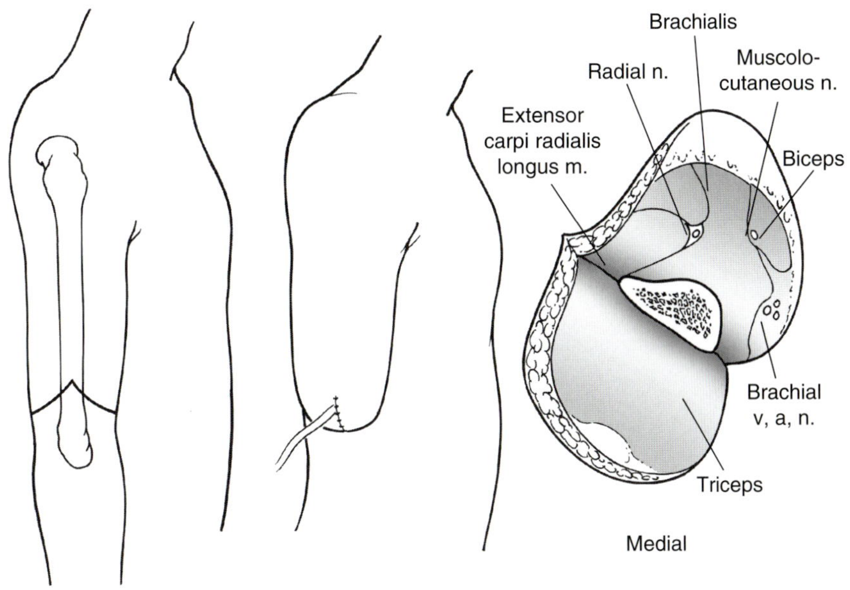

Fig. 59.2 Transhumeral amputation

choice largely depends on the extent and type of soft tissue injury triggering the amputation.

59.3.1.1 Transtibial Amputation (Extended Posterior Flap, Fig. 59.3) [13, 14]

The long posterior flap technique is well established and the rationale for it stems from the fact that the posterior tissues are better vascularized and thicker. However, many prosthetists recommend almost equal flaps, so that the scar is moved distally and posteriorly. With the patient supine, measure distally from the anteromedial joint line the desired length of bone and mark that level over the tibial crest with a skin marking pen. Now fashion an anterior skin flap 5 cm below the desired bone amputation level. Create an extended posterior skin flap 10 cm longer than the anterior incision, covering two thirds of the leg circumference. Longer skin flaps can be trimmed later as necessary. While cutting the flaps, deepen the anterior incision when crossing the tibial crest and mark the periosteum with a cut for future measurement. The posterior incision should be through the deep fascia. Do not separate the skin or deep fascia from the underlying muscle. As a single layer, reflect the deep fascia and periosteum with the anterior flap over the anteromedial surface of the tibia. Continue this dissection proximally to the level of intended bone section, approximately 5 cm higher than the anterior skin line. Use the mark previously made in the tibial periosteum to measure the level of intended amputation and mark the bone at this level with a saw. Section the muscles in the anterior compartment of the leg approximately 0.6 cm distal to the level of bone section so that they retract evenly with the end of the bone. Locate and divide the anterior tibial vessels and deep and superficial peroneal nerves. Ligate and divide these vessels and divide the nerve as

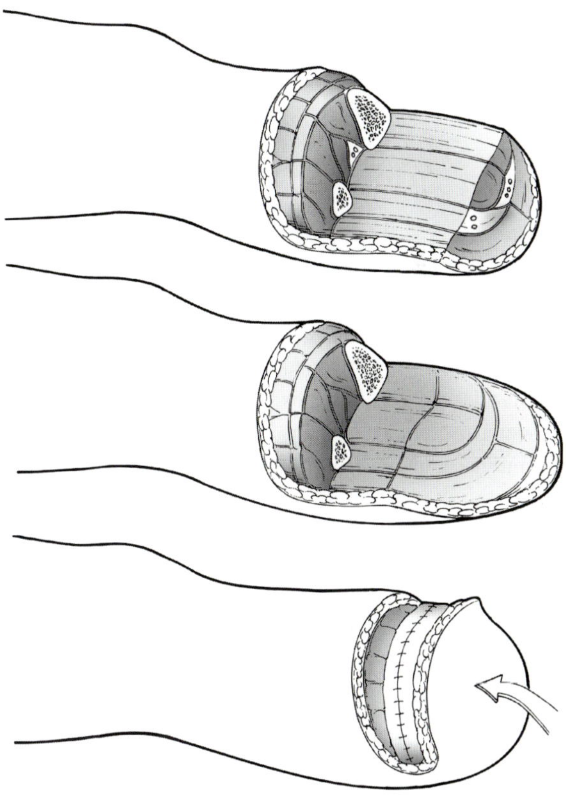

Fig. 59.3 Transtibial amputation, extended posterior flap. Arrow shows how the posterior flap is folded to its final position

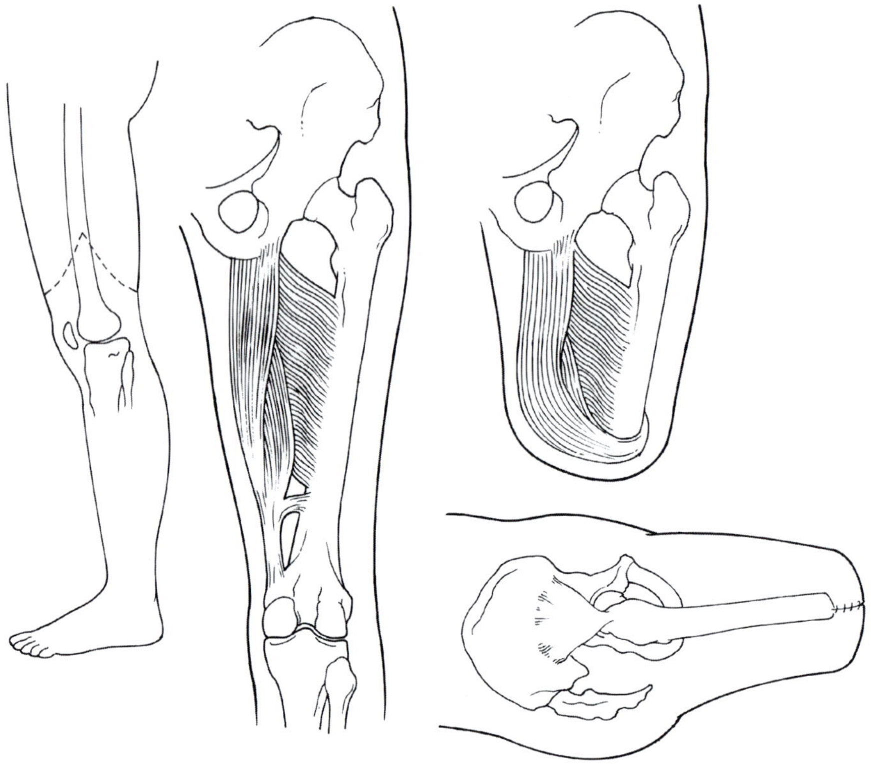

Fig. 59.4 Transfemoral amputation

previously described. Insert a curved hemostat in the natural cleavage plane at the lateral aspect of the tibia so that its tip follows along the interosseous membrane and passes over the anterior aspect of the fibula to emerge just anterior to the peroneus brevis muscle. Using the hemostat, pass the Gigli saw underneath the tibia. Use a tissue protector to retract the soft tissues proximally and then transect the tibia at the amputation mark. Bevel the tibial crest at a 45° angle beginning anterior to the medullary cavity. Transect the fibula 1 cm proximal to this level. Grasp the distal segments of the bones with bone-holding forceps and pull them anteriorly and distally exposing the posterior muscle mass. Transect the muscles in the deep posterior compartment starting 0.6 cm distal to the level of bone section and bevel along the posterior flap. This will expose the posterior tibial and peroneal vessels and the tibial nerve lying on the gastrocnemius-soleus muscle group. Ligate and divide these vessels and divide the nerve as previously described. Bevel the gastrocnemius-soleus muscle mass with a large amputation knife, forming a myofascial flap long enough to wrap around the end of the tibia to the anterior fascia. Rasp the ends of the tibia and fibula to produce a smooth contour. Wash the wound and ensure hemostasis. Wrap the gastrocnemius-soleus muscle flap over the ends of the bones, and suture it to the anterior deep fascia and the periosteum. Place a suction drainage tube deep to the muscle flap and fascia and close the wound in layers.

59.3.2 Disarticulation of the Knee

Although knee disarticulation can result in an excellent end-bearing stump, it requires expertise beyond the training of most general surgeons. Interestingly, a recent study revealed that patients who underwent knee disarticulation after a traumatic lower extremity injury had the highest risk for an overall poor outcome, compared to other types of amputation at a 7-year follow-up [6]. This failure is likely due to injury-associated soft tissue damage, resulting in a lack of viable musculature in the zone of injury. It is also possible that lack of specialized skill or incorrect operative choice in the acute setting may contribute to poor outcomes.

59.3.3 Transfemoral (Above-Knee) Amputations (Fig. 59.4)

Since the patient's knee will be lost, it is essential that the residual limb be as long as possible to provide a strong level arm for control of the prosthesis. However, the standard knee joint on above-knee prostheses extends 9–10 cm distal to the end of the prosthetic socket, so the bone must be amputated at least this far to allow room for the prosthetic joint.

Once you determine the level of amputation, fashion equal anterior and posterior skin flaps ("fish mouth") with the medial and lateral apexes 10 cm above the femoral condyles, if possible. Incise the skin through the subcutaneous tissue and deep fascia. Divide and ligate any superficial veins and divide the quadriceps muscle and its overlying fascia along the line of the anterior flap and reflect this myofascial flap proximally to the level of amputation. Medially, locate, ligate, and divide the femoral artery and vein in the femoral canal on the medial side of the thigh. Circumferentially, incise the periosteum of the femur and divide the bone approximately 5 cm proximal to the lower edge of the skin flaps. Smoothen the edges and flatten the anterolateral aspect of the femur. Use a tissue protector to retract the soft tissues while dividing the bone. Just beneath the hamstring muscles, identify and transect the sciatic nerve under gentle traction and allow the cut end to retract deep into the soft tissues. Transversely, section the posterior muscles starting at the level of amputation and bevel toward the posterior skin line. Remove the leg and irrigate the wound. Attaching the adductor and hamstring muscles under slight tension to the femur, utilizing several small drill holes just proximal to the end of the bone, results in improved functional outcome. Wrap the quadriceps over the end of the bone and suture its fascial layer to the posterior fascia of the thigh. Place a drain beneath the muscle flap and deep fascia and close the wound in layers.

59.4 Conclusion

The incidence of traumatic amputations secondary to penetrating trauma has steadily increased over the past two decades. For this reason, it is essential for trauma surgeons to have a firm understanding of the principles of amputation. Nevertheless, the most difficult aspect of amputation is not the surgical technique, but the actual decision to amputate or salvage a limb. When faced with a patient who may benefit from amputation, it is important to remember that amputation is not a failed attempt to salvage a limb, but rather a therapeutic treatment option for select individuals.

Important Points

1. Decide what you aim for – to get rid of contamination/debris or to create a definitive stump.
2. If a lot of infection or contamination – do a guillotine amputation and revise it in 48 h.
3. A guillotine amputation can be done as low as possible – anywhere and ASAP.
4. A below-knee amputation needs at least a hand width of tibial stump; otherwise it is functionally useless.
5. Save as much upper extremity as you can.

References

1. Heck RK (2008) General principles of amputations. In: Canale ST, Beaty JH (eds) Campbell's operative orthopaedics, 11th edn. Mosby, Philadelphia
2. National Limb Loss Information Center (2008) Amputation statistics by cause: limb loss in the United States. Available at www.amputee-coalition.org accessed on 7th March 2011
3. Arrillaga A, Bynoe R, Frykberg ER et al Practice management guidelines for penetrating trauma to the lower extremity. EAST practice management guidelines group. Eastern association for the surgery of trauma. http://www.east.org/tpg/lepene.pdf accessed on 7th March 2011
4. Bosse MJ, MacKenzie EJ, Kellam JF et al (2002) An analysis of outcomes of reconstruction or amputation of leg-threatening injuries. N Engl J Med 34:1924–1931
5. Busse JW, Jacobs CL, Swiontkowski MF et al (2007) Complex limb salvage or early amputation for severe lower-limb injury: a meta-analysis of observational studies. J Orthop Trauma 21:70–76
6. MacKenzie EJ, Bosse MJ, Pollak AN et al (2005) Long-term persistence of disability following severe lower-limb trauma: results of a seven-year follow-up. J Bone Joint Surg Am 87:1801–1809
7. Sharma S, Devgan A, Marya KM et al (2003) Critical evaluation of mangled extremity severity scoring system in Indian patients. Injury 34:493–496
8. Tisi PV, Callam MJ (2004) Type of incision for below knee amputation. Cochrane Database Syst Rev 1:CD003749
9. Helfet DL, Howey T, Sanders R et al (1990) Limb salvage versus amputation: preliminary results of the mangled extremity severity score. Clin Orthop Relat Res 256: 80–86
10. Archdeacon MT, Sanders R (2004) Trauma: limb salvage versus amputation. In: Smith DG, Michael JW, Bowker JH (eds) Atlas of amputations and limb deficiencies: surgical, prosthetic, and rehabilitation principles, 3rd edn. American Academy of Orthopaedic Surgeons, Rosemont
11. Pinzur MS (2008) Amputations in trauma. In: Browner BD (ed) Skeletal trauma, 4th edn. Saunders, Philadelphia

12. Oliveira IC, Barbosa RF, Ferreira PC et al (2009) The use of forearm free fillet flap in traumatic upper extremity amputations. Microsurgery 29:8–15
13. Khatri VP (2003) Lower extremity amputation. In: Khatri VP, Asensio JA (eds) Operative surgery manual, 1st edn. Saunders, Philadelphia
14. Mihalko M, Martinez S (2008) Amputations of the lower extremity. In: Canale ST, Beaty JH (eds) Campbell's operative orthopaedics, 11th edn. Mosby, Philadelphia
15. American College of Surgeons Committee on Trauma. Management of complex extremity trauma. Ad Hoc committee on outcomes. American College of Surgeons. http://www.facs.org/trauma/publications/mancompexttrauma.pdf. accessed on 7th March 2011
16. Cleveland KB (2008) Amputations of the upper extremity. In: Canale ST, Beaty JH (eds) Campbell's operative orthopaedics, 11th edn. Mosby, Philadelphia

Part VI
Peripheral Arterial Injuries

Peripheral Arterial Injuries from Penetrating Trauma

60

Matthew J. Martin and Ali Salim

Although the incidence of penetrating trauma varies widely between countries and geographic settings, it still represents a minority of overall trauma volume seen in even the busiest inner-city trauma centers. Extremity vascular injuries from penetrating mechanisms are relatively uncommon, with the expected result of a very limited body of experience in evaluation and management of these injuries among trauma and vascular surgeons. This is particularly concerning given the potential for mortality and devastating morbidity if these injuries are not readily identified and properly managed. Having a well thought-out and systematic approach to these injuries can go a long way toward making up for a lack of personal experience.

The keys to success and a good outcome in these patients are (1) rapid and early identification of the arterial injury, (2) control of any ongoing hemorrhage, (3) identification and assessment of associated injuries to major veins, bone, nerve, and soft tissues, and (4) appropriate interventions to restore perfusion and repair the injury. Although this approach appears to be simple and straightforward, each of these steps has potential pitfalls that can lead one astray if not anticipated and appreciated. In addition to the details of the vascular injury, the overall clinical status of the patient must be continuously assessed and considered when deciding on any course of intervention.

Unlike their portrayal in movies and television, the majority of these injuries do not present with dramatic arterial hemorrhage. By the time they have reached a hospital, they often will have stopped bleeding either due to intrinsic hemostatic mechanisms or first-responder interventions such as dressings or tourniquets. All penetrating extremity wounds should be assumed to have injured a major blood vessel until proven otherwise. A thorough physical examination of the injured extremity should focus on identifying the number of wounds, the location, and an assessment for any "hard" or "soft" signs of vascular injury. In addition, the physical examination and plain radiography of the extremity will provide information on the status of the bone, nerves, and soft-tissue structures in proximity to the artery. Most injuries to a major extremity artery do not require any advanced diagnostic studies beyond a good physical exam and measurement of a distal arterial pressure indexed to a normal pressure. If this is strongly suggestive of an arterial injury, then operative intervention can be pursued without further delay. If the physical examination is unrevealing and a clinical suspicion for vascular injury remains, then additional studies such as duplex ultrasonography or CT angiography can be considered.

The basic principles of operative assessment and repair of these injuries has not changed significantly in decades. Proximal and distal control of the affected artery should be obtained prior to exploring the area of injury when possible. Direct manual pressure and proximal tourniquets are important adjuncts to decreasing blood loss while exposing the injured area if it is actively bleeding. Even when full arterial control has

M.J. Martin (✉)
Trauma Service, Legacy Emanuel Medical Center, 2801 North Gantenbein, Portland, OR 97227, USA
e-mail: docmartin2@yahoo.com

A. Salim
Department of Surgery, Cedars Sinai Medical Center, 8700 Beverly Boulevard #8210, Los Angeles, CA 90048, USA
e-mail: ali.salim@cshs.org

G.C. Velmahos et al. (eds.), *Penetrating Trauma*,
DOI 10.1007/978-3-642-20453-1_60,

been obtained, you can expect to encounter significant ongoing bleeding from associated venous and muscle injury that can make the dissection and identification of key structures significantly more difficult than in elective vascular surgery. A detailed knowledge of the local anatomy and arterial position is particularly important when you do not have a readily palpable pulse to guide your dissection and exposure.

Once the exposure and delineation of the vascular injury has been completed, a decision for definitive repair or temporization needs to be made. Estimate the time it will take for a vascular reconstruction, and then double it. If the patient can safely tolerate a procedure of this duration, then proceed. If not, then placement of an intra-arterial shunt and confirmation of distal perfusion can be done rapidly and allow for further resuscitation and repair on a semi-elective basis. Ligation should also be considered as an option for patients in extremis, or in cases where end-tissue perfusion is not significantly compromised by loss of that vessel. The choice of reconstruction should be the simplest appropriate procedure, with primary repairs preferred when there has not been significant segmental loss, and interposition graft reconstruction with either autologous vein or prosthetic in more complex injuries. In addition to repair of the arterial injury, there should be a full assessment of the corresponding vein and nearby nerves which are frequent collateral damage.

Although the surgical exposure and repair principles have not changed significantly over past decades, there has been a revolution in the availability and experience with endovascular therapeutic interventions and repair options. Initially developed and tested in the management of great vessel aneurysmal and atherosclerotic disease, endovascular stents are now being increasingly utilized for the management of traumatic vascular injuries. At the present, these techniques are best utilized in the management of injuries to larger vessels in difficult areas of exposure – such as the subclavian vessels. The role of endovascular stenting for the majority of peripheral vascular injuries remains undefined and should be considered experimental until proven to be as safe, durable, and effective as standard surgical repair. However, endovascular techniques clearly have a major role in treating specific localized vascular injuries or complications, such as coil embolization of pseudoaneurysms, catheter directed clot lysis or thrombectomy/embolectomy, and balloon angioplasty and stenting of postoperative stenoses.

Current and future research in peripheral vascular trauma will focus on the development of techniques, technology, and materials to improve outcomes from these often devastating injuries. This should include significant improvements in diagnostic capabilities, less invasive options for therapeutic interventions, use of biocompatible and removable or biodegradable stents, and development of advanced graft materials that maximize flow properties and infection resistance.

Axillary and Brachial Vessels

61

Ali Salim and Matthew J. Martin

Penetrating injuries to the axillary and brachial vessels are fairly uncommon [1–5]. As with all traumatic injuries, prompt diagnosis and rapid repair provide the best outcomes. A thorough physical examination looking for any "hard" or "soft" signs of vascular injury will identify most injuries. Detailed neurological examination should be performed because of the proximity of these vessels to the branches of the brachial plexus. If an arterial injury is diagnosed on clinical ground, then operative intervention should be performed without further delay. If the physical examination is unrevealing and a clinical suspicion for vascular injury remains, then additional studies such as duplex ultrasonography or CT angiography should be performed. An understanding of the vascular anatomy and the relationships of key structures is critical for any operation, particularly in the emergency setting where anatomy is often distorted and time is of the essence.

A. Salim (✉)
Department of Surgery,
Cedars Sinai Medical Center,
8700 Beverly Boulevard #8210,
Los Angeles, CA 90048, USA
e-mail: ali.salim@cshs.org

M.J. Martin
Trauma Service, Legacy Emanuel
Medical Center,
2801 North Gantenbein,
Portland, OR 97227, USA
e-mail: docmartin2@yahoo.com

61.1 Making the Diagnosis

Although pulsatile arterial hemorrhage from the wound makes for an easy diagnosis, this is seen in only a minority of civilian vascular injuries. A careful and detailed physical examination is often all that is required for diagnosis, and angiography can be reserved for unclear exam findings or multi-level extremity wounds. Pulse examination and pressure measurements (indexed to the uninjured arm) should be performed and documented. Although a normal examination essentially rules out a significant brachial artery injury, injuries to the proximal axillary artery can present with intact pulses due to collateral flow. Hard signs of brachial or axillary artery injury should prompt immediate surgical intervention. Standard or CT angiography may be useful in cases where there is a hard sign of vascular injury but wounds at multiple levels, soft signs only, or a high clinical suspicion (shotgun or multiple fragment wounds, associated nerve injury). The option of an on-table angiogram in the operating room is an excellent but often overlooked alternative.

61.2 Anatomic Considerations

The axillary artery begins as a continuation of the subclavian artery at the outer border of the first rib and ends at the lower border of the teres major muscle (Fig. 61.1). The artery is divided into three parts by the pectoralis minor muscle. The first part lies proximal to the muscle and gives off the superior thoracic artery. The second part lies beneath the muscle and gives off

G.C. Velmahos et al. (eds.), *Penetrating Trauma*,
DOI 10.1007/978-3-642-20453-1_61, © Springer-Verlag Berlin Heidelberg 2012

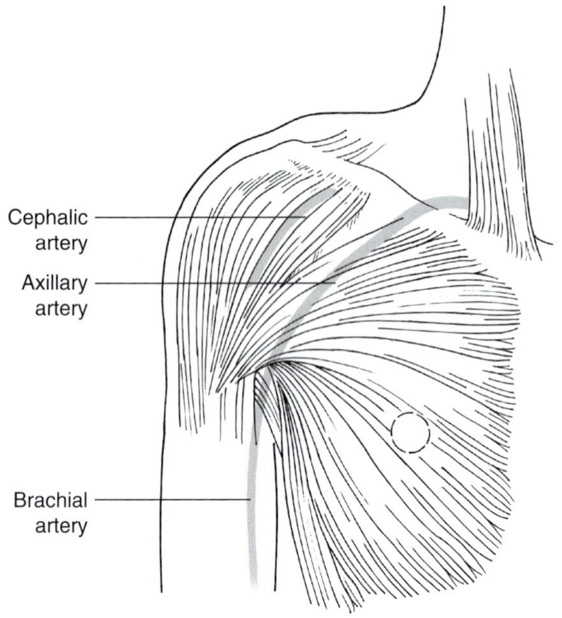

Fig. 61.1 The axillary artery begins as a continuation of the subclavian artery at the outer border of the first rib and ends at the lower border of the teres major muscle

the thoracoacromial and lateral thoracic arteries. The third part lies distal to the muscle and gives off the anterior and posterior circumflex arteries as well as the subscapular artery. These branches of the axillary artery provide a rich collateral circulation to this area in the upper extremity. The axillary vein lies medial and inferior to the artery and branches of the brachial plexus also lie in close proximity. Due to this close relationship, it is not uncommon to have associated venous as well as nerve injuries.

At the lower border of the teres major muscle the axillary artery becomes the brachial artery and ends at the bifurcation of the radial and ulnar arteries approximately 1–2 cm below the elbow. The brachial artery is fairly superficial throughout its course and is easily palpable. Initially, the artery (found medial to the humerus) runs with the median nerve (superior and lateral) and is felt in the groove between the coracobrachialis and biceps muscles, then between the biceps and triceps muscle. The artery courses medially to the front of the arm where it eventually passes in front of the biceps tendon anterior to the elbow. There it is separated from the median antecubital vein by a thick aponeurosis. The brachial artery has three main branches: the profunda brachii, the superior ulnar collateral, and the inferior ulnar collateral, all providing a rich collateral circulation for the upper arm and elbow.

61.3 Exposure and Management of Injuries

61.3.1 Axillary Artery Injuries

Start by placing the patient in the supine position with the arm abducted slightly (no more than 30°). The arm should be supported by a mobile board. Make sure that the chest, neck, shoulder, arm, and hand are included in the sterile field. Also, the ipsilateral or contralateral leg should be prepped in the event a vein conduit needs to be harvested. The incision is placed below, parallel, and at the middle of the clavicle. The incision is then curved down slightly over the deltopectoral groove. You should make a very generous incision, especially if the extent of injury is not known. This will later facilitate obtaining proximal and distal control of the vessel. Electrocautery is used to dissect through subcutaneous tissue and the fascia over the pectoralis major muscle. Use a self-retaining retractor to keep the skin wound open here, especially if you are limited with surgical assistants. The axillary vessels are deep to the pectoralis major and minor muscles. Whether you want to divide the muscle or split the muscle for retraction depends on the status of the injured vessel. If you encounter active bleeding, rapid and wide exposure is absolutely necessary. In this situation, you should divide the pectoralis major muscle with elctrocautery approximately 2 cm from its attachment to the humerus. You can use a tonsil or a Kelly clamp placed deep to the muscle to facilitate its division. Next, you should divide the pectoralis minor tendon close to its insertion into the coracoid process (Fig. 61.2b). The pectoralis minor muscle will withdraw the tendon inferomedially, exposing the axillary vessels as well as the brachial plexus (Fig. 61.2a). You will find the axillary vein below the artery. In the absence of active bleeding, you should split the pectoralis major muscle in the line of its fibers using a Kelly clamp. You can use another self-retaining retractor to keep the muscle split, or have a colleague help retract the muscle with two Army-Navy retractor or two small Richardson retractors. Proceed with dividing the pectoralis minor tendon as described above to achieve adequate exposure to the axillary vessels.

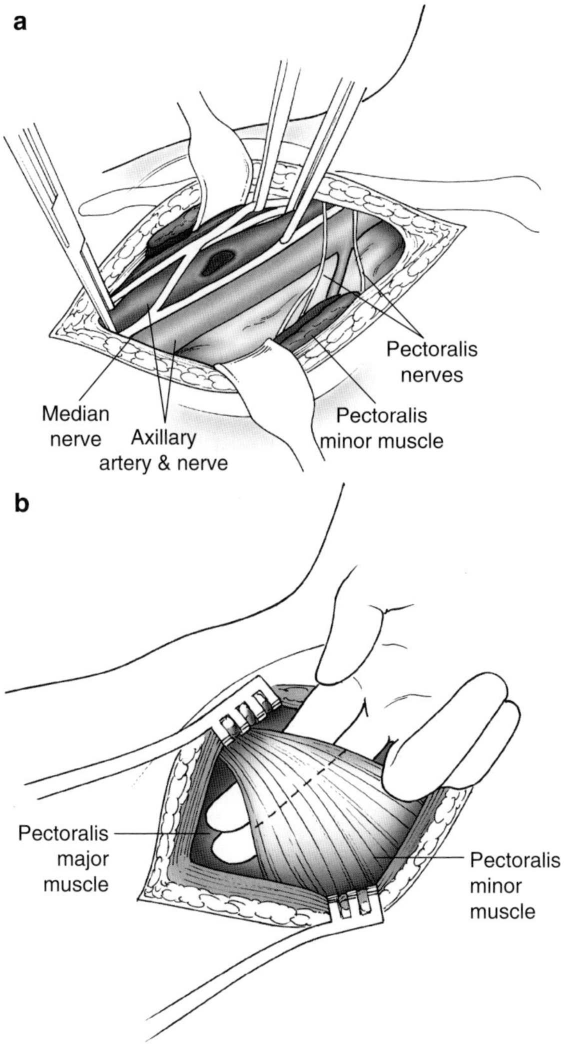

Fig. 61.2 (**a**) The pectoralis minor muscle will withdraw the tendon inferomedially, exposing the axillary vessels as well as the brachial plexus. (**b**) You should divide the pectoralis minor tendon close to its insertion into the coracoid process

Management of the injury depends on the hemodynamic status of the patient and the mechanism of the injury (stab wound versus gunshot wound). Your goals are to stop the hemorrhage and restore arterial flow. For arterial injuries that are actively bleeding, you need to gain proximal and distal control using vascular clamps. Medium size bulldog clamps are very effective and do not take up the same space as traditional vascular clamps. By using a generous incision, a large length of the vessel can be easily exposed and you should have no trouble obtaining control. In patients who are in extremis, a temporary intravascular shunt can be placed easily, followed by wound packing and transfer back to the intensive care unit. There are multiple commercial shunts available; the simplest of these are the flexible PVC tube shunts routinely used in carotid surgery. Choose the largest shunt that fits the vessel lumen and insert it through the injury proximally and distally. Ensure that the shunt is well secured to the artery by a 3-0 silk suture at the proximal and distal end. This maneuver is rarely needed with civilian peripheral vascular injuries. Although it is has been described, ligation of the artery in this setting should be avoided [1, 2].

For the vast majority of patients, you can safely repair the injured vessel. Make sure you have Fogarty catheters available (usually size 3 and 4) and plenty of heparinized saline that can be flushed into the open vessel. For stab wound injuries, simple repair of the vessel without any debridement is all you need to do. First you should remove any distal clot by catheter thrombectomy (start with the 3 Fogarty first, and if it is too small, the 4 Fogarty catheter should suffice) (Fig. 61.3). You should flush the proximal and distal ends of the open vessel with heparinized saline. This local heparinization is adequate enough to preclude the use of systemic heparinization. The vessel is usually not completely transected and you can repair the injury using a 6-0 prolene suture in an interrupted fashion. Even with full transaction of the vessel, you can perform an end-to-end anastomosis either in a running or interrupted fashion using a 6-0 prolene suture (Fig. 61.4a, b). With gunshot injuries, you have to debride the injured artery back to healthy intima (Fig. 61.5), making a simple repair usually impossible and requiring the use of an interposition graft. The choice of whether to use an autologous proximal saphenous vein graft or a prosthetic polytetrafluoroethylene [PTFE] graft is determined by the physiologic status of the patient, the presence of an appropriate size matched vein, and your personal preference as the operating surgeon. To date there is no evidence for the superiority of either one [1]. Once you decide on a conduit, the anastomoses are constructed using a 6-0 prolene suture (Fig. 61.4). Make sure to remember to perform catheter thrombectomy and infuse local heparinized saline as described above. Once the repair is complete, you should perform a completion angiogram to assess the anastomosis and distal runoff. Fill a 20-cc syringe with contrast solution and attach it to a large angiocath. Insert the

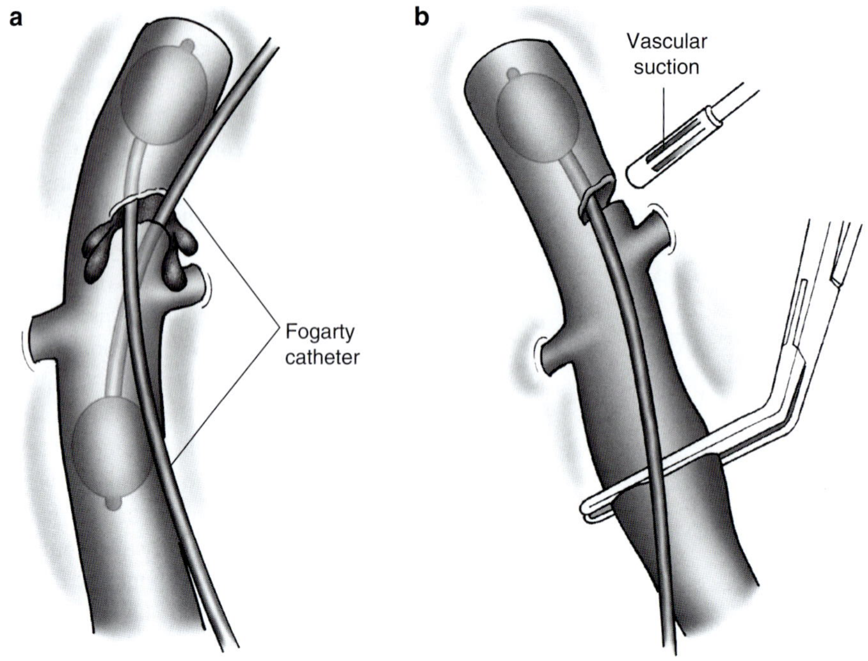

Fig. 61.3 (**a**) First you should remove any distal clot by catheter thrombectomy (start with the 3 Fogarty first, and if it is too small, the 4 Fogarty catheter should suffice). (**b**) Keep distal artery clamped during proximal embolectomy to prevent distal embolization of dislodged clot

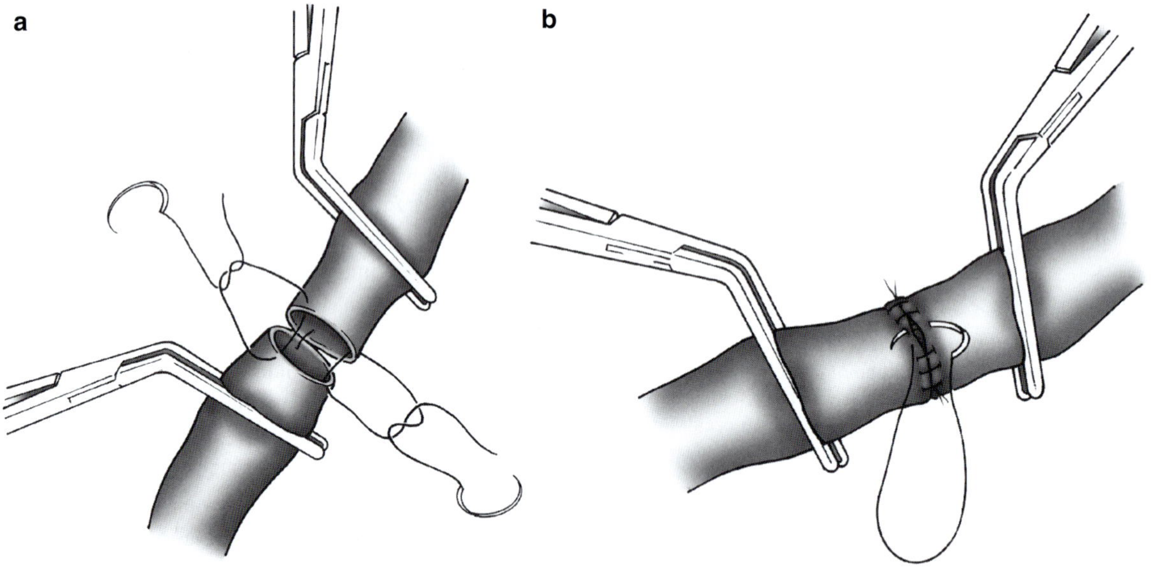

Fig. 61.4 Even with full transaction of the vessel, you can perform an end-to-end anastomosis either in an interrupted (**a**) or running (**b**) fashion using a 6-0 prolene suture

angiocath proximal to the anastomosis and occlude the inflow by placing a bulldog more proximally. Complete the on-table angiogram either using a static x-ray film or fluoroscopy.

Wound closure should be performed meticulously, and a closed suction drain may be used if a large dead space is present. Any necrotic muscle and debris should be removed, and you must always attempt to interpose healthy vascularized tissue over the site of repair or graft. You should reattach the pectoralis minor with a large absorbable suture. If the pectoralis major muscle was divided, you should reattach it

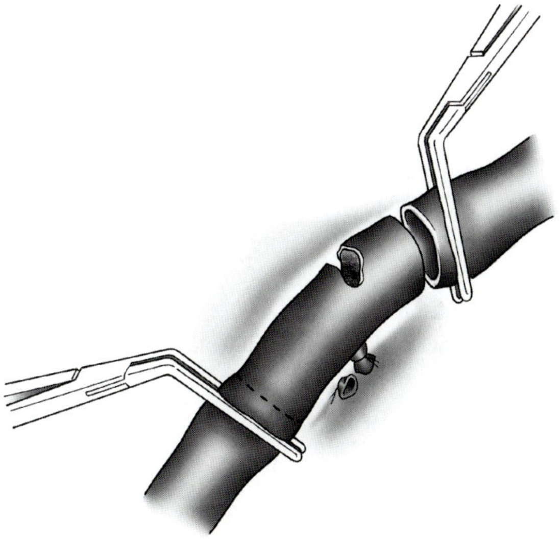

Fig. 61.5 With gunshot injuries, you have to debride the injured artery back to healthy intima, making a simple repair usually impossible and requiring the use of an interposition graft

also with a large absorbable suture. The remaining wound can be closed in two layers also using an absorbable suture. Finally, you can use staples for skin closure.

Just a quick word regarding venous injuries and fasciotomy. You should repair the vein injury only if it can be accomplished with a simple suture repair without narrowing the lumen. Ligation is very well tolerated with minimal complications, but the more proximal the vein the higher the risk of postoperative edema. You should perform a fasciotomy if the patient has an obvious or impending compartment syndrome. Remember that due to the rich collateral circulation around the shoulder, a fasciotomy is rarely needed. Routine or prophylactic fasciotomy should be avoided since fasciotomy on demand has proven to be safe and very effective [6].

61.3.2 Brachial Artery Injuries

With the patient in the supine position, place the arm on a mobile board and keep the arm abducted up to 30°. The entire arm down to the fingers should be included in the sterile field. You should make sure the shoulder and ipsilateral chest are also included in the sterile field in cases of proximal brachial artery injuries where control of the distal axillary artery may be necessary. Make sure that the ipsilateral or contralateral leg is prepped in the event a vein conduit needs to be harvested. You can expose any part of the length of the artery through a longitudinal incision made at the groove between the biceps and triceps muscles. If you need more proximal control, extend the incision to the deltopectoral groove and if you need more distal control, extend the incision to the elbow crease and make an s-shaped curve across the antecubital fossa. Remember that the artery is fairly superficial, so dividing the superficial tissue and investing fascia of the arm with electrocautery will expose the artery. Self-retaining retractors placed in the wound will provide you with an excellent view of the injured artery. The median nerve runs superior and lateral to the artery and may need to be gently retracted to avoid injury.

Management of the injured artery is similar to that described above for axillary artery injuries. Proximal and distal control is best achieved with medium-sized bulldog clamps. You need to remember to perform catheter embolectomy with a small Fogarty catheter (size 3) and flush the open vessel proximally and distally with heparinized saline. You can usually primarily repair stab wound injuries without any need for debridement. Use a 6-0 prolene suture in an interrupted fashion. Make sure to place the sutures in the same axis as the direction of the vessel to avoid significantly narrowing the artery [3]. You can also primarily repair stab wound injuries that cause complete transaction of the vessel. You can perform an end-to-end anastomosis in an interrupted fashion using 6-0 prolene sutures (Fig. 61.4). As far as gunshot injuries, you will need to debride the injured vessel back to healthy intima (Fig. 61.5). You will need to repair the vessel with an interposition graft using either reversed saphenous or cephalic vein, depending on the size match with the artery. There is no role for using a prosthetic graft in this position [3–5]. The anastomoses are constructed using an end-to-end interrupted repair with a 6-0 prolene suture (Fig. 61.4a). Make sure to remember catheter embolectomy using the Fogarty catheter (Fig. 61.3). Usually, two passes of the Fogarty catheter are all you will need. Also, remember to flush the proximal and distal limbs of the artery with the heparinized saline. Once the anastomosis is complete, you need to palpate for distal radial and ulnar pulses. You should perform an on-table angiogram to assess the quality of the anastomosis as well as for distal runoff as described above. Wound closure can be performed in two layers utilizing an absorbable suture followed by staples for the skin closure. A drain is not usually needed.

If there is an associated orthopedic injury, a decision must be made about whether to repair the vascular injury or address the fracture first. In cases of unstable fractures where significant manipulation and stretch will be required, you can restore flow with the use of an intravascular shunt, allow your orthopedic colleague to repair the broken humerus, and then come back for definitive repair as described above. Another option is to perform the definitive repair, allow your orthopedic colleague to come in and address the bony injuries, and then perform a final assessment of your initial repair. It is not unheard of to return and find a clotted vascular graft or repair following orthopedic manipulation.

Finally, just as mentioned above, you should perform a fasciotomy only when the patient has an established or impending compartment syndrome [6].

61.4 Role of Endovascular Therapy

Although the use of endovascular therapy in the setting of acute trauma is increasing, these techniques presently are best utilized in the management of injuries to larger vessels in difficult areas of exposure [7]. The role of endovascular stenting for axillary and brachial artery injuries remains undefined and should be considered experimental until proven to be as safe, durable, and effective as standard surgical repair [8]. As previously mentioned, endovascular techniques clearly have a major role in treating specific localized vascular injuries or complications, such as coil embolization of pseudoaneurysms, catheter-directed clot lysis or thrombectomy/embolectomy, and balloon angioplasty and stenting of postoperative stenoses.

Important Points

- Place the patient in the supine position with the arm abducted at 30°.
- Keep the arm on a mobile board.
- For axillary artery injuries, place the incision below, parallel, and at the middle of the clavicle and curve it down slightly over the deltopectoral groove.
- For brachial artery injuries, make a longitudinal incision at the groove between the biceps and triceps muscles.
- Simple repair is almost always enough for stab wound injuries.
- Debridement, resection, and repair with interposition grafts are almost always required for gunshot wound injuries.
- Never forget catheter thrombectomy and local infusion of heparinized saline prior to any repair.
- Perform an on-table angiogram to assess the repair or anastomosis and distal runoff.

References

1. Demetriades D, Asensio JA (2001) Subclavian and axillary vascular injuries. Surg Clin N Am 81:1357–1373
2. Demetriades D, Chahwan S, Gomez H et al (1999) Penetrating injuries to the subclavian and axillary vessels. J Am Coll Surg 188:290–295
3. Fields CE, Latifi R, Ivatury R (2002) Brachial and forearm vessel injuries. Surg Clin N Am 82:105–114
4. Ergunes K, Yilik L, Ozsoyler I et al (2006) Traumatic brachial artery injuries. Tex Heart Inst J 33:31–34
5. Zellweger R, Hess F, Nicol A et al (2004) An analysis of 124 surgically managed brachial artery injuries. Am J Surg 188:240–245
6. Velmahos G, Theodorou D, Demetriades D et al (1997) Complications and nonclosure rates of fasciotomy for trauma and related risk factors. World J Surg 25:247–253
7. Reuben BC, Whitten MG, Sarfati M, Kraiss LW (2007) Increasing use of endovascular therapy in acute arterial injuries: analysis of the national Trauma Data Bank. J Vasc Surg 46:1222–1226
8. Arthurs ZM, Sohn VY, Starnes BW (2007) Vascular trauma: endovascular management and techniques. Surg Clin N Am 87:1179–1192

Femoral Vessels

62

David R. King

62.1 The "Asymptomatic" Groin Wound

Evaluation of the penetrating wound to the groin in a patient without obvious external hemorrhage or hematoma presents specific challenges. Commonly, patients have no complaints or only report pain at the injury site. These patients can generally be evaluated slowly and carefully; however, you should bear in mind that any sudden or sentinel bleeding event (either externally or manifest by new rapidly expanding hematoma) mandates a rapid transfer to the operating room.

You should begin the investigation of the asymptomatic groin with a careful neurovascular physical exam, which includes a Doppler exam and ankle/brachial indices (ABI). A higher index of suspicion for femoral vessel injury should be exercised if the wound is anteromedial, although proximity alone is not an indication for additional imaging or intervention [1]. If a *normal and bilaterally symmetrical* pulse exam is present, along with an ABI >0.9 in the injured extremity, then you can safely exclude arterial injury and no additional testing or imaging is necessary [1–6]. Hard signs of arterial injury (pulsatile bleeding, expanding hematoma, absent distal pulses, cold pale limb, palpable thrill, audible bruit) remain indications for operative exploration. Patients with abnormal pulse, Doppler, or ABI exam are considered "indeterminate" and this group is addressed in the next section.

You can exclude an injury by a normal physical exam and absence of bleeding or hematoma [7]. In the absence of bleeding, venous injuries rarely represent a significant problem, unless the injury results in thrombosis of the vessel. This, however, usually produces rapid and obvious physical exam findings (unilateral asymmetrical limb swelling, venous congestion, complaint of whole-limb pain in absence of physical findings) prompting additional imaging such as duplex venous ultrasonography or CT (computed tomography) venography to demonstrate thrombosis. Identification of a venous injury with associated thrombosis should prompt operative exploration of the vessel [7, 8]. For penetrating groin injuries producing venous thrombosis alone without identifiable vein disruption, the surgeon may give consideration to therapeutic anticoagulation.

For all penetrating groin wounds, you should remain suspicious, until proven otherwise by careful examination, imaging or exploration, that a stabbing instrument or missile may have penetrated the confines of the infra-inguinal anatomy and involves the intra-abdominal (or rarely intra-thoracic) contents.

62.2 The Indeterminate Groin

This type of patient may present with a prehospital history of bleeding (but no evidence of current ongoing hemorrhage), small nonexpanding hematoma, and minimal additional findings on physical exam. This type of scenario is not uncommon and probably represents the majority of groin wounds [6]. As in the asymptomatic groin, a careful physical and Doppler exam, as well as ABIs, is essential as any abnormalities,

D.R. King
Division of Trauma, Emergency Surgery, and Surgical Critical Care, Massachusetts General Hospital,
165 Cambridge Street, Suite 810, Boston, MA 02114, USA
e-mail: dking3@partners.org

G.C. Velmahos et al. (eds.), *Penetrating Trauma*,
DOI 10.1007/978-3-642-20453-1_62, © Springer-Verlag Berlin Heidelberg 2012

asymmetry, or hard signs should prompt further interrogation of the vessels, either by imaging or operative exploration. Patients with abnormal physical and Doppler findings, in the absence of hard signs, should proceed to have additional imaging of the femoral vessels. CT arteriography has largely replaced formal angiography, although angiography remains the gold standard and absolutely appropriate in the absence of CT availability [6, 9] or in cases of multiply-injured patients who are already in the operating room for associated injuries. CT imaging not only identifies specific vascular injuries, but often allows identification of the projectile path through the tissues. A tract not involving the femoral vessels may reassure you that any subtle abnormal or asymmetric physical or Doppler findings may be chronic and unrelated to the missile [6, 9, 10] or represent vasospasm. Nearly every acute vascular abnormalities attributable to the penetrating injury identified by CT, excepting the isolated hematoma without identifiable vascular injury, will require operative exploration and repair [9].

Local soft tissue injury will sometimes produce vasospasm and an abnormal physical exam (classically asymmetrical pulse exam with slightly abnormal ABI). CT is extremely useful in this population to exclude direct injury to the vasculature and safely permit discharge [6, 9, 10]. Vasospasm usually resolves with gentle intravenous hydration, warming of the extremity, and placing the limb in a neutral or dependent position. Rarely, vasospasm will require pharmacologic intervention, and this should only be undertaken if the vasospasm prevents return to normal function.

62.3 The Bleeding Groin

The bleeding groin dictates the simplest diagnostic approach to femoral vessel injury: operative exploration. No preoperative workup is required and little time should be wasted moving the patient to the operating room after obtaining supradiaphragmatic intravenous access for resuscitation and sending a sample for type and cross to the blood bank. This same approach also applies to a penetrating groin wound with hard signs of injury or an expanding hematoma. You can obtain temporary hemorrhage control with direct pressure, a hemostatic adjunct (a topical hemostatic dressing in a variety of forms), or even a Foley catheter in the wound tract. The principles of hypotensive resuscitation and aggressive use of blood products in appropriate ratios should be applied to the bleeding groin. A patient with a penetrating groin wound that presents in arrest or extremis with profound cardiovascular compromise should undergo emergency anterolateral thoracotomy for aortic cross-clamping and open cardiac massage. Return of vital signs after this procedure will indicate a potentially salvageable casualty, and emergent transfer to the operating theater is required. Commonly, return of vital signs will be accompanied by massive hemorrhage from the groin wound, which requires temporary control as described above. If the supradiaphragmatic aorta has been clamped, impressive venous bleeding may still occur from the groin and local control is indicated.

Once in the operating room, you should prep the entire torso and both lower extremities into the operative field. A penetrating groin wound may give little indication of the direction the penetrating instrument or missile took, and you may quickly find yourself exploring the abdomen or chest if the trajectory of injury proceeds above the inguinal ligament. The entire ipsilateral injured limb should be included in the field to make serial examinations of distal perfusion easy without breaking scrub. You should also include the contralateral lower extremity in the field so that saphenous vein may be harvested for reconstruction if you choose not to use ipsilateral saphenous vein or if the ipsilateral saphenous has also been injured.

Few surgical maneuvers are as satisfying as rapid control of exsanguinating hemorrhage in the groin. Rapid hemorrhage control in the operating room can often very quickly turn a dying patient into a survivor. Control may be obtained by making an aggressive vertical groin incision over the femoral pulsation and extending several centimeters above the inguinal skin crease. In the absence of a palpable pulsation, place your vertical incision equidistant from the anterior superior iliac spine and the pubic tubercle. Quickly dissect down through the hematoma to the site of injury (arterial or venous, sometimes both) and have an assistant control the bleeding with digital pressure. Extend your dissection cephalad to gain proximal control. Stay directly superficial to the vessel and do not stray laterally. There are rarely, if ever, any direct anterior branches of the femoral artery, so this is safe territory to dissect quickly and aggressively with relative impunity. The only exception is a small crossing vein (superficial circumflex iliac vein) that is often present

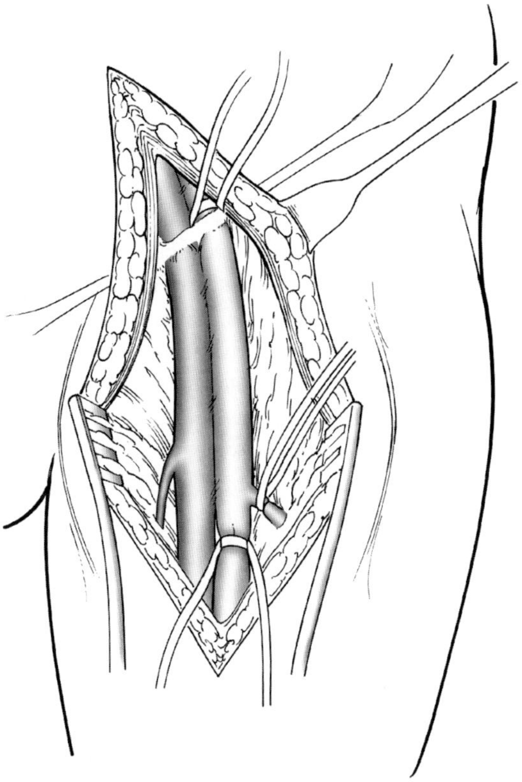

Fig. 62.1 If the injury is high in the groin, exercise little hesitation to dividing the inguinal ligament with scissors in order to expose the very distal external iliac vessels for proximal control

just under the inguinal ligament. This should be divided between ties before taking the dissection higher on the iliac artery. If the injury is high in the groin, exercise little hesitation to dividing the inguinal ligament with scissors in order to expose the very distal external iliac vessels for proximal control (Fig. 62.1). As mentioned above, be careful for the small superficial circumflex iliac vein that seems to be ubiquitous. Alternatively, some surgeons prefer to spare the inguinal ligament and make a horizontal incision in the inguinal ligament 2 cm above its inferior reflection. This allows access to the retroperitoneum. A short simple dissection through fat will reveal the external iliac vessels in uninvolved uninjured tissue. It is the exceptionally rare and fairly destructive injury that requires laparotomy and intra-abdominal proximal control of the iliac vessels; however, this option should never be forgotten because it will become the most useful of maneuvers in the worst of situations, such as is routinely seen in a combined penetrating/blast injury to the groin from an improvised explosive device. You can obtain temporary proximal control with an intraluminal balloon through the artery injury site until surgical control can be effected by dissection. After obtaining proximal control by either an appropriate clamp, vessel loop, or even a double-looped 0 polypropylene suture, distal control should be easier (albeit not simple). Back-bleeding can be impressive, but simply extend your sharp dissection distally from the point of injury until circumferential control is obtained. You can follow the superficial femoral artery distally along its entire course to the adductor canal. The profunda femoral artery should also be controlled without extensive dissection. In general, all of these dissections are done sharply with the scissors. Electrocautery has little role in a blood-filled field.

Once proximal and distal control are obtained, careful dissection of the injury can commence. The complete circumference of the vessel should be inspected with special attention to the often overlooked backwall. Injuries that can be repaired with simple lateral sutures should be fixed immediately, including venous injuries. Massive destruction of the femoral vein, however, should result in ligation rather than a complicated and time-consuming repair, which will likely thrombose soon afterward anyway. Similarly, in a dying patient with massive tissue destruction, the superficial femoral artery may also be ligated with relatively good outcome if the profunda femoral artery is intact.

For anything other than a simple lateral arteriorraphy, you should consider temporary shunting instead of complicated definitive repair in a severely compromised patient. For practical purposes, a complicated repair is any repair that requires graft material or saphenous vein. Your decision to shunt should be based on the patient's physiologic status and the associated injury burden. A very sick patient, as evidenced by hypothermia, acidosis, or coagulopathy, should be shunted and returned to the operating room after these are corrected. Additionally, a heavy injury burden should prompt the surgeon to shunt and move on to treating other injuries. This is particularly helpful strategy in mass casualty events and combat surgery. On the other hand, in a stable patient with good physiology, even the most complicated repairs can be undertaken immediately.

A host of shunts are commercially available, but the Argyle shunt is among the simplest. A size-matched shunt can be placed within the vessel without the need for extensive debridement. Many techniques are used to secure the shunts; however, in a crisis, a simple 0 silk or monofilament tie can be tied around the vessel and shunt proximally and distally, as close to the injury site as possible (after thrombectomy). Upon returning to the operating room, this segment of artery can be excised and appropriately repaired. Patients requiring shunting are usually coagulopathic and no postoperative anticoagulation is required. Shunts may remain safely in place for at least 24 h, and perhaps much longer without risk of thrombosis [11]. Shunting should be followed rapidly by four compartment fasciotomy. Generally, the patients with severely deranged physiology that dictate shunt placement are exactly the same ones at the highest risk for compartment syndrome. There should be a compelling reason to *not* perform fasciotomies after shunting of a proximal groin injury.

The general principles of vascular surgery hold true for complex arterial or venous reconstruction: Autologous conduit is generally better than artificial graft material, especially for the femoral vessels. Reconstruction with reversed saphenous vein (for interposition repairs) or saphenous vein patch for anterior wall injures are simple and, if done well with technical expertise, will last a lifetime. Most complex vascular anastomoses can be easily made with running 4-0 or 5-0 polypropylene suture. You should pay special attention to any combined arterial and venous injuries. Adjacent suture lines should not be allowed to contact one another and a vitalized tissue flap should be placed between these two.

Consideration should be given to placing a muscle flap over any repair done with graft material as well particularly if it is partially or totally exposed. A sartorius muscle flap is a simple and very fast solution. Simply identify the sartorius muscle in the lateral side of the wound and dissect along its circumference superiorly toward the anterior superior iliac spine where the tendinous attachment may be taken down. The muscle can then be rotated over into the groin to provide muscular coverage of vascular repairs. The muscle can be secured in place by tacking it to the inguinal ligament. Alternatively, if the vascular injury is more distal and the incision is already fairly distal, the sartorius can be dissected distally toward its attachment at the medial knee, divided, and placed over the repair. A grossly contaminated wound remains a relative contraindication to use of graft material and this should be a last resort under circumstances where saphenous vein is not available or suitable. If the patient is undergoing a simultaneous laparotomy, for example, a short segment of internal iliac artery can be harvested instead of placing graft material in a contaminated wound.

If the patient as a multiply-penetrated thigh (such as multiple stabs, gunshots, fragmentation from a grenade, or improvised explosive device with shrapnel), then an on-table angiogram should be performed once vascular control has been obtained, but before repair of the femoral injuries. Also completion angiogram is desirable after completion of the repair to confirm good graft proximal and distal anastomosis. The simplest technique is to cannulate the femoral vessel as proximal as possible (but just distal to the point of proximal vascular control) with an 18 or 20 gauge angiocatheter or butterfly. The C-arm x-ray machine can then be brought over the field. The inflow should be occluded while injecting half-diluted intravenous contrast agent. Any commercially available iodinated contrast agent may be utilized that has at least 320 mg/mL of organically bound iodine such that the half-diluted injectate has approximately 160 mg/mL of iodine. Injectate with approximately 160 mg/mL of iodine is all that is required to opacify the femoral outflow from the inguinal ligament to Hunter's Canal. Opacification of the vessels below the knee will require injectate with approximately 320 mg/mL of iodine as contrast agent. Generally, the C-arm should be activated in real time while injecting the contrast and the run recorded for playback. If possible, the digital subtraction technique should be utilized for the best pictures, although adequate imaging is certainly possible without this option. If a C-arm is not available, a simple flat-plate x-ray may be used. Simply position the flat plate below the field and arrange the x-ray machine appropriately over the plate. After occluding the inflow, inject half-diluted contrast agent and shoot the x-ray approximately 6 s after injection. Be sure to include the entire thigh in the x-ray field. A radiolucent table is not necessarily required for this procedure, although it does eliminate the bothersome radiopaque metal bars visualized on most on-table angiograms done on a non-radiolucent table. These bars are generally a simple annoyance and do not affect the utility of the angiogram. If the bar does obscure the area of particular interest on the angiogram, it can simply be re-shot in a slightly different orientation. Once the procedure and injury repair are completed, the femoral vessel can be decannulated and the puncture site closed with a single 5-0 polypropylene stitch. Alternatively, if angiogram capabilities are not available, the entire length of the femoral vessels may be explored surgically with relative ease all the way to the adductor canal, albeit through a somewhat larger incision. In the absence of radiographic capability for a fragmentation wound or multiple penetrating wounds with unilateral pulse discrepancy, this maneuver is mandatory. The only instruments required are scissors and an educated hand.

Postoperatively, groin repairs need not be maintained on any form of anticoagulation or antiplatelet therapy if vein was used as the conduit. Some surgeons will choose to place patients on antiplatelet therapy or vitamin-K antagonism if graft was used in their repair, although the data for this approach is lacking in the trauma population.

Important Points

- Always get proximal and distal control.
- Do fasciotomies early when indicated.
- Do intraoperative angiography after completion of graft anastomosis.
- Avoid venous injury during repair.
- Avoid unnecessary ligations of veins and arteries.

References

1. Shayne PH, Sloan EP, Rydman R, Barrett JA (1994) A case-control study of risk factors that predict femoral arterial injury in penetrating thigh trauma. Ann Emerg Med 24(4):678–684
2. Johansen K, Lynch K, Paun M, Copass M (1991) Noninvasive vascular tests reliably exclude occult arterial trauma in injured extremities. J Trauma 31(4):515–519; discussion 519–522
3. Schwartz MR, Weaver FA, Bauer M, Siegel A, Yellin AE (1993) Refining the indications for arteriography in penetrating extremity trauma: a prospective analysis. J Vasc Surg 17(1):116–122; discussion 122–124
4. Nassoura ZE, Ivatury RR, Simon RJ, Jabbour N, Vinzons A, Stahl W (1996) A reassessment of Doppler pressure indices in the detection of arterial lesions in proximity penetrating injuries of extremities: a prospective study. Am J Emerg Med 14(2):151–156
5. Dennis JW, Frykberg ER, Veldenz HC, Huffman S, Menawat SS (1998) Validation of nonoperative management of occult vascular injuries and accuracy of physical examination alone in penetrating extremity trauma: 5- to 10-year follow-up. J Trauma 44(2):243–252; discussion 242–243
6. Busquéts AR, Acosta JA, Colón E, Alejandro KV, Rodríguez P (2004) Helical computed tomographic angiography for the diagnosis of traumatic arterial injuries of the extremities. J Trauma 56(3):625–628
7. Nitecki SS, Karram T, Hoffman A, Bass A (2007) Venous trauma in the Lebanon War – 2006. Interact Cardiovasc Thorac Surg 6(5):647–650, Epub 2007 Jul 25
8. Quan RW, Gillespie DL, Stuart RP, Chang AS, Whittaker DR, Fox CJ (2008) The effect of vein repair on the risk of venous thromboembolic events: a review of more than 100 traumatic military venous injuries. J Vasc Surg 47(3): 571–577
9. Peng PD, Spain DA, Tataria M, Hellinger JC, Rubin GD, Brundage SI (2008) CT angiography effectively evaluates extremity vascular trauma. Am Surg 74(2):103–107
10. Soto JA, Múnera F, Morales C, Lopera JE, Holguín D, Guarín O, Castrillón G, Sanabria A, García G (2001) Focal arterial injuries of the proximal extremities: helical CT arteriography as the initial method of diagnosis. Radiology 218(1):188–194
11. Taller J, Kamdar JP, Greene JA, Morgan RA, Blankenship CL, Dabrowski P, Sharpe RP (2008) Temporary vascular shunts as initial treatment of proximal extremity vascular injuries during combat operations: the new standard of care at Echelon II facilities? J Trauma 65(3):595–603

Popliteal Vessels

63

Matthew J. Martin and Ali Salim

Penetrating injuries to the popliteal fossa can present a significant challenge to even the most experienced trauma or vascular surgeon. Although injuries to the popliteal vessels are fortunately uncommon, this results in a general lack of experience and expertise even at the busiest trauma centers. Like injuries to the neck, you are dealing with a number of critical anatomic structures that are contained in a relatively small and tight space. Improper early management or a missed injury can result in a devastating functional outcome for the patient, including death or limb amputation. The critical triad of success when you are faced with a penetrating wound to the popliteal fossa is early and accurate recognition of the vascular injury, detailed understanding of the local anatomy and surgical approach, and adherence to the basic principles of emergency vascular surgery.

63.1 Anatomy of the Popliteal Vessels for the Trauma Surgeon

Understanding the popliteal vascular anatomy and the relationships of key structures is critical for any operation, particularly in the emergency setting where anatomy is often distorted and time is of the essence. The crucial factors for the surgeon to appreciate are the location of the artery and vein, the landmarks and easiest routes for exposure, and the important structures (particularly nerves) that need to be protected while attempting to expose or repair the vessels. The popliteal artery and vein lie in the center of the popliteal fossa immediately posterior to the knee. Although they do have multiple collateral vessels at the level of the knee, they should be considered end vessels as ligation or thrombosis of the popliteal artery carries a 75% or higher incidence of amputation and popliteal vein ligation will almost universally result in significant and persistent leg edema [1].

The popliteal artery begins above the knee in the distal thigh as the continuation of the superficial femoral artery at the adductor magnus hiatus. The above-knee popliteal artery is covered by the belly of the semimembranosus muscle, and then courses inferiorly and medially into the popliteal fossa. The artery runs through the middle of the popliteal fossa directly posterior to the knee joint for several centimeters. The below-knee popliteal artery runs between the medial and lateral gastrocnemius muscles, and is also covered distally by the tibial insertion of the soleus. The artery gives off multiple small collateral branches (muscular, sural, geniculate) within the popliteal fossa. Although classically described as a "trifurcation," the below-knee popliteal artery most commonly divides into the anterior tibial artery and the tibio-peroneal trunk at the level of the inferior border of the popliteus muscle. The tibio-peroneal trunk then continues inferiorly and divides into the posterior tibial and peroneal arteries. Multiple anatomic variations exist, the most important for the surgeon being a high

M.J. Martin (✉)
Trauma Service, Legacy Emanuel Medical Center,
2801 North Gantenbein, Portland, OR 97227, USA
e-mail: docmartin2@yahoo.com

A. Salim
Department of Surgery,
Cedars Sinai Medical Center, 8700 Beverly
Boulevard #8210, Los Angeles, CA 90048, USA
e-mail: ali.salim@cshs.org

G.C. Velmahos et al. (eds.), *Penetrating Trauma*,
DOI 10.1007/978-3-642-20453-1_63, © Springer-Verlag Berlin Heidelberg 2012

bifurcation or true trifurcation of the popliteal artery at the level of the knee.

The popliteal vein provides the primary venous drainage for the leg below the knee. The vein forms from the junction of the anterior and posterior tibial veins at the inferior border of the popliteus muscle. Above the knee, the vein is lateral to the artery; in the popliteal fossa, it becomes superficial to the artery; and below the knee, it will be medial to the artery. The vein remains in close proximity to the artery throughout its course, and is encased along with the artery in a thick sheath of connective tissue in the popliteal fossa. The popliteal artery in the fossa is often surrounded by a network of small branches from the popliteal vein, which can make separation of the vessels and exposure of the artery more difficult. The vein then courses superiorly with the artery and enters Hunter's canal at the adductor magnus hiatus. The close relationship of the vein to the artery also makes combined arterial and venous injuries relatively common, and an injury to one should always prompt a thorough search for injury to the other.

The course of the tibial nerve and its relationship to the vessels should always be appreciated, both to identify any associated injury to the nerve and to avoid damage to the nerve during exposure. The nerve begins lateral to the artery and vein above the knee; so it is relatively safe from iatrogenic injury at this point. In the popliteal fossa, the nerve crosses the artery and vein superficially from lateral to medial, making it vulnerable to injury from either the medial or posterior approach. Below the knee, the nerve can be found medial to the artery and should be identified and preserved during a medial approach to the vessels. Other important structures to be appreciated during the vascular exposure are the greater saphenous vein and nerve running superficially along the medial surface of the thigh and the common peroneal nerve coursing through the lateral margin of the popliteal fossa.

63.2 Making the Diagnosis

Any patient with a wound adjacent to or traversing the popliteal fossa should be assumed to have a vascular injury until proven otherwise. You should always approach this workup with the mindset that you need to definitively prove the patient does not have an injury. Fortunately, this is truly one of the few areas left where your physical exam trumps almost any expensive and time-consuming imaging study. Examination of the wounds may give some information about trajectory, but this is never definitive and rarely reliable. You should examine carefully the thigh and popliteal fossa for hematomas, and should perform a good pulse examination including the popliteal, posterior tibial, and dorsalis pedis arteries. Although the presence of strong palpable pedal pulses is highly reliable for ruling out a significant popliteal artery injury, you should always confirm this (for peace of mind and legal documentation) by obtaining an ankle-brachial index with the pressure cuff placed below the suspected level of injury [1, 2]. One of the hardest decisions in trauma, particularly for less experienced surgeons, is making the call to proceed to the operating room without a solid diagnosis. You will much more frequently regret taking a penetrating trauma patient for extensive diagnostic studies than taking them directly to the operating room. Hard signs of a popliteal artery injury should prompt immediate movement to the operating room without undue delay. Soft signs or high clinical suspicion should prompt further evaluation with standard or CT angiography. On-table angiography in the operating room is always a safe and reliable alternative, and should be in the surgical toolbox of all trauma surgeons.

63.3 To the Operating Room

Now that you have passed step one of the "critical triad of success" by making an early and accurate diagnosis, the remaining two steps of the battle are fought and won in the operating room. Emergency vascular surgery is a team sport; so before you start your operation, you should review your capabilities and your operative plan with the anesthesia provider and OR personnel. Table 63.1 lists key factors that should be considered before making the first skin incision. Expect a challenging case with difficult exposure, so you should always call for help earlier rather than later. Unless you are an experienced vascular surgeon, we would recommend bringing an anatomic reference book or chart that details the popliteal anatomy to the operating room. If there is active bleeding from the wound, then a pneumatic tourniquet should be placed immediately on the proximal thigh and inflated to a pressure above the systolic blood pressure. Even in the absence of

Table 63.1 Preoperative checklist for popliteal injuries

Is the patient hemodynamically stable?	Blood products available – how many and what type
Second surgeon or vascular surgeon available	Anesthesia understands the patient status and plan
Vascular instruments and suture	Embolectomy and angiography catheters
Prosthetic vascular grafts	Patient positioning – prone versus supine
Deep self-retaining retractors	Pneumatic tourniquet – sterile if available
Vascular Doppler with sterile probe cover	Heparinized saline and a blunt or "olive" tipped needle
Radiology support for on-table angiography	Orthopedic plan for any fractures – order of repairs

active bleeding, you should always strongly consider placing a sterile pneumatic tourniquet which can be rapidly inflated when there is significant bleeding encountered during the exploration and repair [3].

The vascular approach, exposure, and control in the trauma setting are markedly different from the elective approach. You should not expect nice clean planes of dissection with a dry surgical field and time for leisurely identification of all structures. The anatomy will often be distorted by the wound cavity and foreign debris, particularly with missiles that tumble or fragment. A large hematoma surrounding the vascular injury will often have done some of the dissection and exposure for you, but expect significant combined arterial and venous bleeding if the area of injury is entered prior to obtaining adequate vascular control. The common practice of continually feeling for the arterial pulse may also not be an option if the vessel is transected, thrombosed, or while a proximal tourniquet or clamp is in place. Knowledge of the anatomy becomes even more important in this scenario.

A smooth operation begins with proper patient positioning and the choice of incision. The choice of surgical approach in trauma is always a compromise between optimizing exposure and maintaining options, with the latter often trumping the former. This is clearly evident in popliteal injuries, where the best anatomic exposure of the popliteal structures is obtained via a posterior approach with the patient prone. Although this may be a good option in very select circumstances, it will limit your access to the proximal leg vessels; the contralateral leg for vein harvesting; and the head, neck and trunk for any concomitant procedures. For these reasons the medial approach with the patient supine has become the standard for popliteal exploration in trauma. Both approaches should be understood and will be further detailed and demonstrated.

63.3.1 The Medial Approach

Your standard approach should be the medial approach with the patient positioned supine. The knee should be flexed and supported by pillows and the thigh should be externally rotated as much as possible. Take the time to get the leg as secure as possible in this position so that all hands are free to operate and not having to hold the leg in position. Completely prep and drape both legs and the lower abdomen. Mark an incision starting 1 cm posterior to the medial femoral condyle at the knee, and extend it proximally along the anterior border of the sartorius muscle and distally parallel and 1 cm posterior to the tibia (see Fig. 63.1a). A good rule of thumb is to identify the location of the vascular injury and plan for at least 10 cm of exposure proximally and distally. Leaving a skin bridge across the knee joint may aid in closure and wound healing, but do not sacrifice adequate exposure if needed. The saphenous vein and nerve should be identified in the subcutaneous fat and kept with the posterior flap of the incision. For the above-knee popliteal vessel, divide the superficial fascia longitudinally and then follow the plane between the sartorius and gracilis muscles which should lead directly to the distal superficial femoral artery and above-knee popliteal vessels. The vein will be lateral to the artery at this location. Mobilize the vessels distally into the popliteal fossa (this may require division of the adductor tendon) and note that here the vein changes to a posterior position relative to the artery. For exposure of the below-knee popliteal vessel, retract the medial gastrocnemius posteriorly and then carefully open the deep fascia to expose the vessels. You must be aware that in this position, the vein will be the first structure encountered, with the artery lying lateral to the vein and the tibial nerve posterior to the artery. For more distal exposure of the popliteal and the first bifurcation, divide the soleus muscle from its attachment to the tibia and retract it posteriorly (see Fig. 63.1b) [2, 4].

Have vessel loops readily available to place around the artery and vein, and these can also be used to identify and retract the tibial nerve. Bulldog clamps are often adequate for arterial control, particularly for the

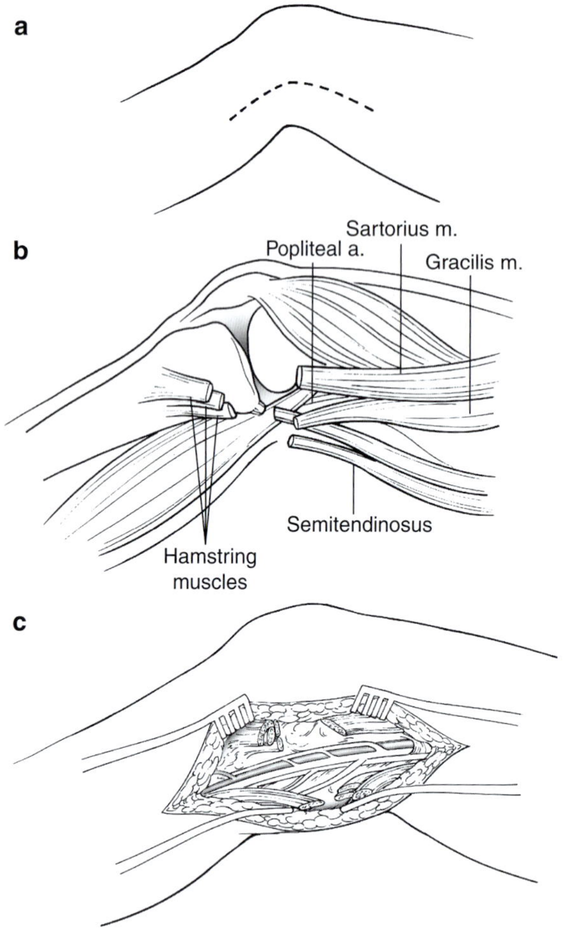

Fig. 63.1 (**a**) Skin incision for the medial approach to the popliteal vessels, patient supine. (**b, c**) Anatomic exposure of the popliteal vessels by the medial approach

distal end of the vessel. Have small and medium clips available as you can expect bleeding from multiple small venous branches. Two self-retaining retractors with deep blades provide excellent hands-free exposure and retraction, and should be placed immediately above and below the knee joint. A dry lap sponge placed into the wound covering the tissue to be retracted can help keep the operative field dry and protect underlying structures from retractor injury.

63.3.2 The Posterior Approach

This approach is much less commonly used in emergency situations for the reasons cited above. However, it does provide superior exposure to the entire popliteal fossa and contents and should be considered as an option for localized wounds in the center of the popliteal fossa. The patient should be placed prone with appropriate padding of the trunk and hips. The opposite leg should also be prepped as saphenous vein can easily be harvested below the knee. You should mark your incision in a "lazy S" pattern beginning 10 cm above the fossa and proceeding longitudinally down the posteromedial thigh. The incision should then cross the posterior knee crease transversely and proceed longitudinally 5–10 cm down the posterolateral calf (see Fig. 63.2a). Skin flaps are then raised superiorly and inferiorly, avoiding injury to the greater saphenous vein (medial) and lesser saphenous vein (lateral). The junction of the lateral and medial gastrocnemius is identified and marks the lower boundary of the popliteal fossa. Retraction of the gastrocs will expose the popliteal fossa, but remember that the most superficial structure will usually be the tibial nerve. The popliteal vein and artery are then easily identified, and division of several small vein branches is usually required to mobilize the artery away from the vein. This approach should allow access to the entire popliteal artery from the adductor canal to the bifurcation of the anterior tibial artery (see Fig. 63.2b) [5].

63.4 Choose Your Arterial Repair Wisely

After gaining adequate exposure and control of hemorrhage, a full exploration should be performed to identify the location and extent of injury. Whenever possible, proximal and distal control should be obtained by exposure of uninjured artery outside the zone of injury and hematoma. Proximal control can also be obtained by a direct cutdown to the femoral artery in the groin or with a pneumatic tourniquet. Similarly, distal control can also be rapidly obtained with a calf tourniquet or with manual compression of the calf by an assistant. Unlike blunt trauma which can result in a wide spectrum of vascular injury, penetrating mechanisms are usually associated with either vessel laceration or complete transection. Occasionally there will be thrombosis of an intact vessel due to local blast effect, but this is uncommon. If the vessel has been completely transected, the ends will usually be retracted and have little to no bleeding due to contraction and clot formation. In contrast, partial lacerations often continue to bleed profusely

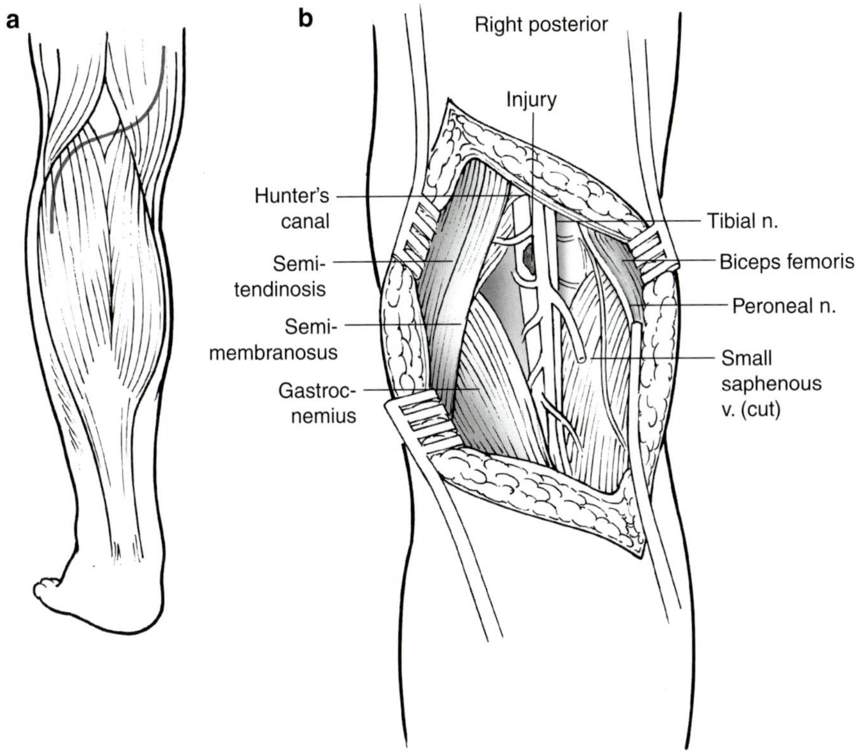

Fig. 63.2 (**a**) Skin incision for the posterior approach, patient prone. (**b**) Anatomic exposure of the popliteal fossa and vessels by the posterior approach

and will require full proximal and distal control. If you cannot identify one or both ends of the transected artery, a useful trick is to make a small arteriotomy on normal proximal or distal artery and pass an embolectomy catheter until it can be seen protruding from the injured vessel.

The type of injury that is identified will determine your options for repair. For small lacerations, a simple running suture repair (lateral or transverse arteriorrhaphy) with 5-0 or 6-0 prolene may be adequate. Care must be taken not to narrow the lumen, and if your repair is going to result in significant stenosis (>25%), then you should choose an alternative method. Most penetrating injuries will not be amenable to this simple method, and will require a more complex repair.

Standard repair options at this point include patch angioplasty with vein or prosthetic, primary end-to-end anastomosis, and placement of a prosthetic or vein bypass graft. Patch angioplasty is an excellent option for a small injury or hole involving <50% of the vessel wall after adequate debridement. All devitalized tissue should be sharply debrided and make sure you inspect the intimal edges for any flaps or tears. A small piece of vein for the patch can usually be found within the incision rather than going to the opposite leg, and larger branches of the saphenous will often suffice. Alternatively, a section of prosthetic material such as a carotid endarterectomy patch can be used. The small patch will be difficult to handle until it is fixed in at least two places, so use two 6-0 prolene sutures to secure the patch to the proximal and distal margin of the arterial defect. The two fixation sutures can then each be run along opposite sides of the defect, taking bites from outside to in on the patch, and inside to out on the vessel wall. You should intermittently flush the operative field and the vessel lumen with heparinized saline throughout the procedure to minimize clot formation. Prior to completing the repair, proximal and distal control should be alternately released to assess inflow and outflow and to flush clot out of the vessel lumen. If there is any question about the adequacy of flow, then one or two careful passes of a fogarty embolectomy catheter proximally and distally should be performed.

In cases of complete or near-complete transection, the vessel ends should be debrided (complete the transection sharply) and mobilized for several centimeters in each direction. To avoid significant retraction when you are completing a near transection, you can place a fixation stitch from normal proximal vessel to normal distal vessel prior to dividing the remainder of the vessel wall. If the vessel ends can be brought together with minimal tension, then a primary end-to-end anastomosis can be performed. This is usually possible with stab wounds, while gunshot wounds most often result in enough vessel loss to require graft placement. The vessel ends should be spatulated with a fresh scalpel blade or fine scissors and a running end-to-end anastomosis performed with 6-0 prolene suture. Simple anterior and posterior fixation sutures between the two ends of the vessel can be placed first, which can then be used to manipulate and roll the anastomosis to maximize exposure and ease of suturing. The more difficult half of the anastomosis (usually the far side) should be done first, followed by the easier half. Alternatively, a three suture triangulating technique for the anastomosis can be performed, equally dividing the anastomosis into three 120° segments. Inflow and outflow should again be assessed prior to completion of the anastomosis, and fogarty catheter embolectomy through the anastomosis performed as needed.

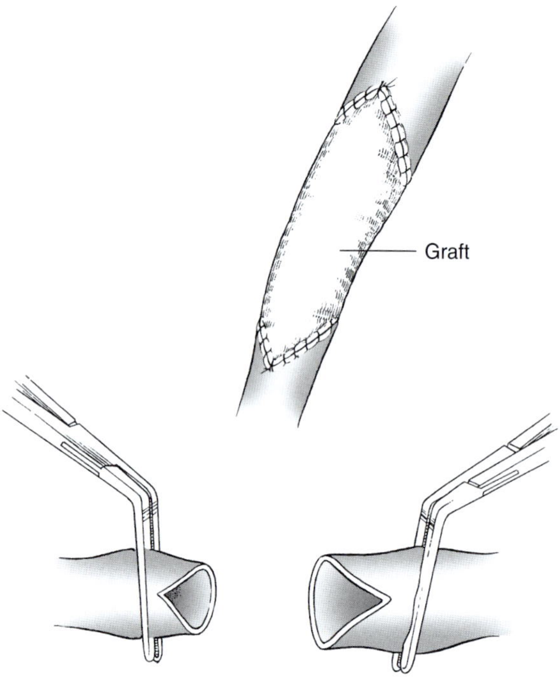

Fig. 63.3 Technique for a saphenous vein or prosthetic interposition graft

The final and most commonly required repair option is replacement or bypass of a segment of the popliteal artery with a vein or prosthetic graft (see Fig. 63.3). Saphenous vein is the preferred conduit, particularly for a repair that crosses the knee joint [6]. Vein should be harvested from the uninjured leg using an anteromedial longitudinal thigh incision. Estimate the length of vein needed and then add an additional 25–50% to ensure adequate final length. Make sure you adequately prepare the vein by reversing the segment to allow flow through the valves, ligating any branches without narrowing the main vessel lumen, and then fully dilating the vein with heparinized saline flush. Stripping the vein of any remaining adventitial bands will allow for greater dilation and better size matching to the injured artery. If adequate length or caliber of vein is not available, then an adequate diameter (usually 6 mm) prosthetic graft can be used. For prosthetic graft that will cross the popliteal fossa, a graft with ring reinforcement may be chosen to avoid kinking with knee flexion.

The bypass graft can most often be placed in the normal anatomic position of the popliteal artery (interposition graft) unless there has been significant tissue loss or contamination. In these situations, you should place the vein or prosthetic graft in a lateral or medial extra-anatomic tunnel to ensure adequate protection and soft-tissue coverage. The length of the interposition graft should always be assessed with the leg near full extension to ensure adequate length, but excess length must be avoided to prevent kinking of redundant vein. There is no absolute rule for the order in which you should perform the anastomoses. The cut ends of the artery and the vein graft or prosthetic should be spatulated as previously described. Due to the usual size mismatch between artery and saphenous vein, the vein graft will often require an additional several millimeter incision at the heel of the spatulation to match the luminal diameter of the artery. The end-to-end anastomoses can be performed with 6-0 prolene as described previously, either using two opposite running sutures or a three suture triangulation technique. When the final anastomosis is near complete, proximal and distal flushing of clot and debris should be performed, as well as fogarty catheter embolectomy if there is inadequate inflow or outflow.

An additional technique that you may find useful in select situations is exclusion and bypass of the injured

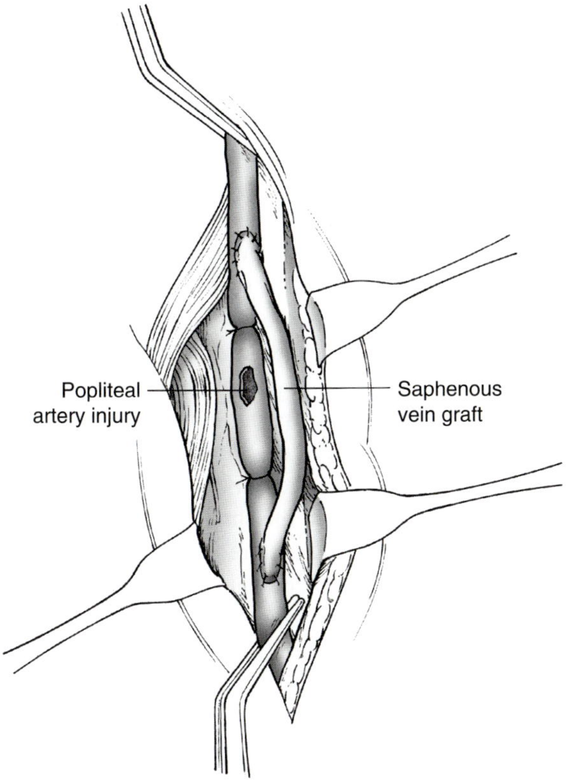

Fig. 63.4 Technique for bypass and exclusion of the popliteal artery injury

segment (see Fig. 63.4). This technique is commonly described for small popliteal aneurysms, but can also be applied in the trauma setting [7]. Rather than diving in to the area of injury, the proximal and distal popliteal artery are mobilized and a vein or prosthetic graft is then placed from the above-knee popliteal artery to the below-knee popliteal artery. Once the bypass graft is in place, the injured segment of artery is then excluded by ligating it above and below the area of injury (see Fig. 63.4).

63.5 Popliteal Vein Injury

Penetrating popliteal vein injuries are less threatening in terms of ischemia and limb loss, but can be as challenging to manage as an arterial injury. Due to the close proximity of the artery and vein, combined injuries are relatively common and remain associated with higher rates of limb loss than any other vascular injury. Unlike pulsatile arterial hemorrhage, bleeding from this large vein is extremely hard to localize and manipulation often results in extension of the injury. Your first priority should be wide exposure of the artery and vein, with direct pressure control of active hemorrhage and control of the artery. Once this is done, control of the venous bleeding is easily done with digital pressure. Bulldog clamps or vessel loops secured around the proximal and distal vein can be used to stop hemorrhage and elevate the vein into the operative field. Another useful technique is to have your assistant use two small sponge sticks to apply direct pressure to the proximal and distal vein, allowing you to visualize and control the area of injury.

In contrast to popliteal artery injuries, the rule for popliteal vein injuries should usually be either a simple repair or ligation [1]. All efforts should be made to maintain some degree of popliteal venous patency, but complex venous repairs in this area should usually be avoided and are associated with a high rate of thrombosis [8]. You can close most lacerations with a running 5-0 or 6-0 prolene suture (lateral venorrhaphy), accepting up to a 50% luminal narrowing. Alternatively, a primary end-to-end anastomosis as described for arterial injuries should be performed for more significant injuries. Although more complex reconstructions have been described for larger injuries with segmental vein loss, they are associated with a high failure rate and no proven benefit over simple ligation. The factors that are critical for you to appreciate are that a popliteal venous injury, even when repaired, will predispose the patient to significant leg swelling, compartment syndrome, and increase the failure rates of an associated arterial repair [9].

63.6 The Post-repair Checklist

As any airline pilot can tell you, a routine or "checklist" approach is the most reliable way to avoid oversights or mistakes, particularly when performing a relatively uncommon task. When your repair has been completed, you should do or at least consider all of the following items. Once flow has been restored, assess the immediate operative field for hemostasis, particularly at the anastomoses. Palpate the proximal and distal vessels in the operative field for a pulse, and then assess the foot for pulses and Doppler signals. Consider performing a completion arteriogram, which can easily be done using a butterfly needle or small catheter in the superficial femoral artery and is best done using fluoroscopy. Any flow limiting problems at the repair or anastomosis should be revised before leaving the operating room. It is not uncommon to have clot accumulate at the repair site or in the distal leg vessels, and this may require catheter embolectomy using a proximal or distal arteriotomy – try to avoid reopening your anastomosis if possible. Ensure adequate coverage of your repair or graft with well-vascularized tissue prior to skin closure. Finally, assess the leg compartments for the need for fasciotomies, and if needed, perform a full four-compartment fasciotomy. Factors that will increase your likelihood of requiring a fasciotomy are longer ischemic times, large resuscitation volumes, systemic shock, associated bony and soft-tissue injury, and the presence of a venous injury. Although fasciotomies can be performed selectively for most arterial injuries, combined popliteal artery and vein injuries should have routine fasciotomies performed.

63.7 Special Situations and Controversies

There currently exists no level 1 or well-controlled data to guide any aspect of the management of popliteal vascular injuries. Although the basic tenets of management are widely agreed upon by most experts, there are multiple finer points or controversial options that remain a matter of opinion. Rather than viewing these as "right or wrong" choices, you should have an appreciation for the heterogeneity of these injuries and when and how to apply some of these techniques.

63.7.1 The Unstable Patient

The first factor that will dictate your operative approach is the hemodynamic and physiologic status of the patient. An unstable patient will not tolerate much additional stress and blood loss, so you should consider this a damage control operation from the start. A proximal tourniquet should be applied immediately to arrest hemorrhage, and direct pressure on the popliteal fossa will control any venous back-bleeding. The historical answer in this scenario has been ligation of the popliteal artery, but this is associated with amputation rates of 75% [10]. If anything more than a simple suture repair of the artery is required, then the best choice is usually placement of an intravascular shunt with a planned return to the operating room when the patient has stabilized [11, 12]. There are multiple commercial shunts available; the simplest of these are the flexible PVC tube shunts routinely used in carotid surgery. Choose the largest shunt that fits the vessel lumen and insert it through the injury proximally and distally. Ensure that the shunt is well secured to the artery by a 3-0 silk suture at the proximal and distal end. More advanced shunts may have inflatable balloons to secure them in the lumen, and often have infusion ports for flushing and administration of heparin. If the popliteal vein is injured, place a shunt in the same manner if it can be done easily and rapidly. Otherwise simply ligate or clip the popliteal vein and get the patient to the Intensive Care Unit for stabilization. In cases of large volume venous hemorrhage and instability, packing or foley balloon tamponade of the popliteal fossa may provide entirely adequate hemorrhage control and delay the need for operative intervention.

63.7.2 Active Hemorrhage

The patient with active hemorrhage presents a significant challenge in both stopping the bleeding and in trying to identify critical structures. A properly inflated proximal tourniquet will provide excellent control of bleeding, but can then make identification of the vessels and nerves more difficult. Bleeding from a deep hole in the popliteal fossa can be tamponaded by insertion of a foley catheter and balloon inflation. Inflate the balloon until bleeding stops, then pull the catheter taut against the skin and clamp it at the skin level with a hemostat. Manual pressure can be applied uniformly to the popliteal fossa using a large kerlex gauze roll placed behind the knee with direct pressure applied or a tight pressure wrap. If the area of injury is inadvertently entered before obtaining proximal and distal control, fogarty balloon catheters can be inserted through the injury or transected end of the vessel and slowly inflated to occlude the vessel.

63.7.3 Associated Fractures

Close coordination with your orthopedic surgeon is required to plan the approach to the injuries and the order of repair. There is ongoing debate about whether the vascular injury should be repaired before or after the fracture, and outcomes with either approach are comparable [13]. If the joint or fracture is unstable, then we favor bony fixation prior to vascular repair to minimize stretch and manipulation of a new vascular graft. A temporary vascular shunt is an excellent option to minimize ischemic time while the fracture is being addressed. If the vascular repair is done first, make sure you fully reassess the status of the repair and distal perfusion after the orthopedic manipulation.

63.7.4 Local Versus Systemic Heparinization

Local flushing of the vessel and any grafts with heparinized saline solution (10 units/mL) should be used liberally. Most traumatic vascular injuries can be safely managed without systemic heparinization, which carries the risk of bleeding from the surgical site and any other wounded area. However, the adverse impact of systemic anticoagulation in the setting of a localized penetrating injury has been largely overstated, and should be considered in high-risk injuries (distal bypass grafts, significant luminal compromise, combined arterial and venous repairs) or if a vigorous clotting response is observed. Trauma patients can be markedly hypercoagulable and if your repair is clotting with no obvious anatomic cause, then administer systemic heparin. You can always transfuse blood and control surgical bleeding, but you cannot heal a dead leg. With the high risk of limb loss associated with popliteal vascular injuries, the use of systemic anticoagulation is safe and may improve limb salvage and functional outcome [14].

63.7.5 Limb Amputation

Amputation is ultimately required in 9% of popliteal vascular injuries, and 38% of combined arterial and venous injuries [9]. Amputation at the first operation is rarely required unless there is an immediate threat to the life of the patient from any attempt at limb salvage. This is usually due to massive reperfusion injury after prolonged (>8h) ischemia, uncontrolled hemorrhage, or non-salvageable bony and nerve injury. In these rare cases, you should perform a rapid guillotine amputation under pneumatic tourniquet control and salvage as much distal skin and muscle as possible [15]. Always attempt to obtain a second expert opinion for these difficult decisions.

63.7.6 Endovascular Techniques in the Popliteal Fossa

No other field of surgery in recent history has undergone such an extensive transformation as vascular surgery due to the advent of endovascular technology and techniques. These methods were developed primarily for the management of aneurismal and atherosclerotic disease but have been successfully extended to traumatic vascular injuries. However, the role of endovascular therapy as the primary modality for penetrating injury to the popliteal vessels remains speculative, and is currently based on case reports and case series mainly from blunt trauma [16]. A good rule of thumb to use is that the more distal the injury, the less of a role there is for current endovascular techniques. This may certainly change and evolve with time and experience. Endovascular techniques are extremely useful for the management of specific injury types, such as arteriovenous fistulae, pseudoaneurysm, or complete thrombosis. In addition, endovascular therapies such as balloon dilation and intravascular stenting can be invaluable in managing post-repair complications such as an anastomotic stenosis [17]. Keep these options in mind as useful adjuncts in the management of challenging popliteal vascular injuries.

Important Points

- Life always takes priority over limb – a prolonged complex vascular reconstruction can result in a perfused limb in a dying patient. Always remember your "damage control" options, particularly at the first operation.
- Call for help and call early – a second pair of experienced hands and eyes can cut hours off of the operative time and mean the difference between limb salvage and limb loss.
- Trust your physical exam – assessment of peripheral pulses is still the best method for detecting a SIGNIFICANT peripheral vascular injury. Check an ABI to document a number that backs up your physical exam.
- Know your anatomy! Review an anatomy text or chart immediately prior to surgery, and bring it with you to the operating room.
- Do not enter the wound cavity until you have proximal control and your operative team is ready – there will always be more bleeding than expected.
- A pneumatic tourniquet provides excellent control of bleeding, but finding the contracted and pulseless artery will be challenging, so see point #4.
- The price of failure is limb loss, so pay attention to detail in handling both the artery and the vein.
- Intravascular shunting can be an excellent option to reduce intraoperative ischemic time or as a damage control maneuver.
- If the patient is unstable, it should be a planned damage control operation from the start. Do not wait until the patient is cold, acidotic, and coagulopathic to switch to a damage control mindset.
- Fasciotomies can be performed selectively, but should be the rule if you have a combined arterial and venous injury.

References

1. Frykberg ER (2002) Popliteal vascular injuries. Surg Clin North Am 82(1):67–89
2. Weaver FA, Papanicolaou G, Yellin AE (1996) Difficult peripheral vascular injuries. Surg Clin North Am 76(4): 843–859
3. Fox CJ, Gillespie DL, O'Donnell SD et al (2005) Contemporary management of wartime vascular trauma. J Vasc Surg 41(4):638–644
4. Hoyt DB, Coimbra R, Potenza BM, Rappold JF (2001) Anatomic exposures for vascular injuries. Surg Clin North Am 81(6):1299–1330, xii
5. Kropman RH, van Santvoort HC, Teijink J et al (2007) The medial versus the posterior approach in the repair of popliteal artery aneurysms: a multicenter case-matched study. J Vasc Surg 46(1):24–30
6. Dorweiler B, Neufang A, Schmiedt W et al (2003) Limb trauma with arterial injury: long-term performance of venous interposition grafts. Thorac Cardiovasc Surg 51(2):67–72
7. Scott BG, Hirshberg A (2004) Exclusion and bypass – a new approach to popliteal artery injuries. J Trauma 57(4):913–914
8. Bermudez KM, Knudson MM, Nelken NA, Shackleford S, Dean CL (1997) Long-term results of lower-extremity venous injuries. Arch Surg 132(9):963–967; discussion 967–968
9. Mullenix PS, Steele SR, Andersen CA, Starnes BW, Salim A, Martin MJ (2006) Limb salvage and outcomes among patients with traumatic popliteal vascular injury: an analysis of the National Trauma Data Bank. J Vasc Surg 44(1):94–100
10. Debakey ME, Simeone FA (1946) Battle injuries of the arteries in World War II: an analysis of 2,471 cases. Ann Surg 123(4):534–579
11. Hossny A (2004) Blunt popliteal artery injury with complete lower limb ischemia: is routine use of temporary intraluminal arterial shunt justified? J Vasc Surg 40(1):61–66
12. Subramanian A, Vercruysse G, Dente C, Wyrzykowski A, King E, Feliciano DV (2008) A decade's experience with temporary intravascular shunts at a civilian level I trauma center. J Trauma 65(2):316–324; discussion 324–316
13. Weaver FA, Rosenthal RE, Waterhouse G, Adkins RB (1984) Combined skeletal and vascular injuries of the lower extremities. Am Surg 50(4):189–197
14. Melton SM, Croce MA, Patton JH Jr et al (1997) Popliteal artery trauma. Systemic anticoagulation and intraoperative thrombolysis improves limb salvage. Ann Surg 225(5):518–527; discussion 527–519
15. Starnes BW, Beekley AC, Sebesta JA, Andersen CA, Rush RM Jr (2006) Extremity vascular injuries on the battlefield: tips for surgeons deploying to war. J Trauma 60(2):432–442
16. Onal B, Ilgit ET, Kosar S, Akkan K, Gumus T, Akpek S (2005) Endovascular treatment of peripheral vascular lesions with stent-grafts. Diagn Interv Radiol 11(3):170–174
17. Criado E, Marston WA, Ligush J, Mauro MA, Keagy BA (1997) Endovascular repair of peripheral aneurysms, pseudoaneurysms, and arteriovenous fistulas. Ann Vasc Surg 11(3):256–263

Part VII
Other Topics

Burns and Inhalational Injury

64

Jennifer Lang and Herb A. Phelan

Burns are one of the most feared and misunderstood traumatic injuries. They are a breed of trauma in which a patient can come in talking and yet succumb to their injuries within 24–48 h if the physician is not diligent. This chapter is meant to provide a guidebook for those who do not treat burns every day. It is for the physician who finds himself or herself in over their head and having to take care of a severely burned patient for the first several days following injury. We will tell you how to stabilize and resuscitate your patient, initiate wound care, and initially treat inhalational injuries so that your patient can be delivered to a burn center with the best possible chance of an excellent outcome.

There are 500,000 burns resulting in 40,000 admissions and 4,000 deaths each year in this country [1]. Fire or flame burns are generally what comes to mind when someone imagines a burned patient. While this is the most common type of burn in adults, do not forget there are several others such as contact, scald, radiation, and electrical and chemical burns. The American Burn Association has developed standard criteria for who can be treated in a community setting and who must be transferred to a specialized burn center (Table 64.1). But what do you do if your area has been the site of a mass casualty event and the regional burn center is over capacity, or weather prohibits any outgoing travel? What do you do if you cannot transfer your patient? How do you care for a patient with an injury you have little to no experience in treating? The following will get you and your patient through the next few frightening days.

Table 64.1 Burn center criteria

• Partial-thickness burn >10%
• Any full-thickness burn
• Burns to face/hands/feet/joints/genitalia/perineum
• Electrical or chemical burns
• Inhalational injury
• Associated trauma
• Significant comorbidities

64.1 Initial Management of the Burned Patient: The Emergency Room

The initial measures in burn care are identical to any trauma situation. Begin by following the ABCs of trauma, which start with airway. Does your patient need to be intubated? As with any trauma patient, someone with a decreased GCS, significant airway trauma, an inability to protect their airway, or respiratory distress with impending respiratory failure warrants intubation. Unfortunately, this algorithm gets a whole lot more complicated when you add in a burn. There are three main reasons why a burn patient may need to be intubated that are in addition to those for

J. Lang
Department of Surgery,
University of Texas Southwestern Medical Center, 5323 Harry Hines Blvd. E5.508A, Dallas, TX 75390-9158, USA
e-mail: jennifer.lang@utsouthwestern.edu

H.A. Phelan (✉)
Division of Burns/Trauma/Critical Care,
Department of Surgery,
University of Texas-Southwestern Medical Center, 5323 Harry Hines Blvd, E5.508A, Dallas, TX 75390-9158, USA
e-mail: herb.phelan@utsouthwestern.edu

G.C. Velmahos et al. (eds.), *Penetrating Trauma*,
DOI 10.1007/978-3-642-20453-1_64, © Springer-Verlag Berlin Heidelberg 2012

any other trauma. The first is swelling and constriction from extensive facial and neck burns. A deep circumferential neck burn is a significant management issue, especially if the patient will require a formal fluid resuscitation. As you resuscitate these patients, the resulting airway edema can compromise their airway. The second is again related to edema and pulmonary compromise. Patients with large burns >40–50% total body surface area (TBSA) require a great deal of intravenous fluid resuscitation. If not electively intubated early, i.e., prior to beginning resuscitation, one can find oneself struggling to intubate a patient who is now in distress with a "difficult" airway due to the edema that comes along with a burn resuscitation. The third is inhalational injury with subsequent pulmonary insufficiency. The mere act of inhaling smoke does not translate into an inhalational injury. Likewise, the presence of singed facial hair and oral soot, while worrisome, do not mandate emergent intubation. However, these findings combined with "hard signs" such as dyspnea, increased work of breathing, stridor, or a feeling of chest tightness indicate a need for immediate airway control [2]. Inhalational injury will be discussed later on at length; suffice it to say for now that the initial management indications for intubation are basically the same as for any trauma patient. If your patient appears to be having symptoms of impending respiratory failure, do not hesitate to intubate them.

OK, now you have made it past one of the most difficult decisions in initial burn care. We will at this point assume that we are dealing with an isolated burn. What comes after the completion of the ABCs? Place the patient on a sterile sheet. Establish two large-bore peripheral IVs preferably through non-burned skin, but if necessary, there is nothing wrong with using a burned extremity. If you choose to do so, however, make sure you suture in the IV! Send some basic labs, and if your patient was trapped indoors, add a carboxyhemoglobin level. Begin warming the patient by placing warm blankets and turn up the temperature in the room to about 90°F. Spend a couple of minutes talking to the paramedics or family members present. Record the time of burn as this will be important later. Ask some questions about the circumstances, particularly if this occurred in a confined space. Find out if the patient is a smoker or has other pulmonary or medical problems. If the patient is a child, ask specific questions about what happened and document what is said.

Now determine the burn size. We cannot emphasize the importance of this step enough. Forget the rule of nines! This is a great way to approach burns in the field, during triage, or perhaps in a hotel room, but a horrible way to start a resuscitation as the rule of nines is notoriously inaccurate. The total body surface area (TBSA) is your starting point for treatment and both underestimation or overestimation can be detrimental. Use specific burn charts such as the chart included at the end of this chapter (Fig. 64.1). How do you tell the depth of a burn based on physical appearance? First-degree burns look like a sunburn. They are red, dry, and painful. Do not count these burns in your percentages! Only second-, third-, and fourth-degree burns count toward TBSA. Second-degree burns are also red and painful but appear blistered or wet. They have a Nikolsky sign which is elicited by rubbing the burn and seeing the outer epidermis peel away. Do not be afraid to touch the burn because knowing the difference between first and second degree is of critical importance. Second-degree burns can be divided into superficial or deep partial-thickness burns. Superficial burns will typically heal in <3 weeks. Deep partial-thickness burns will result in significant scarring if allowed to heal spontaneously. Third-degree, or full-thickness, burns have penetrated through to the level of the nerve endings which are themselves injured which can sometimes result in an insensate burn. When you touch this burn, you will feel that it is hard and leathery, and it will appear deep red, pale pink, or white. Finally, a fourth-degree burn extends past the skin and into the fat and musculature underneath. The burn is hard, insensate, and white/brown. You can sometimes see outlines of thrombosed cutaneous vessels underneath the burn. Do not forget that burned skin does not burn equally throughout. There will be areas of third degree mixed with first and second.

Once you have your burn percentage, you are ready to make some big decisions. Burns that are larger than 20% TBSA for adults or larger than 10% TBSA in children or the elderly need a formal fluid resuscitation. If your patient falls into this category, place a foley catheter and, if intubated, an orogastric tube (OGT). There are several formulae used to estimate resuscitation needs but the one used most frequently and the one we recommend is the Parkland formula. The Parkland formula estimates that a person will need 4 cc/kg/% second- and third-degree burn in the first 24 h post burn (4 cc/kg/%TBSA). This is given as lactated ringer's solution with half given over 8 h and the other half over the next 16 h. Note how much fluid was given prior to your starting point beginning from the

DALLAS COUNTY HOSPITAL DISTRICT
Dallas, Texas

BURN RECORD

To be completd upon admission:

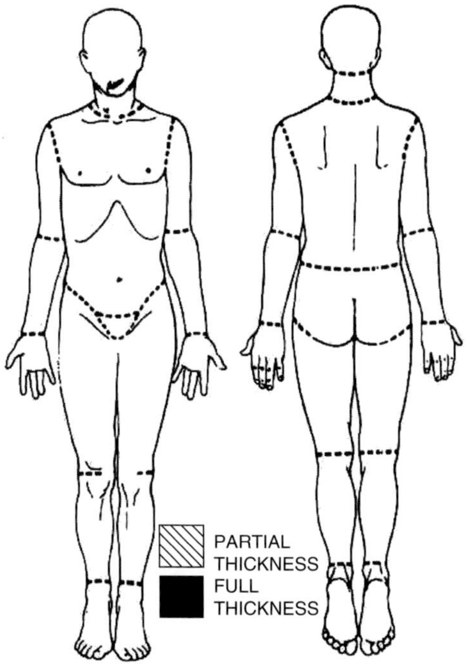

Date: ____________

Height: ____________ Weight: ____________

2° ________ +3° ________ = ________ %

Percent Surface Area Burned
(Berkow Formula)

AREA	1 YR.	1–4 YRS.	5–9 YRS.	10–14 YRS.	15 YRS.	ADULT	2°	3°
Head	19	17	13	11	9	7		
Neck	2	2	2	2	2	2		
Ant. Trunk	13	13	13	13	13	13		
Post. Trunk	13	13	13	13	13	13		
R. Buttock	2½	2½	2½	2½	2½	2½		
L. Buttock	2½	2½	2½	2½	2½	2½		
Genitalia	1	1	1	1	1	1		
R.U. Arm	4	4	4	4	4	4		
L.U. Arm	4	4	4	4	4	4		
R.L. Arm	3	3	3	3	3	3		
L.L. Arm	3	3	3	3	3	3		
R. Hand	2½	2½	2½	2½	2½	2½		
L. Hand	2½	2½	2½	2½	2½	2½		
R. Thigh	5½	6½	8	8½	9	9½		
L. Thigh	5½	6½	8	8½	9	9½		
R. Leg	5	5	5½	6	6½	7		
L. Leg	5	5	5½	6	6½	7		
R. Foot	3½	3½	3½	3½	3½	3½		
L. Foot	3½	3½	3½	3½	3½	3½		
TOTAL								

034

PS 352 7/91

Reprinted with permission of Parkland Health and Hospital Systems

Fig. 64.1 Burns chart

time of burn. Your patient may already be behind the curve or ahead of it depending on how much fluid they have received before getting to you. This will influence your resuscitation. Calculate the rate of IVFs based on burn size and start your resuscitation at that rate. When calculating fluid resuscitation needs, remember that the 8 and 16 h times are from TIME OF BURN and not from the time you start your resuscitation. For example, a 70-kg young male comes in with second- and third-degree burns totalling 60% TBSA burn and has already received 2 L of fluid in the field with a burn time of 2 h prior to arrival.

$$4\text{cc} \times 70\text{kg} \times 60 = 16{,}800\text{cc total resuscitation}$$
$$16{,}800\text{cc} / 2 = 8{,}400\text{cc}$$
$$8{,}400\text{cc} / 6\text{hrs (2hours have already passed)}$$
$$= 1{,}400\text{cc LR} / \text{hr}$$
$$8{,}400\text{cc} / 16 = 525\text{cc}$$

Start your fluid rate at 1,400 cc/h for the next 6 h with the plan being to drop that down to 525 cc/h for the following 16 h. Looking at this fluid amount of 16 L should make the point about intubating large burns a little more clear. If you are caring for a burned patient outside of a specialized center, you should carry out all formal resuscitations in an intensive care unit. The less time spent in the emergency room the better. Quickly get your patient to a more controlled setting where temperature, vital signs, and urine output can be more methodically measured.

64.2 Wound Care and Pain Control

Your patient is now in the ICU. What next? Weigh the patient as soon as possible and go back and recalculate your fluid needs if necessary. Warm the room to 90°F. Wound debridement is one of the first things done after getting to the ICU. Make sure the room has fully warmed and then take a plastic basin with tap water and pour a small bottle of chlorhexidine soap into the water (about 4 oz should be fine). Using gauze pads, begin to wash the patient, debriding away the dead skin in the process. You are basically peeling off the burned blisters. Once fully debrided, apply silvadene cream generously to the wound. Silvadene is a good broad-spectrum antimicrobial, and it will provide some pain relief as burns exposed to air are very painful. If dealing with facial burns, use bacitracin instead of silvadene. Wrap the burns with fine mesh gauze and then a gauze kling wrap to hold it in place. Burns change over time. Go back and revise your diagram after debridement. Things you thought were deep may now appear more superficial. Likewise, burns that initially appeared as second or first degree may evolve into something worse. Revise your numbers if you find that the burn was bigger than you first estimated. Perform these dressing changes twice daily taking care to wash all silvadene off each time so that the actual wound gets cleaned and you do not end up just layering new silvadene on top of old.

Pain control is something that the patient will need starting in the field. Burned patients require enormous amounts of narcotics that most physicians are uncomfortable in giving. Burns are exceedingly painful, and in order to adequately treat them you must step out of your comfort zone. For initial debridement in the non-intubated patient, we generally will use morphine 5 mg IV with repeat dosing in 15 min. You may repeat this multiple times if necessary. Additionally, lorazepam 1 mg IV is used for the initial debridement and then oral lorazepam is given as a 1-mg dose for subsequent dressing changes. The initial dressing change is generally the most painful, but your patient may still require the same morphine dosages for the next few dressing changes. Begin morphine by patient controlled anesthesia (PCA) right away with a setting of 2 mg IV every 6 min with a 40 mg lockout. You may need to bolus more on top of this for breakthrough pain. Remember to watch for signs of narcotic overdose, such as decreased respiratory rate or inability to wake up promptly, and treat accordingly. The intubated patient is much less stressful for the provider. Instead of a PCA, they should be on a narcotic and sedative protocol but will need an additional bolus for dressing changes as well. We recommend the same morphine dosing as the non-intubated patient, but instead of lorazepam we typically use midazolam 5 mg IV.

Elderly patients are a bit different and are much more sensitive to narcotics and benzodiazepines. Therefore, do not use lorazepam or midazolam in a non-intubated elderly patient. Instead of morphine, use hydromorphone with a PCA setting of 0.15 mg every 6 min with a 1 mg 1 h lockout. Dressing changes can be pre-medicated with 1–2 mg of oral hydromorphone.

The principles of early burn excision and grafting are important for reducing burn sepsis and should be a factor in your mind. While definitive burn management is beyond the scope of this chapter, ideally the burn should be excised and grafting begun within the first 3–5 days. Continue to work on getting your patient to a burn surgeon who is better prepared to offer definitive treatment.

64.3 Escharotomies

Particularly concerning is the deep circumferential burn. An eschar has lost all elasticity and once underlying edema from fluid resuscitation sets in, it acts as a tourniquet putting the burned extremity in jeopardy. Careful monitoring for pulse changes with decreasing Doppler signal is important to identify an at-risk extremity. In addition, circumferential burns of the chest can constrict chest wall movements making ventilation more difficult and causing a rise in airway pressures. Escharotomies can be performed at the bedside if your patient is intubated and can be adequately sedated. If not, it may be better to do in the operating room where general anesthesia can be delivered.

64.3.1 Chest

To perform an escharotomy of the chest, use electrocautery to incise the eschar along the anterior axillary line from axilla to the costal margin. Connect the two lines by following along the costal margin and then connect the upper portion with a straight infraclavicular line. If this is still not enough to release tension and decrease airway pressures, you can connect your lateral two lines with multiple transverse incisions and even place more vertical incisions creating a checkerboard appearance. The key is to release the eschar. You will know when that happens because you can actually see the eschar physically spread apart when you reach the subcutaneous fat. It is important with all escharotomies not to incise through non-burned skin!

64.3.2 Lower Extremity

Make sure the patient is in the supine position. Incise the eschar in the midaxial plane both laterally and medially. The incision should extend from the uppermost aspect of the circumferential burn to just above the ankles.

64.3.3 Upper Extremity

Similarly to the lower extremities, the eschar on the arms is incised in the midaxial plane. For the arms, it is important to keep them in the anatomic position as they have a tendency to rotate inward.

64.4 Pulmonary Function

If you have decided not to intubate while in the emergency room, you must continue to reevaluate that decision throughout the resuscitation. Continue to use the criteria that guided your decision previously. Specifically, monitor the patient for signs of respiratory distress and increasing edema (both generalized and localized to the face and neck). Remember that it is always better to err on the side of caution than to struggle later. In patients with circumferential chest burns, the burn can constrict the movements of the chest wall. These patients are usually intubated and you will see rising peak airway pressures and a generalized difficulty ventilating them. Perform escharotomies of the chest as previously described.

If your patient is intubated, you must consider extubation criteria on a daily basis. Use the same criteria you would use to make this decision in any critical care patient. Do they have a cuff leak? Has the resuscitation tapered off? How edematous are they? What is their pulmonary status? Perform spontaneous breathing trials daily and liberate them from the ventilator when they meet extubation criteria.

64.5 When Does the Resuscitation End?

A burn resuscitation typically lasts about 24 h. Burns over 30–35%TBSA cause a release of inflammatory mediators which create systemic vasodilatation leading to capillary leak and extravascular edema with resultant intravascular hypovolemia [3]. This typically lasts for 12–18 h and is the reason why your patient is requiring enormous amounts of fluids. Both underresuscitation and overresuscitation are associated with worsened outcomes. In patients not given enough fluid, their course is complicated by renal failure, progressive organ dysfunction, and death. On the other hand, overshooting the goal will lead to excessive peripheral edema, pulmonary edema, multiorgan failure, and abdominal compartment syndrome [3].

The Parkland formula is an extremely important tool in trying to figure out how much fluid your patient will need. But just as important as its use is the willingness to modify it when necessary. Your patient did not get burned in Charlie Baxter's lab nor did they read what their requirements should be prior to this injury. Every patient is different and they will tell you what they need. You must be prepared to change your resuscitation rates based on their response. At this point, you are monitoring urine output with a foley catheter and recording output every half hour. The goal is 30–50 cc/h of urine output, no more and no less. When you make adjustments to your fluid rate do so in a smooth manner. Do not bolus patients unless you are doing so for hypotension. Instead, if they have made only 15 cc/h, then increase their rate for the next hour. Once you are a few hours into the resuscitation, you can go to hourly urine recordings if they have been making adequate urine.

For the first 24 h, continue to use lactated ringers solution as your resuscitative fluid of choice. Burned patients' sodium levels will decrease and you must be vigilant of hyponatremia in order to avoid complications such as cerebral edema and seizures. After the first 24 h, you should switch to normal saline. Do not use hypertonic saline as the resuscitative fluid since it has been shown to increase rates of renal failure and death [4].

There are situations in which you can be fooled by the urine output. If the patient has intrinsic renal or cardiac disease, urine output will not reflect their intravascular volume status. Hyperglycemia with concurrent glucosuria will cause an osmotic diuresis which will mislead you when trying to interpret the patient's intravascular fluid status. In some of these patients, more invasive monitoring such as central venous pressure monitoring or even pulmonary artery catheters may be needed. A clue to the fact that something else may be going on is if your patient's resuscitative needs are in excess of 150% of predicted [3].

Along the way you may find that the actual amount of fluid the patient requires far exceeds the amount you calculated based on TBSA. There can be several causes for increased resuscitation requirements. Inhalational injuries, electrical burns, deep muscle injury, and delayed resuscitation all increase the amount of fluid required to maintain intravascular volume. By this time you probably know if your patient has an inhalational injury, electrical burn, or if their resuscitation was delayed. But do they have muscular necrosis that you are missing? Beware of circumferential burns. If a patient has a circumferential burn to an extremity, examine the limb for "tightness," pain on passive motion, paresthesias, decreased capillary refill, and decreased pulses or loss of Doppler signal on an hourly basis. The need for escharotomies or even fasciotomies is a clinical decision and must be made early; however, do not mistake early for prophylactic as there is no role for prophylactic escharotomies.

The formal resuscitation typically lasts about 24 h. Fluid requirements can still remain supranormal following this time frame and again the amount of fluid given depends on urine output. There has been much debate about the use of colloid in resuscitative fluids both in burns and critical care. It is not thought to be useful and in fact can be harmful in the first 24 h due to capillary leak. However, in a difficult resuscitation, we will use colloids during the first day if necessary. After the initial 24 h, give 0.1 mL/kg/%burn as 5% albumin solution and then return to a crystalloid solution for maintenance fluids. Change to a dextrose-based fluid such as D5 half NS or D5NS based on individual patient needs. What has their glucose been? Are they on an insulin drip? What is the sodium trend? Are they hyper- or hyponatremic? Give the patient the type and amount of fluid that they are telling you they need. Tailor the amount of IVFs to the urine output keeping the same goal of 0.5 cc/kg/h.

64.6 Altered Hemodynamics

While you are closely monitoring your patient in the ICU, several things will become apparent. They are hemodynamically different from other ICU patients. Cardiac output in a burned patient is initially decreased and then will increase to supranormal levels. This is due to an initial decrease in intravascular volume, increased peripheral resistance, and increased cardiac contractility, all of which lead to decreased cardiac output [3, 5]. Later, a generalized hypermetabolic state will increase cardiac output. All burn patients are tachycardic and this is due to multiple factors including a normal response to the burn injury, pain, and a hypermetabolic response with an increased catecholamine release.

Increased catecholamines, cortisol, and glucagon lead to increased energy expenditure and catabolism with resultant loss of body weight, delayed wound healing, immunosuppression, and a generalized hyperdynamic cardiovascular response. With a burn that has a TBSA >60%, cardiac output and energy expenditure actually double along with increases in protein catabolism, gluconeogenesis, and thermogenesis [6]. The hypermetabolic response can last up to a year after burn, and a negative nitrogen balance can be seen for 6–9 months [6].

Burned skin loses its ability to retain heat. You know this and have already turned up the temperature in the room. But why are your patient's temperature recordings consistently febrile? Burned patients have increased core body temperatures after the first day. Their skin no longer functions as an adequate temperature insulator and the body attempts to compensate for these losses by resetting the hypothalamus to a higher setting. Temperatures of burned patients are about 2°C greater than normal [6]. Fever in a burn victim is 39.0 and not the typical 38.5.

Despite all of these hemodynamic changes occurring in your patient, one thing remains paramount: You must maintain an adequate blood pressure in order to keep your patient from going into shock from their injury. Decreased cardiac output, hypovolemia, and high narcotic use, all contribute to decreased mean arterial pressure. While you are watching the urine output, glance at the mean arterial pressure regularly as well. If you find your patient is hypotensive, it is entirely appropriate to deviate from the "smooth" fluid tailoring and give a fluid bolus to increase blood pressure to normal.

64.7 Nutrition

Nutrition is a critical part of burn survival. Burned patients need more nutrition in order to heal their wounds and their hypermetabolic nature demands caloric amounts greater than the non-burn patient. Feeding your patient earlier rather than later can actually help to decrease this hypermetabolic response [6]. If your patient is intubated, start tube feeds within 6 h of getting to the ICU. If they are not intubated, you will need to actively measure caloric intake and be prepared to place a small bore feeding tube to supplement their intake if necessary.

Table 64.2 Nutritional requirements by patient age

0–1 year	2,100 kcal/m^2 TBSA/day + 1,000 kcal/m^2 TBSA/day
1–11 years	1,800 kcal/m^2 TBSA/day + 1,300 kcal/m^2 TBSA/day
12–16 years	1,500 kcal/m^2 TBSA/day + 1,500 kcal/m^2 TBSA/day
16–60 years	25 kcal/kg/day + 40 kcal/%burn/day
>60 years	25 kcal/kg/day + 65 kcal/%burn/day

Enteral feeding is preferred over parental because of its immunologic benefits. Use high carbohydrate and high protein tube feeds (3% fat, 82% carbohydrate, and 15% protein) [6]. If your patient is not tolerating enteral feeding or has a prolonged ileus, then use parenteral nutrition. We typically measure gastric residuals every 4 h and will hold tube feeding if they are >400 cc. When checking for residuals, make sure to refeed the residuals to the patient so that you do not discard calories (see Table 64.2 for exact caloric requirements). Do not forget that the volume delivered is also part of the resuscitative fluids [3]. Increased protein turnover leads to negative nitrogen balance, and adults need 1.5–2 g/kg/day for burns less than TBSA 20% and 2–2.5 g/kg/day for TBSA >20% TBSA. Use additional protein packets if necessary [6].

Burn patients are on large amounts of narcotics and you must watch for an ileus and stimulate bowel movements. Every patient should be on an aggressive bowel regimen which generally includes colace 100 mg po bid, senna two tabs at night, and then daily dulcolax suppositories if necessary. Prune juice 60 cc TID can also be helpful.

64.8 Other Critical Care Issues

In addition to measures that are specific to the burned patient, there are multiple critical care issues that you need to keep in mind. DVT prophylaxis should begin promptly. We recommend enoxaparin 40 mg SQ bid unless there is evidence of renal insufficiency in which case we use enoxaparin only once daily. Sequential compression devices should also be used in all patients.

Burned patients are at a higher risk for stress ulceration and should all be on GI prophylaxis. For most patients, you can use H_2 blockers such as ranitidine 150 mg po bid. If the patient has a history of prior gastrointestinal (GI) bleed or is on a proton pump inhibitor (PPI) at home, then you should use a PPI as their inpatient GI prophylaxis. Prevention of ventilator associated pneumonia (VAP) is always in the forefront of the mind of every physician who practices critical care. We have no other specific recommendations apart from the generally accepted guidelines for prevention of VAP.

64.9 Inhalational Injury

How do you diagnose an inhalational injury? As previously discussed, a history of being trapped in a confined space, singed facial hair, and carbonaceous sputum are signs that an inhalational injury may have occurred but are not pathognomonic. The actual injury is not due to a "burn" of the lungs because thermal energy is dispersed in the upper airways. The inciting factor is actually inhaled toxins and chemicals which injure type II pneumocytes. This leads to atelectasis, destruction of ciliated epithelial cells, mucosal sloughing, and fibrin cast formation with subsequent obstruction. Following this, there is a significant pulmonary capillary leak leading to ARDS. Irritation of the airways can also cause bronchospasm [2]. This combination of small airway obstruction, edema, and bronchospasm leads to respiratory insufficiency following inhalational injury.

Earlier we recommended checking a carboxyhemoglobin level from the ER. Carbon monoxide poisoning is a lethal component of inhalational injury. Carboxyhemoglobin levels can be 10% in smokers but should be <5% in nonsmokers. Does your patient have an elevated level and an acidosis on their arterial blood gas? If the carboxyhemoglobin level is elevated and your patient has not warranted intubation as of yet, then begin to treat them with 100% oxygen via a non-rebreather mask and some good pulmonary toilet. This will shorten the half-life of carbon monoxide to 40 min. Continue this treatment until their acidosis resolves as evidenced by a bicarbonate level >20 and a normalizing lactate [2].

A patient in whom you have suspicion for inhalational injury AND who is showing signs of respiratory compromise warrants fiberoptic bronchoscopy. Bronchoscopy is the gold standard for diagnosing inhalational injury. What you are looking for is erythema, edema, erosions and ulcerations of the airway, sloughing of mucosa, and carbonaceous material in the lower airways. Be aware that you can see some of these findings in a patient with chronic bronchitis leading to a false-positive diagnosis. On the other hand, if done too early following injury, or your patient is underresuscitated, you may see no abnormalities. It takes some amount of time to develop the findings you are looking for; so if you have a high suspicion but initial bronchoscopy is negative, repeat the endoscopy [7]. Excellent pulmonary toilet is the cornerstone of care for the inhalational injury; however, be aware that aggressive suctioning can create suction catheter artifact.

Once you have diagnosed an inhalational injury, your next concern should be how to treat it. Most of these patients will be intubated if the injury is severe. The respiratory therapists are an integral part of the therapy you will provide. Ask them to perform percussive respiratory treatments, frequent suctioning, and an aggressive pulmonary toilet.

There is no great treatment for inhalational injury and most of what you do will be to support pulmonary function until your patient can recover. Use lung protective ventilation strategies such as a volume control ventilation with a tidal volume of 6 cc/kg ideal body weight. Should you find the peak pressures exceeding 40 cm H_2O, switch to pressure control ventilation with a setting not to exceed 35 cm H_2O. If you are struggling to oxygenate your patient, we recommend high-frequency percussive ventilation (HFPV) as a rescue ventilator mode. HFPV may help decrease pneumonia rates and improve mortality by improving secretion clearance and decreasing alveolar collapse [8]. One retrospective review out of the burn unit at Fort Sam Houston showed that patients treated with HFPV had decreased mortality in bronchoscopically proven inhalational injury when compared to expected death rates [8]. A retrospective review from our own institution looked at 92 patients treated with HFPV as compared with 130 patients treated with conventional mechanical and found a significant survival benefit to HFPV. Interestingly, when subgroups were individually analyzed, this survival benefit was only significant for patients with TBSA <40% [9]. HFPV is only recommended if you have a familiarity with advanced ventilator management.

As far as pharmaceutical treatments for inhalational injury, the majority of treatment consists of pulmonary toilet. For significant inhalational injury, we recommend 5,000 units heparin with 3 cc of 20% *N*-acetylcystine aerosolized with albuterol given every 4 h (HAM therapy). There are mixed opinions in the literature regarding the effectiveness of HAM therapy. One study by Desai et al involving solely pediatric patients found a decrease in reintubation and mortality with the use of HAM [10]. Other studies including children and adults found no benefit. One retrospective review out of the University of Utah Health Sciences Center looked at 150 patients with inhalational injury treated between 1999 and 2005. Sixty-two patients were treated with HAM therapy and 88 patients were not. There were no significant differences found in mortality, length of stay, ventilator days, nor pneumonia rates between the two groups [11]. Do not use steroids for inhalational injury as they offer no additional benefit and have been widely abandoned [2].

64.10 Children

A young child's outcome following a large burn is affected more by the care they receive in the hospital rather than the initial circumstances of the burn. Complicating this is the fact that they have a higher mortality than their adult counterparts and have a whole set of special conditions that make their care more difficult [12]. A child younger than 2 years of age may need dextrose during the resuscitation because of decreased glycogen stores. We recommend using two fluids during resuscitation: a dextrose-based lactated ringer's fluid for maintenance and lactated ringer's for resuscitation fluids. If you are providing tube feeds, then this can serve as your source of glucose. In a child, your urine output goal is higher (1 cc/kg/h). It is also harder to regulate body temperature for children; so make sure and keep the room warm! Children have different body surface area ratios and thus different percentages based on body part burned. The aforementioned charting system for burned patients has columns for children which will account for this difference from adults. A child's nutritional needs are also different (see Table 64.2) as they require 1.5–3 g/kg of protein each day. If your facility has a child life professional, get them involved early to assist with their emotional needs as well as practical concerns regarding schooling and assisting the family.

Finally, we must discuss child abuse. The most important implication of missing a case of child abuse is the potential for continued and escalating harm if the child is returned to the care of the abuser. This is not an easy determination and false accusations can be emotionally detrimental to all involved. The key is to recognize patterns of injury. A "glove and stocking injury" is a symmetric scald-burn of the hands and/or feet, and is highly suspicious. Pay attention to isolated buttock scald burns or contact burns on an infant as they are concerning for a baby who is being placed on a hot surface or into scalding water while being held by his or her arms/legs. Scalds to lower extremities and buttocks are suspicious as children who can crawl out of a hot bathtub generally do. Are they being held there? Was a child who cannot walk or escape the tub being "dunked"? You will see sparing of flexor surfaces as they bend their legs in an attempt to avoid the water. Contact child protective services if the story or patterns of injury are suspicious [13].

64.11 Chemical Injuries

A brief word is due on chemical injuries, which for the most part can be treated just like any other burn. First and foremost make sure to copiously irrigate the burn in a way that rinses the material OFF the patient. A special concern is hydrofluoric acid. While these burns have been reported to cause hypomagnesemia and hypocalcemia, a review of 35 patients with small HF burns (about 2% TBSA) from our institution found no electrolyte abnormalities [14]. Irrigate these wounds with tap water and then treat with calcium gluconate gel which can be made by mixing a 150 g tube of KY-Jelly with one ampule of calcium gluconate.

64.12 Electrical Injuries

Electricity will follow the path of least resistance as it courses through the body, and typically, these burns are worse than they look. Be sure to examine the patient for contact points. They require a formal fluid resuscitation if indicated based on prior mentioned criteria. Be aware that they may need an excess of fluids when compared to the "normal" burn. Watch for rhabdomyolysis by monitoring the color of the urine and CK levels. Pink urine with a urinalysis revealing large blood yet a small number or red blood cells, and creatine kinase levels >15,000 are concerning and treatment for rhabdomyolysis should promptly begin. Treat with increasing fluids to a urine output >100 cc/h. Mannitol and bicarbonate therapy may be useful.

Who needs cardiac monitoring following an electrical injury? Low voltage injuries (<1,000 V) with no

ECG changes, no loss of consciousness, and no arrhythmias can be safely discharged home. All injuries with a witnessed loss of consciousness, EKG changes, or an arrhythmia either in transport or in the ER warrant cardiac monitoring [15]. You can also monitor if they have another indication for admission such as high TBSA or concern for muscular necrosis. CK-MB is not helpful as an indicator of cardiac injury. If they have had no cardiac events for 24 h post-injury or post-resolution of arrhythmia, you can discontinue monitoring [15].

Extremity injuries are difficult to deal with because often you cannot see the injury lying beneath the skin. In the past, surgeons would prophylactically decompress electrically injured extremities. However, the literature does not support the use of immediate decompression in all patients. Selective decompression based on clinical exam leads to decreased amputation rates [15]. Signs of the need for decompression are based on clinical exam and include progressive neurological dysfunction, pain out of proportion to exam, and decreasing pulses or Doppler signal. For these injuries, an escharotomy will not suffice and you must perform formal fasciotomies.

Important Points

- Airway comes first. In general, the indications for intubation in a burn patient are the same as they are in all trauma patients.
- Use a detailed burn chart to establish TBSA and revise after debridement.
- Initial resuscitation fluid is 4 cc/% second- and third-degree TBSA burned/kg of lactated ringer's, one half given over 8 h and the second over the next 16 h. Adjust rate based on patient's urine output.
- Perform escharotomies if clinically warranted. This is based on clinical exam findings such as pulse changes with decreasing Doppler signal of the extremities or increased difficulty ventilating the patient with increased airway pressures.
- Nutrition is crucial to burn survival. Start enteral feeding early.
- Bronchoscopy is the gold standard for diagnosing inhalational injury. Intubation is only necessary if patient also has respiratory distress.
- High-frequency percussive ventilation and HAM therapy may be useful in inhalational injury. However, the most important therapy is good pulmonary toilet.
- Treat carbon monoxide poisoning with 100% FiO_2.
- Be vigilant about the possibility of child abuse when dealing with pediatric burn patients.

Acknowledgments Special thanks to Dr. Gary Purdue and Sharon Lauderbach for their input and assistance in the preparation of this manuscript.

References

1. American Burn Association annual report (2009) http://www.ameriburn.org/
2. Yowler C, Fratianne R (2000) Current status of burn resuscitation. Clin Plast Surg 27(1):1–10
3. Pham T, Cancio L, Gibran N (2008) American burn association practice guidelines burn shock resuscitation. J Burn Care Rehabil 29(1):257–266
4. Huang P, Stucky F et al (1995) Hypertonic sodium resuscitation is associated with renal failure and death. Ann Surg 221:543–554
5. Lee J, Herndon D et al (2008) Burns and radiation injuries. In: Mattox K, Feliciano D (eds) Trauma, 6th edn. McGraw-Hill, New York, p 1051
6. Herndon D, Tomkins R (2004) Support of the metabolic response to burn injury. Lancet 363:1895–1902
7. Pruitt B, Cioffi W (1995) Diagnosis and treatment of smoke inhalation. J Intensive Care Med 10(3):117–127
8. Cioffi W, Rue L, Graves T et al (1991) Prophylactic use of high-frequency ventilation in patients with inhalation injury. Ann Surg 213(6):580–582
9. Hall J, Hunt J et al (2007) Use of high-frequency percussive ventilation in inhalation injuries. J Burn Care Rehabil 28(3):396–400
10. Desai M, Micak R et al (1998) Reduction in mortality in pediatric patients with inhalation injury with aerosolized heparin/N-acetylcystine therapy. J Burn Care Rehabil 19(3):210–212
11. Holt J, Saffle J et al (2008) Use of inhaled heparin/N--acetylcystine in inhalation injury: does it help? J Burn Care Rehabil 29(1):192–195
12. Spies M, Herndon D et al (2003) Prediction of mortality from catastrophic burns in children. Lancet 361:989–994
13. Peck MD, Priolo-Kapel D (2002) Child abuse by burning; a review of the literature and an algorithm for medical investigations. J Trauma 53(5):1013–1022
14. Stuke L et al (2008) Hydrofluoric acid burns: a 15-year experience. J Burn Care Res 29(6):893–896
15. Arnoldo B, Klein M, Gibran N (2006) Practice guidelines for the management of electrical injuries. J Burn Care Res 27(4):439–447

Crush Injuries

65

Herb A. Phelan

Crush injuries represent a special challenge to the trauma surgeon, as they tend to present with attention-grabbing injury patterns that occupy the forefront of the mind. While one is preoccupied in dealing with the mangled extremity or a concomitant solid organ injury, however, other problems silently mount. These complications of a crush injury can kill your patient or endanger the ultimate salvage of their limb every bit as easily as the disfiguring injury pattern that diverts your attention as soon as they roll in the door. If you allow yourself to get distracted by the wound to the exclusion of all else, you will be dealing with arrhythmias, hypotension, and worse before long. If you take nothing else away from this chapter, recognize that it is vital to manage the metabolic and physiologic consequences of the crush syndrome concurrently with the anatomic aspects of the injury itself.

While the energy imparted with a crush injury obviously puts the patient at risk for other severe injuries, trauma to individual organ systems is covered eloquently in other chapters of this book. What this chapter is intended to be is a no-nonsense crash course in dealing with the local as well as the systemic problems you are going to potentially face when managing your patient who has suffered a significant crush injury. Let us get started.

H.A. Phelan (✉)
Division of Burns/Trauma/Critical Care,
Department of Surgery, University of Texas-Southwestern Medical Center, 5323 Harry Hines Blvd, E5.508A,
Dallas, TX, USA
e-mail: herb.phelan@utsouthwestern.edu

65.1 Wound Issues

A young man pinned behind his dashboard after a car wreck; a construction worker on whom a roof collapsed; a city worker struck in the flank by a cross bar after hydraulics break on his garbage truck, and trapped under it when it comes to rest: all are different mechanisms of crush injury, but they all have a common final pathway in terms of the wound issues and problems that arise.

65.1.1 The Mangled Extremity

These dramatic injuries get everyone's attention when they arrive, and are unfortunately an all too common scenario in our Emergency Room. The decision as to whether to amputate primarily or undergo heroic efforts at limb salvage is occasionally straightforward. It can be safely stated that limbs that are completely amputated after a blunt mechanism (which generally involves considerable tissue and bone loss) are not candidates for reimplantation (Figs. 65.1 and 65.2). Frequently the decision is not as clear-cut, however, and the trauma surgeon is left to choose whether or not to commit the patient to a life with a prosthesis. This decision is made even more difficult by the fact that our training as surgeons tends to make us feel like the decision to amputate is somehow a failure or admission of inadequacy, and that some unknown, unnamed surgeon out there would be able to have the patient back to running marathons at the culmination of their treatment course. While this is clearly not true, the decision to amputate is never accompanied by the feeling of satisfaction that a surgeon gets in other instances

G.C. Velmahos et al. (eds.), *Penetrating Trauma*,
DOI 10.1007/978-3-642-20453-1_65,

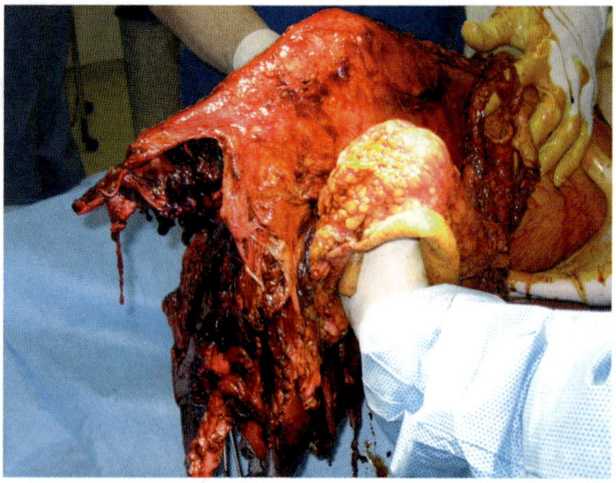

Fig. 65.1 Blunt amputation after a patient attempted to jump onto a train and was dragged under the wheels. This illustrates why blunt amputations are generally not candidates for replantation

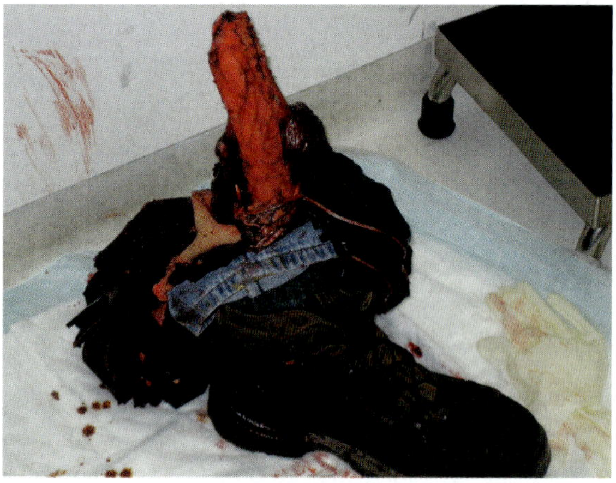

Fig. 65.2 Blunt amputation after a patient attempted to jump onto a train and was dragged under the wheels. This illustrates why blunt amputations are generally not candidates for replantation

when his or her intervention clearly helps a patient. Personally, it was not until I began to get more experience that I began to question the advisability of always adopting the default position of undertaking heroic limb salvage. Embarking on this course commits these patients to undergoing many, many operations with prolonged hospital stays, employment difficulties, and considerable cost. They undertake this endeavor in an effort to salvage a limb which frequently has woefully suboptimal function, and occasionally will request delayed amputation anyway after a considerable expenditure of energy and resources simply out of frustration with their final outcome. So when you are standing there looking at the patient with an injury

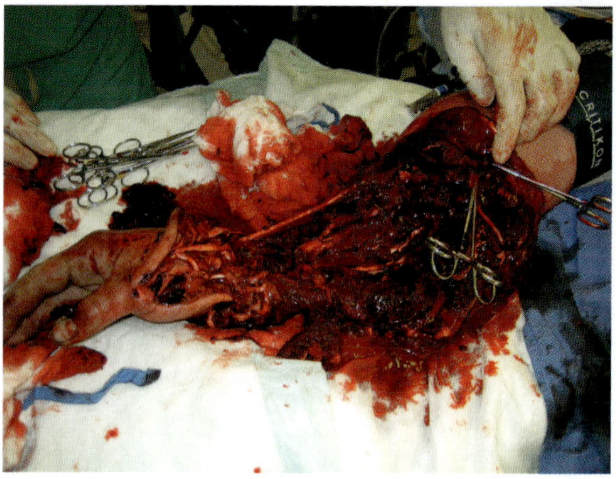

Fig. 65.3 Propellor injury after a patient fell out of a boat

such as Fig. 65.3 on the resuscitation room stretcher trying to decide what to do, do not delude yourself that the "easy" choice to always go all out carries no down side.

The difficulty with this decision has led to a great deal of research in an attempt to come up with objective scoring systems that will predict those patients who will be best served with early amputation. The good news is that there is no shortage of scoring systems from which to choose: the Mangled Extremity Severity Score [1], Hanover Fracture Scale [2], Predictive Salvage Index [3], Limb Salvage Index [4], and others. The bad news is that none of them are that great in terms of answering your question as they tend to lack sensitivity in addressing which limbs should undergo early amputation [5]. While I think that these scoring systems have limited utility when their quantitative scores are used, they are of some use if you look at them qualitatively as they will tell you the variables that need to be factored into your decision.

Let us start with the easy part. This has nothing to do with the crushed extremity, but with the rest of the patient instead. I am referring to the patient's overall trauma burden. How sick are they? With how many organ systems and body cavities are you contending? Are they in shock and not resuscitating well? It can be unequivocally stated that for the patient in extremis, an expeditious guillotine amputation (i.e., rapidly getting the extremity off, ligating the major vasculature involved, and doing nothing else without any attempt at closure) is the procedure of choice at the first operation. For the patient who is hemodynamically stable but has suffered a severe set of injuries, one should keep in mind the tremendous amount of physiologic reserve it takes to try to heal a mangled extremity. Large amounts of traumatized muscle and bone exert profound immunomodulatory effects, and can also serve as a septic source. Given that, one can see that in the massively injured patient it is wise to strongly consider early amputation (remember the old principles of priority in trauma training: life, limb, function, cosmesis). I have had conversations with older, more experienced colleagues who have suggested that an Injury Severity Score greater than 25 is a contraindication to heroic limb salvage. While I think that this number may be a little on the low side, it gives you a frame of reference for the debate. Further, as a patient gets older (and consequently has less in the way of metabolic reserves), one's threshold for amputation due to overall injury burden should lower.

In considering factors associated with the extremity itself, it is interesting to note that a plurality of trauma orthopods interviewed on decision-making factors for amputation in this scenario felt that the single biggest predictor of the need for early amputation was loss of neurologic integrity and/or plantar sensation [6]. Clearly, undergoing limb salvage in the hope of ultimately leaving a patient with an insensate, paralyzed extremity is a questionable course to undertake. One should resist the temptation to be dogmatic about this as an absolute indication, however, because stretch injury, compression, and ischemia can all result in transient nerve deficits. In fact, half of patients who present with an insensate foot and undergo limb salvage will regain sensation at 2 years [7]. If the deficit is felt to be permanent, however (i.e., if the posterior tibial nerve is visualized as transected from a crushing injury), it is defensible to say that amputation should be undertaken early rather than late.

Vascular injuries and ischemia time clearly play a large role in limb viability. After 6 h of warm ischemia time, limb salvage is anecdotal. Of note, one rarely commented upon factor is the importance of the length of an interposition graft in a vascular repair. Long grafts can give rise to the phenomenon of "interstate syndrome." When these high-speed, uninterrupted highway systems were built in the United States, they bypassed many small towns which had previously survived on the business brought to them by visitors passing through on the smaller roads. Just as many of these small towns withered away after potential visitors elected to use the interstates without ever exiting, so to do smaller muscle units wither away as the vascular graft bypasses them without giving off perforators.

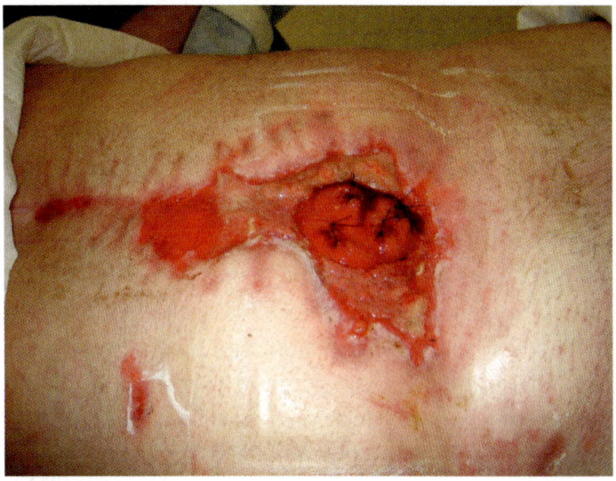

Fig. 65.4 Abdominal wall necrosis with subsequent fistulization after a blow to the right flank by a crossbar on a city garbage truck whose hydraulics broke

The muscular component of the injury is best evaluated by the four "C"s: color, contracture, consistency, and circulation. As a practical matter, the single best predictor of muscle viability is bleeding during debridement. After removing that muscle which is clearly nonviable, the surgeon needs to ask if the crush injury has left the patient with so little viable muscle that the resulting limb is worth continuing to attempt to salvage. If the answer is in the affirmative, it must be asked anew each time the patient goes back to the operating room for further debridement. These issues are not limited to the extremity, as the earlier scenario involving the city worker at the beginning of this section will attest. This man received a massive blow to the right flank, transecting his liver and macerating part of his lower right abdominal wall. His liver was packed, and he subsequently did well. Over a matter of days, however, he required more and more debridement of nonviable muscle wall until only peritoneum remained. He then developed two enterocutaneous fistulae (Fig. 65.4). He underwent a simultaneous fistula resection and abdominal wall reconstruction several months after his initial injury.

Surprisingly, the bony component of the injury is less important than the amount of soft tissue coverage that remains. Simply put, there is no substitute for healthy coverage. This will affect union rates, wound healing, and all of their downstream sequelae.

Finally, we have come to realize that there are social components that go into the likelihood of a successful outcome. Patients with a low frustration threshold, low levels of motivation, and poor social support tend to not do very well with the protracted course entailed with heroic salvage efforts. Before committing the patient to this undertaking, it is wise to have a very frank discussion with them and their family on what can reasonably be expected. They should be made aware of the sobering statistic that at 2 year and 7 year follow-up, functional outcomes are equivalent between amputation and reconstruction, and they are not good [8, 9]. By doing so, the surgeon protects the patient from unrealistic expectations, and consequently him or herself.

65.1.2 Compartment Syndrome

It has been said that paranoia is a healthy attitude in a trauma surgeon, and this is especially true in the diagnosis and management of compartment syndromes. They frequently present in a subtle fashion, and if missed will render the good technical results of an operation moot, inflict serious morbidity on the patient, and potentially serve as a source of litigation. Given the ease with which they can be overlooked, and the serious consequences when that happens, they are accurately viewed as a bear trap by practicing trauma surgeons.

The first step in managing a possible compartment syndrome is to be aware of the clinical scenarios in which they frequently occur. Two broad categories of insult lead to the increase in intracompartmental pressures which characterize the condition. The first is relatively straightforward and generally occurs after direct trauma to the injured portion of the extremity. Here, lacerated muscle and fractured bone bleed into the unyielding fascial compartment and result in the characteristic increased pressure. Crushed and contused muscle will accumulate some degree of hematoma, further exacerbating the condition. The second etiology for compartment syndrome, and the most common one seen in my practice, is after a limb has undergone a period of ischemia typically after a vascular injury. In this setting, the anaerobic metabolites that build up downstream from a site of vascular occlusion accumulate in proportion to the length of time for which a limb has been ischemic. When the limb is reperfused, these toxic by-products of anaerobic metabolism wash out and cause significant capillary leak and cell swelling. In this setting, the syndrome occurs in the compartments downstream from the site of injury. The occlusion can also arise from extrinsic causes, such as when a cast is applied too tightly. Finally, the most insidious presentation of compartment syndrome can occur with the anasarca seen during and after a massive resuscitation. Here, the muscle compartments swell from an accumulation of third-spaced fluid, frequently aggravated by systemic hypotension and hypoperfusion. A limb which has been ischemic for 2 h is at high risk for compartment syndrome, while 4 h of ischemia time will certainly develop a compartment syndrome after reperfusion. By 6 h of ischemia time, not only is a compartment syndrome a certainty, but the neuromuscular deficits are frequently not reversible even after fasciotomy and limb salvage is anecdotal. It is easy to see how a crush injury can put a patient at risk for any of these causes.

Classically, surgical trainees are taught to watch for the five "P"s of compartment syndrome: pain, pallor, paralysis, paresthesias, and pulselessness (occasionally, a sixth is included with poikilothermia). A point that needs to be reinforced is that all are not required for the diagnosis. The earliest sign to be seen is that of pain, particularly if it is out of proportion to what would normally be clinically expected. It is especially pronounced if the muscles within the compartment in question are squeezed or stretched. All of the remaining signs indicate that the condition is in a more advanced stage. Finally, it should be noted that a limb will be in the late stages of compartment syndrome before it loses a pulse. The occlusion of capillary perfusion and venous outflow occurs at much lower pressure levels, and the presence of a pulse in the extremity should not put the surgeon's mind at ease.

Alright, so you have got a patient who has an injury pattern that has you worried and a set of complaints and findings that have got warning bells going off in your head. What do you do now? How do you proceed? Traditional surgical teaching states that compartment pressures should be measured in some way. Some will say that this can be done easily by hooking an IV needle up to a transducer, making sure that it is zeroed, sticking the needle directly into the compartment, and reading the resulting number. This technique is mentioned only to be condemned, however, as muscle can "cork" the end of the needle and artificially elevate the pressure reading. Another option is to use commercially available specialized needles which have their pressure aperture slightly offset in such a manner that they avoid the problem of muscle plugging. This strategy yields a precise pressure value, albeit at the expense of extra, specialized equipment. If a quantitative strategy is undertaken, an absolute intracompartmental pressure of 30 mmHg is diagnostic of a compartment syndrome. Additionally, a pressure value which is within 30 mmHg of the patient's diastolic blood pressure should also be considered to represent a compartment syndrome.

Personally, I prefer to diagnose compartment syndromes clinically. The specialized needles are not always available, and in the few times that I used them early in my training I found them to be problematic (I am reminded of the wisdom of the esteemed surgeon, Chapman Lee, who frequently said of such undertakings, "Remember, a fool with a tool is still a fool."). Further, if you do intend to use quantitative pressure measurements in the management of possible compartment syndrome, you are obligated to believe the number that you get (high or low) and react accordingly as it makes no sense to perform an invasive procedure and disregard its results because they are not to one's liking. Otherwise, why do the test to begin with? Therefore, if I have a patient with a risk factor, significant pain, and a tight compartment on exam, I do not bother checking pressures and proceed to surgery as I trust my judgment more than the ability of the technology to yield an accurate measurement. I will state that I have a low threshold for fasciotomy, as it is not uncommon for these patients to be intubated and sedated at the time of their assessment. The consequences of a nontherapeutic fasciotomy are minimal, and it is much more common to regret not doing a fasciotomy than it is to regret doing one.

Once a diagnosis of compartment syndrome has been made by whatever means, immediate fasciotomy should be performed. Additionally, when taking a patient with a limb that has been ischemic for more than an hour after a vascular injury and external hemorrhage is not an issue, it is prudent to perform a fasciotomy before embarking upon the vascular repair. In the lower leg, a generous skin incision is made halfway between the tibia and fibula (Figs. 65.5 and 65.6). While the fascial incision can be extended under the skin (i.e., while leaving the overlying skin intact), it is absolutely imperative that the skin incision be big enough that it does not cause any compression even in the face of adequate fascial release. If this is at all in question, the skin should be completely opened as concerns for cosmesis are not an excuse for an inadequate fasciotomy. Once the skin incision is completed laterally, the septum between the anterior and lateral compartments is frequently visible as seen in Fig. 65.7. If it is not, a small cross-sectional incision in the fascia and

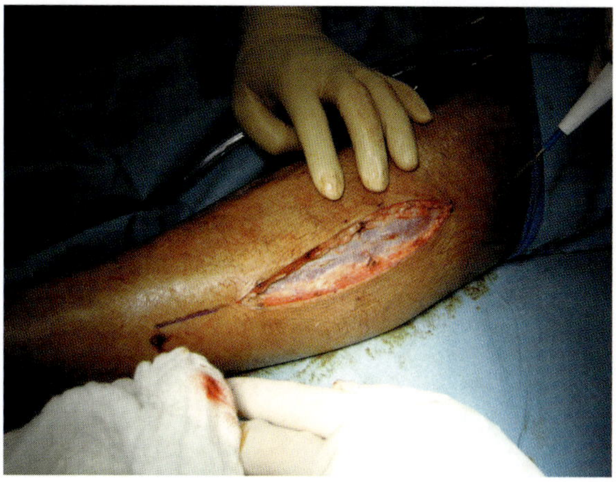

Fig. 65.5 Lateral skin incision for fasciotomy

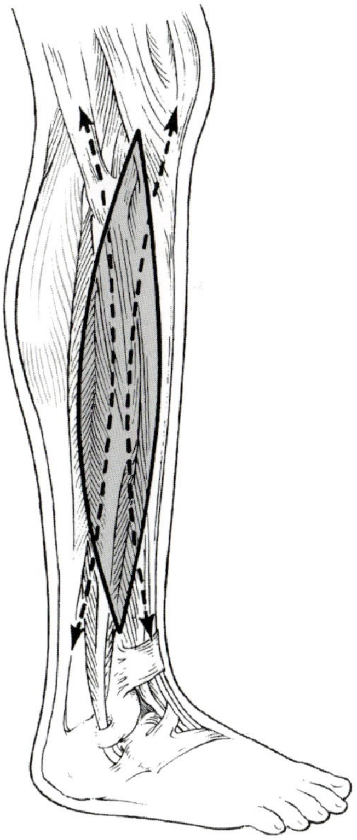

Fig. 65.6 Illustration of lateral skin incision for fasciotomy

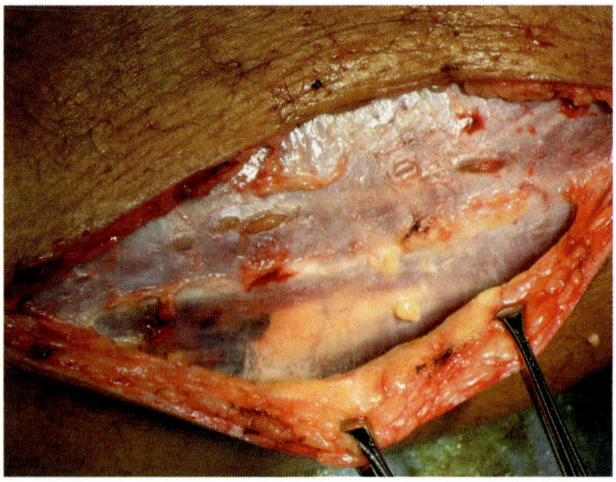

Fig. 65.7 Note the intermuscular septum visible beneath the fascia which separates the *anterior* and lateral compartments

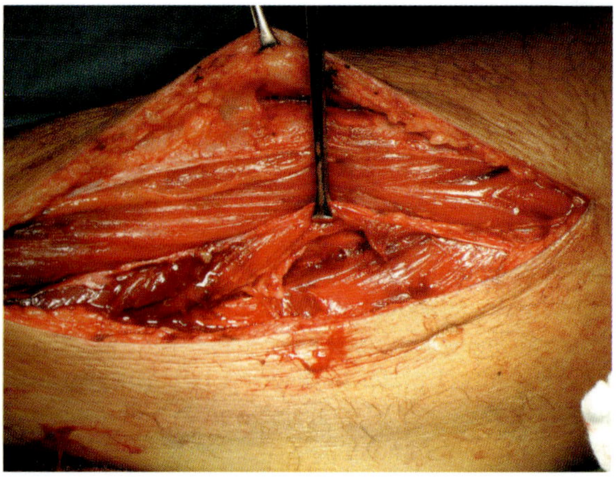

Fig. 65.9 Lateral muscular compartment after fasciotomy

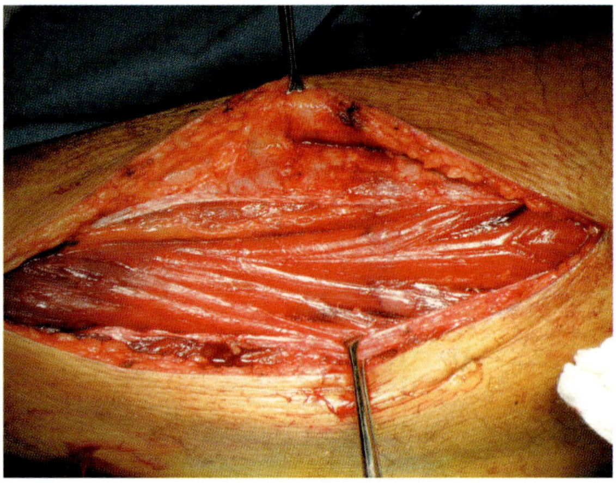

Fig. 65.8 Anterior muscular compartment after fasciotomy

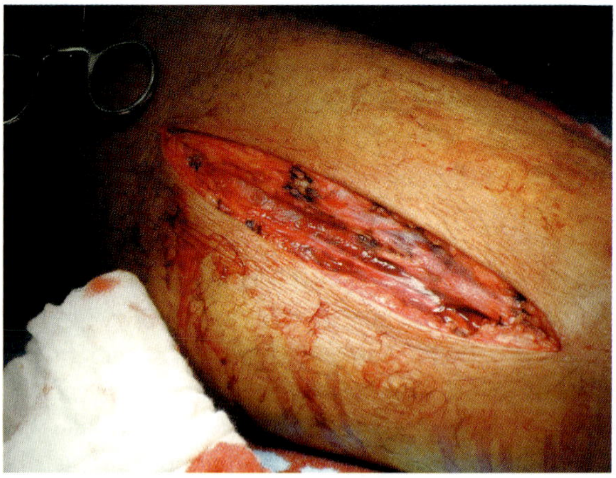

Fig. 65.10 Medial skin incision for fasciotomy

perpendicular to the septum will usually reveal it easily. Once the septum is located, the fascia is completely incised by a push technique with Metzenbaum scissors for the length of the septum (Figs. 65.8 and 65.9). A similar length skin incision is then made on the medial side of the leg one to two fingerbreadths below the edge of the tibia (Figs. 65.10 and 65.11). Care should be taken to avoid the greater saphenous vein if possible as the adequacy of venous outflow is of importance. Once the skin incision is made, the superficial posterior compartment is the only one which is visible, and its fasciotomy can be easily performed a centimeter or two below the edge of the tibia. The next step is a potential trap, however, as anatomical texts and surgical atlases underestimate how easy it is to get lost in the calf and misidentify the fascia of the deep posterior compartment (Fig. 65.12). In order to prevent this from happening, I use the back side of the tibia as my landmark (Fig. 65.13). Since the posterior tibia abuts the deep posterior compartment, I dissect toward this structure and it allows me to reliably identify the fascia of the deep posterior compartment. I have had colleagues who will actually strip the muscle off of the back side of the tibia in order to assure that the deep compartment is released.

It is exceedingly rare to have to do thigh fasciotomies as the greatly increased volumes of the three thigh compartments will accommodate very large amounts of blood or edema. In my experience, when a thigh compartment syndrome does occur it is usually in the setting of a concomitant vascular injury and will

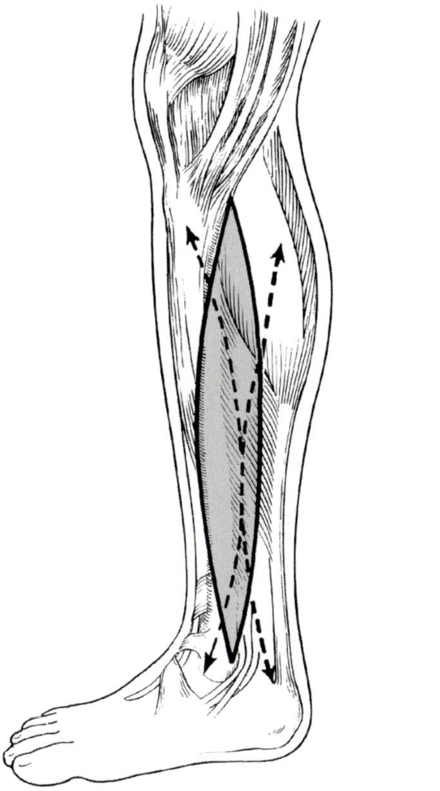

Fig. 65.11 Illustration of medial skin incision for fasciotomy

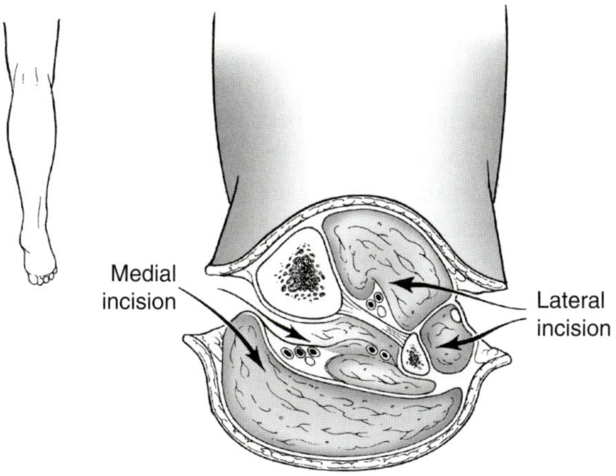

Fig. 65.12 Illustration of compartments released by incision type

be going to the operating room anyway. If fasciotomy is required, the three compartments are released through two incisions. The upper arm only has two compartments, and these are released through two incisions (Fig. 65.14). Finally, the forearm has three

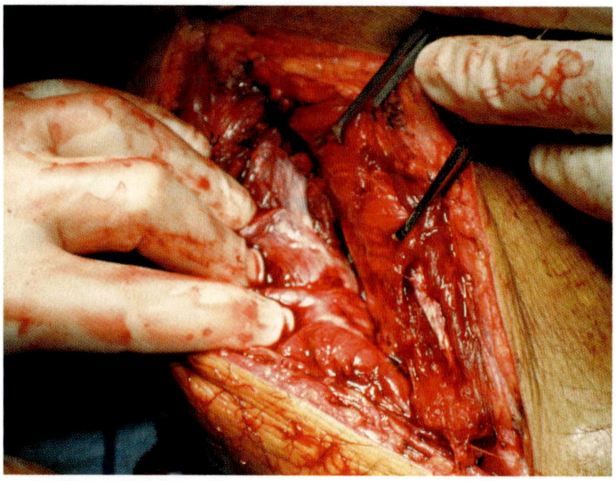

Fig. 65.13 Deep posterior compartment stripped off of back side of the tibia

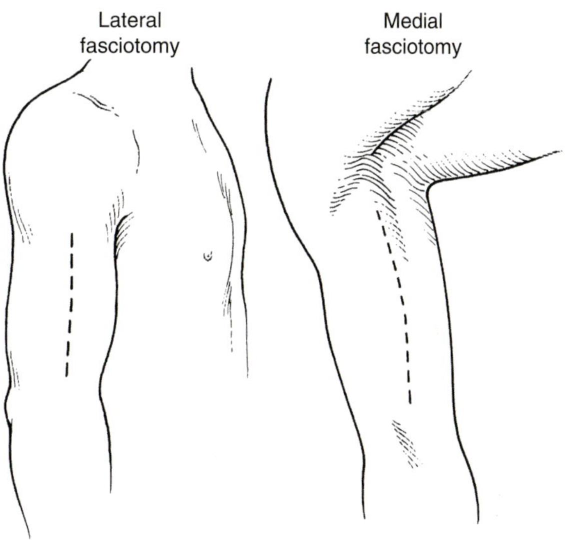

Fig. 65.14 Illustration of upper arm fasciotomy incisions

compartments: anterior, posterior, and lateral (also known as the "mobile wad"). The anterior fasciotomy is accomplished through a skin incision described as a "lazy S" which releases both the anterior compartment and the mobile wad (Figs. 65.15 and 65.16). This incision should also be carried through the carpal tunnel. The posterior release is straightforward (Fig. 65.17).

Assuming that the fasciotomy is adequate, the condition that caused the compartment syndrome to arise generally abates over the course of a few days. Once this happens and the muscle or compartment swelling seems to be improving, one can begin to take steps to

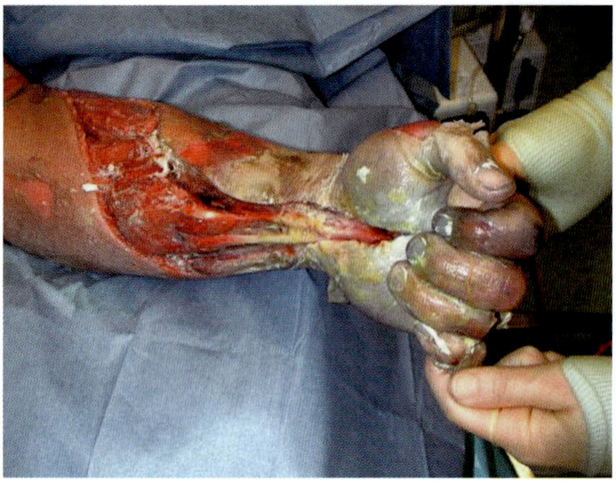

Fig. 65.15 The "Lazy S" incision, releasing the mobile wad and extending through the carpal tunnel

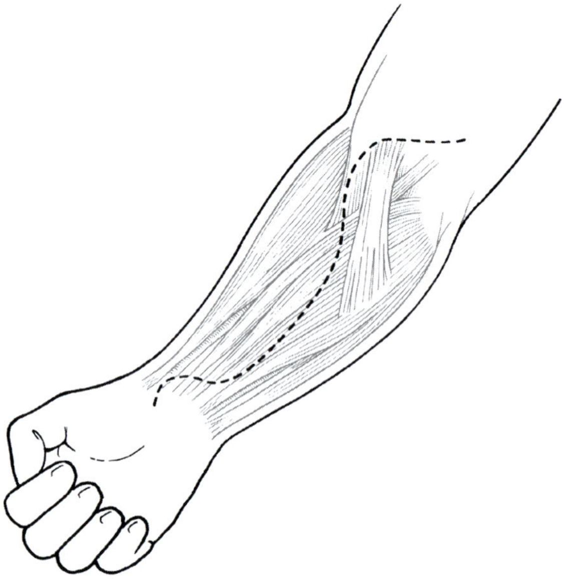

Fig. 65.16 Illustration of "Lazy S" incision

close the fasciotomies. This can be most easily accomplished by crisscrossing a sturdy, elastic vessel loop back and forth across the skin incision. By doing so, tension is maintained across the skin edges and slowly begins to reapproximate them. This can also be done in conjunction with a vacuum-based dressing in order to promote granulation tissue formation. The vessel loops can be tightened every 48 h or so, or whenever laxity is noted in the rubber bands. Once the skin edges are close enough, they can undergo a delayed primary closure. If this does not happen, skin grafting will be required.

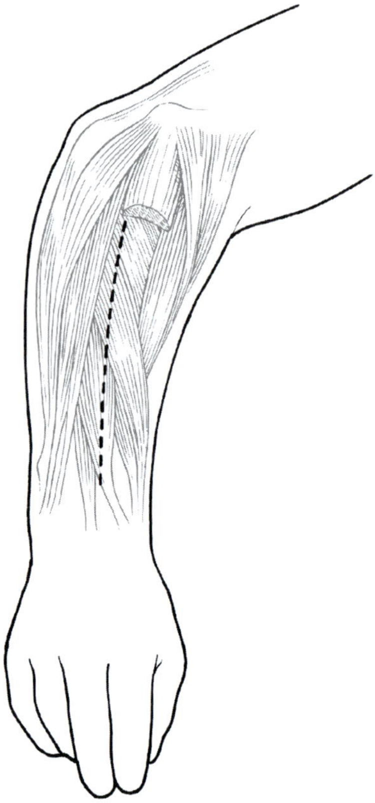

Fig. 65.17 Illustration of incision for posterior forearm fasciotomy

65.2 Systemic Issues

Up to this point, we have been discussing the issues surrounding the anatomy directly affected by the traumatic mechanism. This is satisfying because you can see it, intervene directly, and get tangible results. Now we turn our attention to the sinister portion of the crush syndrome. These interventions are cerebral rather than technical, but no less important. The systemic manifestations of a crush injury present with four problems: hyperkalemia, hypovolemia with metabolic acidosis, nephrotoxicity and acute renal failure, and disseminated intravascular coagulopathy (DIC). They are all interrelated and as we shall see, some of their treatments overlap. The first and most important step, however, is remembering to think about them.

The breakdown of skeletal muscle releases a multitude of intracellular products into the systemic circulation. The most immediately life threatening is potassium. Dangerous levels of hyperkalemia can result, and these should be anticipated and preempted.

Serial potassium measurements are wise at frequent intervals in the early hours after a significant crush injury. If you wait too long and you find yourself dealing with an arrhythmia, start with calcium to stabilize the cardiac myocytes (5 cc of 10% calcium chloride or 10 cc of 10% calcium gluconate, either one given over 2 min). That buys you a half hour but does nothing to fix the underlying problem. My treatment algorithm for severe hyperkalemia consists of starting with an ampule of D50 followed by 10 units of regular insulin, which will drive some of the potassium intracellularly. Make sure you perform frequent finger sticks to assure that you do not bottom out the patient's blood glucose. I then follow this up with oral kayexalate since it has a shorter onset of action than the rectal route. While you will read about other measures such as albuterol or hemodialysis, I have never found them to be necessary. Typically, I will just readminister these agents as needed while I deal with the source of the rhabdo, either through debridement, amputation, or through fasciotomy.

These patients can also get considerable hypovolemia as the damaged muscle will absorb extracellular fluid prior to lysing. This sequestration of volume is frequently in addition to hemorrhagic sources, and as a result patients suffering from a crush injury can have significant volume deficits. These factors contribute to a metabolic acidosis which is multifactorial in origin. Lactate released from dying muscle or elaborated from noninjured tissues during hypoperfusion is frequently seen. Despite the complex interplay of the volume and acid/base dyscrasias, the good news is that the treatment is the same and it is easy. Aggressive crystalloid (and for hemorrhagic sources, blood) resuscitation is a mainstay of therapy.

The myoglobin released by dying and damaged muscle is nephrotoxic. This hit to the kidneys is further exacerbated in the setting of hypovolemia. Finally, acidosis favors the precipitation of myoglobin in the renal tubules. Do not wait for your patient's urine to start turning pink or brown (Fig. 65.18)! You should already be aggressively administering volume to your patient, with a urine output of 100 cc/h as a target if that is achievable. If you are worried, start them on a sodium bicarbonate drip. Just inject three ampules of sodium bicarbonate into a liter of D5W, and start this at a rate of 100 cc/h. Your goal is a urine pH of 6.5 or higher, while making sure that the serum pH is less than 7.5. Under no circumstances, however, should alkalinizing the patient be viewed as an adequate substitute for euvolemia! You will read about mannitol in this setting, but I hesitate to do so in a polytrauma patient in whom the volume status may be questionable. In my experience, these steps should be enough to keep your patient off of the dialysis machine.

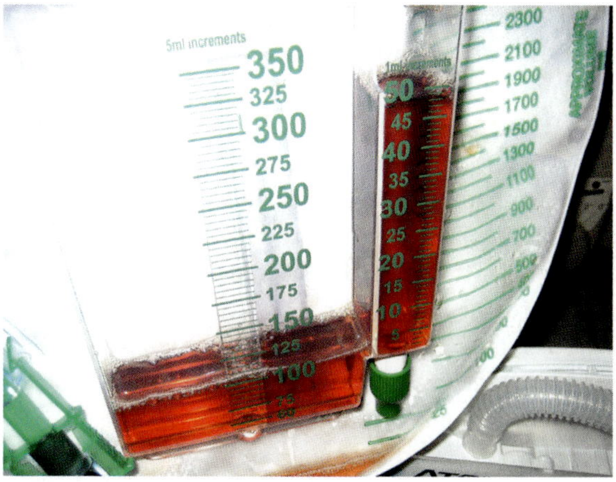

Fig. 65.18 Urine of a patient in rhabdomyolysis

Lastly, muscle necrosis causes the release of tissue thromboplastin. This can in turn lead to DIC. I only transfuse plasma products if I have concerns for surgical hemostasis, largely because the coagulopathy is very difficult if not impossible to fix until the underlying rhabdo resolves. If bleeding is not an issue and the patient does not have an intracranial injury, I just ride the lab value out while I go about fixing the source of the rhabdo through the previously mentioned operative options.

Important Points

- Do not let the dramatic nature of wounds from crush injury distract you from the sinister metabolic component accompanying crush injuries.
- The patient's overall trauma burden is the first and most important determinant in deciding whether to pursue heroic limb salvage.
- For the patient in extremis with a mangled extremity, guillotine amputation is the procedure of choice for the first operation.
- Make sure the patient understands what they are getting in to if they opt for limb salvage in a mangled extremity.

- Diagnose compartment syndromes clinically, not technologically.
- Make sure your skin incisions for fasciotomy are long enough.
- Head toward the back side of the tibia to make sure you release the deep posterior compartment. Strip the muscle off of it if necessary.
- The treatment for many of the systemic symptoms accompanying crush injury: volume, volume, volume.
- Beware hyperkalemia.
- Keep your patient making urine.

References

1. Bosse MJ, MacKenzie EJ, Kellam JF et al (2001) A prospective evaluation of the clinical utility of lower extremity injury severity scores. J Bone Joint Surg Am 83:3–14
2. Bosse MJ, MacKenzie EJ, Kellam JF et al (2002) An analysis of outcomes of reconstruction or amputation of leg-threatening injuries. N Engl J Med 347:1924–1931
3. Bosse MJ, McCarthy ML, Jones AL et al (2005) The insensate foot following severe lower extremity trauma: an indication for amputation? JBJS 87:2601–2608
4. Howe HR Jr, Poole GV, Hansen KJ et al (1987) Salvage of lower extremities following combined orthopedic and vascular trauma. A predictive salvage index. Am Surg 53: 205–208
5. Johansen K, Daimes M, Howey T et al (1990) Objective criteria accurately predict amputation following lower extremity trauma. J Trauma 30:568–573
6. MacKenzie EJ, Bosse MJ, Pollak AN et al (2005) Long-term persistence of disability following severe lower limb trauma: results of a seven year follow-up. JBJS 87:1801–1809
7. Russell WL, Sailors DM, Whittle TB et al (1991) Limb salvage versus traumatic amputation. A decision based on a seven-part predictive index. Ann Surg 213:473–481
8. Suedkamp NP, Barbey N, Veuskens A et al (1993) The incidence of osteitis in open fractures: an analysis of 948 open fractures (a review of the Hannover experience). J Orthop Trauma 7:473–482
9. Swiontkowski MF, MacKenzie EJ, Bosse MJ, LEAP Study Group et al (2002) Factors influencing the decision to amputate or reconstruct after high-energy lower extremity trauma. J Trauma 52:641–649

Blast Injuries

66

Joe DuBose, David S. Plurad, and Peter M. Rhee

Blast injuries are classified as: Primary: due blast wave and is rare in survivors except for tympanic membrane injury, Secondary: due to penetration of fragments from the blast, and the most common injury seen in survivors. Most of the injuries are to soft tissue but the variability of damage and lethality is high. Tertiary is due to blunt trauma from the person being thrown by the blast wave and is rare. Quaternary: everything else such as inhalation injury and crush injury from structures falling on the casualty. The extent of injury depends on size of explosion, proximity to epicenter of the explosion, medium which the blast is transmitted, foreign body/fragmentation burden, protective gear, and open or closed space of the explosion. Some classic sequelae of blast injury, including blast lung injury (BLI) and tympanic membrane rupture, have been well described, but in practical experience are less common than secondary blast injuries due to fragmentation injury. After control of hemorrhage, all wounds should be inspected and examined closely, washed out and debrided. Wounds should be left open as a general rule until the contamination is under control. Soft tissue damage underlying the skin perforation can be severe. A high index of suspicion for injury to all manner of organ systems should be maintained, and the aggressive utilization of comprehensive advanced imaging is highly encouraged.

Blast injuries resulting from explosions are divided into four types:

Primary: injury directly from the propagated blast overpressure.

Secondary: penetrating injury from the blast device fragmentation or objects carried on the blast wave.

Tertiary: injury from the patient being thrown into, onto or against objects.

Quaternary: all other injuries resulting from the explosion.

Explosions can cause both blunt and penetrating injury, the vast majority of the injuries requiring medical attention are actually due to penetrating mechanism. While the injuries are limited only by the imagination, the recent conflict in Afghanistan and Iraq shows that the majority of injuries are straightforward. Large explosions such as nuclear explosions and heavy air bombings are devastating (i.e.: high-order explosives) and can cause lethality from primary blast injuries but the vast majority of those who survive to reach medical care are treated for secondary blast injuries.

Types and severity of injury depend primarily on the following variables:

1. Size of the explosion
2. Proximity to the explosion

J. DuBose (✉)
Air Force/C-STARS, R Adams Cowley Shock Trauma Center, University of Maryland Medical System,
22 South Greene Street, T5R46, Baltimore 21202, MD, USA
e-mail: jdubose@umm.edu

D.S. Plurad
Division of Acute Care Surgery (Trauma, Emergency Surgery, Surgical Critical Care), LAC+USC, 1200 N. State St, Room 1050, Los Angeles, CA 90033, USA

P.M. Rhee
Department of Surgery,
Health Sciences Center, University of Arizona,
1501 N. Campbell Avenue, Rm 5411, Tucson 245063, AZ, USA

G.C. Velmahos et al. (eds.), *Penetrating Trauma*,
DOI 10.1007/978-3-642-20453-1_66, © Springer-Verlag Berlin Heidelberg 2012

3. Medium through which the energy is transferred
4. Fragmentation
5. Use of countermeasures (vehicle protection +/– body armor)
6. Open or closed space explosion

Primary blast injury results from the transfer of energy during alternating under and over-pressurization upon tissues of varied densities. Underwater explosions transmit energy more effectively compared to explosions above the water due to the medium in which the blast wave is propagated. Organs such as the ear, eyes, brain, lungs, and the intra-abdominal gastrointestinal tract are all susceptible to blast effects. Tissue disruption occurs mainly at the interface between tissues of variable density causing local and systemic dysfunction. Patients can be killed due to primary blast injury without any external signs of trauma or with only subtle findings such as tympanic membrane rupture. In addition, secondary injuries typically require more immediate attention while the severity of primary injury may not become apparent until later.

Secondary blast injury results from fragmentation of projectiles contained within the blast device or objects between the explosion and the casualty that are carried at high velocity upon the blast wave. Bomb makers may package any manner of imaginable projectiles around the explosive core of the device. These include various sized metal balls to screws, nails, bolts, and nuts. These projectiles may even be laced with poisons such as arsenic or Coumadin. In the current conflicts in Iraq and Afghanistan, the vast majority of blast injuries are due to improvised explosive devices (IEDs). These may be constructed from antiquated stockpile munitions, modified black-market high explosives, ammunition or even military antipersonnel devices. They may be employed or concealed in various ways; either buried superficially or placed in a variety of objects including dead animals or trash. Even the detonation of IEDs has proven to be highly variable. Direct detonation, heat sensor activation and remote control devices such as cell phones or garage door openers have all been utilized. Vehicular-borne IEDs (VBIED) has also proven a common utilized tactic.

Protecting military personnel from IED attacks remains a significant focus with armoring of troops and vehicles, changes in convoy tactics and the introduction of more effective countermeasures. Despite this, bomb makers have proven to be adaptable. For example, in response to initial up-armoring of military vehicles, insurgents in Iraq began to employ the Explosive Formed Projectile (EFP). This device consists of a conical charge that produces a directed blast that is capable of penetrating the up-armored components. This approach included the detonation of an IED to primarily disable vehicles, then using small arms fire to injure the occupants out of the vehicle as they attempted to escape their incapacitated transport. As this technique evolved, insurgents began to employ a second IED that is detonated in a delayed fashion, after medical and military personnel have secured the area and are attempting to treat and evacuate casualties.

During IED attacks upon dismounted patrols, the majority of casualties have forces applied to unprotected lower extremities that often result in amputations (Fig. 66.1). The amputation was a result of both primary and secondary blast injury but in the survivors secondary injury proved most common threat to life and limb. Often the IED injuries can seem alarming but body armor can be quite protective. The main problem is that body armor does not protect the whole body (Fig. 66.2).

Despite the increase of IED attacks in present zones of conflict, rockets and mortar fire also remain common mechanisms of injury. In the author's experience, injuries due to these weapons most often result in superficial injuries that in most cases require only wound debridement and local care. Many of these types of injuries appear horrific on initial review, with multiple fragmentation injuries covering the entire side of a body. Although appropriate vigilance demands comprehensive evaluation in all of these cases, we have found that in most instances those who survived to reach treatment had injuries confined to the soft tissues, and most often did not penetrate a body cavity. The evaluation and treatment of these injuries should, however, be based on careful examination of each and every single fragmentation injury. The use of radiographs can be used to identify the multiple foreign bodies (Fig. 66.3). Determining intracorporeal penetration remains a challenge and in the battlefield scenario, body

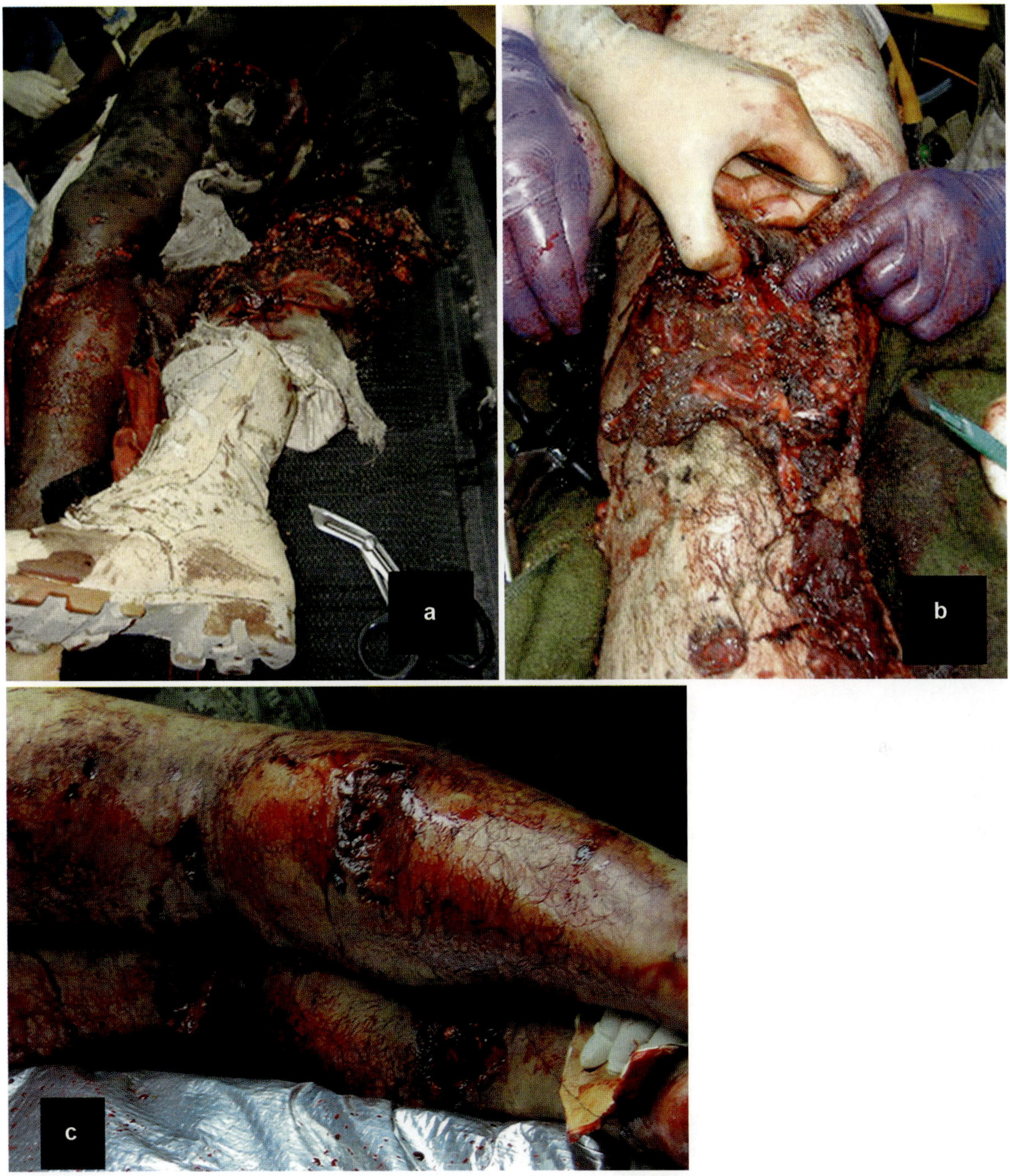

Fig. 66.1 (**a**, **b**, **c**) Lower extremity injuries from improvised explosive devices in Iraq war

cavities often have to be surgically explored. On occasion, fragmentation injuries are also accompanied by burn wounds. Fortunately, in most instances, these burns were relatively minor. Despite our experience, we continue to recommend that a high index of suspicion be exercised in all cases of fragmentation injury (Fig. 66.4). Fragments can be of all types (Fig. 66.5) and this includes dirt, rocks and bone from other casualties.

Tertiary blast injuries occur when the casualty is thrown by the blast wind. This can cause superficial wounds and fractures. Amputation from tertiary blast is not common. Solid organ injuries can occur, but were rarely seen in the authors' experience.

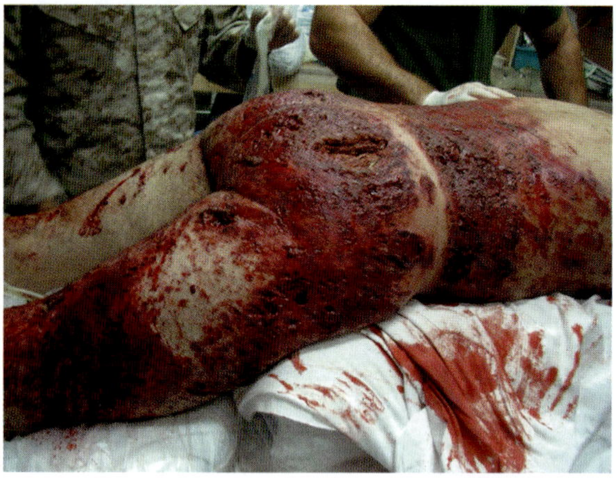

Fig. 66.2 Soldier injured by a buried IED. Note the protection to the torso by the body armor. While the soft tissue injury was dramatic with expectant tissue loss, the injury was limited to the soft tissue without life-threatening injuries or fractures

Quaternary blast injuries include flash burns. Although temperatures from explosions can reach up to 3,000°C, the rise in temperature is rapid and so is the decline in temperature as the fuel is quickly expended. A common example of this type of injury is a propane explosion in a trailer home. These types of flash burn more commonly affect exposed skin. A classic scenario is of a male patient who is minimally clothed in jeans or shorts attempting to light the propane stove after the pilot light has extinguished. Since propane is heavier than air, an enclosed room can fill with propane. If the smell of the accumulating gas is not detected when a match or lighter is ignited, disaster is likely to ensue. In contrast to propane, natural gas is lighter than air and will rise. Subsequently, in a flash explosion of natural gas, curtains or furniture may catch on fire and contribute to the creation of toxic fumes. Inhalation injury occurs if the casualty is in a closed space and there is a concomitant fire. Any fire on clothing or surrounding structures such as parts of a vehicle may result in significant partial or full thickness burns.

Quaternary blast inhalational injuries may also exacerbate underlying asthma or chronic obstructive pulmonary disease. The classic dangers of quaternary injury are from falling debris; from buildings for example. Such debris can cause direct crush injury and cause compartment syndrome and myoglobinemia. These types of injuries may prove common after terrorist attacks on buildings with VBIEDs.

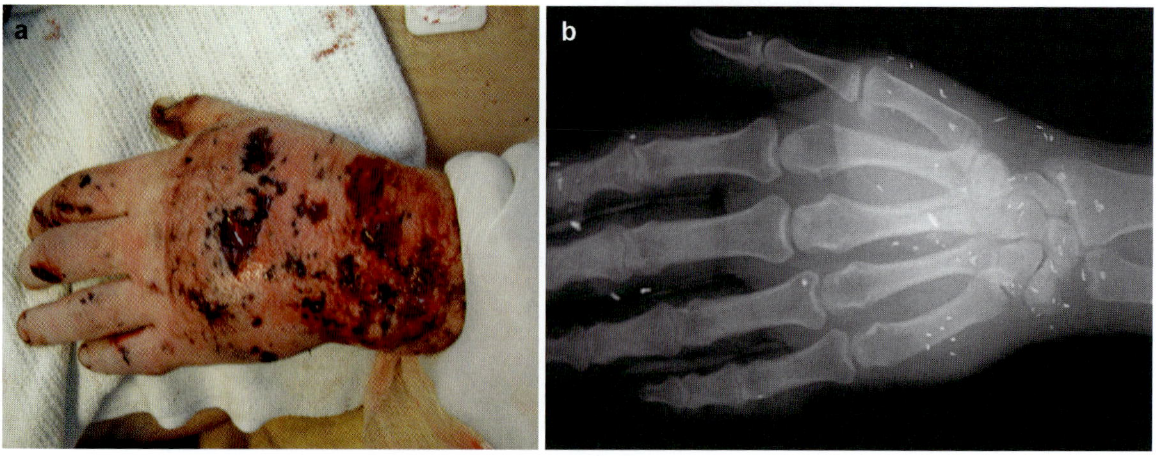

Fig. 66.3 (**a**) Hand injury with multiple fragmentation. (**b**) Plain x-ray of hand

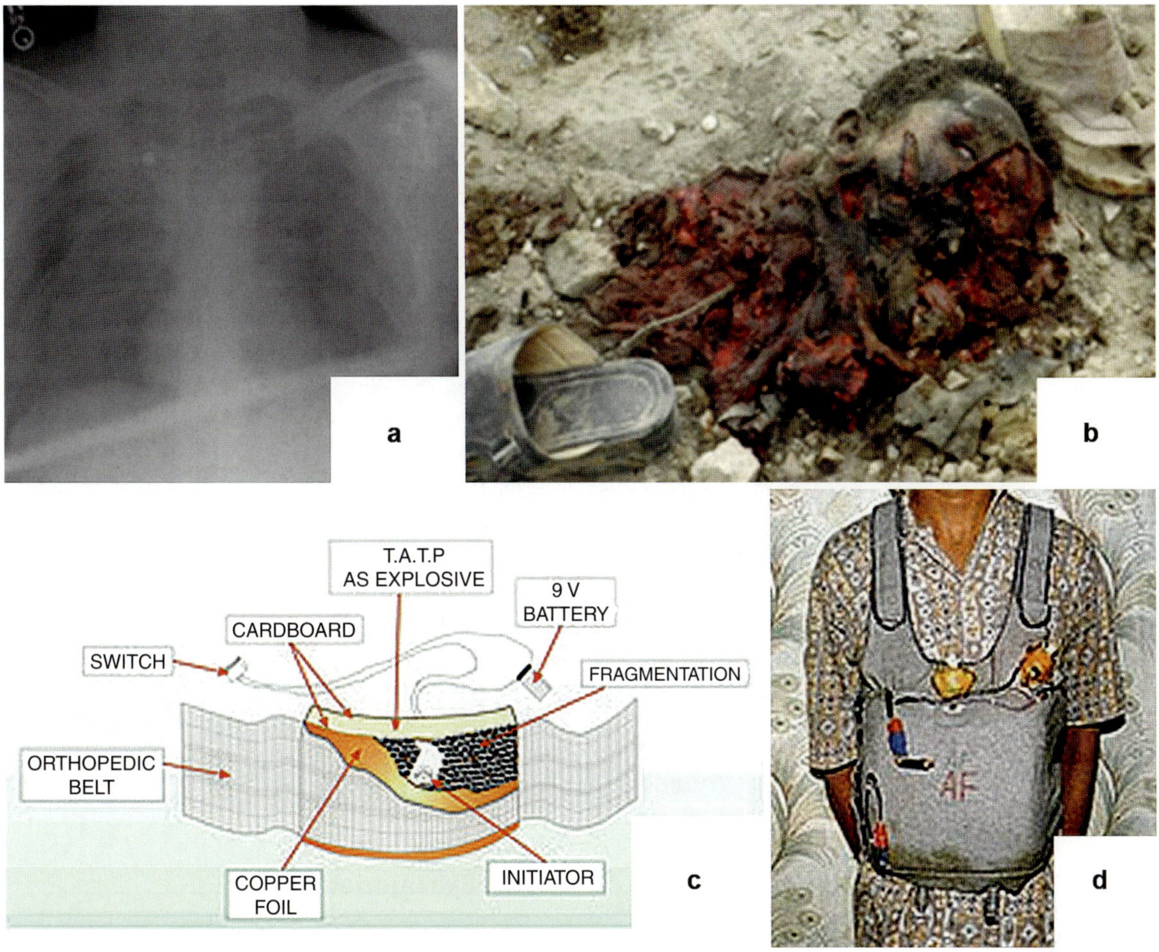

Fig. 66.4 (**a**) One small metal fragment from a suicide bomber that went transmediastinal killing the casualty 1 h after injury; (**b**) the head of the suicide bomber at the scene; (**c**) illustration of the type of bomb used by the suicide bomber which injured over 200 people; (**d**). photo of the type of vest bomb used by the suicide bomber

The mortality from bombings is classically triphasic. Immediate mortality from disruption of bodies, chest injuries, head injuries or rapid exsanguination are the most common. Some immediate deaths will have no external signs of injury, succumbing instead to catastrophic air emboli or fatal cardiac dysrhythmias. The mortality among casualties surviving to reach treatment is lower. It is also important to consider the environment in which the explosion occurs since it may significantly affect the cause of mortality. Explosions in open space tend to produce more secondary blast injuries whereas those occurring in enclosed spaces are more likely to produce primary, tertiary and quaternary injuries. This rationale likely explains the reason for the injury patterns observed in Iraq and Afghanistan, which are largely penetrating secondary blast injuries that occur in open spaces.

66.1 Specific Injury Types

Evaluation of the blast injured patient mandates a comprehensive evaluation, with critical attention for characteristic injury patterns. A high index of suspicion should be utilized throughout this process.

66.1.1 Head Injuries

Tympanic membrane rupture is commonly described as the classic manifestation of blast injury. Injuries to this thin membrane are typically a result of the primary blast wave creating a rapid over-pressurization manifesting in rupture. Certainly all patients suspected to have sustained blast injury should have their tympanic membranes examined and any positive finding in this

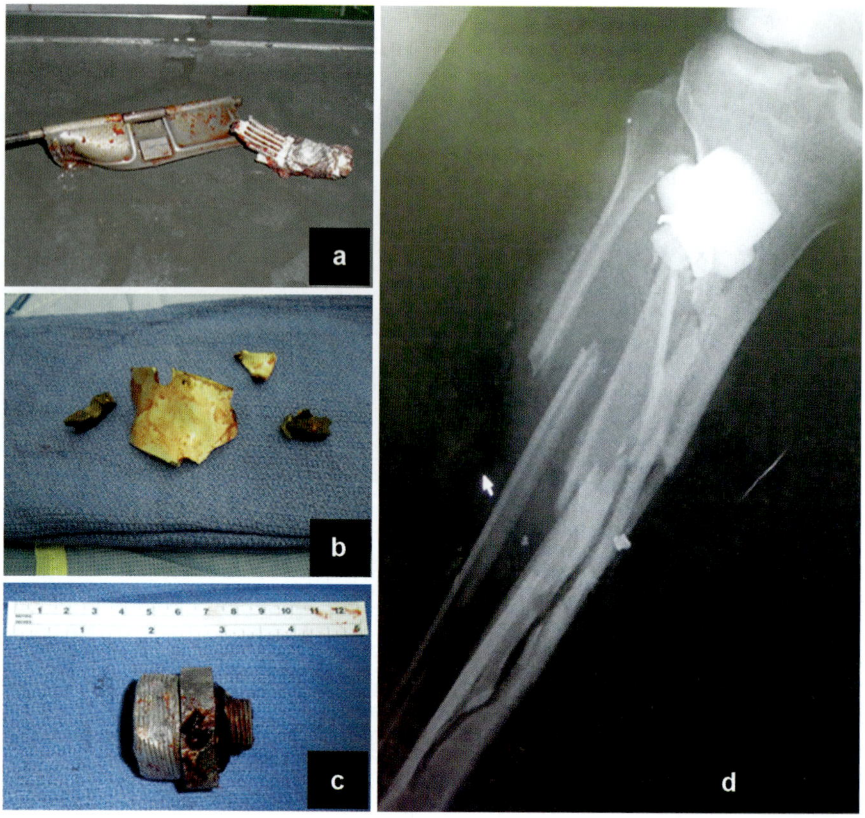

Fig. 66.5 Various fragmentations found in patients: (**a**) dust cover from M-4 rifle, (**b**) various objects, (**c**) bolt, (**d**) fracture caused by bolt in (**c**)

regard must further heighten your suspicion for other over-pressurization injuries (ex: abdominal hollow viscous organs) [1]. Once considered a sensitive indicator of the burden of primary blast injury, recent examination has shown that tympanic membrane perforation occurs in less than 20% of victims of combat explosion-related injuries; and likely does not correlate as well with other injury effects (brain injury, hollow viscous) [2].

Traumatic brain injury (TBI) remains a worrisome and ill-defined sequelae of blast injury. The characteristic effects of primary injury mechanisms and blast wave transmission through the cranium remain poorly understood. All patients in close proximity to a blast injury should be aggressively evaluated for evidence of TBI. The spectrum of injury may range from a post-concussive state to diffuse axonal injury to intracranial hemorrhage or infarct. This topic is among the most actively studied in military medicine today. It is important to emphasize that TBI is a clinical diagnosis. Identification of this entity is aided by the use of computed tomography (CT), but many with TBI will have normal imaging with considerable neurologic deficits. Conversely those with an abnormal head CT scan may have normal neurologic exams.

66.1.2 Eye Injuries

The human eye, a cavity filled with vitreous fluid, is sensitive to blast overpressure events following explosions. The resulting rapid fluctuation of pressure may result in both rupture of the globe or retinal disruption [1]. Injury to the eye due to fragmentation should also remain a strong concern. Ask for formal examination by an ophthalmologist is warranted in all cases in which injuries to the face, changes in gross visual acuity or imaging are suggestive of eye injury.

66.1.3 Chest Injuries

Much discussion regarding blast effects on the body has traditionally emphasized the dangers of blast lung injury (BLI). BLI is a serious, potentially fatal injury to the lungs hypothesized to result from the primary blast wave. A patient with a larger burden of injury to several regions of the body, suggesting more significant exposure to blast forces, should be suspected to have suffered BLI [3]. The clinical spectrum of BLI ranges from slight desaturations to pink frothy sputum and overt pulmonary failure. When it is identified, you should proceed to aggressive efforts to maintain oxygenation and limit secondary injury due to barotrauma associated with the mechanical ventilation [4]. Fortunately, if the acute phase can be survived, most patients surviving BLI will likely regain good lung function [5]. Even more fortunately, this entity is very uncommon. In the extensive combined wartime experience of the two authors of this chapter, we have never seen a case of lung injury that we could attribute directly to blast effect. This includes both soldiers wearing body armor and civilian bombing victims that do not have the benefit of this protection.

66.1.4 Abdominal Injuries

Abdominal injuries following explosions may result from both primary overpressure events that cause distension and rupture of hollow viscous, tearing of solid organs due to their abrupt motion against ligamentous attachments, or as a result of direct fragmentation injury [6]. Given that many patients may not prove evaluable due to loss of consciousness or distracting injuries after these events, you should have a threshold for more aggressive forms of evaluation of the abdominal contents beyond physical exam. Focused ultrasonography for trauma (FAST) exams, plain radiography, computed tomography, diagnostic peritoneal lavage or aspiration should be aggressively utilized whenever an indication exists. Operative exploration is an important and very necessary adjunct when these modalities cannot be utilized or are unavailable.

66.1.5 Musculoskeletal and Soft Tissue Injuries

The largest burden of injury following blast events will fall into this category [6]. These can occur by all of the different types of blast effects. The blast wave associated with the primary injury may shear tissues, creating significant hematoma and laceration. Secondary and tertiary types of injury will contribute to the largest burden of injury with possible heavy fragmentation burden depending upon the type of device. Crush injuries due to falling debris may also lead to significant musculoskeletal injury. Finally, quaternary burns may contribute to the burden of musculoskeletal and soft tissue trauma. All of these forces may even act synergistically to contribute to significant tissue loss and non-viability of limbs. This can be the case in muscle compartment injuries with both fragmentation contamination and primary blast effects contributing to compartment syndrome pathology.

You should consider all soft tissue and musculoskeletal wounds as highly contaminated. In addition to shrapnel of unknown source (Figs. 66.2 and 66.3), the presence of dirt, clothing and other significant infectious sources should always be considered. Minimal skin wounds frequently portend extensive underlying soft tissue and bony injury. You should comprehensively examine, debride and irrigate all these wounds. Various imaging should be utilized to identify foreign bodies, underlying fractures and exclude vascular injury. Appropriate tetanus and antibiotic prophylaxis should be given. It is wisest to avoid the temptation of early wound closure or orthopedic internal hardware utilization until the wound has undergone multiple washouts [7] to avoid subsequent infection.

66.2 The Role of Imaging

Perhaps in no other mechanism of trauma is the liberal use of imaging work-up so important to optimal care. The forces at work are highly variable and unpredictable as are the trajectories of the resulting projectile wounds. The classic sequelae of primary blast injury (BLI, hollow viscous injury, TBI) are commonly difficult to detect by exam alone. All modalities of imaging should be liberally utilized whenever an indication exists. FAST use should be routine. Plain radiography can be used to define the shrapnel burden (Figs. 66.4 and 66.5), identify free air in the abdomen that can be associated with hollow viscous injury, and detect the presence of pulmonary contusion/BLI. Thresholds for advanced imaging, including computed tomography and angiography, should be low. In the treatment of servicemembers injured by a blast-related event, the authors of this chapter have routinely utilized comprehensive CT scan of the head, chest, abdomen, pelvis and axial spine as soon as it was available. In cases of neck injuries or extremity injuries with a suspicious vascular exam, liberal use of computed tomography with angiography (CTA) or traditional angiography is also our practice. Using this approach we have identified injuries to all manner of neurologic, vascular, thoracic and abdominal structures that required subsequent intervention; and that we would not have predicted by lesser means. The projectiles from these events simply do not behave the same as those from a hand gun, or even a high powered rifle [8]. We highly recommend that such injuries be respected and evaluated comprehensively with at least a normal CT on a routine basis. Ultimately, exploration is a mainstay when these technologies are unavailable or indeterminate.

Important Points

- Blast injuries are very unpredictable – a high index of suspicion should always be utilized in these patients.
- Soft tissue and musculoskeletal trauma are the most common injuries encountered after blasts, and secondary blast injury is the most common mechanism of injury among those who survive to reach treatment.
- The skin wound is not a reliable indicator of the havoc fragments can cause to the underlying tissues – or the amount of contamination. Comprehensive exploration, washout and debridement is the rule.
- Tympanic membrane rupture is a classic finding of primary blast overpressure injury and should increase suspicion for hollow abdominal viscous injury – but is most likely not as sensitive a marker for TBI or other injury as once proposed.
- Traumatic brain injury is likely underappreciated after blast injuries – have a high index of suspicion.
- Have a low threshold for optholmalagic examination.
- Blast lung injury is a serious but very rare sequelae of primary overpressure blast injuries. Supportive care is the rule and most patients who survive will regain good lung function.
- Avoid the temptation to close wounds early or put in internal fixation devices for orthopedic injuries until the wound is clean – and this will take several washouts.
- Use comprehensive CT evaluation liberally – it will pick up injuries that you would not have suspected and save you from finding them too late.

References

1. Ritenour AE, Baskin TW (2008) Primary blast injury: update on diagnosis and treatment. Crit Care Med 36(7): S311–S317
2. Ritenour AE, Wickley A, Ritenour JS et al (2008) Tympanic membrane perforation and hearing loss from blast overpressure in operation enduring freedom and operation Iraqi freedom wounded. J Trauma 64(2 Suppl):S174–8; discussion S178
3. Almogy G, Mintz Y, Zamir G et al (2006) Suicide bombing attacks: can external signs predict internal injuries? Ann Surg 243:541–546
4. Pizov R, Oppenheim-Eden A, Matot I et al (1999) Blast lung injury from an explosion on a civilian bus. Chest 115: 165–172
5. Hirschberg B, Oppenheim-Eden A, Pizov R et al (1999) Recovery from blast lung injury. Chest 116:1683–1688
6. Bala M, Rivkind AI, Zamir G et al (2008) Abdominal trauma after terrorist bombing attacks exhibits a unique pattern of injury. Ann Surg 248:303–309
7. Langworthy MJ, Smith JM, Gould M (2004) Treatment of the mangled lower extremity after a terrorist blast injury. Clin Orthop Relat Res 422:88–96
8. Aharonson-Daniel L, Klein Y, Peleg K et al (2006) Suicide bombers form a new injury profile. Ann Surg 244: 1018–1023
9. Depalma RG, Burris DG, Champion HR et al (2005) Blast injuries. N Engl J Med 352:1135–42
10. Ramasay Q, Harrison SE, Clasper JC et al (2008) Injuries from roadside explosive devices. J Trauma 65:910–914

The Elderly Patient

67

Thomas Lustenberger and Kenji Inaba

The geriatric population is the fastest growing age group today, and geriatric trauma accounts for a significant proportion of admissions to trauma centers. Due to functional changes with age, preexisting diseases and pre-injury medications, geriatric trauma patients have limited physiological reserves and therefore require much more aggressive evaluation and treatment than their younger counterparts. A low threshold for field triage directly to a trauma center is warranted in elderly trauma patients. The primary and secondary survey follows ATLS guidelines; however, age-related conditions impact patient evaluation. The treatment algorithms for penetrating trauma in the elderly are no different. In any bleeding elderly patient, consider damage control interventions early. Selective non-operative management of penetrating solid organ injuries, applied in many young trauma victims, is more likely to fail in older patients and, in general, should be reserved for low-grade injuries. When managed successfully, a significant number of elderly patients sustaining penetrating trauma will be able to return to levels of reasonable function and thus justify aggressive management.

T. Lustenberger • K. Inaba (✉)
Division of Trauma and Surgical Critical Care,
LAC+USC Medical Center,
1200 North State Street, IPT-C5L100, Los Angeles,
CA 90033-4525, USA
e-mail: tom.lustenberg@gmail.com; kenji.inaba@med.usc.edu

67.1 Definition and Epidemiology

The definition of the elderly patient varies widely in the literature. There is even data suggesting that patients as young as 45 years old may have a poorer outcome than their younger counterparts; however, the most common cutoff is 65 years old [1].

Currently, trauma is the ninth leading cause of death in the elderly. The most common mechanism is falls, followed by motor vehicle crashes, and automobile versus pedestrian collisions [2]. We analyzed the National Trauma Databank containing patient data from more than 900 trauma centers across the United States. Over 320,000 trauma patients aged 65 years and older were identified, accounting for approximately 17% of the trauma population during a 6-year period. The overall mortality rate was 4.4% with 31% of the deaths occurring in those 65 years or older. Although less common than in younger patients, penetrating injuries still represented 1.4% of the geriatric trauma (GSW 72%; SW 3%) with 30% of these being self-inflicted. This number is even higher in urban settings [3].

67.2 Age-Related Physiology and Effect on Trauma: What You Should Know…

Functional changes with age, preexisting diseases and pre-injury medications result in limited physiological reserves and a decreased ability of the elderly patient to mount an adequate response to stress. A summary of anatomic and physiologic changes with aging is provided in Table 67.1 and Fig. 67.1.

G.C. Velmahos et al. (eds.), *Penetrating Trauma*,
DOI 10.1007/978-3-642-20453-1_67, © Springer-Verlag Berlin Heidelberg 2012

Table 67.1 Age-related anatomic and physiologic changes

Central nervous system
• Brain atrophy
• ↑ Subdural space
• ↑ Tension on bridging veins in subdural space
• Adherent epidural space
Cardiac system
• ↓ Cardiac function/output
• ↓ Maximal tachycardic response
• ↓ Response to intrinsic and extrinsic catecholamines
Vascular system
• Thickening and calcification of vessels
• ↓ Elasticity of vessels
Respiratory system
• ↓ Pulmonary compliance
• ↓ Vital capacity
• ↑ Residual capacity
• ↓ Surface area for gas exchange
• ↓ Cough reflex
• ↓ Mucociliary clearance
• ↑ Chest wall rigidity
Renal system
• ↓ Renal mass
• ↓ GFR
• ↓ Response to ADH/aldosterone
• ↓ Urine concentration ability
• ↑ Renal sensitivity to contrast
• ↑ Urethral outflow obstruction
Skeletal system and soft tissue
• Osteoporosis
• Skin atrophy
• ↓ Subcutaneous fat
• ↓ Cutaneous microcirculation
• ↓ Muscle mass

67.2.1 Cardiovascular System

- Cardiac function declines by 50% between the ages of 20 and 80 years, mainly due to increasing myocardial stiffness, slowing of electrophysiologic conduction, and loss of myocardial cell mass. The cardiac index falls off linearly with age and the maximal heart rate begins to decrease from about 40 years of age. The response of the aging myocardium to circulating catecholamines decreases, limiting its ability to maintain cardiac output in the presence of hypovolemia.
- Baseline hypertension is common in the elderly patient; thus a normal blood pressure may actually indicate significant hypovolemia.
- Medications such as β-blockers and calcium channel blockers limit the normal tachycardic response to shock. Chronic use of diuretics results in intravascular depletion and limited intravascular reserve.

67.2.2 Renal System

- There is a progressive loss of renal mass, with a corresponding decrease in creatinine clearance and urine concentrating ability. Although the serum creatinine level may remain normal because of age-related declines in muscle mass, there is a decreased tolerance to hypotension and nephrotoxic drugs.

67.2.3 Respiratory System

- The pulmonary system demonstrates decreased compliance and vital capacity. There is increased dependence on diaphragmatic breathing, increased work of breathing, impaired mucociliary clearance and a reduced ability to cough, all of which decrease the ability to tolerate even minor chest trauma and increase the propensity for developing complications.

67.2.4 Central Nervous System

- The human brain loses approximately 10% of its weight between the ages of 30 and 70 years.
- A decrease in autoregulation of cerebral blood flow increases the vulnerability to cerebral ischemia associated with systemic hypotension and decreases the tolerance to injury.
- Dementia and other underlying chronic CNS diseases (e.g. degenerative brain disease, hydrocephalus, cerebrovascular disease, etc.) may make the clinical evaluation difficult.

67.3 The Geriatric Patient in the Field: Prehospital Evaluation

The injured geriatric patient should not be exposed to prolonged field stabilization attempts at the expense of transport time. The triage process begins in the field, where prehospital providers must decide on the basis

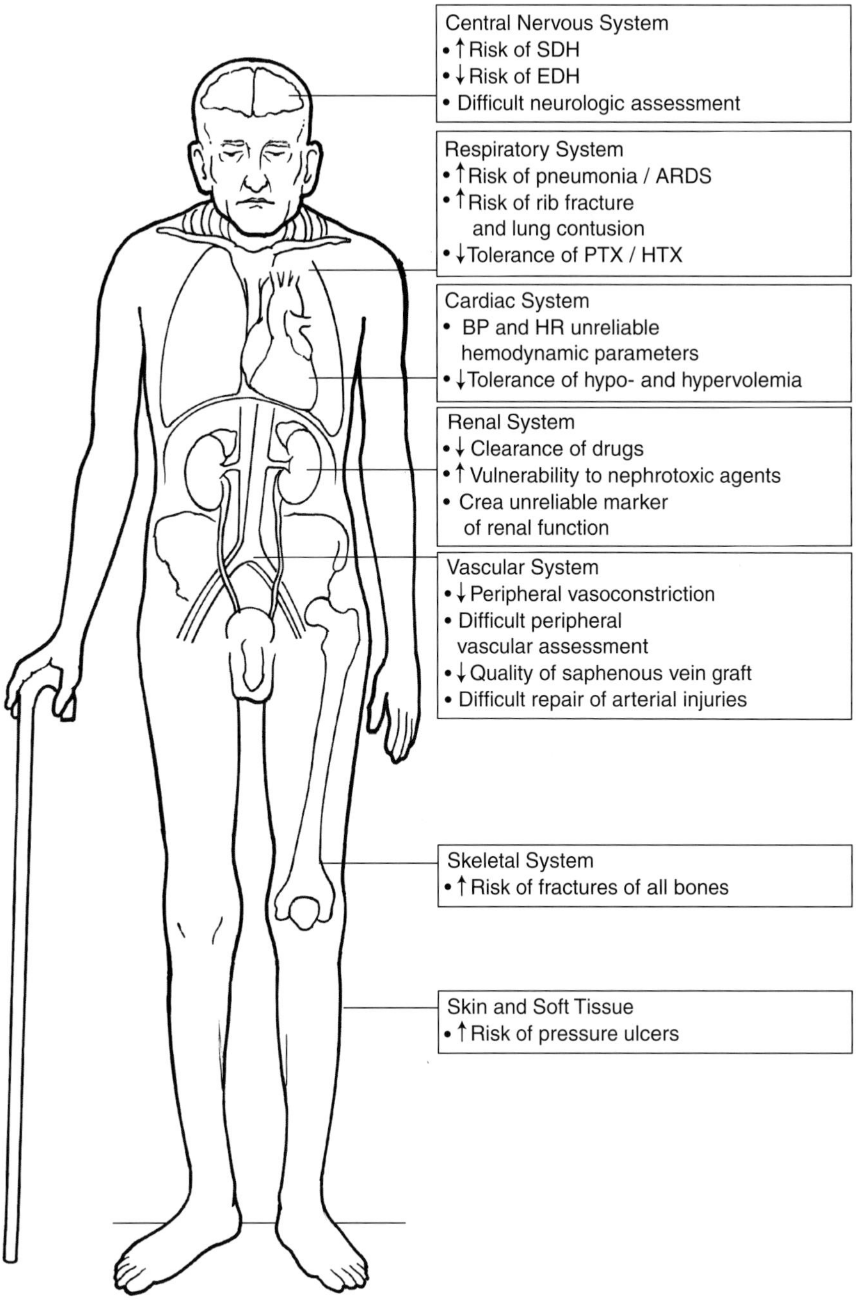

Fig. 67.1 Clinical consequences of age-related changes

of very little clinical information whether a patient should bypass nearby facilities in favor of a designated trauma center. The American College of Surgeons Committee on Trauma recommends patients greater than 55 be considered for transport directly to a verified trauma center, irrespective of the severity of injury [4]. This recommendation is based on the finding that there is a sharp increase in mortality that occurs at this age independent of injury severity, mechanism, and body region involved. Unfortunately, several studies have documented that the opposite may actually be occurring with elderly trauma patients being frequently undertriaged to non-trauma hospitals putting them at risk for admission to a level of care that may be unsuitable [5, 6]. In one study, trauma patients over the age 65 were half as likely as younger patients with similar injuries to be transported to a designated trauma center [5]. In another recent study, undertriage in patients older than 70 years was five times higher than in those younger than 70 years old [6].

67.4 The Geriatric Patient in the Emergency Room: Initial Evaluation and Management

67.4.1 Trauma Team Activation: Be Ready!

On admission, geriatric trauma patients warrant rapid and aggressive evaluation by your trauma team. In a recent clinical series, traditional hemodynamic criteria for mobilizing the trauma team demonstrated 63% of patients aged 70 or above and with an ISS>15 were missed by traditional physiologic criteria [7]. In a follow-up before and after study, for patients older than 70 with an ISS>15, the authors examined the impact of including age alone (>70 years old) as a criteria for activation of the trauma team. This age trigger, resulting in the presence of an attending trauma surgeon and ER physician at patient arrival, continuous cardiopulmonary monitoring and attending or senior resident presence at the bedside at all times, resulted in a significant decrease in mortality from 53.8 to 34.2%, $p = 0.003$ [8]. So for elderly patients, have your trauma team ready when an elderly patient arrives.

67.5 Primary Survey: The "Geriatric ABCs"

In general, the primary survey in the geriatric patient does not differ from that in the younger patient and adheres to the ATLS protocol. However, preexisting comorbidities and medications may impact patient evaluation (Table 67.2).

Airway management: The elderly have a significant loss of protective airway reflexes and therefore aspiration is more common. Mouth opening may be limited, and immobility of the cervical spine, due to stiffening of the atlanto–occipital joint, may make visualization of the glottis during orotracheal intubation difficult. Deterioration of the gums may increase the chance of damage to the teeth. Additionally, many elderly individuals wear dentures. If these become dislodged, airway obstruction may result. Removal of dentures often results in difficulty with mask fit during assisted ventilation. Accordingly, you should leave in place well fitting dentures to assist mask ventilation, but should remove them for intubation.

Breathing: Due to reduced pulmonary reserves, respiratory decompensation may occur rapidly in the

Table 67.2 Preexisting conditions and possible systemic medications and their clinical consequences

Preexisting conditions and comments	Systemic medications and comments
Dementia • Difficult neurologic assessment	*Cholinergics, antidepressants* • ↓ Seizure threshold • ECG changes
Prior stroke • Neurologic deficits	*Aspirin, clopidogrel, warfarin* • ↑ Bleeding
Arterial hypertension • Normal BP may signify hypotension *Heart failure* • Exclude myocardial infarction • Expect arrhythmias	*β-blocker, calcium channel blocker, ACE inhibitor, diuretics, antiarrythmics* • ↓ Tachycardic response • ↓ Peripheral vasoconstriction → ↑ bleeding
Peripheral vascular disease • Difficult vascular assessment and repair	*Aspirin, Clopidogrel, Warfarin* • ↑ Bleeding
Chronic obstructive pulmonary disease (COPD) • Hypoxia, hypercarbia • Early intubation and ventilation	*Steroids* • ↓ PLT function → ↑ bleeding • ↓ Wound healing • ↑ Infection
Chronic renal failure • Fluid overload • Hypertension • Electrolyte disturbance • Contrast induced nephropathy	*Diuretics, antihypertensives* • Exclude electrolyte disturbances • ↓ Intravascular volume → ↓ tolerance of hypovolemia
Diabetes mellitus • Exclude hypoglycemia • Difficult neuro-vascular assessment	*Hypoglycemics* • Check serum glucose
Osteoporosis • ↑ Fractures • Careful intubation (C – spine precautions!)	–
Rheumatoid arthritis • ↑ Difficulty in opening mouth → Difficult intubation	*NSAID, steroids, immunosuppressives* • ↓ PLT function → ↑ bleeding • ↓ Wound healing • ↑ Infection • Monitor renal function closely

geriatric patient. Rule out early penetrating chest injuries resulting in a pneumothorax or hemothorax as they are less well tolerated in the elderly patient. Although the prevalence of COPD is increased in the elderly trauma population, you should not withhold oxygen therapy because of the theoretical concern of CO_2 retention. Consider intubation and respiratory support early in borderline cases, especially prior to inter or intra-hospital transportation. The doses of most sedative agents used to facilitate intubation should be reduced to minimize the risk of cardiac depression and hypotension. On the other hand, the doses of neuromuscular blockers usually remain unchanged.

Circulation: Due to age-related conditions such as hypertension and medications such as β-blockers, the initial blood pressure and pulse rate may be misleadingly "normal" and can give you a false sense of security. Elderly individuals tend to be normally hypertensive. So if they are not, your index of suspicion for blood loss must be high. A hypertensive elderly patient will decompensate far more rapidly than their younger counterparts. It has been shown that a significant number of "clinically stable" geriatric patients are actually in occult cardiogenic shock [9]. Keep in mind that a narrowed pulse pressure or altered mental status may be the only initial signs of serious hemorrhage. In the injured elderly patient, any degree of hypovolemia may be potentially lethal. Severe coronary artery disease in combination with bleeding has a high likelihood of resulting in acute myocardial ischemia, which will exacerbate the hemorrhagic shock. Thus, your initial approach to the geriatric trauma patient should include rapid intravenous access, laboratory evaluation of baseline and trending hemoglobins, base deficit and renal function. Liberal usage of packed red blood cells and autotransfusion of shed pleural blood should be considered. To facilitate this, initiate the crossmatching process early. Because of the risk of potentiating inflammatory complications such as ARDS, and in the elderly patient particularly, the risk of overload, avoid massive crystalloid resuscitation. Although not a reliable marker of fluid status in the elderly, urine output can still provide clinically relevant information and should be monitored. Foley catheter placement is particularly important in males with urethral outflow obstruction. At the same time as the resuscitation, even if hemodynamic monitoring is within normal limits, rapid assessment for hemorrhage is required.

Disability: It may be difficult to establish new neurologic changes from baseline. Many elderly patients have preexisting focal neurologic deficits such as residual weakness from a previous cerebral vascular incident or a more global deficit from dementia. Additionally, glaucoma, prior cataract surgery, and systemic medications can confuse the geriatric ophthalmologic examination. However, never assume that an alteration in mental status is due to chronic or age-related changes. Impending shock or hypoxia as possible causes of a pathologic neurologic examination must be considered.

Exposure: Take the time to obtain and monitor an accurate core temperature. Due to muscle loss and a decrease in subcutaneous tissue, geriatric patients can drop their temperature very quickly. Appropriate steps to prevent this serious complication include warm blankets and warmed fluids, as well as warmed, humidified oxygen. Due to poorly perfused skin, care must be exercised with any direct contact of skin with external heating devices.

67.6 Secondary Survey: Makes a Whole Lot of Difference When Done Properly!

The secondary survey also strictly follows ATLS guidelines. Expose (roll early in penetrating trauma to check the back for wounds), find and catalog all penetrating injuries to determine which body regions are at risk of injury and require treatment. Any hemodynamically unstable patient with a penetrating injury should be taken immediately to the OR. If hemodynamically stable, proceed to a complete incident and past medical history with current medications and allergies. The EMS crew may be the sole source of clinical information and should be interviewed thoroughly while still in the ED. Contact information for family members, neighbors or primary health care providers should be obtained. When possible, advance directives and a legal representative should be documented. Surgical scars may provide you with some basic information in cases where the history is unavailable. For example, a sternotomy scar may be a clue of prior surgery for valvular or coronary disease, and a longitudinal surgical scar on the inner aspect of thigh may be a sign of harvested saphenous vein.

67.7 Laboratory Studies and Corrective Measures

Send blood for a complete blood count, crossmatching, coagulation profile, troponin, and an ABG. Patients on antiplatelet therapy or other anticoagulants are at high risk for bleeding from any given injury. Any patient on a platelet inhibitor with evidence of bleeding requires immediate platelet transfusion. If the patient is on warfarin, start infusing plasma or prothrombin complex concentrate to improve clotting. Additionally, fluid and electrolyte disorders are not uncommon in the elderly patient and should therefore carefully be screened for and corrected.

67.8 General Management

During resuscitation, the geriatric patient may easily go from normotensive to hypotensive with cardiovascular collapse. On the other hand, over-resuscitation may result in overloading and likewise cardiac failure. Given the geriatric patient's decreased physiologic reserves, close monitoring with a low threshold for early invasive monitoring should be considered. In the EAST guidelines, based on data extracted primarily from blunt trauma populations, Jacobs et al. recommend invasive hemodynamic monitoring using a pulmonary artery catheter for any geriatric patient with physiologic compromise, significant injury (AIS > 3), high-risk mechanism of injury, uncertain cardiovascular status, or chronic cardiovascular or renal disease [1]. Early invasive monitoring has been associated with improved survival in the geriatric trauma patient. Scalea et al. compared elderly, multiple injured blunt trauma patients who appeared clinically stable after initial evaluation and who underwent early invasive monitoring with historical controls. Of these, 43% were found to be in cardiogenic shock despite "normal" vital signs. With early aggressive monitoring and intervention, mortality was reduced by half [9]. Consequently, at our center, all patients ≥70 years of age, irrespective of injury mechanism, are immediately transferred to the surgical ICU for monitoring, with liberal use of pulmonary artery catheterization and echocardiography.

67.9 Surgical Management: No Patient Is "Too Old" for Surgery

The specific management of penetrating injuries to the chest, abdomen, neck and extremities follows the same principles as for younger patients. For penetrating injuries to the abdomen, age is not a contraindication for non-operative management. In the elderly patient however, you should have a low threshold for surgical intervention as they will not be able to tolerate the delayed diagnosis of clinically significant injuries as well. In addition, because peritonitis on clinical examination is a contraindication to non-operative management, care must be taken in the elderly because altered pain perception may make peritoneal signs less prominent after hollow viscus or vascular injury. For penetrating injury to the extremity, underlying peripheral vascular disease may make the clinical assessment difficult. On your examination include the contralateral extremity. This includes the presence and strength of peripheral pulses, warmth of the extremity, presence of capillary filling and the ankle-brachial index. If the examination is not completely normal or is asymmetric, CT angiography, duplex or traditional angiography depending on local resources is mandated. Collateral flow is important in the elderly patient and while often poorly appreciated may mitigate certain injury patterns in this age group.

Despite their diminished physiologic reserve and the greater incidence and severity of concomitant disease, never consider a patient as "too old" for anesthesia or surgical intervention based on age criteria alone. The comorbidities and physiologic status may, however, make the anesthesia and surgical stress more challenging. In addition, previous surgeries may result in significant anatomic distortion or adhesions. A laparotomy, sternotomy or thoracotomy scar means that access may be difficult, especially in the bleeding patient. Vessels with atherosclerotic lesions may be fragile, posing an increased risk of intraoperative hemorrhage and iatrogenic injury.

In general, consider damage control early in any bleeding elderly patient! This may be life saving. Quick termination of hemorrhage and contamination, aggressive resuscitation, temporary closure, and normalization in the surgical ICU should be your algorithm by default. All elderly patients sustaining moderate or severe injury should be admitted to the surgical ICU.

67.10 The "Old, Injured Solid Organ" and Non-operative Management: A Matter of Controversy

In younger evaluable trauma victims, selective non-operative management (SNOM) of penetrating solid organ injuries is evolving after vascular and hollow viscus injuries have been ruled out [10, 11]. It has been shown that almost 30% of penetrating injuries to the liver can safely be managed non-operatively in the appropriate trauma center environment. Likewise, 15% of penetrating injuries to the kidney can be successfully managed non-operatively. Even high-grade solid organ injuries (grades III–V) did not preclude non-operative management [10]. However, for elderly patients, there is very little literature regarding the optimal management strategy for penetrating solid organ injuries. The elderly patient with limited reserves is most likely not an ideal candidate for SNOM if there is a known solid organ injury.

In blunt trauma, age >55 years has been demonstrated to be a predictor for failure of non-operative management of splenic trauma. Anatomically, older spleens have a weakened capsule and fragile vasculature secondary to a decrease in the amount of smooth muscle and elastin fibers. A large, multicenter study concluded that older patients fail SNOM more often than their younger counterparts, and those who do suffer increased mortality and morbidity [12]. Therefore, for penetrating trauma, we are hesitant to attempt SNOM in anything but low-grade injuries.

67.11 Diagnostic Imaging

In general, imaging considerations for the elderly penetrating trauma patient are similar to those for younger patients, driven by the injury and management plan rather than by age. Different modalities including ultrasound, plain radiography and CT are all utilized with the same indications. One issue that you need to consider, however, is contrast induced nephropathy (CIN). The elderly are often volume depleted, enhancing the impact of IV contrast administration. Well-identified risk factors for CIN include preexisting renal insufficiency, diabetes mellitus, hypotension, heart failure, and age greater than 75 years. Thus, if contrast is required, take precautions to reduce the risk of CIN with volume expansion, premedication with bicarbonate or *N*-Acetylcysteine, minimizing the dose of contrast media, and maximizing the time interval between procedures [13]. In selecting the imaging modality, for example in the assessment of penetrating injuries to the lower extremity, rather than using traditional catheter-based angiography, use CT angiography (CTA) whenever possible. With equivalent sensitivity, the CTA allows bilateral extremity runoff views with less contrast and no damage to the fragile elderly groin vasculature. Finally, when you send an elderly trauma patient to the radiology suite for multiple investigations, monitor the patient closely and continuously – even if it is a patient with "fairly minor" injuries. A sudden deterioration may occur in this suboptimal environment.

67.12 Outcomes

Both short- and long-term outcomes after trauma are worse in geriatric patients when compared with their younger counterparts. Their reduced physiologic reserves, as well as the higher prevalence of preexisting medical conditions, are thought to account for these poor outcomes. Although the data are predominantly from blunt trauma patients, age itself seems to have some value for predicting outcome. Kuhne et al. observed an increase in mortality with age 56 years and above, independent of injury severity [14]. However, to date, there is not enough literature to support a specific age cut-off beyond which hospital mortality rises with any degree of confidence. Preexisting conditions such as liver disease, renal dysfunction, malignancy, heart disease, and chronic obstructive pulmonary disease have all been shown to increase the risk of death in elderly trauma patients [15]. However, since the frequency of preexisting conditions does increase with age, it is difficult to separate these two factors and determine their independent relationship with adverse outcomes. Although very little data on outcomes in penetrating trauma are available, in a study from the Cook County group, patients ≥65 years old had a mortality rate of 8.2% when compared to matched younger patients with a rate of 3.5% [3].

When looking at specific injuries and outcome, have these additional points in mind:

- For patients that sustain both penetrating injury and a concomitant head injury, elderly patients with traumatic brain injury have an increased mortality and a worse functional outcome when compared to their younger counterparts with the same or less severe injuries [1].

- Mortality and pneumonia rates following thoracic trauma are high in the elderly. A retrospective analysis studying patients ≥65 years with rib fractures after blunt chest trauma demonstrated twice the mortality and thoracic morbidity than younger patients with similar injuries. For each additional rib fracture, mortality increased by 19% and the risk of pneumonia by 27% [16]. For penetrating chest trauma, the collateral data from blunt patients have forced us to be very vigilant in the elderly patient.

Following penetrating trauma, it has been shown that older patients arriving alive at the hospital are as likely to survive as their younger counterparts who have injuries of similar severity. However, these results are usually achieved at the expense of more resources due to longer intensive care unit and hospital length of stays [3, 17]. The long-term outcome after trauma in the geriatric patient has been the subject of several studies. McGwin et al. showed that the increased risk of death in elderly trauma patients persists for up to 6 years from the time of hospitalization for injury [18]. Furthermore, trauma has a significant impact on long-term quality of life in geriatric trauma survivors. Most importantly, a loss of independence was seen at long-term follow-up [19]. Nevertheless, a significant number of elderly patients who survive their acute injury are able to return to levels of reasonable function, and often the help of home care agencies, spouses, and family members allows these patients to remain living at home. Therefore, aggressive treatment of elderly patients after penetrating trauma with the goal of discharge to home is warranted.

Important Points

- Advanced age should lower the threshold for field triage directly to a trauma center.
- Never underestimate the risks of seemingly insignificant trauma in geriatric patients. The geriatric trauma victim has limited physiologic reserves and, as such, "minor" injuries may prove life-threatening.
- Always obtain a detailed medical history from the paramedics, the family and the patient. Ask specifically about β-blockers, cardiac or antihypertensive medication, anticoagulants, and antiplatelet agents.
- Consider a liberal policy of endotracheal intubation and respiratory support in patients with severe trauma and "normal" respiratory function. Elderly patients often decompensate rapidly.
- Blood pressure and pulse may not be reliable hemodynamic parameters due to preexisting heart disease and cardiac medications.
- Early aggressive hemodynamic monitoring in the geriatric trauma patient is critical and can improve outcomes.
- The abdominal examination is more difficult in the elderly trauma patient due to a blunting of peritoneal signs. Consider liberal use of CT-scanning with renal protection.
- Never underestimate the importance of "minor" head injuries. There is a high incidence of intracranial pathology. Subdural hematomas may manifest clinically later than in younger patients. Consider liberal head CT scanning.
- Many aged patients have preexisting neurologic deficits that can interfere with the physical examination.
- Never send a geriatric trauma patient even with fairly "minor" injuries, from the emergency department to the radiology suite without close continuous monitoring. Sudden deterioration may occur in a suboptimal environment.
- The geriatric trauma patient is at special risk for contrast-induced nephropathy. Take appropriate precautions.
- Non-operative management of penetrating solid organ injuries may be less successful than in younger trauma patients.
- Do not give up because of age; a significant proportion of elderly patients survive after penetrating trauma and are successfully discharged home.

References

1. Jacobs DG, Plaisier BR, Barie PS et al (2003) Practice management guidelines for geriatric trauma: the EAST practice management guidelines work group. J Trauma 54:391–416
2. United States Census Bureau (2008) Age groups and sex 2008. United States Census Bureau, Washington, DC
3. Nagy KK, Smith RF, Roberts RR et al (2000) Prognosis of penetrating trauma in elderly patients: a comparison with younger patients. J Trauma 49:190–193; discussion 193–194
4. American College of Surgeons, Committee on Trauma (1999) Resources for optimal care of the injured patient. American College of Surgeons, Chicago
5. Chang DC, Bass RR, Cornwell EE et al (2008) Undertriage of elderly trauma patients to state-designated trauma centers. Arch Surg 143:776–781; discussion 782
6. Rehn M, Eken T, Kruger AJ et al (2009) Precision of field triage in patients brought to a trauma centre after introducing trauma team activation guidelines. Scand J Trauma Resusc Emerg Med 17:1
7. Demetriades D, Sava J, Alo K et al (2001) Old age as a criterion for trauma team activation. J Trauma 51:754–756; discussion 756–757
8. Demetriades D, Karaiskakis M, Velmahos G et al (2002) Effect on outcome of early intensive management of geriatric trauma patients. Br J Surg 89:1319–1322
9. Scalea TM, Simon HM, Duncan AO et al (1990) Geriatric blunt multiple trauma: improved survival with early invasive monitoring. J Trauma 30:129–134; discussion 134–136
10. Demetriades D, Hadjizacharia P, Constantinou C et al (2006) Selective nonoperative management of penetrating abdominal solid organ injuries. Ann Surg 244:620–628
11. Velmahos GC, Toutouzas KG, Radin R et al (2003) Nonoperative treatment of blunt injury to solid abdominal organs: a prospective study. Arch Surg 138:844–851
12. Harbrecht BG, Peitzman AB, Rivera L et al (2001) Contribution of age and gender to outcome of blunt splenic injury in adults: multicenter study of the eastern association for the surgery of trauma. J Trauma 51:887–895
13. Callaway DW, Wolfe R (2007) Geriatric trauma. Emerg Med Clin North Am 25:837–860
14. Kuhne CA, Ruchholtz S, Kaiser GM et al (2005) Working group on multiple trauma of the German Society of Trauma. Mortality in severely injured elderly trauma patients-when does age become a risk factor? World J Surg 29:1476–1482
15. Grossman MD, Miller D, Scaff DW et al (2002) When is an elder old? Effect of preexisting conditions on mortality in geriatric trauma. J Trauma 52:242–246
16. Bulger EM, Arneson MA, Mock CN et al (2000) Rib fractures in the elderly. J Trauma 48:1040–1046; discussion 1046–1047
17. Roth BJ, Velmahos GC, Oder DB et al (2001) Penetrating trauma in patients older than 55 years: a case-control study. Injury 32:551–554
18. McGwin G Jr, Melton SM, May AK et al (2000) Long-term survival in the elderly after trauma. J Trauma 49:470–476
19. Inaba K, Goecke M, Sharkey P et al (2003) Long-term outcomes after injury in the elderly. J Trauma 54:486–491

The Pediatric Patient

68

Graeme Pitcher

The landscape of penetrating pediatric injury will vary depending on the community in which you practice surgery. In developing countries especially those characterized by civil strife and political change for example South Africa, Central Africa and the Middle East, children get caught up in the vortex of violence and are injured by bullets, shrapnel from explosives and blast injury. The pattern of injury in these groups may be similar to the injuries seen in adult victims but are often much more severe due to the greater injuring capacity of weapons on such small bodies.

In most developed countries, children are injured in two discrete patterns (Table 68.1): as adolescents usually in inner city areas where they get caught up in the crime and drug culture; and younger children who are usually the victims of accidental injury although deliberate homicide attempts are occasionally seen. These children (usually boys!) are sometimes injured by a bizarre array of different missiles and devices, sometimes of their own making such as homemade bombs and explosives. An accurate history of the injuring agent is essential to understand and treat the patient when they present.

G. Pitcher
Division of Pediatric Surgery, Department of Surgery, University of Iowa Children's Hospital, Iowa City, USA

Department of Surgery, Roy J. and Lucille A. Carver College of Medicine, 200 Hawkins Drive, Iowa City, IA 52242-1086, USA
e-mail: graeme-pitcher@uiowa.edu

68.1 Resuscitation

Resuscitation should be performed in a swift and goal-oriented manner. One of the worst errors you can make is spending too much time with a bleeding patient in the emergency room and delaying operative hemostasis. In unstable patients, an airway should be secured, good venous access (Table 68.2) obtained by the quickest and simplest technique applicable and resuscitation commenced. It is usually clear to an experienced surgeon that the patient is not responding to resuscitation and the trip to the operating room should be undertaken without further delay. The patient must be kept warm and packed red blood cells and other hematological products should be prepared for. The decision as to which body cavity or limb needs to be explored is usually clear after examination and initial resuscitation. Chest tubes can be placed with local anesthetic even in uncooperative children and should be placed as resuscitative measures to avoid tension pneumothorax or hemothorax. Because of the thin anterior abdominal wall of most children, a large hemoperitoneum is usually clinically obvious. Trips to the CT scanner are hazardous in this situation and you will almost always regret them – rarely will you regret the absence of imaging information!

68.2 Resuscitative Thoracotomy

The place of emergency department thoracotomy is an ongoing controversy in the management of the injured patient. I prefer to think of it as a resuscitative thoracotomy (RT), indicating its role as an adjunct to resuscitation when the patient does not respond to conventional

G.C. Velmahos et al. (eds.), *Penetrating Trauma*,
DOI 10.1007/978-3-642-20453-1_68, © Springer-Verlag Berlin Heidelberg 2012

Table 68.1 Patterns of penetrating injury in children and adolescents

Adolescents	Children
Gunshot wounds homicidal	Accidental gunshot injuries
Gunshot wounds suicidal	Gunshot wounds homicidal
Stab injuries usually with knives or similar	Penetrating stab injuries
	Arrows and other missiles
	Nonpowder gun injuries
	Blast injuries
	Impalements

Table 68.2 Stepwise approach to venous access in severely injured child

Stepwise approach to venous access in severely injured child
• Peripheral IV with the largest size needle possible
– Long saphenous vein
– Cephalic or basilic veins
– External jugular vein
• Percutaneous central line by Seldinger stick
– Subclavian vein
– Internal jugular vein
– Femoral vein
• Intraosseous access
• Direct venous cutdown as a last resort

resuscitation. Previously, children were assumed to have greater physiological reserve and hence RT was applied liberally in an attempt to salvage desperate situations but this usually failed or, even worse, produced survivors with neurologic compromise. Cumulative experience to date indicates that RT should be reserved for the following categories of pediatric patients after penetrating trauma:

1. Penetrating thoracic injury with deterioration or poor response despite vigorous resuscitation.
2. Patients with penetrating thoracic injury who present with no signs of life to the emergency room but with a recently witnessed cardiac arrest.

Under these circumstances, salvage rates of between 4% and 26% can be expected depending on the mechanism of injury and local circumstances. Children with penetrating abdominal injuries who do not respond to resuscitation should be transferred immediately to the operating room for laparotomy. It is my experience that children who receive a thoracotomy followed by laparotomy under these circumstances have a dismal prognosis and are best treated by laparotomy alone.

68.2.1 Technique

The technique is essentially the same as in the adult. The patient is positioned in the supine position with the selected side (usually left to facilitate direct cardiac massage) elevated on a bolster and the arm on that side elevated. After skin preparation an incision is made with a cold knife as an anterolateral thoracotomy below the line of the nipple. The incision is carried through all layers and the pleura is opened with a scissors to avoid injury to the lung. A Finochetto retractor or rib spreader is placed. The pericardium is picked up between hemostats, taking care to avoid injury to the phrenic nerve and opened with a scissor if necessary to release tamponade or to allow internal cardiac massage. Aortic clamping is best achieved with a gently curved aortic clamp. Bleeding from hilar vessels can be controlled temporarily by the firm application of an angled vascular clamp. If it is necessary to cross the sternum and perform a clamshell incision [1] to improve access to the heart or to enter the other side, this can be done quite easily in a child by using a strong curved scissors or bone cutting shears due to the incompletely calcified bone.

68.3 The Abdomen

Whereas one may sometimes deliberate over the decision of the best incision for abdominal access for other conditions, in penetrating trauma the answer is easy (even in small children) – the *midline laparotomy* (Fig. 68.1). This will give you the best access to the entire abdominal cavity including the aortic hiatus and pelvis; can be easily extended when you inevitably encounter the unexpected (into a sternotomy or thoracoabdominal incision); and heals in a durable and acceptable fashion. If necessary you can leave the incision open in the context of abdominal compartment syndrome, leaving you the easiest closure later. Remember to prepare and drape the patient from knees to chin to allow access to the femoral vessels, neck and chest if required. Make sure that the operating room is heated to at least 26–28°C and keep the patient warm with active warming devices. Mechanical retractors can make the difference between success and failure and should be available from the start. In cases of vigorous bleeding, autotransfusion appears to be a helpful adjunct to these patients care.

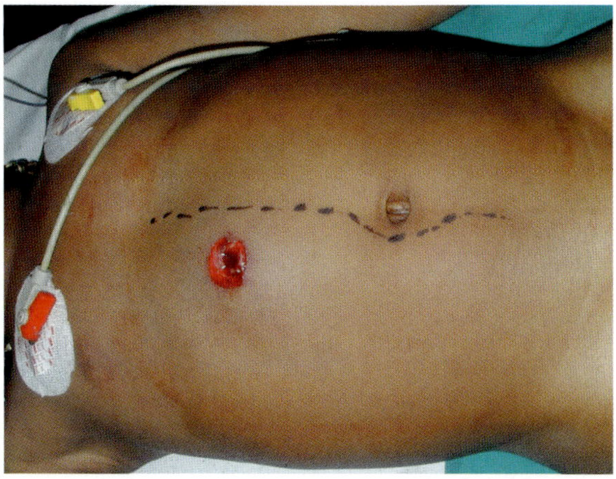

Fig. 68.1 Midline laparotomy gives you best access to the child's abdomen

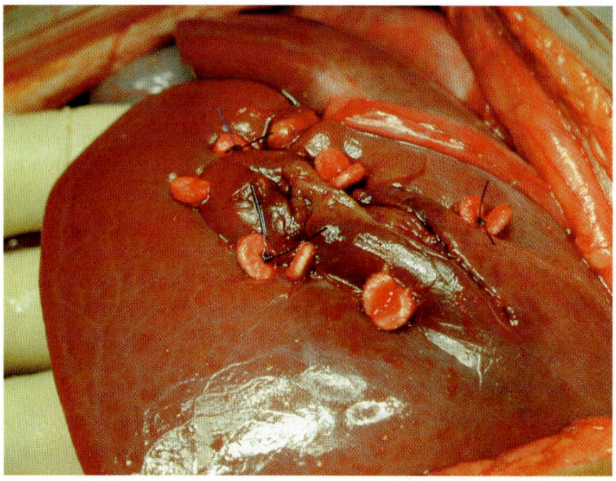

Fig. 68.2 In most peoples' hands and in most circumstances, bleeding from liver wounds is most safely treated by packing or by simple suture techniques

In most cases, definitive surgery can be performed in children with penetrating abdominal injuries as they are less likely to develop a systemic inflammatory response syndrome (SIRS) or organ dysfunction than their similarly injured adult counterparts and will generally have the physiological reserves to tolerate the additional time on the operating table. In cases with an established coagulopathy and hypothermia, damage control techniques can be life saving [2].

68.3.1 Practical Advice and Pitfalls with the Abdomen

1. Ensure you use an adequate sized foley catheter to allow for good drainage – not the smallest size available!
2. When stomas are necessary, always ensure meticulous parastomal closure between the fascia and the bowel – the small bowel of a young child is like a puppy and can escape through the smallest defects!
3. Drain as little as possible – only for anticipated bile, urine or pancreatic leak and ongoing bleeding from parenchymal organs – not for bowel anastomoses.
4. In most peoples' hands and in most circumstances, bleeding from liver wounds is most safely treated by packing or by simple suture techniques (Fig. 68.2). Major liver resections in the context of hypovolemia are dangerous and usually unnecessary.
5. Splenic injury can be treated by salvage in many cases but do not compromise the safety of your operation, particularly in an older child (>12) who will tolerate having their spleen out with a low risk of overwhelming infection.
6. Nonexpanding renal hematomas can be left alone. If you enter them you will probably end up removing the kidney!
7. Do the simplest operation to achieve your goal.
8. Do not make two bowel anastomoses to preserve a short segment of bowel in a patient with normal length – resect it and do a single anastomosis.
9. Close with continuous monofilament suture of adequate size (1 for adolescents, 0 for 7–12 years, 2/0 for 3–7 years, 3/0 for 0.5–3 years and 4/0 for small infants and neonates).
10. Use a headlight and optical magnification – 2.5× loupes allow you a broader field if you wish, but also allow you to see exactly what you are doing.

68.3.2 The Place for Laparoscopy

We (almost) all strive to treat our patients with the smallest incision and the least invasive approach. The laparoscope can be a useful tool but *only in the stable patient*!

The main role in my opinion is diagnostic: to assess in cases *where it is clinically not clear* whether:

1. There has been penetration of the abdominal cavity by a missile or sharp object.

2. There has been diaphragmatic injury (with the potential to present many years later with strangulation in a diaphragmatic hernia).

Laparoscopy in such patients will avoid many unnecessary explorations and avoid the embarrassment of missed diaphragmatic injuries.

Its role as a therapeutic intervention is increasing as surgeons become more practiced. You can certainly start an exploration of a patient with a worrisome abdomen by the placement of a port and laparoscopy. You can run the bowel to search for injury with reasonable confidence and you can even repair intestinal injuries intracorporeally or exteriorize them for anastomosis extracorporeally. Ultimately what you do will depend on how well you can visualize the abdominal cavity and how confident you are in repairing the injuries that you find. For most surgeons laparotomy remains the gold standard to deal with injuries in most patients.

68.3.3 The Place for Selective Conservatism

For the vast majority of children who are shot in the abdomen with a rifle or handgun, laparotomy is mandatory and the incidence of negative explorations is low once missile penetration has been established. Stab wounds or other impalement injuries can be managed conservatively if patients are stable, if there are no signs of peritonitis and no omental or intestinal evisceration. The relative large size of the blade in a small child makes this scenario uncommon and frequently wounds will need to be closed in the operating room to repair evisceration. That is a good time to use laparoscopy to ensure there are no serious intra-abdominal injuries.

68.4 Penetrating Thoracic Injury

As in adults, most children with injuries penetrating the thoracic cavity can be managed by tube drainage alone [3]. The indications for thoracotomy are essentially the same as for the adult patient. Patients with gunshot injuries may require operation more frequently especially in the younger age groups [4]. Accepted indications for thoracotomy include:

1. Brisk thoracic hemorrhage and ongoing hemodynamic instability or deterioration
2. Evidence of cardiac tamponade or post-traumatic pericardial effusion
3. Evidence of major airway injury
4. Evidence of esophageal injury

Table 68.3 Recommended chest tube sizes by age

Age	Size (Fr)
0–3 months	10–12
3–18 months	12–16
18–24 months	18
2–4 years	20–22
4–6 years	22–24
6–8 years	24–28
8–12 years	28–30
12–16 years	30–34

Ongoing bleeding requiring blood transfusion of greater than 50% of blood volume or at a rate of greater than 1–2 mL/kg/h may be an indication for thoracotomy depending on the circumstances. You need to carefully consider which incision to use for access. If you need to get to both pleural cavities or the central mediastinal structures including the great vessels and their immediate branches, then median sternotomy is preferable.

68.4.1 Technique of Insertion of a Chest Tube

The standard position recommended for intercostal drain placement is the fifth intercostal space in the anterior axillary line. You can be sure that the young child will be uncooperative with regard to the drain in the recovery period! For this reason the drain should be well secured by both suture and skin strapping to ensure that it stays put. The skin incision should be placed one intercostal space below the intended space of chest entry to ensure a tunneled subcutaneous tract. When the drain is removed, direct pressure on the subcutaneous tract prevents iatrogenic pneumothorax in a crying child. The drain should be placed primarily by blunt dissection and trocars are not used to avoid iatrogenic injury. The recommended size of intercostal drains at various ages is shown in Table 68.3

68.4.2 Practical Advice and Pitfalls with the Chest

1. Secure tubes diligently. Even then the child can pull them out.
2. Always create a tunneled tract to limit the risk of post-removal pneumothorax.
3. When removing a drain in an uncooperative child, clamp drain closed with a hemostat, surround exit site with paraffin gauze dressing and pull drain

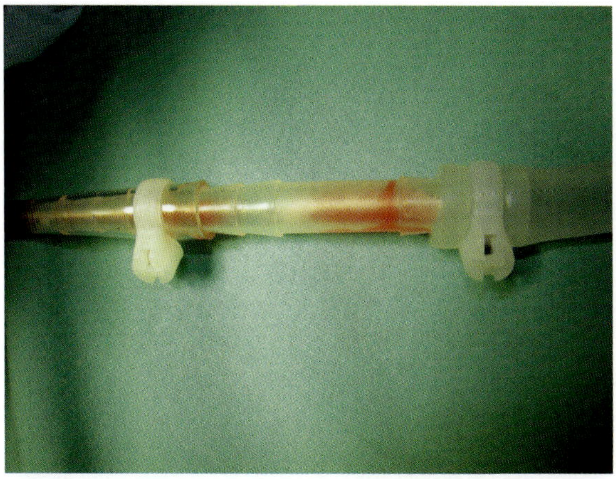

Fig. 68.3 Cable ties used to secure chest tube to drainage tube

swiftly while applying pressure with gauze on track. Apply an occlusive dressing. Attempts to tie sutures will often result in iatrogenic pneumothorax.
4. Secure chest tubes to the drainage tubing with cable ties (Fig. 68.3) or something similarly secure.
5. Median sternotomies give good access in small children and are useful if you need access to both pleural cavities or the mediastinal structures.
6. Clamshell incisions must be closed by careful re-alignment of the sternum with wires to ensure an acceptable cosmetic result.
7. Pulmonary lacerations in children are easily controlled by the application of a linear cutting stapler device.
8. Whenever there is an unexplained pleural collection suspect esophageal injury – you will be surprised (horrified?) at how often you are right.

68.5 Penetrating Neck Injuries

The approach to penetrating cervical injuries in children is essentially the same as in adults.

68.5.1 Practical Advice and Pitfalls with the Neck

1. Small children are more likely to experience airway compromise as a result of swelling or hemorrhage into the airway and surrounding tissues.
2. If you need to place a tracheotomy, take particular care to select the size correctly. If you select too *large* a catheter it will tend to be too *long* as well and may intubate the right main bronchus. Also as with all tubes in children – secure it thoroughly.
3. The transverse collar incision can be useful for trans-cervical injuries of Zone 2, particularly when good access to the larynx and pharynx are needed and when access to the base of the skull is unlikely to be necessary. The apron (vertical anterior sterno-mastoid bilateral incision with inferior transverse bridge) incision is also useful in selected cases.
4. Selective conservatism can be used. Suitable investigations to exclude injuries include CT angiography [5], esophagogram (Fig. 68.4), in all cases and esophagoscopy and bronchoscopy where indicated.

68.6 Peripheral Vascular

Penetrating injuries causing major peripheral vascular injury are fortunately uncommon in children. The under-five age group is challenging with poor patency rates being the historical norm. If you are unfortunate to encounter these injuries, best results are achieved when these tiny vessels are repaired with the aid of the operating microscope. Angiography can be a dangerous intervention in small children with higher rates of iatrogenic injury than seen in adults. Use angiography sparingly – to avoid the scenario of the patient with a traumatic injury on one side and iatrogenic occlusion of the femoral artery on the other! Clinical assessment of a vascular injury is sufficient grounds for exploration. Consider carefully whether to perform angiography to look for subclinical lesions – even if you find an abnormality you will probably treat these expectantly in any event.

You should treat all major vascular injuries in childhood where there are signs of ischemia or where there is ongoing bleeding or traumatic arteriovenous fistula by prompt exploration and repair with revascularization. In rare cases even when complete vascular occlusion has occurred there may be no signs of acute ischemia. In these cases, efficient collateral circulation is maintaining the viability of the limb (commonly in the axillary and brachial arteries). Some children can present with evidence of an arterial injury but no evidence of ischemia or limb threat. If you operate these patients in an attempt to restore flow, you may do harm by interfering with the collateral circulation and converting a stable situation to one of limb threat (especially in the young child where the vascular anastomosis is most technically challenging). These patients are sometimes best treated by close observation and follow up. The Doppler Ankle Brachial Index (ABI) is helpful under these circumstances. An index of greater than 0.6 indicates sufficient arterial perfusion by collaterals. If the patient develops growth

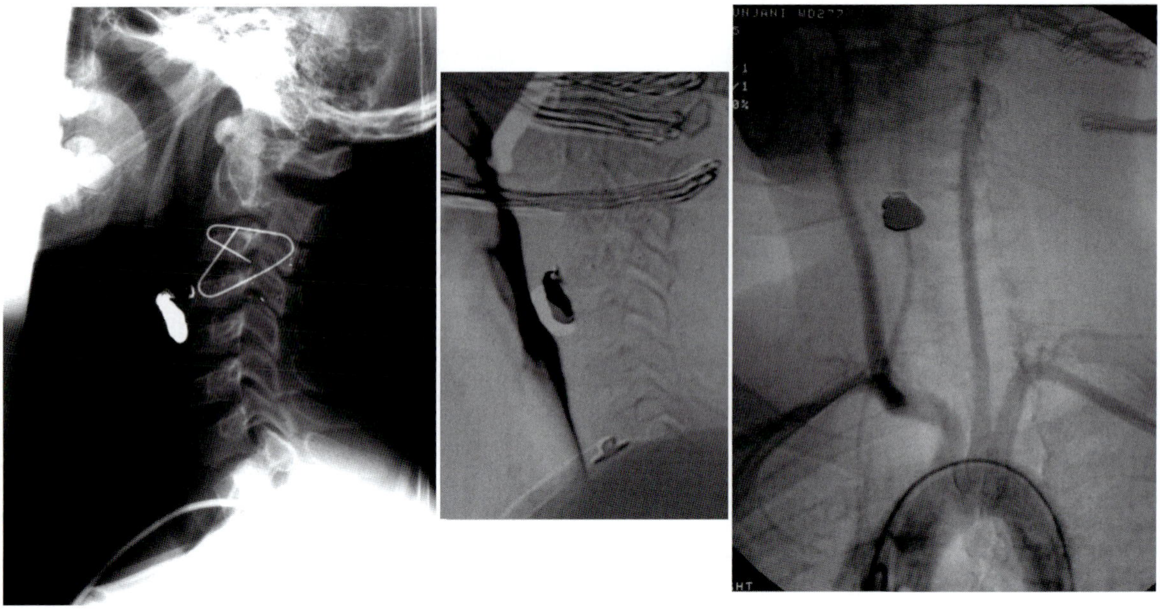

Fig. 68.4 Suitable investigations to exclude penetrating neck injuries include CT or conventional angiography and esophagogram (as shown here) in all cases. Esophagoscopy and bronchoscopy can be applied where indicated

retardation of the affected limb, elective vascular repair can be performed at a later date but this will rarely be necessary. An ABI of greater than 0.90 is a useful screening test for the presence of significant arterial injury.

Arterial spasm occurs more commonly in children than in adults. Vasospasm is thought to occur when there is a shear injury or contusion to a blood vessel. This results in anatomical or functional separation of the endothelium and the media. The constant vasodilatory effect maintained by endothelial production of nitric oxide is therefore lost and the vessel goes into prolonged spasm. The small caliber of pediatric vessels makes them particularly vulnerable. The role of spasm in penetrating arterial trauma is not clear. Most vessels explored for angiographically diagnosed spasm after penetrating injury reveals a clearly injured vessel. Do not assume that poor arterial supply is due to spasm and therefore self-limiting. This may delay exploration and repair of the vessel and decrease the chances of successful revascularization.

68.6.1 Practical Advice and Pitfalls with Vascular Injuries

1. Ligate all veins if repair is not possible except for the superior vena cava, suprahepatic inferior vena cava and popliteal vein.

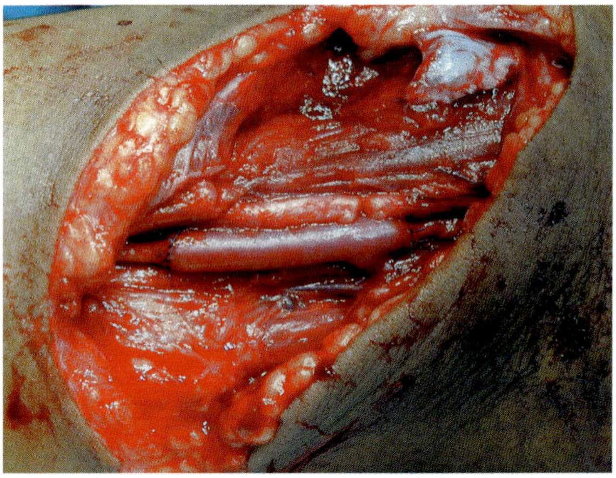

Fig. 68.5 Avoid prosthetic grafts if at all possible in children. Best patency rates are achieved by autologous vein grafts

2. Avoid prosthetic grafts if at all possible in children. Best patency rates are achieved by autologous vein grafts (Fig. 68.5).
3. Use the operating microscope in small children under 5 years of age.
4. Interrupted suturing and the use of absorbable material such as polydiaxanone allows for growth.
5. No preoperative angiography in patients with obvious injuries.

68.7 Nonpowder Gun Injuries

These are weapons which propel the missile by compressed air, either created by a mechanical spring or compressed air. The array of weapons sold as "toys" has become increasingly impressive in recent years. Many of these weapons are capable of muzzle velocities in the 400–1,200 fps range, comparable to powder guns. Although the missile fired is generally smaller and lighter, significant injuries can occur especially to the globe of the eye, intracranial structures, the trachea in the neck and the peripheral vascular tree. Penetration into the chest and abdominal cavity occur less commonly but deaths in these scenarios have also occurred. If you treat lots of children in a developed country, especially in the "gun friendly" countries such as the United States, you will see these injuries! Treat them with due respect – they can cause almost the same array of injuries that traditional gunpowder propelled missiles do [6].

68.8 Summary

Children should not have to suffer penetrating injuries. When they do, an approach based in principle on the adult approach to these injuries will yield good results. The best place to treat a severely injured and unstable patient is the operating room – do not delay in getting your patient there! In general, selective conservatism of injuries to body cavities is less useful (but still perfectly applicable) for pediatric patients because of the greater incidence of injuries. The operating microscope is an essential tool for repairing very small blood vessels. The pellet fired by a "toy" gun can sometimes cause injuries in excess of what you might expect.

Important Points

- The treatment of the unstable child with a penetrating injury needs to occur in the operating room and not in the emergency room. Delays can be fatal!
- Resuscitative thoracotomy should only be used in the context of penetrating thoracic trauma.
- For trauma, a midline laparotomy affords the best access for all sizes and shapes of children.
- Laparoscopy and thoracoscopy may be very useful additions to your armamentarium *in stable patients*.
- Selective conservatism of penetrating abdominal injuries is less useful in small children because the rate of organ injury is generally high and abdominal defects need to be repaired anyway.
- Tunnel all chest tubes, fix them thoroughly and pull them out under gauze to ensure that you do not cause pneumothorax in uncooperative children.
- Unnecessary angiography carries a real risk of contralateral vessel injury. Request it only if it will change your management in a significant way.
- Do not embark on repair of limb vessels in small children who have an injury but good ABIs and no limb threat – you could interfere with the collaterals that are sustaining that limb and cause limb loss if your anastomosis fails.
- If a limb is threatened due to what you assume to be spasm – explore it to rule out injury. You will usually find it.
- Nonpowder gun injuries are becoming more common – treat them with respect they are powerful!

References

1. Doss M, Woehleke T, Wood JP, Martens S, Greinecker GW, Moritz A (2003) The clamshell approach for the treatment of extensive thoracic aortic disease. J Thorac Cardiovasc Surg 126(3):814–817
2. Cotton BA, Nance ML (2004) Penetrating trauma in children. Semin Pediatr Surg 13(2):87–97
3. Inci I, Ozcelik C, Nizam O, Eren N, Ozgen G (1996) Penetrating chest injuries in children: a review of 94 cases. J Pediatr Surg 31(5):673–676
4. Nance ML, Sing RF, Reilly PM, Templeton JM Jr, Schwab CW (1996) Thoracic gunshot wounds in children under 17 years of age. J Pediatr Surg 31(7):931–935
5. Bell RB, Osborn T, Dierks EJ, Potter BE, Long WB (2007) Management of penetrating neck injuries: a new paradigm for civilian trauma. J Oral Maxillofac Surg 65(4):691–705
6. Laraque D (2004) Injury risk of nonpowder guns. Pediatrics 114(5):1357–1361

The Pregnant Patient

69

Dimitrios Theodorou and Andreas Larentzakis

Consider pregnancy always when dealing with a female trauma patient of reproductive age. The changes in anatomy and physiology, as well as the trauma care of two individuals, represent issues that must be considered, beyond the well-established principles of the injured patient management.

Penetrating trauma during pregnancy is the result of gunshot wounds, followed by stab wounds. Gunshot wounds are more lethal for both mother and fetus [1, 2]. The subgroup that most likely suffers penetrating trauma is pregnant teenagers, between 15 and 19 years old [3]. Mother's and fetus's morbidity and mortality are significantly different. Maternal mortality is less than 5%, while perinatal fetal mortality rate ranges between 40% and 71%, in the setting of maternal abdominal penetrating trauma [1, 2, 4–8].

69.1 Alterations During Pregnancy

When you have to deal with an injured pregnant patient, you have to be aware of the changes in its physiology and anatomy, because they alter maternal response to trauma requiring subsequent treatment adaptations [6, 9]. Most changes occur as early as the beginning of the 1st trimester of pregnancy but are evident by the end of it, while the peak effects are noted during the 2nd or 3rd trimester [10, 11].

69.1.1 Changes in Anatomy

When you evaluate the abdomen of a pregnant patient, it is important to remember that the abdominal organs are displaced upwards by the growing gravid uterus [10]. The bladder is also displaced superiorly along with the growing uterine fundus and should be no more considered as a pelvic visceral organ in the second trimester. This predisposes to bladder injury in the latter stages of pregnancy [11]. After 20 weeks of gestation, the uterus can provoke aortocaval compression, which can reduce venous return to the heart, as well as cardiac output. About 10% of pregnant women will experience the supine hypotensive syndrome. If compensation from paravertebral collaterals is not sufficient, the patient can experience pallor, sweating, nausea, vomiting, hypotension, tachycardia and even mental status changes. So, remember placing the pregnant patient in the left lateral decubitus position during the evaluation, because it maximizes blood flow to the uterus and releases aortacaval pressure [1, 10]. The diaphragm is raised approximately 4 cm, and the thoracic anteroposterior diameter increases [1, 12]. The dextrorotation of the enlarging uterus produces a predilection for right-sided ureteral dilation [11], but also bilateral ureteral dilation may be apparent, as bladder is displaced superiorly [10].

D. Theodorou (✉)
Unit of Foregut Surgery, Department of Surgery, School of Medicine, University of Athens, 24 Myron Str, Athens 10434, Greece
e-mail: dimitheod@netscape.net

A. Larentzakis
Department of General Surgery, School of Medicine, 1st Propaedeutic Surgical Clinic, University of Athens, 3rd September 1843 Street No 11, Egaleo, Attiki 12242, Greece
e-mail: alarentz@med.uoa.gr

G.C. Velmahos et al. (eds.), *Penetrating Trauma*,
DOI 10.1007/978-3-642-20453-1_69, © Springer-Verlag Berlin Heidelberg 2012

Table 69.1 Alterations in physiology during pregnancy

Parameter	Alteration	Amount
Heart rate (beats/min)	↑[a]	By 10–15
Systolic blood pressure (mmHg)	↓[b]	By 5–15
Diastolic blood pressure (mmHg)	↓	By 10–20
Central venous pressure (mmHg)	↓	Up to 5
Stroke volume (mL)	↑	By 5–10
Cardiac output (L/min)	↑	Up to 50%
Systemic vascular resistance (dynes·cm/s^5)	↓	Varies
Pulmonary vascular resistance (dynes·cm/s^5)	↓	Varies
Total blood volume (Lt)	↑	By 30–50%
Plasma volume (Lt)	↑	By 30–40%
Erythropoiesis	↑	By 10–15%
Hemoglobin (g/dL)	↓	10 is still normal
Hematocrit (%)	↓	30 is still normal
White blood count (×1,000 per mm^3)	↑	5–25 is normal
Platelets	No change	No change
Clotting factors (II, VII, VIII, IX, X)	↑	Varies
Fibrinogen (mg/dL)	↑	Up to 400
Functional residual capacity	↓	By 20%
Residual volume	↓	Varies
Expiratory reserve volume	↓	Varies
Tidal volume (mL)	↑	By 40%
Respiratory rate	↑	Changes minimally
Minute ventilation	↑	Up to 50%
$PaCO_2$ (mmHg)	↓	By 5–10
Oxygen consumption	↑	Up to 20%
PaO_2 (mmHg)	↑	100 or more
pH	No change	No change
Serum bicarbonate (m Eq/L)	↓	By 2–7

[a]Increment
[b]Decrement

69.1.2 Changes in Physiology (Table 69.1)

69.1.2.1 Circulatory

The most prevalent changes during pregnancy occur in the cardiovascular system. Why all these alterations are important to you when you try to resuscitate a pregnant woman suffering a penetrating trauma? The increase in total blood volume, plasma volume, heart rate, stroke volume, and cardiac output, as well as the decrement in blood pressure, and central venous pressure can interfere with assessment of the hemodynamic status of your patient.

Blood pressure is lower during pregnancy due to the decreased systemic vascular resistance owing to progesterone-induced vasodilation and due to the low resistance of the placental bed [1, 11].

The increase in heart rate is the result of the estrogen-mediated increases in myocardial alpha receptors [13]. The normal ECG changes in pregnancy include sinus tachycardia, left axis deviation, ectopic beats, Q wave in leads III and aVF, inverted or flattened T waves in leads III, V1 and V2, and unspecific ST changes [14, 15].

Volume loss may be underestimated and hemodynamic instability signs may not be apparent until your patient has lost over 30% of her total blood volume [10, 12, 16–18]. If blood loss excides 2,500 mL, then pregnant patient's condition can deteriorate extremely rapidly. Also, uterine blood flow comprises about 20% of cardiac output, has no autoregulation, and is dependent on maternal mean arterial blood pressure [1], but you have to keep in mind that the fetus may be at risk even with no maternal signs of hypovolemia, while after their appearance the fetus is in jeopardy. So, you cannot rely on hemodynamic stability as an indicator of maternal blood loss, and it is reasonable to overhydrate in order to prevent hypoperfusion of the uteroplacental circulation [2, 19].

The confusion can be even greater if you do take into consideration the "physiologic anemia" of pregnancy, as maternal erythropoiesis increment does not keep pace with the increase of plasma volume [2, 11, 19]. Hematocrit and hemoglobin values of 30% and 10 g/dL, respectively, are considered normal. A smart enough approach is to compare, if available, the most recent laboratory exams, as a lot of pregnant women have hematocrit levels obtained as a part of routine care.

Also, colloid osmotic pressure declines progressively with advancing gestational age owing to the falling level of serum albumin [10].

69.1.2.2 Respiratory

The respiratory system also undergoes changes. Oxygen consumption is increased due to the augmentation of the metabolic demands of the growing breasts, uterus, placenta, and fetus [11], and the partial pressure of oxygen (PaO_2) rises in order to maintain adequate oxygen delivery to all these tissues and fetus

[16, 19]. Under this hypermetabolic status, you should always supply supplemental oxygen to the pregnant patient, even before you start your evaluation.

The growing uterus elevates the diaphragm. Subsequently, the respiratory reserve and residual volumes decline and result to the decrease of the functional residual capacity [11]. So, you do not have as much time as you may think in case your pregnant patient has depressed respiration or is apnoeic [20].

These respiratory changes lead to an increase of the tidal volume and a slight increase of the respiratory rate, resulting to an upgrade of minute ventilation and lowering of the partial pressure of carbon dioxide levels ($PaCO_2$). So, you must consider any $PaCO_2$ levels between nonpregnant values. The pH remains, however, between normal values, because of the compensatory renal excretion of bicarbonate. As you already know, this is called compensated respiratory alkalosis. Keep in mind that this means that the pregnant patient has, already, a component of metabolic acidosis before her injury.

69.1.2.3 Renal

The renal perfusion is markedly increased during pregnancy, resulting in an increase in glomerular filtration rate [16]. This leads to a drop in both serum creatinine and blood urea nitrogen levels, and values above 0.8 and 13 mg/dL, respectively, should be considered abnormal [11]. Also, serum sodium is reduced [10]. It is important if you want to evaluate a pregnant patient's kidney function in trauma setting. Hydronephrosis, hydroureter, and urinary stasis are not uncommon owing to the relaxing effects of progesterone on smooth muscle, as well as to the growing uterus, predisposing to urinary infections [11].

69.1.2.4 Progesteron-Mediated Smooth Muscle Relaxation

Progesteron-mediated smooth muscle relaxation results to a decreased lower esophageal sphincter tone, and also the gastric empting is prolonged. In addition, stomach is displaced cephalad. Because of these changes, the risk of aspiration increases in a pregnant patient who cannot protect her airway in case of trauma [1, 12]. Remember that normal confusing complaints of the pregnant patient include nausea, vomiting, and abdominal discomfort. Bowel peristalsis is declined, too. As a consequence of this, there may be a prolonged period of postoperative ileus, nausea, and vomiting. Also, stasis of both gastric and gallbladder contents is common in pregnancy. Chronic distention of the parietal peritoneum by the expanding uterine contents produces less acute symptoms in cases of intraperitoneal bleeding, while the stretching of the peritoneum makes localizing pain difficult late in pregnancy [10, 11].

69.1.2.5 Laboratory Variants

Maternal white blood count increases in pregnancy, with levels between 5,000 and 25,000 per cubic milliliter (mm^3) considered normal. Platelets ranges as in the nonpregnant status, while at the lowest values. The levels of fibrinogen upgrade twofold times compared with nonpregnant measurements [11], and most procoagulant factors are increased, too. This seems to be beneficial for the pregnant patient in achieving hemostasis after trauma [1]. But, also, you should carefully evaluate normal or low values of fibrinogen, with elevated fibrin degeneration products, and below normal values of platelets, as suggestive of disseminated intravascular coagulation (DIC). Another issue needed to be considered is that the increased procoagulant factors, in addition to the venous stasis in the lower extremities during pregnancy, places pregnant patient at risk for deep venous thrombosis and pulmonary embolism. Therefore, when not contraindicated, thromboembolic prophylaxis should be considered.

69.2 Patterns of Injury

Pregnancy alters the pattern of injury as gestation advances. The risk of trauma of fetus increases with gestation age. Fetal death is the result of direct fetal injury or preterm delivery [21]. Before 13 weeks of gestation, the uterus is not yet an abdominal organ and is protected by the pelvic bones [6]. Fetal loss in the first trimester is the result of maternal hypotension or death rather than a result of direct trauma. As the uterine enlarges, it and its contents occupy more and more space in the abdominal cavity, and it displays the bowel cephalad. This is protective regarding the bowel, but the uterus and fetus are more vulnerable to injury [2]. The incidence of visceral injury with penetrating trauma in pregnancy is 16–38%, compared with 80–90% in nonpregnant population [2, 9]. Also, there is a thinning of the uterine wall and relative decrease in amniotic fluid volume with gestation age advancement, contributing to fetal vulnerability. Penetrating injuries in their majority involve uterine wall or uterine wall and fetus. The density of the uterus dissipates the energy of low-velocity traumas, but high-velocity ones are more devastating to mother and fetus. Maternal penetrating trauma in the upper abdominal area or posterior entry wounds are, however, associated with bowel or other visceral injuries [4, 11]; therefore, these injuries are explored surgically more often [4, 9].

The bladder is displaced cephalad, too, making it susceptible to direct injury. So, you have to remember that in case of hematuria.

69.3 Peri-operative Management

It is recognized that most pregnant trauma victims should be transported to a trauma center [9]. Prehospital findings such as tachycardia (>110 beats/min), chest pain, loss of consciousness, and third trimester pregnancy have been independently associated with the need for care in a trauma center [9, 22]. The evaluation and management of these patients requires a multidisciplinary approach. The trauma surgeons, the obstetricians, as well as maternal-fetal medicine specialists, emergency medicine technicians, emergency room physicians and nurses, anesthesiologists, and pediatricians are all members of a large collaborating team with the same intent, the rescue of mother and fetus [1]. Treatment protocols regarding penetrating injuries are the same for the pregnant patient. Between your treatment options are immediate laparotomy and surgical exploration, laparoscopy, local wound exploration, diagnostic peritoneal lavage, CT imaging, observation in an intensive care setting with continuous fetal monitoring and serial evaluations [15].

The guidelines regarding the prehospital trauma care and the Advanced Trauma Life Support of the pregnant patient are the same with those for non-pregnant trauma victims.

The main principle in the care of the pregnant trauma patient is the resuscitation and rescue of the mother, in order to provide the best chance for a favorable outcome for both mother and fetus. While it is important to monitor both mother and fetus, your only way to give better chances to the fetus is to adequately resuscitate mother. Time is one of your enemies. Rapid assessment and treatment are of paramount importance, while patient's management must be performed under a thorough understanding of the changes in maternal anatomy and physiology that occur in pregnancy.

69.3.1 Primary Survey

The ABCDEs of the initial assessment are the same as for the nonpregnant trauma patient. Life-saving procedures, medications, and diagnostic imaging are the same, too. Immediate administration of high-flow oxygen is very important. Remember the increased risk for aspiration of gastric content. Laryngoscopy and intubation is not an easy task in pregnant patients [23]. In rapid sequence intubation, remember to apply cricoid pressure, and that both depolarizing and nondepolarizing agents cross the placentoembionic barrier, resulting in a transient depression of the fetus.

When a chest tube is needed, the insertion point has to be moved one or even two intercostal spaces higher than in the nonpregnant patient. The reasons for this are the substernal angle increment in about 50%, the upward displacement of the diaphragm, and the augmentation of the anteroposterior diameter of the chest [15].

The fluid resuscitation of the pregnant trauma patient must be aggressive, according to the principles of ATLS. Transfusion, if indicated, should be done with typed-cross-matched packed red blood cells; however, if you don't have the luxury of time O-Rh-(−) blood is used. During the resuscitation process, particularly if gestation age is beyond 20 weeks, it is important to place your patient on her left side, in order to displace the uterus laterally and increase the cardiac preload and output.

In your list of causes for altered mental status in a trauma patient you should also add eclampsia.

69.3.2 Secondary Survey

The head-to-toe physical examination, the search for any entry or exit wounds, the history regarding the injury, as well as past medical and surgical history are the same as for the nonpregnant patient, but there are some more issues. Do not forget to ask about the obstetric history of the current and any past pregnancies. Keep always in mind the location of the uterine fundus according to the gestational age. A simple rule of thumb is that the distance of the uterine fundus from the pubic symphysis measured in centimeters corresponds to gestational age in weeks [9]. Palpate the uterus to asses for contractions, rigidity, and tenderness. However, signs might be absent because the gradual distention of the peritoneum provoked by the growth of the uterus desensitizes patient to the peritoneal. You have to continue with a sterile-speculum vaginal examination in order to assess for rupture of membranes or vaginal bleeding. The latter may indicate preterm labor, uterine rupture and/or abruption, in the setting of penetrating pregnant trauma patient. Digital cervical examination should be avoided in the presence of vaginal bleeding, until the placenta previa is excluded. Something you should never forget is to do a rectal examination to evaluate for bleeding and/or hematoma.

The fetus should be evaluated at this time. Fetal heart rate should be assessed as soon as possible during the secondary survey. Keep in mind that the normal range of fetal heart rate is from 120 to 160 beats/min. Use your stethoscope if the fetus is older than 20 weeks of gestation, but you are going to need a Doppler ultrasound between 10 and 14 weeks. Continuous monitoring is needed when the fetus is viable and gestational age is greater than 24 weeks [1]. You must remember that abnormal heart rate (i.e., tachycardia, bradycardia, loss of beat-to-beat variability, or recurrent declarations) may be the only sign of maternal hemodynamic instability [24]. Another warning sign of premature labor in pregnant patients with trauma is uterine contractions more than four per hour [10].

Laboratory studies are the same as for the nonpregnant patient. Just remember that Kleihauer-Betke test may be indicated [25, 26].

X-ray studies should be performed as for nonpregnant patients, and be limited if possible. The uterus must be shielded as indicated. The accepted maximum dose of ionizing radiation during the entire pregnancy is 5 rad (0.05 Gy), while the fetus is at highest risk during first and early second trimester. Table 69.2 shows fetal radiation exposure involved in diagnostic radiology. As it is evident, doses are much lower than the threshold and present no substantial risk of fetal death, malformation, or mental impairment [27].

Table 69.2 Fetal radiation exposure in several radiographic examinations

Examination	Fetal exposure (rad)	Fetal exposure (Gy)
Chest X-ray	0.000045	0.00000045
Pelvis X-ray	0.04	0.0004
Cervical spine X-ray	0.002	0.00002
Abdomen CT[a]	1–4	0.01–0.04
Head CT	<0.05	<0.0005

[a]Computed tomography

What other options do you have in order to evaluate a pregnant patient suffering penetrating trauma? You have focused abdominal sonography for trauma (FAST), which can detect intraperitoneal fluid with a 85% sensitivity and 99% specificity, as well as pericardial fluid with a 100% sensitivity and 99% specificity [15, 28]. Also, you can use ultrasound to assess fetal heart rate or gestational age. Finally, diagnostic peritoneal lavage (DPL) is rarely indicated.

69.3.3 Emergency Cesarian Delivery

The indications for emergency cesarean delivery (ECD) in a pregnant patient suffering penetrating trauma are:

- Unsuccessful maternal cardiopulmonary resuscitation after 4 min or recent maternal death (perimortem cesarean delivery).
- Compromise of a viable fetus with a hemodynamically stable mother.
- Need for surgical interventions to the uterus [29].

The ECD should be performed under the rule of "5 min," which means that the fetus has to be delivered in a no more than 5 min time interval, after maternal death, as this is the time described to have the optimum fetal survival. In the setting of cardiopulmonary resuscitation (CPR), this rule is applied as 4 min spent for CPR, and 1 min for fetus delivery [15].

Even if all these are well understood, here are some more questions for you:

- What is the gestational age beyond which you should attempt an ECD?

  Generally, you should not perform an ECD if the gestational age is less than 24 weeks, depending on the neonatal intensive care facilities you have available.

- Should you perform an ECD if you are not in the rule of "5 min"?
  You must be very cautious doing this. Despite the fact that fetus survival has been reported in the setting of more than 4 min CPR, Katz et al. [29], however, reported that between infants born by perimortem cesarean delivery, the 70% of the delivered into 5 min from maternal death survived, without neurologic deficit, while only the 13% of the delivered beyond 5 min from maternal death survived, and all had neurologic deficit.
- Should you proceed with ECD when there are no fetal heart beats heard?
  It has been reported no fetal survival in the absence of fetal heart beats before the ECD.
  Emergency delivery is performed through a vertical midline incision from the xiphoid to the pubic symphysis. Sterility is a luxury, so do not miss time. Then you have to proceed with a longitudinal incision in the uterus. Care should be taken to avoid the bladder at the lower margin of the uterus. A 5- to 7-cm incision from the fundus to the mid-uterine level is adequate. The next step is to enter the amniotic membranes, and the fetus is delivered. After the fetus has been delivered, you have to remove the placenta from the uterine wall with blunt dissection using your hand. The uterus is then closed with continuous absorbable suture in a run-and-lock fashion. Do not forget to administer oxytocin, in order to eliminate postpartum hemorrhage from the placental implantation site.

69.3.4 Non-operative Management

Non-operative management should be considered if the following criteria are satisfied:

1. Stable maternal vital signs.
2. No evidence of fetal distress in the case of a viable fetus.
3. Anterior entry wound below the level of the uterine fundus.
4. Radiographic visualization of the foreign body, if any.

Ultrasonography can be an excellent modality for determining the location of metal projectiles owing to the acoustic "shadowing" created by these objects.

Close monitoring of both mother and fetus in an intensive care setting is required. A viable fetus demonstrating evidence of distress is an indication for immediate cesarean delivery regardless of the site of injury. Such an approach should be carried out only in high-level trauma centers.

69.3.5 Prophylaxis

Tetanus toxoid (0.5 mL) should be administered if the previously immunized pregnant patient has not received a booster in the 5 years prior to an episode of penetrating trauma, in conjunction with tetanus immune globulin if the patient has not been previously immunized. Broad-spectrum antibiotics are indicated to prevent fetal infection when conservative management is undertaken [11].

The American College of Obstetrics and Gynecology has recommended that consideration be given to administering D-immunoglobulin to all unsensitized D-negative pregnant patients who are evaluated for abdominal trauma [30]. One ampule containing 300 mug of D-immunoglobulin protects against fetal-maternal hemorrhage of less than 30 mL. Additional ampules may be administered to patients experiencing more than 30 mL of fetal-maternal hemorrhage as defined by the Kleihauer-Betke test [2].

69.4 Operative Management

An aggressive approach to laparotomy for the management of gunshot wounds to the abdomen is usually followed during pregnancy. Selective laparotomy may be contemplated in the pregnant woman with stable vital signs when the entry site is anterior and subfundal and when imaging techniques demonstrate that the missile has not crossed the posterior uterine wall. Laparotomy for maternal indications is not also an indication to perform a cesarean section. You may, however, to do so if there is a fetal indication (fetal distress) or if the gravid uterus prevents adequate exposure for any needed and appropriate intra-abdominal exploration and repair of maternal injuries or the uterus displays a significant injury requiring extensive debridement and repair. In case it is known, at the time of laparotomy, that the fetus has expired secondary to penetrating trauma, you should follow the same principles, regarding the cesarean delivery. It is preferable, if possible, to proceed with vaginal delivery with prostaglandin induction of labor several hours later, because cesarean delivery spends blood and time. If you note uterine perforations during the exploratory laparotomy, you should proceed with excisional debridement and simple closure with absorbable sutures.

Another issue is extreme prematurity, in order to assess the need of any interventions for fetal indications (distress or injury). You have to weigh the viability of the delivered fetus against the risk of retaining the fetus in utero. Keep in mind that fetal viability is observed with increasing predictability after 23 weeks of gestation. Your non-operative option is close fetal surveillance.

Important Points

- Make sure you do not miss an incidental pregnancy.
- Remember that some of your drugs can cause complications to a pregnancy.
- Appropriate management of the mother will give a chance of survival to the fetus.
- But if the mother is dying because of injuries incompatible with life and the fetus is mature and still alive, consider emergency cesarean section.

References

1. Hill CC, Pickinpaugh J (2008) Trauma and surgical emergencies in the obstetric patient. Surg Clin North Am 88: 421–440
2. Stone IK (1999) Trauma in the obstetric patient. Obstet Gynecol Clin North Am 26:459–467
3. Greenblatt J, Dannenberg A, Johnson C (1997) Incidence of hospitalized injuries among pregnant women in Maryland, 1979–1990. Am J Prev Med 13:374–379
4. Awwad JT, Azar GB, Seoud MA (1994) High-velocity penetrating wounds of the gravid uterus: review of 16 years of civil war. Obstet Gynecol 83:259–264, Trauma in Pregnancy
5. Knudson MM, Rozycki GS, Paquin MM (2004) Reproductive system trauma. In: Feliciano D, Mattox K, Moore E (eds) Trauma. McGraw-Hill, New York
6. Mattox KL, Goetzl L (2005) Trauma in pregnancy. Crit Care Med 33:S385–S389
7. Sandy EA, Koemer M (1989) Self inflicted gunshot wound to the pregnant abdomen: report of a case and review of the literature. Am J Perinatol 6:30–31
8. Theodorou DA, Velmahos GC, Souter I et al (2000) Fetal death after trauma in pregnancy. Am Surg 66:809–812
9. Shah AJ, Kilcline BA (2003) Trauma in pregnancy. Emerg Med Clin North Am 21:615–629
10. Dodo SM, Johnson VS (2000) Evaluation and care of the pregnant patient with minor trauma. Clin Fam Pract 2: 707–722
11. Moise KJ Jr, Belfort MA (1997) Damage control for the obstetric patient. Surg Clin North Am 77:835–852
12. Rozycki G (1993) Trauma during pregnancy: predicting pregnancy outcomes. Arch Gynecol Obstet 253:S15–S20
13. Norwitz ER, Robinson JN, Malone FD et al (2004) Pregnancy-induced physiologic alterations. In: Clark SL, Cotton DB, Hankins GDV (eds) Pregnancy-induced physiologic alterations, 4th edn. Blackwell Scientific, Malton
14. Anderson RN (2002) Trauma and pregnancy: prehospital concerns. Emerg Med Serv 31:71–75, 79
15. Tweddale CJ (2006) Trauma during pregnancy. Crit Care Nurs Q 29:53–67
16. Cruikshank D, Wigton T, Hays P (1996) Maternal physiology in pregnancy. In: Gabbe SG, Neibyl JR, Simpson JL (eds) Obstetrics: normal and problem pregnancies, 3rd edn. Churchill Livingstone, New York
17. Gazmararian J, Lazorick S, Spitz A et al (1996) Prevalence of violence against pregnant women. JAMA 275: 1915–1920
18. Greiss FC Jr (1966) Uterine vascular response to hemorrhage during pregnancy, with observations on therapy. Obstet Gynecol 27:549–554
19. Esposito TJ (1994) Trauma during pregnancy. Emerg Med Clin North Am 12:167–199
20. Archer GW, Marx GF (1974) Arterial oxygen tension during apnoea in parturient women. Br J Anaesth 46:358–360
21. Buchsbaum H (1979) Penetrating injury of the abdomen. In: Buchsbaum H (ed) Trauma in pregnancy. WB Saunders, Philadelphia, pp 82–100
22. Goodwin T, Breen M (1990) Pregnancy outcome and fetomaternal hemorrhage after noncatastrophic trauma. Am J Obstet Gynecol 162:665–671
23. Kuczkowski KM (2004) Trauma in the pregnant patient. Curr Opin Anaesthesiol 17:145–150
24. Baerga-Varela Y, Zietlow SP, Bannon MP et al (2000) Trauma in pregnancy. Mayo Clin Proc 75:1243–1248
25. Dhanraj D, Lambers D (2004) The incidences of positive Kleihauer-Betke test in low-risk pregnancies and maternal trauma patients. Am J Obstet Gynecol 190:1461–1463
26. Muench MV, Baschat AA, Reddy UM et al (2004) Kleihauer-Betke testing is important in maternal trauma. J Trauma 57:1094–1098
27. International Commission on Radiological Protection (2000) Pregnancy and medical radiation. Ann ICRP 30:1–43
28. Ma OJ, Mateer J, Ogata M et al (1995) Prospective analysis of a rapid trauma ultrasound examination performed by emergency physicians. J Trauma 38:879–885
29. Katz VL, Dotters DJ, Droegemueller W (1986) Perimortem cesarean delivery. Obstet Gynecol 68:571–576
30. Pearlman MD, Viano D (1996) Automobile crash simulation with the first pregnant crash test dummy. Am J Obstet Gynecol 175:977–981

Anticoagulation in Penetrating Trauma

70

David R. King

Coagulopathy after trauma remains significantly associated with complications and death [1–5]. If co-existing traumatic brain injury is present, there is a dramatic increase of all-cause mortality [6] compared to non-brain-injured patients. As an extension of this concept, the use of anticoagulants following severe injury may be associated with worsened outcomes. Anticoagulation following penetrating trauma may be considered under some select circumstances; however, careful evaluation of these patients should be undertaken to exclude contraindications. Injury burden will dictate the decision to consider the use of anticoagulants, if they are indicated for a particular injury.

Vascular reconstruction following penetrating injury is commonly accomplished by either primary repair, interposition, bypass or patch with autologous vein, or interposition, bypass or patch with prosthetic. The type of reconstruction and the patient's existing medical comorbidities may influence the decision to use anticoagulants and antiplatelet agents.

In the absence of severe existing ischemic vascular disease, arterial and venous injuries repaired with autologous vein do not require postoperative systemic anticoagulation or antiplatelet therapy [7, 8]. Additionally, if the popliteal vein is ligated at time of surgery, postoperative anticoagulation does not influence rate of thrombosis or recannalization [9]. If no contraindications exist (such as traumatic brain injury or existing trauma-related coagulopathy), intraoperative anticoagulation during reconstruction (regardless of conduit) may improve rate of limb salvage [7, 8]. Shunting with anticoagulation may also improve limb salvage if definitive reconstruction needs to be delayed [10, 11]. The use of intraoperative angiography (as opposed to preoperative CT angiogram or formal angiography) may also improve chances of saving a limb [12].

Reconstruction with polytetraflouroethylene (PTFE) has been shown to be effective when autologous vein is not available, especially the heparin bonded variety [13, 14]. Limb salvage rates are comparable to autologous vein reconstruction, although there may be increased infection risk in contaminated wounds [10, 12, 15, 16]. Similar to autologous vein reconstruction, PTFE reconstruction after trauma does not require long-term postoperative anticoagulation or antiplatelet agents [7, 8, 15–17] unless there is existing severe ischemic vaso-occlusive disease.

Early, or prophylactic, fasciotomy should be carefully considered for traumatic vascular reconstructions, particularly of the lower extremity. The military experience suggests higher limb salvage rates with aggressive prophylactic fasciotomy [10, 15, 16], although the civilian literature suggests a selective approach be utilized [8, 11, 18, 19]. Factors contributing to likely benefit from early or prophylactic fasciotomies include long interval from presentation to repair, prolonged operative time, complex reconstruction, and existing peripheral vascular disease [18, 19]. If the surgeon feels a limb is at particularly high risk for compartment syndrome, then intraoperative anticoagulation may offer benefit. There is some evidence that the use of intraoperative heparin may prevent compartment syndrome and obviate the need for fasciotomy

D.R. King
Division of Trauma, Emergency Surgery, and Surgical Critical Care, Department of Surgery,
Massachusetts General Hospital, Harvard Medical School,
55 Fruit Street, Boston, MA 02114, USA
e-mail: dking3@partners.org

G.C. Velmahos et al. (eds.), *Penetrating Trauma*,
DOI 10.1007/978-3-642-20453-1_70, © Springer-Verlag Berlin Heidelberg 2012

[20]. Consequently, this should be considered when contraindications do not exist.

In conclusion, early aggressive revascularization should be undertaken for penetrating vascular injuries. The use of intraoperative angiography is associated with improved limb salvage, as is use of intraoperative anticoagulation. Primary lateral repair or autologous vein graft remains the preferred option for reconstruction; however, PTFE should be used liberally if autologous vein is not available, even in a potentially contaminated field. The use of prophylactic fasciotomies is controversial; however, the surgeon should carefully weigh the risk and benefits for each patient. Heparin anticoagulation during surgery may help avoid compartment syndrome. Finally, unless there is co-existing ischemic vascular disease, no postoperative or long-term anticoagulation or antiplatelet therapy is required for vascular repairs following penetrating trauma.

Important Points

- Heparin anticoagulation should be used intraoperatively for all vascular reconstructions when contraindications do not exist. This will improve limb salvage rates and may avoid need for fasciotomy.
- Regardless of conduit used for reconstruction, no long-term postoperative anticoagulation or antiplatelet therapy is required in the absence of existing ischemic vascular disease.
- Traumatic brain injury remains an absolute contraindication to anticoagulation even for complex vascular reconstructions.

References

1. Allard CB, Scarpelini S, Rhind SG, Baker AJ, Shek PN, Tien H, Fernando M, Tremblay L, Morrison LJ, Pinto R, Rizoli SB (2009) Abnormal coagulation tests are associated with progression of traumatic intracranial hemorrhage. J Trauma 67(5):959–967
2. White NJ, Martin EJ, Brophy DF, Ward KR (2010) Coagulopathy and traumatic shock: characterizing hemostatic function during the critical period prior to fluid resuscitation. Resuscitation 81(1):111–116
3. Sawamura A, Hayakawa M, Gando S, Kubota N, Sugano M, Wada T, Katabami K (2009) Disseminated intravascular coagulation with a fibrinolytic phenotype at an early phase of trauma predicts mortality. Thromb Res 124(5):608–613
4. Gando S, Kameue T, Matsuda N, Hayakawa M, Ishitani T, Morimoto Y, Kemmotsu O (2002) Combined activation of coagulation and inflammation has an important role in multiple organ dysfunction and poor outcome after severe trauma. Thromb Haemost 88(6):943–949
5. MacLeod J, Lynn M, McKenney MG, Jeroukhimov I, Cohn SM (2004) Predictors of mortality in trauma patients. Am Surg 70(9):805–810
6. Talving P, Benfield R, Hadjizacharia P, Inaba K, Chan LS, Demetriades D (2009) Coagulopathy in severe traumatic brain injury: a prospective study. J Trauma 66(1):55–61; discussion 61–62
7. Frykberg ER (2002) Popliteal vascular injuries. Surg Clin North Am 82(1):67–89
8. Huynh TT, Pham M, Griffin LW, Villa MA, Przybyla JA, Torres RH, Keyhani K, Safi HJ, Moore FA (2006) Management of distal femoral and popliteal arterial injuries: an update. Am J Surg 192(6):773–778
9. Smith LM, Block EF, Buechter KJ, Draughn DC, Watson D, Hedden W (1999) The natural history of extremity venous repair performed for trauma. Am Surg 65(2):116–120
10. Gifford SM, Aidinian G, Clouse WD, Fox CJ, Porras CA, Jones WT, Zarzabal LA, Michalek JE, Propper BW, Burkhardt GE, Rasmussen TE (2009) Effect of temporary shunting on extremity vascular injury: an outcome analysis from the Global War on terror vascular injury initiative. J Vasc Surg 50(3):549–555; discussion 555–556
11. Mullenix PS, Steele SR, Andersen CA, Starnes BW, Salim A, Martin MJ (2006) Limb salvage and outcomes among patients with traumatic popliteal vascular injury: an analysis of the National Trauma Data Bank. J Vasc Surg 44(1):94–100
12. Callcut RA, Acher CW, Hoch J, Tefera G, Turnipseed W, Mell MW (2009) Impact of intraoperative arteriography on limb salvage for traumatic popliteal artery injury. J Trauma 67(2):252–257; discussion 257–258
13. Daenens K, Schepers S, Fourneau I, Houthoofd S, Nevelsteen A (2009) Heparin-bonded ePTFE grafts compared with vein grafts in femoropopliteal and femorocrural bypasses: 1- and 2-year results. J Vasc Surg 49(5):1210–1216
14. Sala F, Hassen-Khodja R, Lecis A, Bouillanne PJ, Declemy S, Batt M (2003) Long-term outcome of femoral above-knee popliteal artery bypass using autologous saphenous vein versus expanded polytetrafluoroethylene grafts. Ann Vasc Surg 17(4):401–407
15. Vertrees A, Fox CJ, Quan RW, Cox MW, Adams ED, Gillespie DL (2009) The use of prosthetic grafts in complex military vascular trauma: a limb salvage strategy for patients with severely limited autologous conduit. J Trauma 66(4):980–983
16. Woodward EB, Clouse WD, Eliason JL, Peck MA, Bowser AN, Cox MW, Jones WT, Rasmussen TE (2008) Penetrating femoropopliteal injury during modern warfare: experience of the Balad Vascular Registry. J Vasc Surg 47(6):1259–1264; discussion 1264–1265
17. Brown J, Lethaby A, Maxwell H, Wawrzyniak AJ, Prins MHE (2008) Antiplatelet agents for preventing thrombosis after peripheral arterial bypass surgery. Cochrane Database Syst Rev Oct 8;(4):CD000535

18. Davidovic LB, Cinara IS, Ille T, Kostic DM, Dragas MV, Markovic DM (2005) Civil and war peripheral arterial trauma: review of risk factors associated with limb loss. Vascular 13(3):141–147
19. Sagraves SG, Conquest AM, Albrecht RJ, Toschlog EA, Schenarts PJ, Bard MR, Powell CS, Rotondo MF (2003) Popliteal artery trauma in a rural level I trauma center. Am Surg 69(6):485–489; discussion 490
20. Guerrero A, Gibson K, Kralovich KA, Pipinos I, Agnostopolous P, Carter Y, Bulger E, Meissner M, Karmy-Jones R (2002) Limb loss following lower extremity arterial trauma: what can be done proactively? Injury 33(9):765–769

Care Under Austere Conditions: Unlimited Restraints

71

Terence O'Keeffe

There are many reasons why you as a surgeon could find yourself practicing under adverse or austere conditions. This is clearly to be expected in the case of a military deployment, or a volunteer mission to an underdeveloped nation, but recent events have shown us that we can find ourselves in these circumstances much closer to home. The events surrounding the evacuation of patients from Charity Hospital in New Orleans following Hurricane Katrina in 2005 amply demonstrate that we can rapidly find ourselves with unanticipated problems without even leaving our home institutions [1, 2].

Natural disasters, wars, pandemics, and terrorism can all lead to sufficient numbers of injured patients that exceed the capabilities of the routine medical system. Some medical networks are already at breaking point, with extremely limited resources, and may be unable to cope with even the day-to-day provision of routine surgical care. Examples from the last few years where surgeons have practiced under adverse conditions might include Haiti, Zimbabwe, and Sri Lanka from among the developing nations, and Italy and the United States from the industrialized world.

We must also be clear what we mean by adverse or austere conditions, and although the Oxford English Dictionary gives a total of six definitions of "austere" it is in the sense of "severely simple in style, unadorned; without any luxury" that we are trying to define these circumstances. We should also remember that Webster's also has a definition of austere as "giving little or no scope for pleasure," which would certainly be the case for many of the patients who find themselves in these unfortunate circumstances. There are no accepted definitions of austere *conditions*, but there is a reason that this chapter is subtitled "unlimited restraints," as you as the surgeon will find yourself faced with a myriad of limiting factors that will impede your ability to provide excellent care.

This chapter aims to give some broad advice to surgeons who have never practiced under these conditions, and to help provide a framework on which to organize your thoughts and actions in the field.

71.1 Identify Your Resources

One of the first and most important things to do is to identify what resources you have at your disposal. These resources may be thought of in terms of personnel, actual medical equipment, physical plant and/or location, medications, what options you have to refer patients from your facility and what transportation options are available both to bring patients to you and return them to their homes (Table 71.1). The complexity of care that you will be able to provide will be very much influenced by the resources you have available. A good example of this comes from the military with their forward surgical teams that have been deployed widely in Iraq, which have only limited resources and personnel. After initial stabilization of the injured soldier, which may or may not include surgery, the patient is then transferred to field hospitals which are much more liberally equipped with greater man-power, equipment, personnel, intensive care units and facilities for onward transportation [3].

T. O'Keeffe
Division of Trauma/Critical Care and Emergency Surgery, University of Arizona, 1501 N Campbell Avenue, Rm 5411, P. O. Box 245063, Tucson, AZ 85724-5063, USA
e-mail: tokeeffe@surgery.arizona.edu

G.C. Velmahos et al. (eds.), *Penetrating Trauma*,
DOI 10.1007/978-3-642-20453-1_71, © Springer-Verlag Berlin Heidelberg 2012

Table 71.1 Resource identification at different levels

Resource	Pre-hospital	Hospital	After discharge
Equipment	Are there resources available to the patients?	Surgical instruments, radiology	Prosthetic limbs
			Walking aids
			Dressing changes
Physical plant	Not applicable	Physical building, electricity, water supply, clinics, OR, wards, etc.	Do rehab facilities exist? Will the patient be safe in their own house?
Personnel	Paramedics, local healthgivers	Nurses, ancillary staff, cleaners, cooks, etc.	Are supportive family available?
Language	Do you speak the local language?	Do the staff speak the same dialect as the patient?	Can you communicate with the family?
Medications	Self-medication inc. inappropriate	Do you have the medications that you need?	Are there other resources that have medications?
Nutritional	Is the local population well-nourished?	Does the hospital have a secure source of food for the patients?	Will the patient be able to get enough food for their post-op recovery?
Local expertise	Treatment by local "healthgivers" e.g., herbalists, bonesetters	Ethnically appropriate care	Community health care workers
Referral options	How do patients get to you or your hospital? Self-referral?	See below	Can the patient go to a regional referral center? How?
Specialists and/or subspecialists	Are you being referred patients by other doctors?	Ortho, neurosurgery, plastics, medicine, or just you?	Can you refer on to subspecialists? Who does the follow-up?
Transportation	Ambulances?	How do you transport patients in hospital?	How do the patients get home?

Once an accurate assessment of the available resources has been made, it is easier to make an appraisal regarding the level of care that you can provide to each patient. For example, if there are no critical care facilities or trained personnel, it is will be extremely challenging to deal with severely injured patients post-operatively. To take a specific instance, damage control laparotomy has become part of standard practice for the forward surgical teams military in Iraq and Afghanistan, but this would be highly challenging in a clinic or hospital run by non-governmental organization (NGO) in many African nations, for example. The military has an extensive onward transportation network to send patients to referral centers, often outside the country, an option that is often not available to other organizations.

71.2 What Do I Really Need? Plan Accordingly

A necessary part of this assessment is to evaluate what you as a surgeon really need, as it is very unlikely that you will have the resources and facilities available that you normally have in your daily practice. We work in an increasingly technological world with easy access to CT, laboratory testing as well as readily available specialist consults. If you are performing complex vascular surgery in an industrialized nation, then you will want the ability to perform angiography, balloon thrombectomy and IV heparinization. However, providing vascular surgery in an austere environment may involve only shunting of injured vessels and transferring them to a facility that can provide definitive care, if available. Similarly, as surgeons we all have our favorite sutures and instruments, but it is very clear that with a modicum of improvisation good surgery can be performed without our favorite #1 PDS suture or a Bookwalter retractor.

A good example of this is split-thickness skin grafts. You will probably have had experience with an electric dermatome, and a mesher, but in an austere environment you may be faced with only a Humby knife (or Weck blade) for the very first time. This is a long blade that is used to literally shave off the skin graft from the donor site. It is an acquired skill to be able to obtain a large, uniform piece of skin that will serve as a graft. Also, meshing will need to be done by hand by making small incisions in the skin graft, a time-consuming and tedious, but necessary process. Something as simple as a skin graft takes on a whole new complexity under these conditions. If you are able to familiarize yourself with this equipment in your usual practice, this will make this endeavor much easier when you perform it under less than ideal circumstances.

The placement of chest tubes is another area where it is likely you will have to contend with different equipment, as you may be using the classic "Three-bottle" system to drain air or blood from the thoracic cavity. The self-contained disposal systems that we are so familiar with are usually not available in this setting, and so familiarity with the intricacies of a three-chamber system is important. Similarly, a Heimlich valve should be placed in the system to prevent back-flow of fluid, as the bottles may not possess one-way valves. Heimlich valves may also form the primary treatment for broncho-pleural fistulas under these conditions.

You should also carefully consider the implications prior to creating a stoma in a patient in this environment. The majority of patients suffering a colonic injury from trauma can be primarily repaired [4], and committing a patient to a stoma that you may not be around to reverse is a huge burden on that patient especially if they are not going to have access to help learning how the stoma functions, and they may not be able to afford stoma supplies even if they are available. Serious consideration should be given to early closure of a stoma during the patient's initial hospital stay, as this has been shown to be safe and efficacious [5].

When it comes down to it, our clinical skill and surgical expertise may be really the most important factors in providing excellent care to these patients. In adverse conditions, the surgeon will have little back-up and needs to be able to work with the resource constraints that exist. There is no use planning an operation that cannot be successful because of the limitations placed upon you, but sometimes a short period of waiting can be beneficial for both the patient and the surgeon. For example, if the operation may entail significant blood loss from the patient and no compatible blood is available, it may be prudent to delay the surgery if it is non-urgent until a source of blood for transfusion can be found. Similarly, if a specific piece of equipment or medication is required that can be sourced in a short period of time, temporizing surgical therapy may be appropriate. However, being able to find a Fogarty embolectomy catheter in the middle of a war zone is highly unlikely, and surgery should not be delayed.

71.3 Improvisation

It is clear that a surgeon should go into these kinds of situations knowing ahead of time, that he/she will have to improvise using only the equipment that is available. A wise orthopedic surgeon working in Africa once said, "The secret to a good surgeon is an ability to improvise," and nowhere is this more true than in situations where there is limited expertise or equipment. There is a big difference between going from using a different type of mesh that you are comfortable with for a hernia repair, to having to perform surgery with the patient under a Ketamine anesthetic and without proper OR lighting or ventilation. I would encourage physicians who are going to work in this kind of environment to familiarize themselves with some of the older textbooks as well as an atlas of surgical procedures, as they may find themselves performing operations which have fallen by the wayside in most modern surgical practices. Ulcer surgery would be just one example. An older edition of Zollinger's surgical atlas makes both a great reference for unfamiliar operations and a fantastic and useful gift to the hospital or medical staff when you depart. The World Health Organization has a publication entitled "Surgical Care at the District Hospital," which while very simple for the practicing surgeon still has a number of useful tips and can be downloaded online [6]. The International Committee of the Red Cross has also produced a downloadable book called "War Surgery" that may also be of use to the surgeon [7]. In addition, a number of the NGOs have developed courses that are specifically designed to help broaden the expertise of surgeons to enable them to deal with the different management techniques that need to be employed for wound and burns management, orthopedic injuries, and neurological trauma.

It goes without saying that all surgeons operating under these conditions should be able to competently perform an emergency cesarean section, as this may be required in either civilian or military settings.

71.4 Triage

It is necessary to revisit the concept of triage in this discussion. This concept, which originally came from the military, of treating only the most life-threatened, but also most salvageable of patients, has slightly different connotations in the civilian sector. Once again, the availability of certain resources will greatly influence how we provide medical care. For example, in a patient with a traumatic brain injury there is little that a surgeon can offer in the absence of a CT scanner or neurosurgical expertise, and care may be limited to merely providing respiratory and basic life support, which may or may not be successful without an intensive care unit. Triage is more often associated with mass casualties or battlefields and will be more difficult if there is a single surgeon acting as both a triage officer and the operating surgeon.

Nevertheless, although the surgeon is often viewed as a team leader, he/she requires a team. Anesthesia, OR staff, nurses and ancillary personnel are all a vital part of the regular function of a surgical unit, but under austere circumstances, the members of this team may need to play many different roles. Other members of the team may be called upon to provide triage assessment if the surgeon is occupied operating on a patient. In rare circumstances, some surgeons have been required to play the role of both anesthesiologist and surgeon, by providing both services to the same patient, which is certainly less than ideal. Additionally in many cases, the anesthesia provider may not be a doctor, but will have experience in providing that service. It may also be a luxury to have both a circulating and a scrub nurse, and it is imperative that the surgeon is able to "think on his feet," and work well with the personnel that he has available.

71.5 Specific Resource Shortages: No Air, No Suction, No Blood

Special mention needs to be made of a few very particular resources: Air, i.e., oxygen, suction and blood, as all are usually in very short supply in austere conditions.

Oxygen at therapeutic concentrations may be difficult to come by in war zones, disaster areas, and less developed nations. The distillation of gaseous oxygen into liquid form in portable canisters is a very technical process, which requires functioning industry to be able to provide. In the event of a disaster or war, bottled oxygen may become increasing hard to find. This is therefore a resource that should be used judiciously and conserved. Oxygen concentrators can provide a good back-up but are very limited in their scope; they can provide flow rates of up to 5 L/min with concentrations from 50% to 95%, are semi-portable, but require a secure source of electricity (Fig. 71.1). Unfortunately, they are relatively expensive ($400–$1,500) and may simply not be available. Although the archetypal trauma patient is a young, healthy male, not all patients fall into this category, and the surgeon may find himself unpleasantly surprised by dealing with patients with significant co-morbidities especially respiratory in a challenging environment with few resources. Oxygen or a lack thereof is therefore another impediment that would otherwise not be an issue under regular conditions.

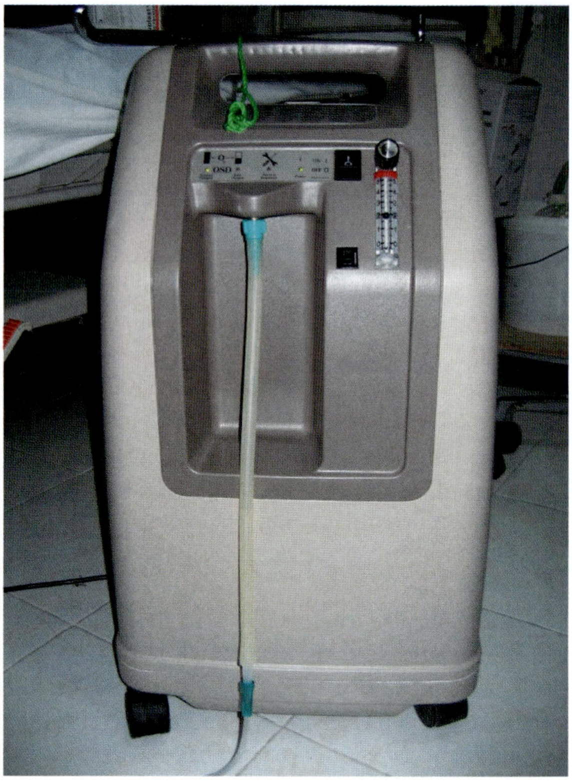

Fig. 71.1 An electric powered oxygen concentrator (Photo: O'Keeffe)

You will find even the easiest of operations difficult to perform without a source of aspiration for the fluids encountered. However, in many places, wall suction does not exist and electricity may be in very short supply. If you are lucky, a small electric or battery-powered suction device will be available to assist you, but the tubing will in all likelihood be too short or the level of suction provided too weak. If you are less lucky, you will be forced to use a foot-pump to generate suction

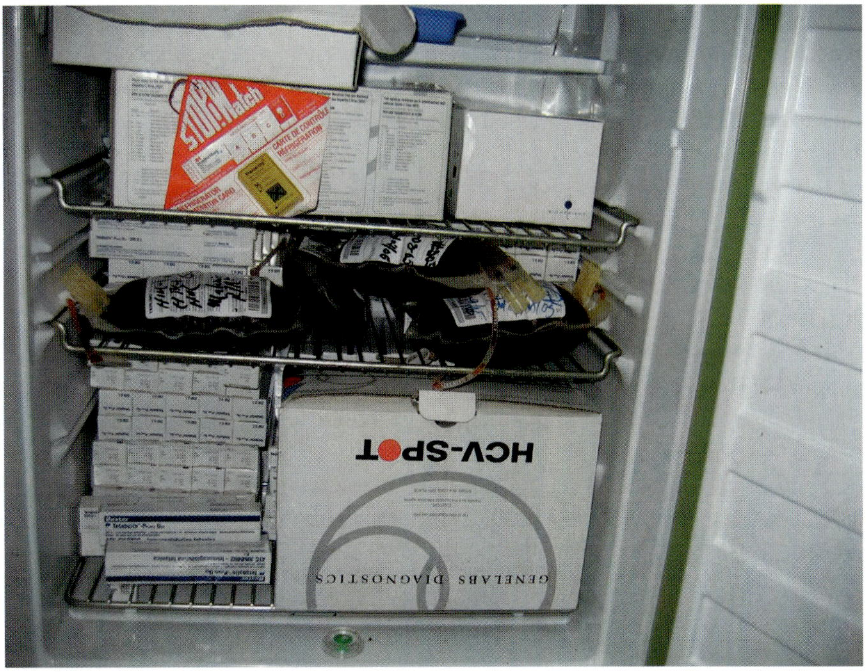

Fig. 71.2 "Blood bank" in austere conditions (Photo: O'Keeffe)

so that you are exercising at the same time as you are operating. Even if you have a reliable source of suction, you will often need to instruct your assistant how to use it and where to apply it, as they may not have much experience in this role. Thus even something as basic as suction presents a new challenge in less well-equipped settings.

With the advent of rapid HIV screening, it has been easier for less well-equipped hospitals to be able to provide blood for transfusion. However, it still needs to be stored, and this requires provision of a refrigerator as well as an uninterrupted supply of electricity with which to power it, both of which may be hard to find. It should be remembered, however, that when fresh whole blood is refrigerated, the platelets will become inactivated.

It is also unlikely that under these conditions, a ready supply of altruistic donors will be easily available. In a civilian setting, family members may be approached and asked if they would consider donating blood to aid in the care of their loved one. Even if the blood is not compatible it can be stored and used for future patients, and in this way a small "blood-bank" can be created that allows for some flexibility in subsequent patients. Figure 71.2 shows an example of such a blood bank used at a NGO hospital in Haiti.

The US military has adopted a similar approach, often termed a "walking blood bank" where soldiers whose blood group is already known donate fresh whole blood to be transfused to their wounded colleagues. This represents the best possible resuscitation fluid: warm, whole blood that is without storage lesions, and this has no doubt contributed in some part to the reduction in mortality seen in this conflict. Some NGOs even ask their volunteer staff members to know their blood group so that they may be used as a similar "walking blood bank" in cases of severe shortage.

71.6 Critical Care

The provision of critical or intensive care under limited or austere conditions can be extremely challenging, if not almost impossible. There are two different ways in which this can be addressed. The first is to accept the lack of resources that exist and try to do the best that you can with what exists. The second is to "bring everything with you," which is the model more often employed by military or disaster field hospitals, that seek to provide as close to modern critical care as possible. This can be a mammoth undertaking, as one paper showed which described setting up a field hospital with 12 intensive care beds required 5 Hercules aircraft to transport its equipment [8]. With the exception of the military, in most cases this is beyond the scope and/or ability of an organization to and the physician is left to manage critically ill or injured patients with a fraction of the means that are usually at their disposal. However, field hospitals have been successfully employed in many disaster zones in the past, although most authors have made the point that a significant proportion of their workload was from non-traumatic illnesses [9, 10]. Military supplies and equipment may not necessarily be suited for the many medical conditions that may therefore be encountered.

Venticinque has published a good review of critical care in the austere environment in 2008 [11], which the reader is referred to.

71.7 Be Culturally Sensitive

Most of us train in medical systems where the rapid throughput of patients is seen as desirable from both the system standpoint in terms of efficient use of resources and also from the patient perspective who will be more comfortable at home with his or her loved ones. You need to be mindful if working in a foreign country that this cultural viewpoint is not universal. Many patients in different parts of the world have the expectation that when they go to hospital, they will not be leaving it until they are completely cured of whatever was their presenting problem. It can be easy for the medical staff to become frustrated dealing with patients who they clearly feel are ready for discharge, but for some indefinable reason do not want to leave the hospital. This can lead to a breakdown in the doctor–patient relationship, as well as the obvious consequences for the medical facility if patients do not wish to leave. This needs to be approached with some degree of cultural sensitivity, based on the local customs and expectations, although it is not always easy to reconcile what is medically appropriate with the wishes of the patient and/or their family.

Similarly, there are some parts of the world where it is difficult for male physicians to examine female patients and vice versa. If you are not sufficiently aware of the local mores and display a lack of understanding, then it will be very difficult to gain the trust of the people you are treating. A few hours studying the local history, customs and tradition before arriving time well spent. Even a few words of the local dialect can be exceptionally useful; a well-timed joke in their language at the end of a long day can help lift the spirits of your operating room staff to get everyone to the end of the day and help maintain rapport.

71.8 Knowing Your Own Limitations

Although it would be a cliché to claim that there is a certain "breed" of surgeon that wishes to practice surgery under these conditions, it would be fair to say that not everyone would wish to find themselves in these circumstances, even if this is not of their own making. It is important that the surgeon remains humble and does not fall into the trap of their own hubris because of the role that they are playing in whatever natural or manmade disaster that has led to the breakdown of medical care, or the expertise that they may bring to an underdeveloped system. It remains important to know one's own limits and not to practice outside the scope of this. The temptation will always exist that if there is nothing to lose, then anything is "worth a try," even if the doctor has never previously performed this procedure. While this may indeed lead the surgeon to perform lifesaving surgery, e.g., a burrhole for an acute epidural hemorrhage, the potential exists for causing harm. We should always try to adhere to the dictum of *primum non nocere* or "do no harm," and this should not be suspended just because of the adverse circumstances that we may find ourselves in. The patient may be better served by waiting to undergo a procedure, being transferred or not even undergoing the procedure at all.

It is a good general rule that routine day-to-day medical care should be followed as closely as possible, including the roles of medical and other personnel, even if the conditions are not ideal. This will ensure that all staff are practicing medicine in a way that they are used to, which will inherently make things smoother, as well as ensuring that we continue to adhere to evidence-based guidelines for best practice. It would be very easy, considering the stressful and challenging times that the physicians and other staff face, to be tempted to cut corners and abandon usual standards, but this should be resisted and guarded against as much as is feasible. Providing substandard medical care under the excuse of limited capabilities may be worse than providing no help at all.

71.9 Conclusions

Much time and effort has been spent in the last decade planning and practicing for medical care emergencies and natural disasters, with some limited success. In all likelihood they will continue to occur, both at home and overseas. Hopefully we can learn from previous mistakes, and the lessons can be shared throughout the medical community, to allow us to improve the care that we provide patients who find themselves victims of austere conditions. This is a highly rewarding area of surgery, one that allows us to give of ourselves without asking for the usual compensations, but it needs to be approached with forethought and preparation.

Important Points

- Take the time to assess what resources you have.
- Use local expertise wherever possible.
- If there is an item you must have, take it with you.
- Identify what options you have for referral/transfer.
- Ask family members to donate blood and build up a blood bank.
- Think hard before committing patients to a stoma.
- Practice some orthopedic, maxillofacial operations and caesarian sections before you leave.
- Learn some of the local language and do not forget to be culturally sensitive.
- Take some useful books with you, and leave them behind when you leave.
- Know your own limitations, do not just "have a go."

References

1. Eastman AL, Rinnert KJ, Nemeth IR, Fowler RL, Minei JP (2007) Alternate site surge capacity in times of public health disaster maintains trauma center and emergency department integrity: Hurricane Katrina. J Trauma 63:253–257
2. Brevard SB, Weintraub SL, Aiken JB et al (2008) Analysis of disaster response plans and the aftermath of Hurricane Katrina: lessons learned from a level I trauma center. J Trauma 65:1126–1132
3. Eastridge BJ, Stansbury LG, Stinger H, Blackbourne L, Holcomb JB (2009) Forward Surgical Teams provide comparable outcomes to combat support hospitals during support and stabilization operations on the battlefield. J Trauma 66:S48–S50
4. Demetriades D, Murray JA, Chan L et al (2001) Penetrating colon injuries requiring resection: diversion or primary anastomosis? An AAST prospective multicenter study. J Trauma 50:765–775
5. Velmahos GC, Demetriades D, Stewart M et al (1998) Open versus closed diagnostic peritoneal lavage: a comparison on safety, rapidity, efficacy. J R Coll Surg Edinb 43:235–238
6. World Health Organization (1998) Surgical Care at the District Hospital – The WHO Manual. Available at http://www.who.int/surgery/publications/scdh_manual/en/index.html. Accessed Sept 2009
7. International Committee of the Red Cross (2009) War surgery: working with limited resources in armed conflict and other situations of violence. Available at http://www.icrc.org/web/eng/siteeng0.nsf/htmlall/p0973/$File/ICRC_002_0973.PDF. Accessed Sept 2009
8. Halpern P, Rosen B, Carasso S et al (2003) Intensive care in a field hospital in an urban disaster area: lessons from the August 1999 earthquake in Turkey. Crit Care Med 31:1410–1414
9. Pesola G, Bayshtok V, Kvetan V (1989) American critical care team at a foreign disaster site: the Armenian experience. Crit Care Med 17:582–585
10. Bar-Dayan Y, Leiba A, Beard P et al (2005) A multidisciplinary field hospital as a substitute for medical hospital care in the aftermath of an earthquake: the experience of the Israeli Defense Forces Field Hospital in Duzce, Turkey, 1999. Prehosp Disaster Med 20:103–106
11. Venticinque SG, Grathwohl KW (2008) Critical care in the austere environment: providing exceptional care in unusual places. Crit Care Med 36:S284–S292

The Impact of Trauma on the Psyche

72

F.Y. Jeenah and M.Y.H. Moosa

Physical trauma refers to harm inflicted on the body by an injury. It is defined by the World Health Organization as "a suspected bodily lesion resulting from acute over-exposure to energy (mechanical, thermal, electrical, chemical and radiant) interacting with the body in amounts or rates that exceed the threshold of physiological tolerance." A number of characteristics influence the nature and severity of the resulting effects of physical trauma viz. mechanism of injury, activity and intent, location at time of injury, severity, and the location and extent of damage. A common acute impact on the psyche is the development of delirium. Delirium is a syndrome consisting of impairments in consciousness, arousal, cognition, perception, and emotion. The clinical picture results from disruptions of normal brain function due to biochemical, electrical, or mechanical disturbances.

Physical trauma is often accompanied by psychological trauma. *Psychological trauma refers to psychological damage resulting from an injury (including sexual abuse, violent attack, natural disaster, or act of warfare), which may overwhelm a person's ability to emotionally cope with the experience and/or causes the person to believe that his/her life is in danger.* However, different people will react differently to similar events. One person may experience an event as traumatic while another person would not suffer trauma as a result of the same event [8]. People's reactions could be considered "traumatic" if their reactions include intense fear, helplessness, or horror, and if they develop clinically significant impairment in social, occupational, or other important areas of functioning that last more than a few weeks [1]. The incidents would typically be unexpected and, in context, would be considered significant enough to be associated with significant distress in most people [2].

The problems and disorders that arise in the aftermath to exposure to trauma have three main features. Firstly, the onset of problems or disorders is clearly linked to a significant and identifiable event (and presumably problems and disorder would not have developed without exposure to the event). Secondly, the problems must cause significant impairment in functionality. Thirdly, they share characteristic symptoms, which can include elevated physical and emotional reactivity to reminders of the event, attempts to avoid exposure to reminders, symptoms of depression and anxiety, and possible dissociation. Identified acute trauma-related disorders include Acute Stress Reaction, Acute Stress Disorder, and Posttraumatic Stress Disorder [1, 2].

This chapter attempts to provide the reader with some of the clinical features and emergency room management of:

(a) Delirium
(b) Common trauma-related psychological disorders

F.Y. Jeenah (✉)
Division of Psychiatry, University of the Witwatersrand, Johannesburg, Republic of South Africa and
Department of Psychiatry, Chris Hani Baragwanath Academic Hospital, University of the Witwatersrand Medical School, 7 York Road, Parktown, 2193, Johannesburg, Republic of South Africa
e-mail: fatima.jeenah@wits.ac.za

M.Y.H. Moosa
Division of Psychiatry, University of the Witwatersrand, Johannesburg, Republic of South Africa and
Department of Psychiatry, District Health Services, University of the Witwatersrand Medical School,
7 York Road, Parktown, 2193, Johannesburg, Republic of South Africa

G.C. Velmahos et al. (eds.), *Penetrating Trauma*,
DOI 10.1007/978-3-642-20453-1_72, © Springer-Verlag Berlin Heidelberg 2012

72.1 Delirium

A delirious state should be recognized as a medical emergency – it can rapidly progress to death if not managed appropriately. It is of paramount importance to distinguish this state from primary psychiatric conditions so as to avoid mismanagement of the patient with possible devastating consequences. The majority of cases are reversible with rapid improvement when the underlying pathology is remedied.

72.1.1 Clinical Features of Delirium

- Onset and course: Usually sudden and develops over hours or days, course is brief and fluctuating.
- Impairment in:
  (a) Level of consciousness: This feature is universal; can range from lucid intervals to barely perceptible dulling of awareness to profound coma. Characteristically, this impairment fluctuates often worsening at night, with fatigue, and decreased environmental stimulation.
  (b) Arousal, alertness, and psychomotor behavior: The patient may be hypoactive with diminished alertness, and appear depressed, demented, or even catatonic. In contrast, there may be hyperactivity with increased alertness The picture may be mixed – it is common to see rapid changes from phases of overactivity to periods of apathy and aspontaneity. The hyperactive restless patient may present with noisy disturbing behavior. Such overactivity typically consists of purposeless, repetitive behaviors such as groping or picking movements.
  (c) Cognitive function: Thought processes are slowed. The patient has difficulty focusing thoughts and mental fatigue occurs readily. Reasoning becomes less clear and coherent, logic is impaired, and thinking is concrete. Trains of thought become chaotic (presents as fragmented and incoherent speech). Comprehension of events is impaired – the patient may be unaware of the most obvious features of a situation, e.g., whether he is indoors or outdoors. Bizarre thoughts and fantasies intrude into awareness. Thought content becomes disturbed – ideas of reference and delusions, involving themes of persecution, develop. Delusions in this context are vague, poorly elaborated, transient, and inconsistent. There is disturbance of registration, retention, and recall. Recent memories are faulty, long-term memory is generally intact. The patient is clearly disoriented for time, often for place, and rarely for self.
  (d) Perception: Perceptual changes are often present, but are not essential to the diagnosis. There may be hallucinations, most commonly in the visual modality, but auditory, tactile, and olfactory hallucinations can exist. These may be simple or complex. Illusions are very common.
  (e) Emotions: There are clear alterations in affect and mood. Early there may be mild depression, anxiety, and irritability with shallow affect and later apathy, indifference, and emotional withdrawal. Intense anxiety and fear are common, often progressing to terror and panic.
- Associated Signs. Sleep–wake cycle is characteristically disturbed. There is often exacerbation of symptomatology at bedtime – "sundowning." Neurological – tremor, incoordination, dysphasia, urine incontinence, nystagmus, ± focal signs.

72.1.2 Investigations for Delirium

The delirious patient must be investigated as follows:

- Blood glucose – dextrostix
- Urine examination – dipstix
- Urine toxicology
- Blood urea and electrolytes
- Serum calcium and magnesium
- Full blood count
- Liver function tests
- Lumber puncture, X-ray, and radio-imaging if indicated.

72.1.3 Management of Aggression in a Delirious Patient

Delirious patients may be aggressive and very difficult to handle, especially to obtain a history or to physically examine them. They must be managed as follows:

- De-escalating process

Do not approach the patient alone. Do not issue threats and keep comments simple. Attempt to reassure the patient. Be polite and calm but firm. Keep calm, and keep everyone else calm. Ask the aggressive person how you can help them. He/she may calm down and cooperate if treated with respect and given an opportunity to express his/her concerns. Explain who you are and what you are going to do, i.e., talk to the patient to find out what the problem is. Introduce yourself courteously. Respect the person's body space – do not get too close or touch the person unnecessarily. Ensure that there are sufficient people around to restrain the person if he/she fails to respond to talking. Encourage the person to talk. Treat him/her with dignity but also with firmness. Threatening the person very often escalates the situation. You can say things like: "We are here to help you. Your behavior is not allowing us to give you help. We cannot allow you to hurt yourself or other people. Can you tell us more calmly what the problem is?"; "Why don't you tell me how angry you feel rather than hitting me?"; "I am listening to you."

- Physical restraint

  Physical restraint refers to the use of physical force to prevent a person from taking part in an action that could have negative consequences. It is to "place under control when necessary to prevent serious bodily harm to the patient or to another person, by the minimal use of such force as is reasonable, having regard to the physical and mental condition of the patient." The inclusion of the word "serious" requires that the risk to the patient or other persons not be slight, negligible, or frivolous. Consequently, there must be a real risk of harm to the patient or others before restraint is employed. If attempts at calming the aggressive person by talking fail, physical restraint of the individual may become necessary. The goal here is to contain the aggressive individual by using the least amount of force necessary. Physical restraining should not be done alone. It is important to use a team approach when restraining an aggressive person. Ideally, five people are needed – this would allow one person to hold each limb of the aggressive person, and the fifth person to hold the head and direct the restraining procedure. Moreover, the mere demonstration of there being enough people to contain him/her is often enough to calm an aggressive person down. Important: Beware not to use excessive force – one does not want to injure the ill person.
- Chemical restraint

  Several drugs are available which can be used to sedate the acutely psychotic/aggressive patient. If the patient has a medical condition/delirium, then lower doses of medication must be given.
  1. Benzodiazepines
     - Lorazepam (Ativan): 0.5–2 mg PO, IMI or IVI (slowly).
     - Diazepam: 5–10 mg PO, IVI (slowly) – Do not use IMI – poor absorption
     - Clonazepam (Rivotril): 1–2 mg PO, IMI, or IVI slowly

       A Word of Caution
       - Benzodiazepines can cause respiratory depression.
       - The safest route of administration is oral followed by intramuscular (except for diazepam which has erratic absorption intramuscularly) with the intravenous route having the highest risk of respiratory depression and arrest.
       - The safest route should be used wherever possible.
       - Monitor vital signs closely during and after administration.
  2. Antipsychotics

     If hallucinations, delusions, disorganized thought, and behavior are present:
     - Haloperidol: 2.5–5 mg orally, IMI or IVI (slowly). This can be given in combination with Lorazepam. In a medically ill psychotic patient, use lower doses (0.5–2 mg).
     - Risperidone (if available): 0.5–2 mg daily.
     - Zuclopenthixol Acetate (Clopixol Acuphase): 50–150 mg IMI. The effect will last 2–3 days.

       Caution
       - Chlorpromazine should not be used for emergency situations/sedation. It can worsen the confusion because of its anticholinergic effects.
       - Do not give combinations of antipsychotics (e.g., Haloperidol + Zuclopenthixol Acetate. However, the combination of an antipsychotic and a benzodiazepine can be useful (as above). Avoid Clothiapine

Table 72.1 Types of mechanical restraints and how they are used

Type	Description	How to use mechanical restraint
Anklet	A soft leather band around the ankle or leg	Secure to a stationary object.
		Acceptable fasteners include Velcro and buckle-type devices.
		The devices must not be secured tightly as to interfere with circulation or so loose as to permit skin chafing. (Two-finger widths should fit between the cuffs and patient).
		Padding the inside of the device aids in preventing chafing.
Wristlet	A soft leather band fastened around the wrist or arm	Secure to a stationary objects.
		Acceptable fasteners include Velcro and buckle-type devices.
		The devices must not be secured tightly as to interfere with circulation or so loose as to permit skin chafing.
Chair fixation	A soft leather material put across the chest.	Secure to the back of the chair.
		Acceptable fasteners include Velcro and buckle-type devices.
		The devices must not be secured tightly as to interfere with respiration.
Bed fixation	A soft leather material put across the bed.	Secure on both sides of the bed.
		Acceptable fasteners include Velcro and buckle-type devices.
		The devices must not be secured tightly as to interfere with respiration
Mitten	A covering for the hand.	The device must be the proper size for the patient.

(Etomine) – causes severe hypotension and is epileptogenic.

- Acute, dangerous side effects: acute laryngeal dystonia, hypotension, arrhythmias, and neuroleptic malignant syndrome.
- ACUTE DYSTONIA is an emergency! Clinical Presentation – Fixed, abnormal posture of head, neck, tongue, or other muscles. Could also present as occulogyric crisis. Breathing could be obstructed. Management
  - Akineton (Biperidine) 1 ampoule = 5 mg given IMI or IVI – May be repeated once if ineffective.
  - IM Benzodiazepines may be used in addition to achieve muscle relaxation.

- Mechanical restraints
  Mechanical restraints are any mechanical device applied to a person's body for the primary purpose of restricting movement of any part of that person's body. Mechanical restraints would not be used as a planned intervention, but rather in an emergency situation to meet a duty of care. In such a situation, intervention is reasonably required and not intervening could be considered a breach of duty to care. Mechanical restraints (Tables 72.1 and 72.2) are indicated when all other attempts at de-escalation have failed.

Table 72.2 Method of restraint and how it is applied

Method	How restraint is applied
2 point	One arm and one leg on the opposite side of the body
	Both arms
3 point	One arm and both legs
	Both arms and one leg

72.1.4 Management of Alcohol Withdrawal in a Delirious Patient

Often patients afflicted with trauma may be suffering from comorbid alcohol and drug use disorders and may present with nervousness, physical complications of drug use (e.g., ulcer, gastritis, liver disease, hypertension), evidence of self-neglect (e.g., poor hygiene). During the time in the emergency department, they may present with signs of withdrawal from alcohol (e.g., sweating, tremors, sickness, hallucinations [usually visual] seizures), opioids (nausea, sweating, restlessness, goose bumps, diarrhea (cold turkey), hallucinations); sedatives (anxiety, tremors, insomnia, hallucinations), and stimulants e.g., cocaine, crack, amphetamine, ecstasy (depression, moodiness, irritability).

- For patients with mild alcohol withdrawal symptoms, frequent monitoring, support, reassurance,

Table 72.3 Diazepam regimen

Days 1 and 2:	20–30 mg qds
Days 3 and 4:	15 mg qds
Day 5:	10 mg qds
Day 6:	10 mg bd
Day 7:	10 mg nocte

adequate hydration, and nutrition are sufficient treatment without medication.

- Patients with a moderate withdrawal syndrome may require benzodiazepines and vitamins in addition. Most can be detoxified, with a good outcome, as outpatients or at home. Community detoxification should only be undertaken by practitioners with appropriate training and supervision.
- Patients at risk of a complicated withdrawal syndrome (e.g., with a history of fits or delirium tremens, very heavy use and high tolerance, significant polydrug use, benzodiazepine dependence, severe comorbid medical or psychiatric disorder) who lack social support or are at a significant suicide risk may require specialist input and likely inpatient detoxification by the physicians in liaison with specialist alcohol services.
- Diazepam is recommended. The initial dose should be titrated against withdrawal symptoms, within a range of 5–30 mg 4 times a day. This requires close, skilled supervision. The following regimen is commonly used, although the dose level and length of treatment will depend on the severity of alcohol dependence and individual patient factors (e.g., weight, sex, and liver function); Table 72.3:
- Naltrexone may decrease alcohol consumption in people with alcohol dependency but their compliance with treatment appears problematic.
- Dispensing should be daily or involve the support of family members to prevent the risk of misuse or overdose. Confirm abstinence by checking the breath for alcohol, or using a saliva test or breathalyzer for the first 3–5 days.
- Thiamine (150 mg per day in divided doses) should be given orally for 1 month. Transfer patient immediately to a general hospital or clinic with appropriate resuscitation facilities for parenteral supplementation if any one of the following is present: ataxia, confusion, memory disturbance, delirium tremens, hypothermia and hypotension, ophthalmoplegia, or unconsciousness.
- Daily supervision is essential in the first few days, then advisable thereafter, to adjust dose of medication, assess whether the patient has returned to drinking, check for serious withdrawal symptoms, and maintain support.
- Patients requiring management of alcohol withdrawal with any of the following complications should be managed in an inpatient setting (see Table 72.4).

Table 72.4 Reasons for admission to a General Medical Hospital/Ward

Admission to a General Medical Hospital/Ward	
Complication Category	Specific Element
Complication obtained from the previous history	• Previous complicated withdrawal (e.g., delirium tremens, alcohol hallucinosis)
	• Previous convulsions or other complications during withdrawal
	• Recent loss of consciousness
	• Comorbid psychoactive substance abuse
Complications related to alcohol	• Severe state of intoxication
	• Markedly excessive alcohol use: the more potent the alcohol, the more frequent the use, and the longer it lasted, the more likely is complicated withdrawal
	• No, or insignificant relief 2 hours following the first outpatient benzodiazepine dose
Complicating physical features	• Malnutrition
	• Fever
	• Hypothermia
	• Dehydration
	• Jaundice
	• Severe tremors
	• Signs of significant trauma, especially head trauma
	• Specific organ failure
	• Acute abdominal signs
	• Gastrointestinal bleeding
	• Localizing neurological features
	• Wernicke's encephalopathy
	• Presence of other medical or surgical conditions or use of medication likely to complicate withdrawal management
Complications related to the mental status examination	• Clouding of consciousness
	• Delirium
Complications related to the financial/socioeconomic status of the patient	• Patients who do not have the financial/social resources to cope with outpatient detoxification.

72.2 Common Trauma-Related Psychological Disorders

72.2.1 Trauma-Related Psychological Disorders

(a) Acute stress reaction

For acute stress reaction (ASR), symptoms develop within minutes of a traumatic event and last up to hours or days. Although ASR is identified as a diagnosable disorder in ICD-10, it could more appropriately be considered a normal response to psychological trauma (as it remits naturally within hours or days), whereas acute stress disorder (ASD) and posttraumatic stress disorder (PTSD) are more abnormal responses.

(b) Acute stress disorder

Acute stress disorder may be diagnosed within the first 4 weeks following a traumatic incident. It is characterized by:

1. Intrusive symptoms (reliving the event in memories, dreams, and images)
2. Avoidance symptoms (avoiding things that remind the victim of the trauma and having difficulty remembering the event)
3. Arousal symptoms (hypervigilance, sleep disturbances, irritability, etc.)
4. Dissociation symptoms (a sense of detachment or numbness, decrease in awareness of surroundings, depersonalization, etc.)

   If these symptoms persist past 4 weeks, posttraumatic stress disorder is diagnosed [9, 12, 13].

A person may be described as having acute stress disorder if other mental disorders or medical conditions do not provide a better explanation for the person's symptoms. If symptoms persist after a month, the diagnosis becomes posttraumatic stress disorder. Symptoms include:

- Lack of emotional responsiveness, a sense of numbing or detachment
- A reduced sense of surroundings
- A sense of not being real
- Depersonalization or a sense of being dissociated from self
- An inability to remember parts of the trauma, "dissociative amnesia"
- Increased state of anxiety and arousal such as a difficulty staying awake or falling asleep
- Trouble experiencing pleasure
- Repeatedly re-experiencing the event through recurring images and/or thoughts, dreams, illusions, flashbacks
- Purposeful avoidance of exposure to thoughts, emotions, conversations, places, or people that remind them of the trauma
- Feelings of stress interfering with functioning; social and occupational skills are impaired affecting the patient's ability to function, pursue required tasks, and seek treatment

(c) Posttraumatic stress disorder

Types of symptoms exhibited in PTSD include those listed above for ASD (although dissociation symptoms are emphasized more in diagnosing ASD compared with PTSD). PTSD is considered chronic if symptoms last for 3 months or more, but may last for years or even decades, especially if untreated.

(d) Panic disorder

It is very common for trauma victims to experience panic attacks during the traumatic experience, and traumatic experiences appear to increase the risk of later development of panic disorders. Panic attacks occur suddenly, with symptoms that include rapid heartbeat, feelings of fear or terror, dizziness, and difficulty breathing.

(e) Depression

Depression is characterized by feelings of hopelessness, helplessness or despair, lethargy, lack of interest in former interests, difficulty concentrating, and other symptoms. It often occurs as a comorbid symptom with PTSD, but can occur on its own following a traumatic experience. Victims who are diagnosed with depression (without PTSD) following a traumatic event are less likely than those diagnosed with PTSD to have chronic mental health effects.

72.2.2 Management of Psychological Trauma

(a) Early intervention strategies

It is essential to examine accepted principles of mental health early interventions that can be adapted to psychological trauma. The Australian Government Department of Health and Ageing (DHA) define early intervention as: … timely interventions which target people displaying the early signs and symptoms of a mental health problem or a mental disorder. Early intervention also encompasses the early identification of patients suffering from a first episode of disorder [3]. Early intervention overlaps between prevention and treatment and is part of a continuum of care, not a "stand-alone" approach.

Early intervention aims to prevent emerging signs and symptoms for people developing or experiencing a first episode of mental disorder from progressing into diagnosable disorders, and reduces the need for recovery interventions. Early intervention aims to reduce the effect of the disorder in both its duration and the damage it may cause to a person's life [4]. Early intervention should include three broad strategies: indicated prevention, case identification, and early treatment.

(b) Indicated prevention

Indicated prevention strategies are aimed at "at-risk" individuals who are identified as having minimal signs and symptoms that could foreshadow or warn of a developing mental illness. For psychological trauma, interventions should be considered when some of the diagnostic criteria for ASR or ASD are appearing, usually in the hours and days following exposure to traumatic events, and should aim to prevent the progression of ASR to ASD, or the development of ASD. Exposure to traumatic events alone could be regarded as enough to trigger indicated prevention strategies, as exposure alone can satisfy one of the diagnostic criteria for ASR or ASD. Common indicated prevention strategies include "psychological first aid," psychoeducation, reinforcement of coping and resilience, maximizing social support and cohesion, and cognitive, emotional, and behavior strategies to mitigate symptoms. Also included may be strategies to increase therapeutic alliance, maximize engagement with therapy if required, advocate for mental health treatment, provide education to destigmatize, maximize assistance-seeking, create a positive expectation of recovery, and aid self-recognition of symptoms and appropriate self-referral.

(c) Case identification

Case identification in early intervention aims to recognize signs and symptoms of emerging disorders, even when the signs and symptoms are fewer, of shorter duration, or less intensive and disruptive than necessary for full diagnosis [4].

(d) Early treatment

Early treatment for ASD and sub-threshold ASD aims to prevent the development of PTSD-Acute and to restore functionality. First-line treatment for ASD or PTSD-Acute is generally psychotherapy. The basic criteria for use of psychotherapeutic treatments for acute trauma are that they are evidence based and appropriate. Standardized Cognitive Behavioral Therapy (CBT) strategies for ASD are available [7, 10]. They show promise in ameliorating ASD and preventing the subsequent development of PTSD, and should be considered as first-line options [6, 7, 11].

72.2.3 Counseling the Family

Trauma is not only profoundly distressing but also bewildering – to patients, their family members, and, at times, even mental health professionals. Persons in close relationships with traumatized patients are exposed to emotional contagion and vicarious trauma.

In the early stages of trauma, families will benefit from being informed of the seriousness of the trauma, management plan, and the prognosis and possible long-term outcomes of the trauma.

Families need to be also informed of the psychological consequences of trauma. When psychological disorders set it, it is usually the family members who notice that the traumatized person is jumpier, anxious, depressed, or not sleeping well and withdrawing from people. During these times, family members and friends are in a very good position to offer support and recovery. Secure and stable relationships are the foundation for healing. Therefore, an early positive working alliance needs to be established between the treating physician and the family. Providing education and an understanding of the consequences of trauma to the family is a platform for future treatment and hope.

It is important to inform the family that trauma-related problems may undermine attachments, often creating a vicious circle of spiraling distress wherein the traumatized person feels increasingly alienated from sources of support – and further traumatized. Family members may be impacted by the traumatized person's emotional crises. They become sensitive to small mood changes or other risks to stability; find it difficult to relax and feel as if they are "walking on eggshells"; become fearful if their loved one is angry or aggressive; are reluctant to talk about the trauma or avoiding situations that might upset the patient; angry or resentful toward the patient; tired because of worry; isolated if the patient refuses to socialize. Eventually family members may become depressed or angry about the changes in family life, with resultant emotional distance from the patient. They may need to be referred for counseling and/or therapy.

Recommended Reading

1. American Psychiatric Association (1994) Diagnostic and statistical manual of mental disorders, 4th edn. American Psychiatric Association, Washington, DC
2. World Health Organization (1994) International classification of diseases and related health problems, 10th revision. World Health Organization, Geneva
3. Australian Health Ministers (2003) National mental health plan 2003–2008. Australian Government Department of Health and Ageing, Canberra
4. Commonwealth Department of Health and Aged Care (2000) Promotion, prevention and early intervention for mental health. A monograph. Commonwealth Department of Health and Aged Care, Canberra
5. Bryant RA, Harvey AG (2000) Acute stress disorder: a handbook of theory, assessment, and treatment. American Psychological Association, Washington, DC
6. Bryant RA, Harvey AG, Dang ST et al (1998) Treatment of acute stress disorder: a comparison of cognitive-behavioural therapy and supportive counselling. J Consult Clin Psychol 66:862–866
7. Bryant RA, Moulds ML, Nixon RV (2003) Cognitive behaviour therapy of acute stress disorder: a four-year follow up. Behav Res Ther 41:489–494
8. DePrince AP, Freyd JJ (2002) The harm of trauma: pathological fear, shattered assumptions, or betrayal? In: Kauffman J (ed) Loss of the assumptive world: a theory of traumatic loss. Brunner-Routledge, New York, pp 71–82
9. American Psychiatric Association (2000) Diagnostic and statistical manual of mental disorders: DSM-IV-TR. American Psychiatric Association, Washington, DC
10. Foa EB, Riggs DS (2001) Brief recovery program (BRP) for trauma survivors. University of Pennsylvania, Philadelphia
11. Foa EB, Hearst-Ikeda D, Perry KJ (1995) Evaluation of a brief cognitive behavioral program for the prevention of chronic PTSD in recent assault victims. J Consult Clin Psychol 63:948–955
12. Kaplan HI, Sadock BJ. Synopsis of Psychiatry. Behavioural Sciences/Clinical Psychiatry. 8th edition. Lippincott Williams and Wilkins
13. Robertson B, Allwood C, Gagiano C (eds) (2001) Textbook of psychiatry for Southern Africa. Oxford University Press, Southern Africa

Early Neurotrauma Rehabilitation

73

Ronald E. Hirschberg

Recovery and repair begin with injury. This continues during the acute care stay and onward to the rehabilitation floor or hospital, as the environment and surrounding expertise adapt to the changing medical and functional needs of the patient. Just as early resuscitation and treatment of trauma patients has advanced the field of trauma surgery, early rehabilitation is of key importance in reducing morbidity and improving functional outcome. Emphasis on early rehabilitation intervention strategies in acute care has been studied in traumatic brain injury (TBI), spinal cord injury (SCI), and stroke rehabilitation, showing the great need for these services following acute trauma or disease [1, 2]. The injuries and impairments that affect the trauma patient are of broad scope. This chapter will highlight the two main categories of neurotrauma rehabilitation, traumatic brain injury, and spinal cord injury.

Following both primary and secondary injury to the brain and spinal cord, restoration of residual function ensues. The term "plasticity," the idea that neuronal tissue is both modifiable and capable of recovery, is a relatively new phenomenon within the field of neuroscience, and over the past 10–15 years, a large collection of preclinical and human studies show that indeed repair, restoration, and regeneration of neuronal tissue are possible. Both functional reorganization (uninjured tissue subserving needs for injured tissue) and neuronal regeneration (neuronal sprouting within the traumatic lesion) are the two basic mechanisms by which neuroplasticity are proposed to occur. Environmental enrichment, practice, and repetition are all fundamental principles of neuroplasticity underlying neurotrauma restoration and thus provide rationale for physical rehabilitation [12].

R.E. Hirschberg
Department of PM&R, Massachusetts General Hospital, Harvard Medical School, 55 Fruit Street, Ruth Sleeper Hall, 3rd Floor, Boston, MA 02114, USA
e-mail: rhirschberg@partners.org

73.1 Acute Traumatic Brain Injury Rehabilitation

TBI is the third leading cause of death by injury in the United States 550,000 persons hospitalized each year with TBI, and more than 80,000 persons per year developing long-term disability. In 2003, in the USA, 32% of TBIs were attributed to falls, 19% by traffic accidents, and 18% from other trauma [3]. The majority of persons with TBI are male and less than age 30. Younger age at injury amounts to devastating consequences on social, financial, emotional, and familial development. Since the advancement of earlier in-field care (i.e., "Jaws of life"), and more recent neurosurgical guidelines, people are surviving severe TBI more than ever before. This has implications on rehabilitation of TBI patients given the shear volume of patients, and with respect to the low levels of function, these patients begin their recovery with, once medically and surgically stabilized.

The TBI rehabilitation plan begins with establishing the major impairments specific to the injury itself. The patient with polytrauma or concomitant spinal cord injury poses unique challenges for the patient and the team, which will be discussed within this chapter. General impairments in TBI encompass three main groups: Cognitive, physical, and behavioral.

G.C. Velmahos et al. (eds.), *Penetrating Trauma*,
DOI 10.1007/978-3-642-20453-1_73,

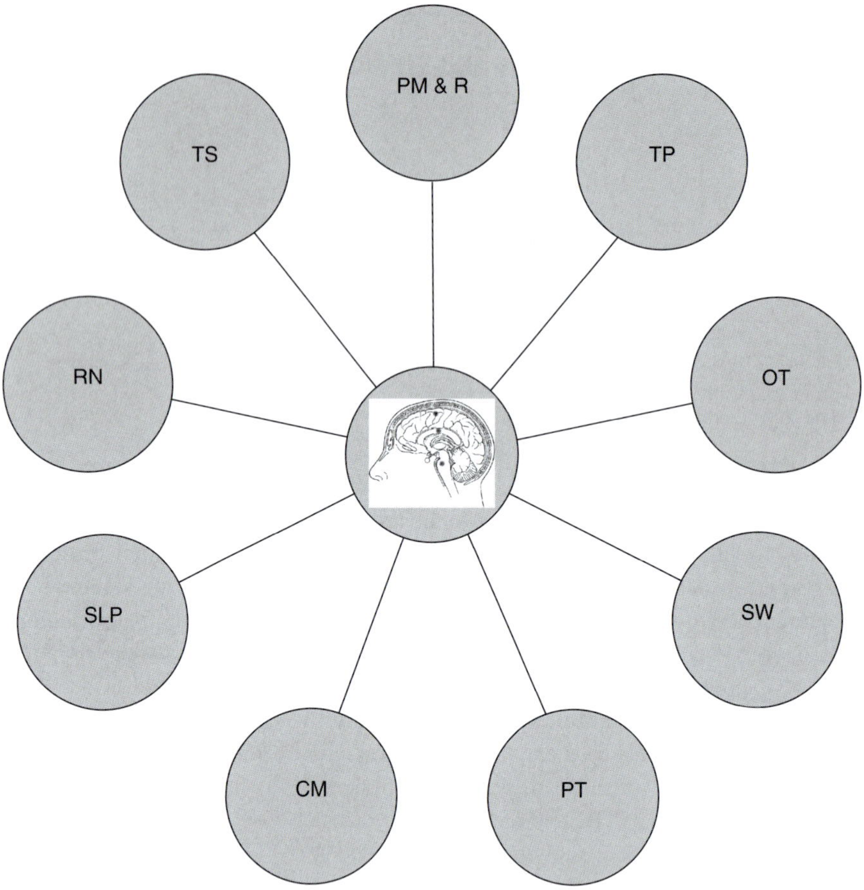

Fig. 73.1 Due to the enormous complexity of physical, cognitive, and behavioral dysfunction, in the setting of potential premorbidy such as alcoholism, mental health disorders, and/or social challenges, regular communication among trauma team members is paramount to optimizing recovery

Cognitive deficits are first manifested in problems with communication and comprehension which have profound impact on the rehabilitation plan of care. Typical cognitive sequelae that affect all aspects of both early and later rehabilitation include memory, concentration, and attention deficits. Diffuse injury, commonly occurring in closed head injuries from acceleration-deceleration mechanism, classically results in cognitive-related language problems (due to executive dysfunction) rather than linguistic-related problems (i.e., aphasia) [6]. Physical impairments range from upper and lower extremity and trunk motor dysfunction to speech and swallowing dysfunction. The behavioral impairments of moderate-to-severe TBI include impulsivity, distractibility, aggression, and agitation as a person with acute TBI emerges through the stereotypical levels of cognitive functioning (Ranchos Los Amigos, or RLA scale of Levels of Cognitive Functioning I-VIII).[1]

The patient with moderate-to-severe TBI especially requires a multidisciplinary approach including members of surgery, physiatry (physical medicine and rehabilitation specialists), psychiatry, nursing, physical and occupational therapy (PT, OT), speech and language pathology (SLP), social work, and case management. Due to the enormous complexity of physical, cognitive, and behavioral dysfunctions, in the setting of potential premorbidity such as alcoholism, mental health disorders and / or social challenges, regular communication among trauma team members is paramount to optimizing recovery (Fig. 73.1). The collaboration should begin in the intensive care unit with carry-over throughout acute care. Admission to the inpatient rehabilitation center is a major step upward with respect to intensity and frequency of rehabilitation; however, it should ideally serve as a continuation of TBI rehabilitation as persons go from "coma to community," rather than the *initiation* of rehabilitation.

[1]Original Scale co-authored by Chris Hagen, Ph.D., Danese Malkmus, M.A., Patricia Durham, M.A. Communication Disorders Service, Rancho Los Amigos Hospital, 1972.

73.1.1 Projections and Prognosis

TBI rehabilitation is incomplete without discussions of prognosis. This is begun in the initial stages of recovery and continues during acute rehabilitation, depending on the individual patient's trajectory of gains. Rehabilitation plans with the entire team are carved out on the basis of outcome expectations and goals. All TBI characteristics, including CT and MRI findings, age, Glasgow Coma Scores (GCS), comorbidities, and premorbid psychosocial aspects, play a significant role in realistic prognostication.

Interstingly, prognostic guidelines have supported use of "threshold values" rather than percentages of "good outcome" or "poor outcome," as families have noted positive response to this. Even with twenty-first century research and technology in the expanding field of TBI, posttraumatic amnesia (PTA), or the time between injury and the time at which ongoing new memories are made, has actually been the strongest predictor to date for outcome in TBI patients. Threshold values for PTA include: "Severe disability is unlikely when PTA last less than 2 months," and "Good recovery is unlikely when PTA last longer than 3 months" [22]. The trauma physiatrist collaborates with the primary trauma team, neurosurgery, and neurology, offering caregivers and families potential expectations for outcome and explaining the dynamic course of recovery and rehabilitation toward realistic goals.

Diffuse axonal injury (DAI), commonly seen concomitant with focal cerebral injuries, poses a unique challenge to the rehabilitation team given its classic injury pattern manifestations of arousal, behavior, and cognitive impairments. Deeper lesions to the brainstem or cerebellar peduncles (grade III DAI), middle-regions to subcortical structures like the corpus collosum (grade II DAI), and surface regions such as the frontal convexity (grade I DAI), all correspond to these impairments, respectively (Fig. 73.2). Although no evidence supports need for MRI to detect these injuries in the hyperacute phase of injury given that there is no change in medical or surgical management, these findings can have rehabilitation treatment and prognostic relevance [5].

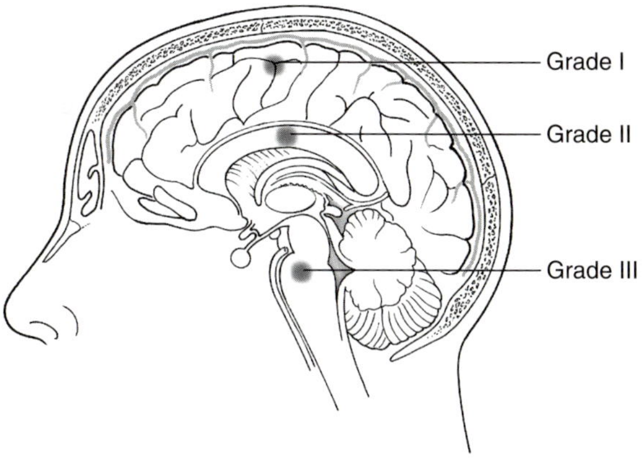

Fig. 73.2 Deeper lesions to the brainstem or cerebellar peduncles (grade III DAI), middle-regions to subcortical structures like the corpus collosum (grade II DAI), and surface regions such as the frontal convexity (grade I DAI), all correspond to these impairments, respectively

73.1.2 Function and Participation

Once hemodynamically stable, the patient with acute moderate-to-severe TBI embarks on rehabilitation with increasing duration and frequency of treatments over weeks. PT, OT, and SLP interactions begin first with assessments, followed by extensive work on engagement of the patient. As patients emerge, they generally fall into three categories with respect to overall function: the confused-agitated patient (delirious state within PTA), the low-functional-state patient, and the confused-participatory patient. Although some portion of rehabilitation is passive, much depends on active participation, and therefore creating both environmental and pharmacological plans in order to optimize daily engagement for the specific patient is crucial.

The acute TBI patient can have several reasons to be agitated and restless, including pain, infection, fear, and substance withdrawal, and therefore isolating the primary cause is important. Interestingly, recovery following acute TBI (specifically those with DAI) will usually follow a natural progression through levels of cognition, and the RLA level IV indicates the "confused and agitated state." This is usually followed by confused and non-agitated states and can often be both a hurdle for the patient and family to move beyond, but at the same time a positive marker of continued functional gains. During this stage, nursing staff and therapists strive to incorporate environmental and behavioral modification tactics (controlled stimulation in the environment, small numbers of visitors, sleep–wake cycle adherence) [7].

Medications are usually required for optimizing participation and improving safety of the patient and staff. Opiates, typical antipsychotics (haloperidol), and benzodiazepines may be required initially for severe pain, extreme agitation, and confounding alcohol withdrawal; however, on serial review of the patient, he or she should be transitioned to other agents. Although the data is not clear as to the negative effects of chronic atypical antipsychotic use, studies have indicated that ongoing typical antipsychotic treatment (largest amount of dopamine [D2] blockade) results in deleterious motor effects in animal models [8]. Interestingly, a Cochrane Database Study in 2003 covering all to-date trials in agitation and aggression after acquired brain injury revealed that the only reasonable evidence for positive treatment response were trials using beta-blockers (inderal and pindolol) [9].

Low-functional-state patients represent persons in coma (lack of wakefulness), vegetative states (VS) (wakefulness), and those in minimally conscious states (MCS) (environmental awareness). These neurological stages correspond to the aforementioned recovery scale RLA levels I, II and III, respectively. During these low functioning states following severe TBI, rehabilitation focuses on: (1) optimizing daily participation, (2) fostering sleep–wake cycles, (3) minimizing all complications of immobility, and (4) realistic short-term goal setting for mobility, communication, and cognition.

Preparedness of the patient in VS (or RLA II) and MCS (or RLA III) for ongoing rehabilitation efforts is of key importance during the initial stages of recovery. The team emphasizes early mobilization to encourage practice-dependent neuroplasticity with daily stimulation from all therapy and other staff modalities. As medical stability improves, strong emphasis on nutrition, avoidance of infections, and layering off all sedating medications (especially daytime) are placed by the physiatrist and/or the primary surgical team. It is the job of the trauma physiatrist to always re-assess what medications are potentially not necessary as the patient transitions, not only through acute care but inpatient rehabilitation. Antiepileptic medication courses are monitored closely, in addition to other potentially neurologically deleterious medications like metoclopramide, antihistiminergic agents, benzodiazepines, and others.

The amount of level I evidence for the use of neurostimulants to augment the recovery process in TBI patients emerging from low-level states is slim. However, there is some evidence that the dopaminergic medication Amantadine accounts for heightened arousal, cognitive and overall functional scores in several studies. Amphetamines, (methylphenidate) utilized for arousal and attention deficits, and another agent for arousal originally indicated for narcolepsy (modafinil) have had reasonable efficacy in this population. The rationale for using these agents during rehabilitation and restoration is twofold: (1) increased arousal and attention provide the environment for increased quantity and quality of physical and cognitive rehabilitation treatments, and (2) there are inherent positive properties of neuroactive medications which can affect neuronal growth factors, antagonize NMDA receptors, and improve lipid peroxidation, etc. [10, 11].

73.1.3 Complications and Rehabilitation Challenges

The complications and sequelae of TBI directly affect optimal rehabilitation of the patient, and therefore outcome. DAI, brainstem injury, and associated hypoxia are all associated with dysautonomia, or “storming” which is a clinical entity involving labile cardiac function, pyrexia, sweating, and decorticate or decerebrate posturing, and is associated with prolonged acute care and rehabilitation stays and worse functional outcomes. Management during both acute and rehabilitation settings involves identifying primary triggers (pain, fractures, infection, other noxious stimuli), which in the patient with polytrauma has clear relevance (pelvic, spinal, and/or extremity fractures). Pharmacological treatment with beta-blockers, bromocriptine, dantrolene, and even intrathecal baclofen has been utilized during both acute care and the rehabilitation setting.

Upper motor neuron dysregulation following TBI results in velocity-dependent increased muscle tone (spasticity) which can interfere with mobility, positioning, hygiene, and becomes a pain generator. Initial treatment includes early maintenance of passive and active range of motion, stretching programs and serial casting or splinting upon collaboration with physical and occupational therapy. Common pharmacological treatment consists of baclofen (GABA-B agonist) which has more sedating effects and may be less desirable of first agent, dantrolene (blocks calcium release at the sarcoplasmic reticulum) which offers direct effects at the muscle belly. Focal motor point blocks with Botox intramuscularly and neurolysis with phenol offer localized treatment and can also be effective with concomitant serial casting of the patient [13, 14].

Some degree of immobility is unavoidable in patients with moderate-to-severe TBI and many organ systems are affected. Deconditioning results in muscle atrophy and weakness, osteopenia with lack of weight-bearing, postural hypertension, dehydration, constipation, gastric reflux, etc. In combination with various problems specific to the TBI patient (associated polytrauma, posturing and spasticity of limbs and trunk, need for tracheostomy and gastrostomy, dysphagia, sensory dysfunction and communication impairments), the effect of deconditioning on function is that more challenging to the patient and to rehabilitation teams. Attempting to attenuate and reverse the cycle with early mobilization is therefore of key importance in these patients [13, 14].

As with all dramatic functional changes encountered after trauma, family involvement and education cannot be underemphasized as patients proceed through rehabilitation phases. The entire family is "injured" in acute TBI in many complex ways and is modified by premorbid dynamics among members or caregivers. During both acute and rehabilitation care settings, it is essential that the rehabilitation team direct, educate, and counsel the family. As mentioned, trauma physiatrists can play a key role as "interventionalists," guiding patients and families with realistic prognostication, as well as ongoing education as patients recover at various stages during recovery and rehabilitation.

73.2 Acute Spinal Cord Injury Rehabilitation

Traumatic spinal cord injury affects roughly 10,000 persons per year in the USA which has surprisingly remained the same over 30 years, with about 50% due to motor vehicle accidents, 25% due to falls, 10% from sports, and 12% from violence. Falls have increased steadily, and violence has decreased over the past three decades. The ratio of male to female is 4:1 and unchanged over the years [15, 16]. To date, there has been no solid evidence for the use of medical treatments at the acute stage of injury, including high-dosed methylprednisolone which has now been considered a "treatment option" rather than the standard of care. Therefore, much emphasis on proper recovery has been on early stabilization and mobilization as to begin the rehabilitation process as soon as possible [17].

Following acute SCI, physiatry should assist with diagnosing injury severity and discussing functional relevance, management of specific spinal cord related impairments, patient education including communication of the diagnosis and long-term expectations, and prevention of physical and medical complications associated with SCI. Classification of injury is typically performed within 72 h from injury and repeated at roughly 1 month, usually during the initial stages of one's inpatient rehabilitation stay. The American Spinal Injury Association (ASIA) has developed the reliable and standardized classification system, most recently updated in 2003, which offers physicians and therapists specific guidelines for treatment and rehabilitation with respect to a patient's neurological level and completeness of injury. (Completeness of injury is defined by ASIA standards as SCI with no sparing of sensation or voluntary motor activity of the sacral segments S4-S5 on rectal examination) [17, 18].

The initial rehabilitation of the patient focuses on prevention of the complications of immobility (contractures, decubitus ulcers, thromboembolism, infections), vigilant pulmonary toilet, and bowel and bladder management. PT and OT, along with RN and family members, can incorporate plans for daily passive- and active-assisted range of motion to prevent contracture in vulnerable flexor muscle groups at the hips, knees, ankles, shoulders, and elbows. Of key importance is ongoing stretching and strengthening of the *intact* muscle groups, as to avoid atrophy and deconditioning. Patients with cervical injuries may require evaluation by SLP to ensure safety of swallowing, especially after tracheostomy, and communication devices are initiated in order to medically and physically treat the patient as he or she begins to participate in the rehabilitation program [18].

73.2.1 The SCI Review of Systems

Spinal cord injury rehabilitation and medical management are largely dictated by the level of injury, and many of the "SCI-review of systems" are similarly affected in both tetraplegia and paraplegia. These include bowel, bladder, renal, skin, hematologic, nutrition, musculoskeletal, and psychological manifestations. A distinction should be made however with respect to the cardiopulmonary systems, which are discussed in more detail below.

Cervical injuries are highly prone to pulmonary complications (atelectasis, hypoventilation, and secretions), affecting 84% of all C1-C4 level of injury patients, and 60% of all C5-C8 patients. Rehabilitation efforts at all stages post-injury should focus on maintenance of secretion clearance with assisted cough, including mechanical insufflator-exsufflator (M-IE) device (positive pressure immediately followed by negative pressure), and manually assisted cough or "quad cough" with abdominal thrusts on expiration. During active weaning of ventilatory support during the recovery and rehabilitation phase for tetraplegics, titration of high tidal volumes is encouraged while chest x-rays are followed toward the resolution of atelectasis [17].

Autonomic dysreflexia (AD) can occur occasionally in the acute care setting and should be recognized. It will typically manifest following resolution of spinal chock. AD is caused by dysregulation of the autonomic nervous system with both unopposed sympathetic and parasympathetic responses to noxious stimuli and results classically in hypertension, bradycardia (compensatory response to hypertension), and usually with associated headache. This occurs in patients with levels of injury of T6 and higher and is more commonly associated with complete injury. The noxious stimulus is typically the result of impacted bowel, or obstructed outflow from the bladder, but can certainly include pain stimuli; thus polytrauma patients have more relative risk. Treatment includes addressing the underlying cause or stimulus and if unable to do so, lowering blood pressure with nitrate medications. Suboptimal management of AD can result in less rehabilitation duration and frequency, and is potentially harmful to the patient, with extreme prolonged systolic blood pressures greater than 200 posing risk for intracerebral hypertension [14, 15, 19].

Orthostatic hypotension due to loss of sympathetic tone is common in SCI patients of all levels of injury and initiates with onset of spinal shock, or loss of spinal reflexes (including sympathetic responses) below the level of injury. Initial management strives to encourage patient participation with therapies without becoming symptomatic, and includes ace-wrapping or thigh-high TEDs, abdominal binders to decreased splanchnic vascular pooling, introducing tilt table and progressive postural exercises in order to gradually retrain carotid baroreceptors. If needed for mobilization of the patient, salt tablets, midodrine, and/or fludrocortisone should be utilized [15, 19].

Spasticity is a part of the "upper motor neuron syndrome" in patients with SCI, and is commonly encountered during recovery and rehabilitation, with the resolution of spinal shock. As previously defined, it is velocity-dependent increases in muscle tone, and in SCI, it typically includes clonus, increased tendon reflexes, muscle spasms, and/or UMN signs such as the Babinski reflex. Roughly 80% of SCI patients experience spasticity, and treating spasticity is indicated only when it interferes with function of the patient (mobility, transfers, ambulation), impedes hygiene, causes pain, or leads to contractures of the joints.

Early rehabilitation management should include 1–2 times per day stretching (can reduce motoneuron excitability for hours), posture maintenance avoiding extensor bias at the trunk and hips, and serial casting in a prolonged stretch. Medications commonly used are Baclofen, Clonidine, and Tizanidine. Benzodiazepines are effective as well; however they are ideally avoided as to minimize sedation and cognitive effects during active rehabilitation. Neurolysis with phenol injection and intramuscular Botox are not as commonly used in SCI as in stroke and TBI in that the pathology is usually more diffuse; however, there are certainly cases where SCI patients benefit from focal blocks, especially in patients with incomplete SCI [18, 20].

73.2.2 Functional Goals

Functional goals for motor complete tetraplegia and paraplegia during rehabilitation are based on the level of motor impairment. Motor levels of injury are defined as the most caudal key muscle group at least 3/5 strength (antigravity) bilaterally, with the segments cephalad to this level being of normal strength (5/5). Injury level, depending on confounding factors such as age and comorbidities, is predictive of basic goals of feeding, grooming, dressing, bathing, bed mobility, transfers, wheelchair propulsion, and driving at 1 year post injury.

The two fundamental goals for motor levels C1-C4 are that of learning to instruct and manage one's own care with caregivers and family, and to learn the use of assistive technology (i.e., power wheelchairs with "sip

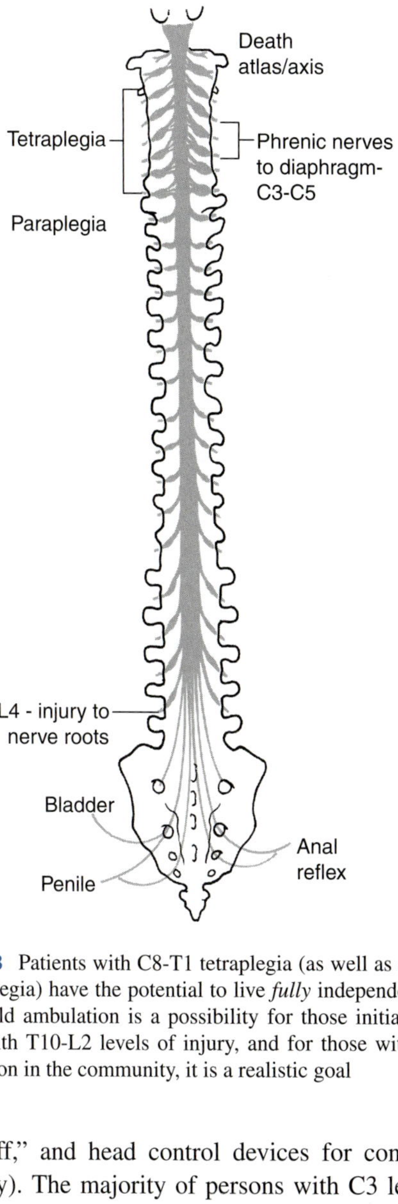

Fig. 73.3 Patients with C8-T1 tetraplegia (as well as all levels of paraplegia) have the potential to live *fully* independent lives. Household ambulation is a possibility for those initially diagnosed with T10-L2 levels of injury, and for those with L3-S5 ambulation in the community, it is a realistic goal

and puff," and head control devices for controlling mobility). The majority of persons with C3 levels or higher will require long-term ventilatory support. However, with intact phrenic nerve function, these patients become potential candidates for diaphragmatic pacing systems. For the most part, patients with C4 levels will be able to wean off the ventilator [18].

Persons with both C5 and C6 levels of injury at 1 year have the potential for independence with respect to feeding, grooming wheelchair propulsion, as the key muscle groups of elbow flexors (biceps) and wrist extensors (extensor carpi radialis) are functional, respectively. Those with C7 levels of injury possess the most significant leap in independence for tetraplegics in that the triceps muscle enables one to perform transfers, weight-shifts, and bed mobility. Patients with C8-T1 tetraplegia (as well as all levels of paraplegia) have the potential to live *fully* independent lives. Household ambulation is a possibility for those initially diagnosed with T10-L2 levels of injury, and for those with L3-S5 ambulation in the community, it is a realistic goal [16, 18] (Fig. 73.3).

73.3 The "Dual-Diagnosis"

The Spinal Cord Model Systems data report that 28.2% of SCI patients have at least mild TBI (loss of consciousness) and that 11.5% have TBI resulting in significant behavioral and/or cognitive disturbances. Adding to the extreme functional challenges that follow post-SCI alone, the classic impairments of memory, attention, insight, and judgment experienced in TBI can greatly complicate rehabilitation for the patient and pose more challenges to the team. Posttraumatic amnesia (inability to retain new information), as one might imagine, can be devastating for optimal participation.

Clinicians should be cognizant of the low threshold of sedation and cognitive disturbance in those with TBI of all severities when treating spasticity with benzodiazepines, baclofen, and clonidine or tizanidine as mentioned above. Also, casting and splinting efforts may not be tolerated in those with TBI given propensity for restlessness and agitation from pain and sensory disturbances [18, 20]. There is limited work emphasizing outcomes for "dual-diagnosis" patients; however clinical opinion demonstrates that early identification of these particularly challenging patients is necessary to better utilize proper clinicians and resources during acute care and inpatient rehabilitation in hopes of better quality of the recovery process for the patient and family, and overall cost reduction [19, 21].

Important Points

- Environmental enrichment, practice, and repetition are all fundamental principles of neuroplasticity and provide rationale for physical rehabilitation.

- Cognitive deficits after TBI manifest in problems with communication and comprehension which have profound impact on the rehabilitation plan of care.
- TBI rehabilitation is multidisciplinary and begins in the intensive care unit. Inpatient rehabilitation provides increased intensity and should ideally serve as a continuation "coma to community," rather than the *initiation* of rehabilitation.
- The trauma physiatrist collaborates with other consultants offering families potential expectations for outcome and explaining the dynamic course of recovery toward realistic goals.
- The low-functional-state patient, the confused-agitated patient, and the confused-participatory patient are the three categories of emerging patients with severe TBI, dictating specific medical and rehabilitative management.
- Dysautonomia, spasticity, and the complications of immobility following acute TBI are the key challenges for the rehabilitation team as the patient emerges and recovers.
- After acute SCI, physiatry should discuss functional relevance of neurologic level of injury, help manage specific spinal cord related impairments, and communicate long-term expectations to the patient and the family.
- The "SCI-review of systems" includes the major organ systems affected by the injury. Managing the SCI-ROS optimally will provide the environment necessary for ongoing rehabilitation.
- Functional goals are based primarily on the neurologic level of injury from C1 to S5. For tetraplegia, the levels of C7 and below implicate potential for full functional independence.
- Almost 30% of patients sustaining SCI have concomitant TBI with more than 10% having significant behavioral or cognitive impairments, having large effects on the overall rehabilitation process.

References

1. Cifu DX, Stewart DG (1999) Factors affecting functional outcome after stroke: a critical review of rehabilitation interventions. Arch Phys Med Rehabil 80:S35–S39
2. Wagner AK, Zafonte RD, Goldberg G et al (2003) Physical medicine and rehabilitation consultation: relationships with acute functional outcome, length of stay, and discharge planning after traumatic brain injury. Am J Phys Med Rehabil 82:526–536
3. Centers for Disease Control and Prevention (1999) Traumatic brain injury in the United States: a report to Congress. Centers for Disease Control and Prevention, Atlanta
4. Brown AW, Elovic EP (2008) Congenital and acquired brain injury. 1. Epidemiology, pathophysiology, prognostication, innovative treatments, and prevention. Arch Phys Med Rehabil 89(3 Suppl 1):S3–S8
5. Manolakaki D, Velmahos GC (2009) Early magnetic resonance imaging is unnecessary in patients with traumatic brain injury. J Traum Inj Inf Crit Car 66(4):1008–1014
6. Mills V, Cassidy JW, Katz DI (1997) Neurologic rehabilitation: a guide to diagnosis, prognosis, and treatment planning. Wiley-Blackwell, Malden
7. Cherney L, Gillam R, Kennedy M, et al (2005) American Speech-Language-Hearing Associated Roles of speech-language pathologists in the identification, diagnosis, and treatment of individuals with cognitive-communication disorders. Position statement. ASHA Supplement 24:200
8. Feeney DM, Gonzalez A, Law WA (1982) Amphetamine, haloperidol, and experience interact to affect rate of recovery after motor cortex injury. Science 217:855–857
9. Fleminger S, Greenwood RJ, Oliver DL (2003) Pharmacological management for agitation and aggression in people with acquired brain injury. Cochrane Database Syst Rev (1):CD003299
10. Whyte J et al (1997) Effects of methylphenidate on attentional function after traumatic brain injury. A randomized, placebo-controlled trial. Am J Phys Med Rehabil 76(6): 440–450
11. Zafonte RD (2006) Neuropharmacology: a rehabilitation perspective. In: Zasler ND, Katz DI, Zafonte RD (eds) Brain injury medicine. Demos, New York
12. Stein D (2006) Concepts of CNS plasticity and their implications for understanding recovery after brain damage. In: Zasler ND, Katz DI, Zafonte RD (eds) Brain injury medicine. Demos, New York
13. Flanagan SR, Kwasnica C et al (2008) Congenital and acquired brain injury. 2. Medical rehabilitation in acute and subacute settings. Arch Phys Med Rehabil 89(Suppl 1):9–12
14. Bell K (2006) Complications associated with immobility after TBI. In: Zasler ND, Katz DI, Zafonte RD (eds) Brain injury medicine. Demos, New York
15. DeVivo M (2002) Epidemiology of traumatic spinal cord injury. In: Kirshblum S, Campagnolo DI, DeLisa JA (eds) Spinal cord medicine. Lippincott Williams & Wilkins, Philadelphia

16. Ho CH, Wuermser L et al (2007) Spinal cord injury medicine. 1. Epidemiology and classification. Arch Phys Med Rehabil 88(Suppl 1):49–54
17. Wuermser L, Ho CH et al (2007) Spinal cord injury medicine. 2. Acute care management of traumatic and nontraumatic injury. Arch Phys Med Rehabil 88(Suppl 1):55–59
18. Kirshblum S, Ho CH et al (2002) Rehabilitation of spinal cord injury. In: Kirshblum S, Campagnolo DI, DeLisa JA (eds) Spinal cord medicine. Lippincott Williams & Wilkins, Philadelphia
19. Campagnolo D, Geno M (2002) Autonomic and cardiovascular complications of spinal cord injury. In: Kirshblum S, Campagnolo DI, DeLisa JA (eds) Spinal cord medicine. Lippincott Williams & Wilkins, Philadelphia
20. Zafonte RD (2002) Spasticity following spinal cord injury. In: Kirshblum S, Campagnolo DI, DeLisa JA (eds) Spinal cord medicine. Lippincott Williams & Wilkins, Philadelphia
21. Zafonte RD (2002) Traumatic brain injury in a person with spinal cord injury. In: Kirshblum S, Campagnolo DI, DeLisa JA (eds) Spinal cord medicine. Lippincott Williams & Wilkins, Philadelphia
22. Katz DI, Alexander MP (1994) Traumatic brain injury: predicting course of recovery and outcome for patients admitted to rehabilitation. Arch Neurol (51):661–670

74 Rehabilitation

Amy H. Phelan

For many surgeons, the role of the Rehab team is somewhat of a mystery and the criteria for what qualifies for transfer to the inpatient rehabilitation unit arbitrary and somewhat random. This leads to confusion and frustration in dealing with the Rehabilitation team, but it does not have to be that way. Ideally, rehabilitation of the trauma patient begins during the initial hospitalization. During the acute hospitalization, the Rehabilitation team can initiate functional assessments and help prevent secondary disability. An example would be initiating proper splinting to avoid heel cord contractures that may delay ambulation and mobilization once the patient is out of the ICU. Frequently during these assessments and therapies, injuries or conditions that may impair recovery and return to function may be identified. Small hand fractures or traumatic rotator cuff tears, that may not been detected during initial triage, can impair the use of ambulatory aids and also delay return to ambulatory status. There may also be any number of musculoskeletal issues or conditions present prior to injury as well as psychological issues that may impair return to function. The Rehab team is uniquely able to assess and address these issues and thus expedite your patient toward the goal of disposition. Perhaps one of the Rehab Team's most valuable contributions is the ability to maximize function during the acute hospitalization and determine and arrange appropriate disposition, whether that be home, skilled nursing facility, inpatient unit, or other venue. In short, we can make them go away once your work is done! In the absence of a Rehab team, this responsibility usually falls to you and an overworked Social Worker, and in my experience, most surgeons find this aspect of patient care their least favorite and this the Rehab specialists most appreciated talent.

In Rehab, we use the word "team" a lot. That is because this is the approach we use when working with patients. The patient is always the most important member of the team; however, the Rehabilitation team is led by the physiatrist, who coordinates and directs the other members of the team and consults on medical issues. Physiatrists are trained in neurologic/musculoskeletal evaluation and functional assessment as well as the various treatment options and modalities. The Rehab consultant is frequently called on to assist the primary team in coordination of care and addressing acute care issues such as spasticity and bowel/bladder management, as well as prevention of secondary injury including skin breakdown and contractures. Most importantly, and I cannot emphasize this enough, is the assessment of function and the anticipation of future needs once definitive care of the trauma team is completed.

All of the members of the Rehab Team have their roles. Members of the rehabilitation team include nursing, physical therapy, occupational therapy, speech therapy, recreational therapy, vocational therapy, psychology, and social work. They each function in their own area of expertise, as well as in conjunction with the other team members. Not all patients will require treatment from all of the various disciplines; that is for the Physiatrist to determine. (i.e., who needs PT, who needs speech therapy, etc.) Rehabilitation nurses function pretty much as nurses on other services. They are

A.H. Phelan
Physical Medicine & Rehabilitation,
UT Southwestern Medical Center,
5323 Harry Hines Blvd, Dallas, TX 75390, USA
e-mail: amy.phelan@utsouthwestern.edu

G.C. Velmahos et al. (eds.), *Penetrating Trauma*,
DOI 10.1007/978-3-642-20453-1_74,

the "Moms" of the team. They assist in care of the patient and education of the patient and family. This can range from education regarding medications and wound care, to self-catheterization and bowel programs for neurogenic bowel and bladder injuries. They play a vital role in patient monitoring and prevention of secondary disability, specifically skin breakdown and pressure sores. Frequent position changes and hygiene are critical in these patients, and if not already in place, proper protocols should be in place for the care and monitoring of skin integrity. Physiatrists are experts at developing these protocols in conjunction with nursing staff. Pressure sores can significantly impair return to function and may delay wheel chair training and mobilization of any patient but especially the spinal cord patient. They may even be significant enough to keep the patient from qualifying for inpatient rehab and/or require further surgery.

Physical therapists are the Gym teachers or Coaches. They work to maintain strength, mobility, and coordination. They frequently function in the acute care setting in maintaining range of motion in the limbs, prevention of contractures and ambulation, when appropriate. Initiation and progression of therapy is directed by the Physiatrist. The therapists can look to the Physiatrist for guidance in treatment protocols and advancement of therapies. This allows for continuity of care even if therapy personnel change. Included in the scope of the physical therapist is appropriate bracing of the lower extremities to prevent contractures and pressure sores. These may be an "off-the-shelf" item or custom-made item depending on the needs of the patient.

Occupational therapists focus on life skills. They assist with activities of daily living (ADLs) and self-care, such as eating, bathing, oral-facial hygiene, and dressing. Some patients may require adaptive equipment and special utensils to perform these tasks, and OTs are excellent at problem solving these issues. They also work on advanced ADLs such as cooking, laundry, and housekeeping. They focus on the skills and functions that the patient will need in order to achieve independent living. The OT focus is mainly on upper extremity/hand function in regards to these tasks. Another treatment they can provide is appropriate splinting to prevent contractures and dynamic splinting to assist with functional tasks.

Speech therapists are the communicators. Their area of expertise is in communication, both verbal and nonverbal. They are a vital team member for patients with all kinds of aphasia and traumatic brain injury. They can also assess for dysphagia and cognitive/communication deficits. In the acute care setting, when patients are ready to resume oral intake, the Speech therapist can perform swallow evaluations and make dietary recommendations, if there is any doubt as to the patient's ability to protect his/her airway. In the area of cognitive function, the Speech therapist can assess for cognitive deficits and possible brain injury which may or may not be obvious, but whose diagnosis may require intervention and possible inpatient Rehab therapies. There are many reasons for cognitive impairment following trauma, both related to mechanism of injury and subsequent treatment and assessment of these deficits while on the acute care service can expedite care, lead to identification of resources available and possibly speed recovery.

The Social Worker is also an important member of the acute care and rehabilitation team. Once the functional status and needs of the patient are identified, the Social Worker helps to navigate the system in regards to resources and support. Their focus is on financial need, funding, and disposition issues. They are experts in identifying resources and helping patients and families make application for various support programs, such as Social Security disability.

Not necessarily part of the acute rehabilitation team but important members of the inpatient rehabilitation team are the Recreational and Vocational rehabilitation specialists. The Vocational Rehab specialist addresses return-to-work issues and, if needed, job retraining. They work with the Social Worker as patient advocates with employers to assist with getting patient back to work as soon as possible. Then education and job retraining is requiring for eventual placement. The Vocational Rehab specialist advocates for the patient to make sure that the patient's rights to fair treatment and reasonable accommodation in the workplace are upheld.

The Recreational therapist brings the fun back in life. They focus on avocational activities that are important to the patient. Seeing the possibilities for resuming or discovering activities they love helps to motivate the patient during recovery, fight depression associated with loss of function, and help them feel "normal" again. The Recreational Therapist is an expert in adaptive equipment for sports such as skiing, sailing, and just about any sport imaginable.

Rehabilitation psychologist addresses behavioral and cognitive issues, mood disorders, and adjustment to loss/change in functional status. They carry out neuropsychology testing to determine any cognitive deficits and design treatment plans for adaptation and compensation for these deficits. Issues such as impulsivity, aggression, and motivation are just some of the areas these professionals work with. In addition, there are frequently psychological and adjustment issues specifically related to the trauma which brought them to the hospital. Acute stress disorder, posttraumatic stress syndrome, reactive depression, and anxiety can all occur after penetrating trauma and subsequent loss of function.

For many non-physiatrist, the criteria for admission to inpatient rehabilitation seem mysterious and arbitrary, and it is true that there are variations based on insurance, region, and facilities as to what patients can be best served in an inpatient rehab unit. In general, candidates include patients suffering acute physical, cognitive, behavioral, and/or functional deficits that are candidates for inpatient rehabilitation. Although they may still require medical care, patients must be medically stable and have completed definitive care of their injuries before transfer. Most inpatient units can accept patients with tracheostomy, feeding, and chest tubes. Patients with ventilator dependence must be transitioned to a portable ventilator and be relatively stable with their settings. Medical issues addressed on the inpatient unit include, but are not limited to, DVT prophylaxis, nutritional support, bowel/bladder management, pain control, skin/wound care, trach/peg care, and spasticity management. In general, patients should demonstrate a capacity and motivation to learn and improve their functional status. They should be able to physically tolerate at least 3 h of therapy per day. Patients who do not meet these criteria may be transferred to a skilled nursing facility until such time as they are appropriate for inpatient rehab.

This is a broad outline of the Rehabilitation process in trauma patients with details depending on the nature of the injury and the individual involved. I encourage you to incorporate the Rehabilitation team into your acute care routine. Early intervention can be critical in assuring a smooth transition into recovery and return to function. Once you have saved their life, they must return to life and that is what Rehabilitation is all about.

Important Points

- The Members of the Rehabilitation Team: Physiatrist, Nursing, Physical Therapy, Occupational Therapy, Speech Therapy, Recreational Therapy, Vocational Therapy, Psychology, and Social Work.
- Think Rehabilitation Consult for acute loss of function due to neurologic and musculoskeletal injury.
- Think Rehabilitation Consult for assessment of functional status and prevention of secondary disability.
- Rehabilitation Consult can assist with disposition, funding issues, and return-to-work issues.
- In short: After you save their life, we get them get back to living!

Trauma Rehabilitation Recommended Reading

Robinson LR (2006) Trauma rehabilitation. Lippincott Williams & Wilkins, Philadelphia

Braddom RL (2007) Physical medicine & rehabilitation, 3rd edn. Saunders/Elsevier, Philadelphia

Penetrating Injury Prevention 75

David S. Plurad

> A good plan executed today is better than a perfect plan executed tomorrow.
>
> –George S. Patton

In 2006, there were 30,034 deaths related to firearms violence in the United States with 3,026 fatalities occurring in victims less than or equal to 19 years [1]. Between 2007 and 2009, there were 2,603 homicides in the Los Angeles County. Of those, 1,935 (74.3%) were due to firearms [2]. The concept of penetrating injury as a health problem and not only a crime problem is cornerstone to application of preventative medicine techniques [3]. An analysis of 753 consecutive deaths at a level I center reveals that 13% were potentially preventable with changes in treatment; however, greater than 50% of deaths may have been avoided with changes in pre-injury behaviors including reductions in alcohol abuse, and restraint and helmet use [4]. In penetrating trauma, decreasing recidivism is a particular urgency. Recidivists whose first injury was penetrating are at greater risk that their second admission will also be penetrating and mortality significantly increases with second and third admissions [5].

Primary prevention measures seek to avert disability and disease in addition to promote general good health. Immunizations, insuring a clean water supply with fluorination, and laws requiring certain automobile safety devices are examples whereas education regarding smoking, sun exposure, and regular exercise are activities aimed at promoting general good health. The reach of these programs is intended for widest dissemination to the general population. The main objective of secondary prevention is detection of disease at its earliest stages before symptoms occur. Screening is considered a secondary prevention maneuver. Examples include mammography and cervical exams. Early treatment can also take place in conjunction with this phase. Cogent secondary prevention programs also identify populations at risk, maximizing the cost-effectiveness of screening. Identification of these groups grants an opportunity to modify these factors and reduce the incidence of overt disease. Reliable identification of these groups can be difficult. Tertiary prevention activities are intended to improve quality of life, reduce the severity of progression of symptoms, and, if needed, provide rehabilitation after disease has been diagnosed. This phase is considered treatment.

On March 30, 1981, John Hinckley Jr. attempted to assassinate President Ronald Reagan outside the Park Central Hotel in Washington DC. President Reagan, police Officer Tom Delahanty, and Secret Service agent Tim Mc Carthy sustained gunshot wounds while Press Secretary James Brady sustained a severe traumatic brain injury resulting in paralysis. Investigation would later show that Mr. Hinckley owned a multitude of firearms and used "Devastator" bullets designed to explode on impact. Later, sale of this type of munitions was restricted and on November 30, 1993, President William Jefferson Clinton signed the Brady Bill restricting firearms purchases in states that did not have restrictions already in place. The signing of the Brady Bill represents one strategy of primary injury prevention in the form of handgun control. Preventative

D.S. Plurad
Division of Trauma and Surgical Critical Care,
Harbor-UCLA Medical Center,
1000 W. Carson Street, D9, Room 112,
Torrance, CA 90509, USA
e-mail: plurad@usc.edu

G.C. Velmahos et al. (eds.), *Penetrating Trauma*,
DOI 10.1007/978-3-642-20453-1_75, © Springer-Verlag Berlin Heidelberg 2012

legislative measures include but are not limited to denial of purchase for those with felony convictions, age restriction bans, waiting periods, strict registration and licensing, concealed weapon legislation, zero tolerance for firearms at schools, and combinations of laws [6]. Since firearms availability is linked to significant increases in associated injury and mortality in several series, it would stand to reason that laws restricting access would similarly be related [3]. Indeed, data would suggest that this legislation decreases the incidence of handgun-related violence, particularly suicides [7–10] and the effect seems to be more pronounced when high-risk individuals are refused purchase [8, 10, 11]. Further, regardless of manner of procurement, storage, type, or number of weapons, the presence of a firearm significantly increases the risk of homicide or suicide in that household [12]. However, data is mixed and there is no conclusive evidence that these measures decrease violent firearms-related deaths overall [6]. Results of Brady Act passage does show benefit in certain groups (i.e.,: age ≥55 years) but not uniformly across all demographics [9]. Even so, these legislative measures do generally relate to decreased incidence of violent handgun-related acts and continue to be considered effective primary prevention in many communities.

Another primary prevention measure for penetrating injury would be community firearm buyback or exchange programs. Typically, these events are thought to decrease the firearms density in high-risk areas, thereby decreasing the incidence of violent crime. The media heavy aspect of these events produces visually effective messages, but, like the impact of handgun legislation, the results of buyback programs are variable. Buyback weapons tend to be older (many times nonfunctional), small caliber, and of the revolver type whereas firearms used in crimes tend to be newer and semiautomatic [13]. Additionally, in a series of persons relinquishing firearms, almost 50% reported the reason for participation was so that a child would not find the firearm but 60% continued to be gun owners. In this series, 23% of the weapons were nonfunctional. Those who remained gun owners were just as likely as the national average to keep a loaded gun in the house or carry the weapon with them [14]. Despite these results, buyback programs are a highly public form of primary injury prevention. Also on the supply side of the gun control issue is identification of high-risk dealers. Those merchants with a high rate of denial of gun sales and pawnbrokers have a higher incidence of having a crime-related handgun traced to them [15]. It is apparent that improved methods of firearm tracing are needed. In a study of gun violence perpetrated by or victimizing juveniles in the Oakland, CA area, only 55% of weapons could be traced to a dealer and only 39% could be traced to an owner [16]. The authors noted great need for comprehensive tracing programs to include federal registration of ownership and changes in ownership, mandatory reporting of stolen weapons, and intervention services to juveniles involved in handgun violence upon their first contact with the justice system.

On April 20, 1999, two high school students, Eric Harris and Dylan Klebold, entered Columbine High School in Littleton Colorado. Using two sawed-off shotguns, a 9MM carbine and a TECH 9 machine pistol, they killed 15 students and teachers and injured another 23 [17]. School programs seek to intervene in high-risk groups before violent injury occurs. Secondary prevention of violent assault is difficult since interventions must be meaningful, timely, targeted, culturally relevant, and durable. The effects of these programs are variable. In a review of school-based randomized controlled trials of secondary prevention programs, there was a decrease in violent behavior but no series compared rates of violent injury [18]. Further, in a study of multicenter holistic programs, there was little effect on rates of aggressive behaviors or missed classes due to violence or fear of violence [19]. The Youth Alive project currently active in Oakland and Los Angeles, CA, seeks to intervene in student groups in high-risk locales. The secondary prevention arm of their efforts is the "Teens on Target" program. This advocacy group trains peer educators to interact with disenfranchised students to provide coping skills and other assistance as needed. Among other tangible effects, these programs seem to greatly increase graduation rates among participants compared to their respective school's norms [20]. Additionally, these groups work with community leaders to facilitate related legislation. Notably is involvement with Oakland's gun tracing project which revealed deficiencies in current measures [16]. The ability for these school programs to reduce violent crime rates is indeterminate but, overall, these efforts do have other salient effects for these high-risk youth.

Trauma recidivism can be as high as 50% in some series and is of particular importance since patients experience increasing mortality with re-injury [5, 21]. In preventative medicine terms, these patients have had evidence of disease progression since they have been admitted to the hospital, treated in the Emergency Department, or have had involvement with the justice system. Risk factors for re-injury are substance abuse (especially alcohol), mental illness, urban habitation, male gender, homelessness, and history of perpetration of or victimization by a violent act [21–27]. Caught in the Crossfire (CinC) is an advocacy program active under the auspices of Youth Alive. In an attempt to decrease retaliatory violence, "Intervention specialists" who have been admitted in the past as a result of penetrating injury are trained to advocate for patients between the ages of 12 and 20 years who have likewise been injured [28]. Clients who volunteer to participate are provided with assistance as needed for themselves and their families. These include assistance with victim-of-violence restitution funds, assistance for medical costs, job/school placement assistance, referral for mental health treatment, and even transportation to court appointments. In 2008, CinC Los Angeles treated 89 clients and 220 family members [29]. There were no readmissions and 50% of clients who were not enrolled in school began or returned to coursework. Participants tended to demonstrate a significantly decreased incidence of criminal involvement of any type but no difference in recidivism rates or mortality even in a prospective randomized trial [28, 30, 31].

Interpersonal violence causes over 1,300 deaths and 2 million injuries per year. Since 33% of fatalities have had a previous victimization and there is a 20% 5-year mortality rate after repeat attacks, it is a priority to develop hospital-based programs for identification and intervention [32, 33]. In a program of interpersonal violence intervention, substance abuse in the perpetrator generally trended toward higher re-injury in the victims while involvement in seeking legal action was protective [33]. However, similar to other prevention measures, results are varied. In a case control observational series of victims of interpersonal violence, there was a significant decrease in self-reported re-injury at 6- and 12-month follow-up but no difference in state-reported injuries or perpetrator/victim incarcerations.

Recidivism reduction associated with alcohol abuse may represent a more productive endeavor since it is widespread. Up to 40% of trauma patients are (+) for alcohol on admission and up to 60% screen (+) for any intoxicant [25]. Also, chronic use is easily identified objectively using simple survey instruments [25, 26, 34]. Alcohol use is associated with behaviors that increase the risk of traumatic events. In a review of patient population who screen (+) for acute and chronic use, 77% engaged in one or more high-risk driving and 40% engaged in violence-related behaviors [26]. Intervention is particularly warranted since alcohol use at initial injury portends to greater mortality on re-injury [21]. The brief alcohol intervention can be performed by physician and physician extenders alike with equal effectiveness. It involves a patient oriented, non-confrontational discussion regarding their patterns of usage and relationship to the injury event [25]. Data comparing patients who participated in the programs vs. those that did not show a significant decrease in DUI arrests after discharge but did not show decreased rates of recidivism [34]. However, a prospective randomized trial describes a 47% decrease in Emergency Department visits and a 48% decrease in hospital readmissions [27]. The American College of Surgeons Committee on Trauma recognizes the importance of the Alcohol Screening and Brief Intervention (SBI) program for trauma centers to reduce recidivism and provides specific guidance [35].

Penetrating trauma, similar to many disease states, can be approached using preventative medicine concepts as violent injury is more widely accepted as a health problem rather than a crime problem. Data would suggest that resources would be better expended on prevention rather than new treatments. Similar to many preemptive health programs, the effect of legislation is difficult to define. Also, it is difficult to determine who would benefit most from screening and what strategies would be most effective at what time. Though decreases in penetrating trauma are not uniform across the vast majority of programs, the success of these strategies must be defined by overall favorable community effects rather than only rates of injury or re-injury.

Important Points

1. Injury due to violence is as much as a health problem as it is a crime problem.
2. Preventative medicine concepts are and should continue to be applied to trauma.
3. Handgun density is associated with rates of homicide and suicide while the effect of legislation and community activities to reduce accessibility is variable.

4. Physicians who care for the injured are uniquely positioned to decrease recidivism.
5. Institution of the ACS-COT recommendations for Alcohol Screening and intervention is a promising measure in preventing trauma.

References

1. CDC website, Div. of Violence Prevention, Available at: www.cdc.gov/ncipc/dvp/dvp.htm. Accessed 25 Jan 2010
2. http://projects.latimes.com/homicide/causes/. Accessed 26 Jan 2010
3. Christoffel KK, Longjohn MM (2002) gun injury prevention comes of age. J Trauma 53:213–218
4. Stewart RM, Myers JG, Dent DL et al (2003) Seven hundred fifty-three consecutive deaths in a level I trauma center: the argument for injury prevention. J Trauma 54:66–71
5. Brooke BS, Efron DT, Chang DC et al (2006) Patterns and outcomes among penetrating trauma recidivists: it only gets worse. J Trauma 61:16–20
6. Hahn RA, Bilukha OO, Crosby A et al (2003) First reports evaluating the effectiveness of strategies for preventing violence: firearms laws. Findings from the Task Force on Community Preventive Services. MMWR Recomm Rep 52(RR-14):11–20
7. Frassel KM, Wintemute GJ, Wright MA et al (2003) Association between handgun purchase and mortality from firearm injury. Inj Prev 9:48–52
8. Wright MA, Wintemute GJ, Rivara FP (1999) Effectiveness of denial of handgun purchase to persons believed to be at high risk for firearm violence. Am J Public Health 89:88–90
9. Ludwig J, Cook PJ (2000) Homicide and suicide rates associated with implementation of the Brady Handgun Violence Prevention Act. JAMA 284:585–891
10. Wintemute GJ, Wright MA, Drake CM et al (2001) Subsequent criminal activity among violent misdemeanants who seek to purchase handguns: risk factors and effectiveness for denying handgun purchase. JAMA 285:1029–1026
11. Wintemute GJ, Parham CA, Wright MA et al (1998) Weapons of choice: previous criminal history, later criminal activity, and firearm preference among legally authorized young adult purchasers of handguns. J Trauma 44:155–160
12. Dahlberg LL, Ikeda RM, Kresnow M (2004) Guns in the home and risk of a violent death in the home: findings from a national study. Am J Epidemiol 160:929–936
13. Kuhn EM, Nie CL, O'Brien ME et al (2002) Missing the target: a comparison of buyback and fatality related guns. Inj Prev 8:143–146
14. Romero MP, Wintemute GJ, Vernick JS (1998) Characteristics of a gun exchange program, and assessment of potential benefits. Inj Prev 4:206–210
15. Wintemute GJ, Cook PJ, Wright MA (2005) Risk factors among handgun retailers for frequent and disproportionate sales of guns used in violent firearm related crimes. Inj Prev 11:357–363
16. Calhoun D, Dodge AC, Journel CS (2005) The supply and demand for guns to juveniles: Oakland's gun tracing project. J Urban Health 82:552–559
17. http://fioa.fbi.gov/foiaindex/columbinehigh.htm. Accessed 20 Jan 2010
18. Mytton JA, DiGuiseppi C, Gough DA et al (2002) School-based violence prevention programs: systematic review of secondary prevention trials. Arch Pediatr Adolesc Med 156:752–762
19. Orpinas P, Kelder S, Frankowski R et al (2000) Outcome evaluation of a multi-component violence-prevention program for middle schools: the Students for Peace project. Health Educ Res 15:45–58
20. http://www.youthalive.org/tnt/index/#how. Accessed 26 Jan 2010
21. Dischinger PC, Mitchell KA, Kufera JA et al (2001) A longitudinal study of former trauma center patients: the association between toxicology status and subsequent injury mortality. J Trauma 51:877–886
22. Caulfield J, Singhal A, Moulton R et al (2004) Trauma recidivism in a large urban Canadian population. J Trauma 57:872–876
23. O' Donnell ML, Creamer M, Elliott P et al (2009) Prior trauma and psychiatric history as a risk factor for intentional and unintentional injury in Australia. J Trauma 66:470–476
24. Wan JJ, Morabito DJ, Khaw L et al (2006) Mental illness as an independent risk factor for unintentional injury and injury recidivism. J Trauma 61:1299–1304
25. Gentilello JM (2005) Alcohol interventions in trauma centers: the opportunity and the challenge. J Trauma 59:S18–S20
26. Field GA, Claassen CA, Keefe O' (2001) Association of alcohol use and other high-risk behaviors among trauma patients. J Trauma 50:13–19
27. Gentilello LM, Rivara FP, Donovan DM et al (1999) Alcohol interventions in a trauma center as a means of reducing the risk of injury recurrence. Ann Surg 230:473–480
28. Shibru D, Zahnd E, Becker M et al (2007) Benefits of a hospital-based peer intervention program for violently injured youth. J Am Coll Surg 205:684–689
29. http://www.youthalive.org/cinc/#results. Accessed 26 Jan 2010
30. Becker MG, Hall JS, Ursic CM et al (2004) Caught in the crossfire: the effects of a peer-based intervention program for violently injured youth. J Adolesc Health 34:177–183
31. Cooper C, Eslinger DM, Stolley PD (2006) Hospital-based violence intervention programs work. J Trauma 61:534–540
32. Zun LS, Downey L, Rosen J (2006) The effectiveness of an ED-based violence prevention program. Am J Emerg Med 24:8–13
33. Crandall ML, Nathens AB, Kernic MA et al (2004) Predicting future injury among women in abusive relationships. J Trauma 56:906–912
34. Schermer CR, Moyers TB, Miller WR et al (2006) Trauma center brief interventions for alcohol disorders decrease subsequent driving under the influence arrests. J Trauma 60:29–34
35. http://www.facs.org/trauma/publications/sbirtguide.pdf. Accessed 30 Jan 2010

The Economics of Trauma Care

76

Frederick Millham

A common aphorism recited in hospital boardrooms and in departments of public health goes something like this: "The answer is money, now remind me what the question is." Trauma care requires highly skilled surgeons working in a highly technical environment in a time-constrained manner. This is an expensive proposition. In many areas, trauma patients are, on the whole, less well insured than patients in other surgical domains. At a time when the number of well-trained general surgeons appears to be diminishing [1], attracting and retaining the best surgeons may be a formidable task. The success of any trauma program director requires that he or she have an understanding of the economics of trauma care. Trauma directors need an understanding of the macroeconomic issues in trauma care to justify investment in their programs by hospitals and governments. More importantly, surgeons must master the microeconomics of trauma care: how to design programs that have appropriate scope and scale to generate income both for the participants in the business, the surgeons, and for their sponsoring institution. This chapter will review the macroeconomic impact of injury, and present a microeconomic approach to trauma service structure. Unlike the other chapters in this book, this financial analysis will not focus on care of penetrating trauma patients alone, but will assume that trauma centers and surgeons care for a mix of penetrating and blunt trauma victims.

F. Millham
Department of Surgery, Harvard Medical School,
Boston, MA, USA

Department of Surgery, Newton Wellesley,
Green 664, 2014 Washington St, Newton, MA 02462, USA
e-mail: fmillham@partners.org

76.1 Macroeconomics of Trauma

The World Health Organization reports that 8 of the 15 leading causes of death in young people are related to injury [2]. The data for the USA are even more dramatic: Between the ages of 1 and 45, 60% of all deaths in the USA are attributable to injury [3]. Yet, the tremendous burden posed by injury is not limited to the developed world. Though data are sparse, it appears trauma is an even more significant public health issue in the poorer countries; for example, it is estimated that 1.6% of the Gross Domestic Product of Ghana is consumed by the care of victims of vehicular trauma alone [4]. As these data illustrate, unlike heart disease and cancer, trauma kills at a younger age, removing wage earners from the economy during or before their most productive years. While estimating the real cost of the death of a 30 year old cannot be done, one can estimate what the value of future earnings of a 30-year-old American, earning the median income for an American worker for 35 years of productive employment. Assuming a 4% discount rate (cost of capital), the death of this 30 year old sacrifices \$3.6 million in future earnings. Even if one assumes the victim will earn only \$25,000 per year, the economic loss amounts to \$1.8 million. Considering that over 14,954 Americans of between the age of 25 and 34 die due to injury each year, the economic cost, in terms of lost income, resulting from these deaths is between \$1.8 and \$3.7 billion per year. Given that around 150,000 people die due to injury in the USA each year, certainly,

G.C. Velmahos et al. (eds.), *Penetrating Trauma*,
DOI 10.1007/978-3-642-20453-1_76, © Springer-Verlag Berlin Heidelberg 2012

the cost of injury, in terms of lost income and productivity, is immense.

76.2 Microeconomics of Trauma

Over the past decade, the economics of trauma care at the hospital or group level has been a topic of a number of excellent analyses. Several factors are responsible for this high level of academic interest; first, the shift to nonoperative or nonsurgical management of many common traumatic injuries reduced the amount of billable work per year in many centers. The second factor has been the increasing trend to specialization among general surgeons as a group. Many centers historically rounded out trauma call rosters with "non-trauma" faculty allowing for fewer core trauma surgeons to manage busy centers. The absence of these "FTEs" from the trauma roster means that more core trauma faculty have to be added to the center payroll. The third factor affecting the economic viability of trauma care has been the concordant dawn of the era of "in-house attending call" and the "80-h resident work week." These factors further increase the number of faculty required to operate a service. Finally, the increased time trauma-attending surgeons devote to care of non-operative patients diminishes the time available to devote to elective surgical practice which is usually more financially rewarding. These forces are all occurring at a time of decreasing overall reimbursement and a rising percentage of uninsured or underinsured patients arriving in ambulances. Since most trauma services in the USA operate in an environment of "no margin, no mission," it is incumbent upon the trauma center director to find ways to scratch out a nonnegative bottom line in spite of these forces arrayed to produce a negative one.

Designing a financially productive trauma service is, indeed, a challenge, but there are viable approaches. In 1994, Peter Drucker, a world-renowned professor of business and writer, proposed the concept of "The Theory of Business" [5]. Though his subject was the predicament of failing corporations, his thesis applies well to the present economic challenges facing trauma surgeons and trauma centers. Drucker's theory of business has 3 components which I have adapted to our subject:

1. *Strategy*: Trauma Directors must understand the relationships between the trauma service and the system in which it exists. The trauma surgeon must understand the sources of patients, potential sources of patients, and the Trauma Center's relationship with competitors for these patients. What sort of patients is the center likely to receive? What is the mix of penetrating to non-penetrating mechanism among patients the center expects to receive? It also involves the relationship of the Trauma Center with its payers. Specifically, what is the expected reimbursement per relative value unit worked? Are surgeons relatively well reimbursed per RVU or are the surgeons relatively disadvantaged? The prospect of a bundle payment reimbursement system in the USA dramatically changes the assumptions behind this part of the theory of the trauma service. In other countries, this part of the Theory of the Business might involve providing a key resource to regional or national public health authorities, who have been educated to see trauma as a major public health issue.
2. *Tactics*: The Trauma Director must understand the specific mission of his or her trauma service. The structure of this mission is, of course informed by the assumptions that are made in the above strategic domain. A trauma service managing marginally insured blunt trauma patients will inevitably need to do more than "trauma care" to be financially viable. This requires an understanding the service mix the team will provide. Recently many trauma services have added emergency surgery to their service offering as a way of enhancing revenue and operative experience. Other trauma services provide critical care services in their hospitals. Some trauma services provide both. It is essential for trauma leadership to understand exactly how the local environment will support or impede the mission of the trauma service. At the tactical level, the trauma director may have to choose his or her battles carefully, seeking to expand the scope of the service while maintaining key relationships with colleagues.
3. *Core Competencies*: In order to succeed on the tactical level above, trauma team leadership must understand and deliver the core competencies necessary to accomplish the mission. This component includes not just clinical competencies such as added competency in critical care, but also competency in documentation, medical coding, and billing specific to the mission domains the service will be working in.

It is a mistake to believe that one theory of the trauma business will work in every setting. Rather, *each trauma service* must develop its own theory of its business. This theory must be known to all members of the team and must be frequently reevaluated and adjusted as conditions demand.

One thing is certain, the traditional theory that trauma surgery could stand alone as a clinical enterprise is no longer valid. There is concern in North America about an impending shortage of general surgeons [1]. Many believe that this shortage will be felt most acutely in the field of trauma care [6].

76.3 Developing a "Theory of Business" for Trauma Care

The design of any medical service should begin with an understanding of the salary market for providers in the specialty, and the average reimbursement per relative value unit this service will expect. In the USA, there are several national reference databases where regional estimates of median, upper, and lower quartile salaries can be found. The American Medical Group Association is one such source of information about physician salaries for various regions of the USA [7]. For our purposes, we can start by looking at the median salary for a trauma surgeon in the USA for 2007: $465,773 [7]. This value is slightly higher than that reported in the peer-reviewed literature [8]. I will use 400,000 as a convenient value for the purposes of discussion. Average reimbursement per relative value unit can be calculated from historical performance. This value varies considerably across regions of the country. Medicare reimburses at around $36.50 per RVU. A surgical practice in New England might expect around $55 per RVU. Practices in other areas, with higher indemnity insurance penetration, might expect $75 per RVU. These data will allow the director to estimate the number of relative units per provider that will be necessary to cover salaries and overhead (one usually assumes a 40–60% overhead rate, but again, historical performance can inform this assumption.) This calculation will usually work out to 7–9,000 RVU per year [8]. Looking at service volume and service mix will then allow the director to determine if the RVU per year goal is reasonably achievable. In some settings, grant support, funds from medical education, or other payment may reduce the total number of RVU the service must generate per year to meet its goal.

Figure 76.1 outlines a simplified model that might inform one's theory of the trauma service. This model makes a number of assumptions and vastly simplifies the patient revenue projections to assume that the 200 patients of 2,000 admissions will require surgery, and the average procedure will yield the number of RVU provided by a splenectomy (optimistic). The model assumes every admission is billable as a critical care admission (very optimistic). Furthermore, the model assumes nonoperative patients stay an average of 3 days, the second two of which are billed as mid-level hospital care. An actual analysis would require a good deal more modeling, but this analysis is sufficient for demonstration purposes. At the bottom of the figure, the proportion of the RVU required to meet the needs of the service is listed. Even when RVU's are reimbursed at $75 each (a utopian assumption), the service is able to generate only 61% of the required revenue. Clearly, in this environment, either a subsidy will be required, or the trauma service will need to do more than manage trauma patients. A parallel model of RVU return for emergency surgery and critical care for a particular hospital can be constructed to predict which components will be required to fill the reimbursement gap.

This approach can be modified to work in settings beyond the USA. All medical systems have some method of reimbursement, whether that is from fees for services rendered, or government payments to individuals or institutions. Every system has rules from which one can estimate the financial return for particular activities or services. One must determine what service output is required to generate the financial return necessary to keep surgeons happily employed. If the math does not work out, the trauma director will have a good estimate of what subsidy will be required from either the institution or extramural funding source to balance the budget.

76.4 Strategy

From a strategic standpoint, most hospitals, even those with the most unfavorable patient payer mixes, find trauma care to be a profitable service. Trauma surgeons are not always well reimbursed for their care, but the hospital where the care occurs usually makes a

Fig. 76.1 A Simplified Model of Potential Trauma Service Revenue

I. Finance Assumptions:			
Target / Surgeon	$ 400,000.00		
Overhead / Surgeon	$ 200,000.00		
Total Revenue per Surgeon	$ 600,000.00		
Total Revenue required	$ 3,000,000.00		
II. Clinical Assumptions:			
Group Size	5		
Admissions	2000		
Average LOS	3		
Trauma Procedures	200		
Overhead	50%		
III. Service Mix Assumptions:	CPT Code	RVU	RVU per year
RVU/Adm	99291	5.99	11980
RVU/LOS	99232	1.89	6804
RVU/Operation	38100	28.74	5748
Total			24532
IV. Financial Return		**$/RVU**	
	36.5	55	75
Required Break Even RVU	82,191.78	54,545.45	40,000.00
Actual RVU Yeild	24,532.00	24,532.00	24,532.00
Actual/Required RVU	**30%**	**45%**	**61%**

reasonable margin on each admission [9, 10]. The trauma director can use this fact to his or her advantage in negotiating issues with administrators. In terms of the Theory of the Trauma Business, the Strategy becomes: "The trauma surgeons will provide 24-h yearlong coverage of this profitable service line, coordinating disparate services, managing the details of patient care and placement." This service may require either a subsidy from the institution or, more effectively, access to alternative practice zones such as critical care or emergency surgery.

76.5 Tactics

Most trauma directors will find that there are insufficient RVU's available taking care of trauma patients alone to balance the books [11, 12]. It is this reality that has led to a revolution in trauma care. Many trauma services now expand their focus to include non-trauma patients: the Acute Care Surgery model. The acute care surgery service, in addition to managing all the trauma admissions to the institution, also manages traditional general surgery emergencies such as bowel obstruction or appendicitis, i.e., any abdominal visceral inflammation, obstruction or perforation fall under the prevue of the "Trauma and Acute Care Surgeon" [13]. Surgical Critical Care can be an important component of this model as well. Since many of the patients in the surgical ICU "belong" to the trauma service anyway, it makes good sense from both a patient care and a financial standpoint for the trauma service to manage these cases. Many trauma/acute care surgery programs find it advantageous to perform as much of the procedural work their patients need as possible, including procedures such as percutaneous gastrostomy and IVC filter placement, which may, in many institutions "belong" to others.

76.6 Core Competencies

To accomplish the tactical missions outlined above, the trauma acute care surgeon must not only be an expert visceral surgeon, but also must be a skilled, fellowship trained, intensivist. He or she must also maintain the procedural skill necessary to perform all the procedures on the menu the director establishes. It is better to eschew procedures one cannot master. In fact, there is some evidence of a learning curve in services adopting the acute care paradigm [14].

In addition to clinical excellence, the trauma acute care service must establish impeccable and focused business practices. To maximize the team's profitability, and therefore its viability, all clinical activity must be accurately documented and appropriately billed. This usually requires the addition of skilled, nonphysician team members. Physician extenders such as physician's assistants and nurse practitioners, carefully deployed, can multiply the work throughput of the trauma acute care surgeon. In addition, a business manager to attend to the details of coding and billing is essential for efficient charge capture and compliance with billing regulations.

An approach to trauma care involving the addition of acute care surgery and critical care medicine can provide a "balanced portfolio" providing patients with excellent, team-oriented continuity of care, while providing surgeons with a challenging and profitable work environment. Creating such a balanced portfolio may be the key to success for trauma center directors and their administrative champions.

Important Points

1. Trauma Care returns more years of productive life per intervention than most other medical specialties.
2. Trauma Care is generally profitable to the hospital.
3. An effective trauma service should have a "Theory of the Business" encompassing three related domains:
   (a) Strategy: How will the trauma service fit into its home institutions mission and system needs?
   (b) Tactics: How will the trauma service function to meet its strategic requirements? What services will it provide? How will this plan work to pay the bills?
   (c) Core Competencies: What clinical and business skills will the trauma service need to master to succeed both clinically and financially.
4. A Balanced Portfolio of trauma care, management of acute surgical emergencies, and critical care can provide for a practice environment that is satisfying and profitable.
5. With careful planning, a trauma/critical care/emergency surgery service can be a financially and professionally rewarding enterprise for the general surgeons of the future.

References

1. Fischer JE (2007) The impending disappearance of the general surgeon. JAMA 298(18):2191–2193
2. Butchart A, Harvey AP, Krug E, Meddings D, Peden M, Sminkey L (2007) Preventing injuries and violence: a guide for ministries of health. WHO Press, Geneva
3. National Center for Injury Prevention and Control (2009) Top 10 leading causes of Death in the United States, Atlanta [updated 04/23/09; cited 2009 8/21/2009]; Available from: http://webapp.cdc.gov/sasweb/ncipc/leadcaus10.html
4. Anon (2007) Road incidents cost Ghana 1.6% of GDP. Inj Prev2007 13(6):408
5. Drucker PF (1994) The theory of the business (cover story). Harv Bus Rev 72(5):95–104
6. Rotondo MF (2007) At the center of the "perfect storm": the patient. Surgery 141(3):291–292
7. Association AMG (2009) Physician compensation survey. 2009 [12/13/2009]; Available from: http://www.cejkasearch.com/compensation/amga_physician_compensation_survey.htm
8. Cohn SM, Price MA, Villarreal CL (2009) Trauma and surgical critical care workforce in the United States: a severe surgeon shortage appears imminent. J Am Coll Surg 209(4):446–452.e4
9. Taheri PA, Butz DA, Greenfield L (1999) Paying a premium: how patient complexity affects costs and margins. Ann Surg 229(6):807–814
10. Taheri PA, Butz DA, Watts CM, Griffes LC, Greenfield LJ (1999) Trauma services: a profit center? J Am Coll Surg 188(4):349–354

11. Aucar JA, Hicks LL (2005) Economic modeling comparing trauma and general surgery reimbursement. Am J Surg 190(6):951–960
12. Rogers FB, Osler T, Shackford SR, Healey MA, Wells SK (2003) Charges and reimbursement at a rural level I trauma center: a disparity between effort and reward among professionals. J Trauma 54(1):9–15
13. Esposito TJ, Rotondo M, Barie PS, Reilly P, Pasquale MD (2006) Making the case for a paradigm shift in trauma surgery. J Am Coll Surg 202(4):655–667
14. Schenarts PJ, Phade SV, Goettler CE, Waibel BH, Agle SC, Bard MR et al (2008) Impact of acute care general surgery coverage by trauma surgeons on the trauma patient. Am Surg 76(6):494–502

Organ Donation

77

Eric J. Ley and Ali Salim

77.1 Identifying Donors

Transplanted organs are harvested from three major sources: cadaveric "brain-dead" donors, cadaveric "cardiac death" donors (donation after cardiac death), and living (related and unrelated) donors. Cadaveric, brain-dead, donors account for approximately 54% of all donors and the most common causes of death in this group are cerebrovascular accident /stroke (CVA), head trauma, and anoxia [1]. Traumatic brain injury (TBI), once the most common cause of brain death, has been surpassed by CVA and this has important implications. As such, organs from younger and healthier trauma patients have been replaced by older, sicker stroke patients. Both TBI and CVA will continue to contribute a significant number of organs as nearly 50,000 US residents die from TBI and nearly 142,000 citizens die from CVA per year [2].

77.2 Consent

Consent is the single largest impediment to donation. Every effort should be made to assign a surrogate prior to brain death. In general, the typical choice for surrogate decision maker starts with the appointed legal guardian and runs in descending order to spouse, adult children, parents, siblings, and then more distant relatives. The best predictor of donation success is the family's response to the initial request by the healthcare provider [3]. This initial interaction is paramount to the process of consent, and requires emphasis in the development of a protocol for consent. Fifty-three percent of families that deny donation did not receive an adequate explanation of brain death, and the next of kin who decided against donation had less understanding of brain death than those who agreed to donation [4].

Senior physician or experienced health care provider involvement with family interactions is particularly important. One component of these interactions is defining the role of the physician. The physician and other members of the health care team should establish themselves as allies of the grieving family and purveyors of information regarding organ donation, as opposed to de facto agents of the health care system or organ procurement organization.

Education of all health care providers is important, as is the involvement of uniquely trained and experienced individuals. Transplant coordinators, in the form of a dedicated physician or other specially trained health care provider, demonstrate their effectiveness in coordinating efforts to facilitate both consent and transition of care to aggressive organ preservation and harvest. These coordinators should be an established component of the hospital as they are responsible for identifying donors, managing their hospital course, and consenting family members. Throughout the process, the coordinators spend a significant amount of time with family members, providing education and attending to the unique social and ethical concerns of each individualized situation. Implementation of

E.J. Ley (✉) • A. Salim
Department of Surgery, Cedars Sinai Medical Center, 8700 Beverly Blvd, Suite 8215NT, Los Angeles, CA 90048, USA
e-mail: eric.ley@cshs.org; ali.salim@cshs.org

G.C. Velmahos et al. (eds.), *Penetrating Trauma*,
DOI 10.1007/978-3-642-20453-1_77,

in-house coordinator (IHC) programs has led to significant improvements in conversion and consent rates even maintaining consent and conversion rates as high as 67% [5]. Early success was replicated in several Level I trauma centers throughout the United States [6]. The use of IHC's has proven particularly effective in trauma centers with a primarily minority donor population [5–7].

The increased donation resulting from an IHC program has been attributed to several factors: [1] a consistent donation process based on early and intensive family support; [2] more extended interaction and support with donor families; and [3] sustained relationships with key medical, nursing, and hospital leadership [6, 7]. By spending significantly more time with families and ensuring that donation becomes a hospital priority, the IHC program differentiates itself from the conventional OPO referral method. Not surprisingly, total time spent with families was found to be significantly associated with favorable consent [6].

77.3 Intensive Care Unit Admission and Protocols

Early intensive care unit (ICU) admission with an aggressive donor management (ADM) protocol results in a reduced incidence of cardiovascular collapse in the donor and improved organ recovery and function in the recipient [8]. Of note, 92% of organs that were initially thought unacceptable for transplantation were successfully transplanted with good results [8]. In one center, adoption of a protocol of ADM was associated with an 82% increase in the number of actual donors, a 71% increase in the number of organs recovered, and an 87% decrease in the number of donors lost from hemodynamic instability [9]. The net result was a significant increase in the number of organs available for transplantation. An ICU with an ADM protocol for invasive monitoring, steroids, vasopressors, fluid restriction, and diuretics resulted in successful transplantation of "unacceptable" lungs without compromise of 30-day or 1-year graft survival [10]. In a prospective pilot study involving 10 organ procurement organizations and 88 critical care units, a 10.3% greater number of organs recovered per 100 donors was observed when an ADM protocol was implemented [11]. When a rapid brain death determination protocol was implemented and aggressive resuscitation was guided by invasive monitoring, a significant increase in the number of organs per donor and a decrease in medical failures was observed [12]. With the emergence of more effective noninvasive monitoring modalities to guide fluid resuscitation and vasopressor use, newer technologies may also prove beneficial in the resuscitative management of this unique population.

Preventing, or even decreasing, the number of donors lost from cardiovascular collapse increases the number of organs available for transplantation. Other proposals for interventions to optimize organ function prior to potential donation include the use of high-frequency chest wall oscillation for pulmonary optimization [13] and inhaled nitric oxide to support cardiopulmonary function and improve solid organ optimization [14].

77.4 Declaration of Brain Death

Considerable confusion and misconceptions exist about declaration of brain death. When brain death is suspected, discussion with family and friends needs to be caring but direct. In rare instances, families may not accept the diagnosis. After declaration of brain death is completed, the physician is under no moral or legal obligation to continue medical support, although, reasonable requests to spend time with the body should be accommodated. The acceptance of death by neurologic criteria is accepted by every major religion, with the exceptions of selected orthodox Jewish sects. In New York and New Jersey, state laws do not allow the declaration of death by neurologic criteria if the family or individual previously objected to the concept of brain death based on religious beliefs. Under these isolated circumstances, the physician is required to continue medical support [15].

Declaration of brain death begins with a neurological evaluation that includes response to pain, pupillary response, oculocephalic reflex, corneal reflex, the cold caloric reflex test, and assessment of spontaneous respirations. Bronchial suctioning rather than endotracheal tube movement should be used to assess for a cough reflex. Painful stimuli to the extremities should be significant because this examination must not be misinterpreted.

The apnea test is an evaluation of a brainstem reflex. Apnea tests are not benign and can be associated with cardiopulmonary death and loss of recoverable organs if not performed properly. Preoxygenation and normalization of the partial pressure of carbon dioxide (pCO_2) is important before starting the test. The examiner must be aware of any reflexive-type movements, which can mimic respiration. The examination should be discontinued if there is significant hypotension or hypoxia during the testing. Vasopressors may be necessary to support a patient's blood pressure. If the patient is unable to tolerate or complete the examination, a confirmatory test is required.

Although there are slight variations in the apnea test, the authors favor the following guidelines which are summarized from the American Academy of Neurology Practice for determining Brain Death in Adults. The test begins when the core temperature is 36.5°C or 97°F. Systolic blood pressure must be maintained above 90 mm Hg with fluid/vasopressor if necessary or the apnea test is ended. The patient is preoxygenated with 100% oxygen for 10 min and an arterial blood gas (ABG) is drawn. A normal arterial pCO_2 of 35–45 mm Hg is necessary prior to beginning the test. Slide a cut nasal cannula to approximately the level of the carina and deliver 100% oxygen at 8 L/min. Verify function of pulse oximeter and disconnect the ventilator. During the test, confirm the lack of respiratory movements. If the patient's pulse oximeter falls below 90% or if the systolic blood pressure falls below 90 mm Hg, then the test is ended, ventilatory support is resumed and an ABG is drawn. If the patient tolerates the test for 10 min, then the test is also ended and the patient is placed back on the ventilator and an ABG is drawn. Regardless of time drawn, if the ABG measures a pCO_2 above 60 or 20 mm Hg above the pCO_2 measured on the initial ABG, the apnea test result is positive, and the diagnosis of brain death is established. All paperwork or legal documents that need to be completed should list the time of death as the time of death by neurologic criteria and not the time of circulatory or cardiopulmonary arrest.

77.5 Aggressive Resuscitation

Brain death is associated with profound physiologic alterations that result in diffuse regulatory disturbances and widespread cellular injury. Severe alterations in metabolism, endocrine function, and coagulopathy are commonly observed. These disturbances frequently lead to multiorgan system failure, cardiovascular collapse, and asystole in up to 60% of patients if not appropriately managed [16].

Upon ICU admission, placement of a pulmonary artery catheter improves donor treatment. Donor management with a pulmonary artery catheter led to significantly greater recovered organs compared to donor management without such a catheter [17]. Provide fluid resuscitation to maintain a mean arterial pressure greater than 70 mm Hg (Fig. 77.1). Utilize Vasopressors and inotropes if the mean arterial pressure (MAP) remains less than 70 mm Hg despite adequate fluid resuscitation. Donors who require a combined vasopressor need of greater than 10 mcg/kg/min (either epinephrine or dopamine alone, or in combination) are given a "T4 protocol" consisting of 1 ampule 50% dextrose, 2 g of solumedrol, 20 units regular insulin, and 20 mg of thyroid hormone (T_4), followed by a continuous infusion of 10 mcg/h. Therapeutic replacement with thyroid hormone has been associated with complete reversal of anaerobic metabolism and subsequent stabilization of cardiac function when applied to human brain-dead subjects [18]. In addition, the use of thyroid hormone has been associated with significant improvements in cardiovascular status, reductions in inotropic support, and decreases in donors lost from cardiac instability [19, 20].

77.6 Brain Death–Related Complications

Early identification and management of brain death–related complications such as disseminated intravascular coagulation (DIC), diabetes insipidus (DI), neurogenic pulmonary edema (NPE), hypothermia, and cardiac arrhythmias is required [21]. DIC-related coagulopathy can be corrected with FFP, Factor VII, and Factor XI. DI treatment is with desmopressin or vasopressin if vasopressors are otherwise required. NPE may require high-frequency percussive ventilation, or lung-protective pressure-controlled ventilator management. Salt replacement with hypertonic saline is helpful for SIADH. The complex hemodynamic, endocrine, and metabolic dysfunction associated with brain death is frequently associated with major complications in the potential donor. If inappropriately treated, these complications can progress to cardiovascular collapse with loss of valuable organs for transplantation.

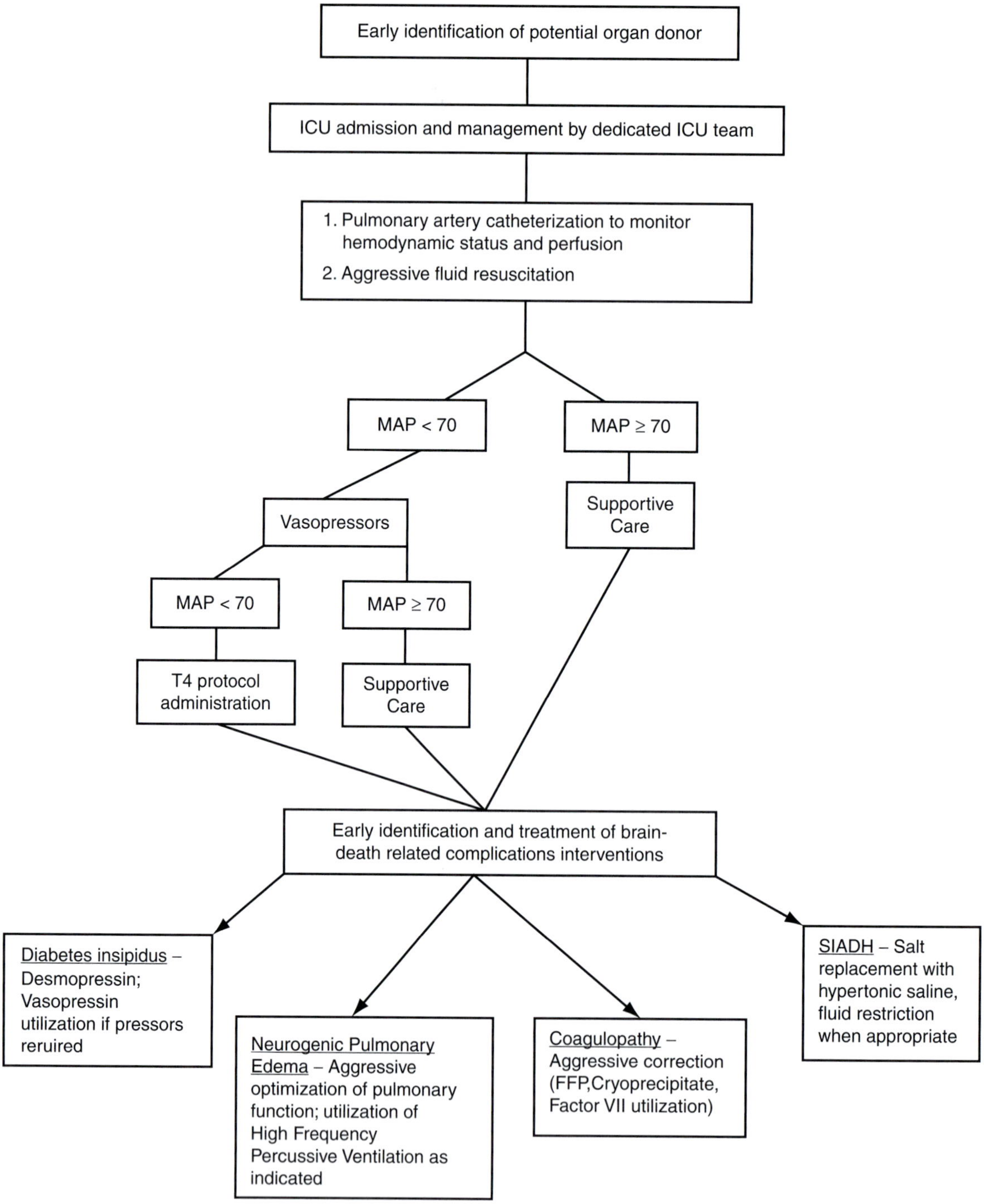

Fig. 77.1 Algorithm for optimizing recovered organs

In conclusion, identify potential donors early with the expectation that organ recovery will primarily occur in the CVA and TBI population. Optimize consent for donation by involving senior surgical staff (Fig. 77.1). Early admission of critically ill patients to the ICU with aggressive management even in cases of terminal injury will increase recovered organs. Brain death is associated with profound physiologic alterations that result in diffuse vascular regulatory disturbances and widespread cellular injury. As such, donor management with a pulmonary artery catheter leads to significantly greater recovered organs. Fluid resuscitation, vasopressors, and inotropes are utilized to maintain a MAP greater than 70 mmHg. With increased vasopressor requirements, start a "T4 protocol." Aggressive management of brain death–related complications such as disseminated intravascular coagulation, diabetes insipidus, neurogenic pulmonary edema, hypothermia, and cardiac arrhythmias will increase recovered organs.

Important Points

- Optimize consent for organ donation by involving senior surgical staff and implementing an in-house coordinator.
- Early potential donor admission to the ICU with aggressive management will increase recovered organs.
- Donor management with a pulmonary artery catheter leads to significantly greater recovered organs.
- Provide fluid resuscitation to maintain a mean arterial pressure greater than 70 mm Hg.
- Vasopressors and inotropes are utilized if the mean arterial pressure (MAP) remains less than 70 mm Hg despite adequate fluid resuscitation.
- With increased vasopressor requirements, start a "T4 protocol."
- Aggressive management of brain death–related complications such as disseminated intravascular coagulation, diabetes insipidus, neurogenic pulmonary edema, hypothermia, and cardiac arrhythmias will increase recovered organs.

References

1. U.S. Department of Health and Human Services. Organ donation breakthrough collaborative: from best practice to common practice. http://www.organdonationnow.org/. Accessed 26 July 2007
2. Department of Health and Human Resources. Centers for disease control and prevention. http://www.cdc.gov/nchs/injury.htm. Accessed 26 July 2007
3. Siminoff LA, Mercer MB (2001) Public policy, public opinion, and consent for organ donation. Camb Q Healthc Ethics 10:377–386
4. Franz HG, DeJong W, Wolfe SM et al (1997) Explaining brain death: a critical feature of the donation process. J Transpl Coord 7:14–21
5. Shafer TJ, Davis KD, Holtzman SM, Van Buren CT, Crafts NJ, Durand R (2003) Location of in-house organ procurement organization staff in level I trauma centers increases conversion of potential donors to actual donors. Transplantation 75:1330–1335
6. Shafer TJ, Ehrle RN, Davis KD et al (2004) Increasing organ recovery from level I trauma centers: the in-house coordinator intervention. Prog Transplant 14:250–263
7. Salim A, Brown C, Inaba K et al (2007) Improving consent rates for organ donation: the effect of an inhouse coordinator program. J Trauma 62:1411–1414
8. Wheeldon DR, Potter CD, Dunning J et al (1992) Haemodynamic correction in multiorgan donation. Lancet 339:1175
9. Salim A, Martin M, Brown C, Rhee P, Demetriades D, Belzberg H (2006) The effect of a protocol of aggressive donor management: implications for the national organ donor shortage. J Trauma 61:429–433; discussion 433–435
10. Straznicka M, Follette DM, Eisner MD, Roberts PF, Menza RL, Babcock WD (2002) Aggressive management of lung donors classified as unacceptable: excellent recipient survival one year after transplantation. J Thorac Cardiovasc Surg 124:250–258
11. Rosendale JD, Chabalewski FL, McBride MA et al (2002) Increased transplanted organs from the use of a standardized donor management protocol. Am J Transplant 2:761–768
12. Jenkins DH, Reilly PM, Schwab CW (1999) Improving the approach to organ donation: a review. World J Surg 23:644–649
13. Braverman JM (2002) Increasing the quantity of lungs for transplantation using high-frequency chest wall oscillation: a proposal. Prog Transplant 12:266–274
14. Prodhan P, Casavant D, Medlock MD, Yager P, Kim J, Noviski N (2004) Inhaled nitric oxide in neurogenic cardiopulmonary dysfunction: implications for organ donation. Transplant Proc 36:2570–2572
15. Manno EM (2006) The declaration of death and the withdrawal of care in the neurologic patient. Neurol Clin 24:159–169
16. Salter DR, Dyke CM, Wechsler AS (1992) Triiodothyronine (T3) and cardiovascular therapeutics: a review. J Card Surg 7:363–374
17. Hadjizacharia P, Salim A, Brown C et al (2010) Does the use of pulmonary artery catheters increase the number of organs available for transplantation? Clin Transplant 24:62–66
18. Novitzky D, Cooper DK, Reichart B (1986) Value of triiodothyronine (T3) therapy to brain-dead potential organ donors. J Heart Transplant 5:486–487
19. Cooper DK, Novitzky D, Wicomb WN (1989) The pathophysiological effects of brain death on potential donor organs, with particular reference to the heart. Ann R Coll Surg Engl 71:261–266
20. Salim A, Vassiliu P, Velmahos GC et al (2001) The role of thyroid hormone administration in potential organ donors. Arch Surg 136:1377–1380
21. Salim A, Velmahos GC, Brown C, Belzberg H, Demetriades D (2005) Aggressive organ donor management significantly increases the number of organs available for transplantation. J Trauma 58:991–994

Index

G.C. Velmahos et al. (eds.), *Penetrating Trauma*,
DOI 10.1007/ 978-3-642-20453-1, © Springer-Verlag Berlin Heidelberg 2012

B